GRAINGER & ALLISON'S DIAGNOSTIC RADIOLOGY

SIXTH EDITION

Neuroimaging

GRAINGER & ALLISON'S DIAGNOSTIC RADIOLOGY

SIXTH EDITION

Neuroimaging

EDITED BY
H. Rolf Jäger, MD, FRCR

Jonathan H. Gillard, BSc, MA, MD, FRCP, FRCR, MBA

ELSEVIER

London New York Oxford Philadelphia St Louis Sydney Toronto

ELSEVIER

Notices

ISBN: 978-0-7020-6937-6

Executive Content Strategist: Michael Houston
Content Development Specialist: Louise Cook
Project Manager: Andrew Riley
Design: Christian Bilbow
Marketing Manager: Rachael Pignotti

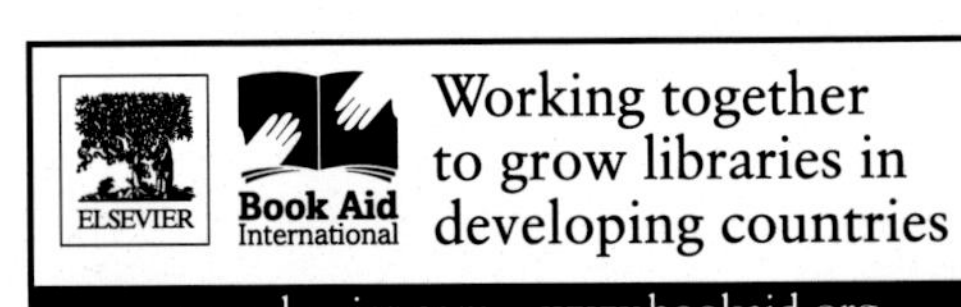

Contents

Preface

The 8 chapters in this book have been selected from the contents of the Neuroimaging section in *Grainger & Allison's Diagnostic Radiology, Sixth Edition*. These chapters provide a succinct up-to-date overview of current imaging techniques and their clinical applications in daily practice and it is hoped that with this concise format the user will quickly grasp the fundamentals they need to know. Throughout these chapters, the relative merits of different imaging investigations are described, variations are discussed and recent imaging advances are detailed. Please note that imaging techniques of the spine are considered in the separate section 'The Spine' in *Grainger & Allison's Diagnostic Radiology, Sixth Edition*.

Grainger & Allison's Diagnostic Radiology has long been recognized as the standard general reference work in the field, and it is hoped that this book, utilizing the content from the latest sixth edition of this classic reference work, will provide radiology trainees and practitioners with ready access to the most current information, written by internationally recognized experts, on what is new and important in the radiological diagnosis of disorders of the brain.

List of Contributors

Joti Jonathan Bhattacharya, MBBS, MSc, FRCR
Consultant Neuroradiologist, Department of Neuroradiology, Institute of Neurological Sciences, Southern General Hospital, Glasgow, UK

Frederik Barkhof, MD, PhD
Professor of Neuroradiology, Alzheimer Center and Department of Radiology, VU University Medical Center, Amsterdam, The Netherlands

Timothy Beale, MBBS, FRCS, FRCR
Consultant Head and Neck Radiologist, University College Hospital, Royal National Throat Nose and Ear Hospital, London, UK

David J. Bowden, MA, VetMB, MB, BChir, FRCR
Senior Registrar, University of Cambridge, Addenbrooke's Hospital, Cambridge, UK

Jackie Brown, BDS, MSc, FDSRCPS, DDRRCR
Consultant Dental and Maxillofacial Radiologist, Guy's and St Thomas' Hospitals Foundation Trust; Senior Lecturer at King's College London Dental Institute of Guy's, King's College and St Thomas' Hospitals, London, UK

Indran Davagnanam, MB, BCh, BMedSci, FRCR
Consultant Neuroradiologist, National Hospital for Neurology and Neurosurgery, Lysholm Radiological Department; Radiology, Moorfields Eye Hospital; Honorary Research Associate, The Brain Repair and Rehabilitation Unit, Institute of Neurology, London, UK

Kirsten Forbes, MB BChir, MD, MRCP, FRCR
Consultant Neuroradiologist, Department of Neuroradiology, Institute of Neurological Sciences, Southern General Hospital, Glasgow, UK

Julia Frühwald-Pallamar, MD
Assistant Professor of Radiology, Medical University of Vienna, Department of Biomedical Imaging and Image-Guided Therapy, Subdivision of Neuroradiology and Musculoskeletal Radiology, Vienna, Austria

Massimo Gallucci, MD, PhD
Professor of Neuroradiology, Neuroradiology Service, San Salvatore University Hospital, L'Aquila, Italy

Beatriz Gomez Anson, MD, PhD, FRCR
Clinical Head of Neuroradiology, Unit of Neuroradiology, Department of Radiology, Hospital Santa Creu i Sant Pau, Universitat Autonoma, Barcelona, Spain

H. Rolf Jäger, MD, FRCR
Reader in Neuroradiology, Department of Brain Repair and Rehabilitation, UCL Institute of Neurology, UCL Faculty of Brain Sciences; Consultant Neuroradiologist, Lysholm Department of Neuroradiology, National Hospital for Neurology and Neurosurgery, and Department of Imaging, University College London Hospitals, London, UK

Brynmor P. Jones, BSc(Hons), MBBS, MRCP, FRCR
Consultant Neuroradiologist, Imperial College Healthcare NHS Trust, Charing Cross Hospital, London, UK

Ruchi Kabra, MBBS, BSc, MRCS, FRCR
Neuroradiology Fellow, King's College Hospital, London, UK

Amrish Mehta, MBBS, BSc(Hons), FRCR
Consultant Neuroradiologist, Department of Imaging, Imperial College Healthcare NHS Trust, London, UK

Caroline Micallef, MD, FRCR
Consultant Neuroradiologist, National Hospital for Neurology and Neurosurgery, University College London Hospitals, London, UK

Katherine Miszkiel, BM(Hons), MRCP, FRCR
Consultant Neuroradiologist, Lysholm Department of Neuroradiology, The National Hospital for Neuroradiology and Neurosurgery; Honorary Consultant Neuroradiologist, Moorfields Eye Hospital, London, UK

John Rout, BDS, FDSRCS, MDentSci, DDRRCR, FRCR
Consultant Oral and Maxillofacial Radiologist, Radiology Department, Birmingham Dental Hospital, Birmingham, UK

Alex Rovira, MD
Head of Magnetic Resonance Unit (IDI), Department of Radiology, Vall d'Hebron University Hospital, Barcelona, Spain

Daniel J. Scoffings, BSc(Hons), MBBS, MRCP(UK), FRCR
Consultant Neuroradiologist, Department of Radiology, Addenbrooke's Hospital, Cambridge, UK

John M. Stevens, MBBS, DRACR, FRCR
Consultant Radiologist (retired), formerly at Lyshom Department of Neuroradiology, Radiology Department, The National Hospital for Neurology and Neurosurgery, London, UK

Pia C. Sundgren, MD, PhD
Professor of Radiology; Head, Department of Diagnostic Radiology, Clinical Sciences Lund, Lund University; Center for Medical Imaging and Physiology, Skåne University Hospital, Lund, Sweden

Majda M. Thurnher, MD
Associate Professor of Radiology, Medical University Vienna, Department of Biomedical Imaging and Image-Guided Therapy, Vienna, Austria

Stefanie C. Thust, MD, FRCR
Neuroradiology Fellow, National Hospital of Neurology and Neurosurgery, London, UK

Peter Zampakis, PhD, MSc, MD
Consultant Neuroradiologist, Radiology, University Hospital of Patras, Patras, Achaia, Greece

CHAPTER 1

Overview of Anatomy, Pathology and Techniques; Aspects Related to Trauma

Joti Jonathan Bhattacharya • Kirsten Forbes • Peter Zampakis • David J. Bowden • John M. Stevens

CHAPTER OUTLINE

OVERVIEW OF ANATOMY, PATHOLOGY AND TECHNIQUES

Modern imaging techniques depict the brain in ever more exquisite detail in all three orthogonal planes. Since neuroradiology forms an important part of radiology training and a substantial part of most radiologists' daily work, familiarity with some of the intricacies of neuro-anatomy becomes increasingly important; radiology remains in large part applied anatomy. The brain, at the macroscopic level, is a largely symmetric structure aiding the identification of abnormalities. Here we offer an overview of brain and vascular anatomy as shown on current imaging techniques, beginning with a brief summary of brain development. Imaging techniques for the brain and vasculature are then reviewed.

ANATOMY OF THE BRAIN AND VASCULAR SYSTEM

Embryology

The brain derives from the rostral end of the embryonic neural tube, formed of neural ectoderm. The initially fairly uniform neural tube develops three swellings, the primordial cerebral vesicles (prosencephalic, mesencephalic and rhombencephalic), which subsequently give rise to five vesicles.[1] At this stage it remains one cell thick, with a pseudostratified epithelium containing the neural stem cells. The cavity of the neural tube represents the future cerebral ventricles and the central canal of the spinal cord, ending anteriorly at the membrane of the lamina terminalis. Thus the anterior wall of the third ventricle (lamina terminalis) represents the rostral end of the neural tube (Fig. 1-1).

Bulges appearing on either side of the prosencephalic vesicle represent the developing telencephalic vesicles and, subsequently, cerebral hemispheres, and their opening, the future interventricular foramen (of Monro). With growth, the wall of the neural tube thickens and nutrition, which was initially by simple diffusion from the amniotic fluid to the neural plate, and after closure of the tube by diffusion from the surrounding primordial vascular plexus, is no longer sufficient. a depression appears in the roof of the developing third ventricle and adjacent cerebral hemispheres, invaginating a layer of ependyma and vascular pia mater, to form the choroid plexus (Fig. 1-2).

Thus the original function of the choroid plexus appears to be oxygenation and nutrition of the deep portions of the brain.[2] Subsequently, penetrating vessels grow into the brain substance. With growth of the cerebral hemispheres, neuronal proliferation occurs in the periventricular zone, followed by migration of neurons along radially oriented glial cells to reach the pallial surface of the brain. This results in formation of the cerebral cortex, with its characteristic lamination. Over most of the hemispheric surface a six-layer neuronal structure can be identified: the isocortex (neocortex). Paul Broca traced the isocortex to its medial edge (Latin: *limbus*), thus identifying a medial limbic lobe (the hippocampus and associated structures) which was found to have a simpler three-layer structure, the allocortex. An intermediate band of cortex between the isocortex and allocortex can be discerned, termed the mesocortex. Other

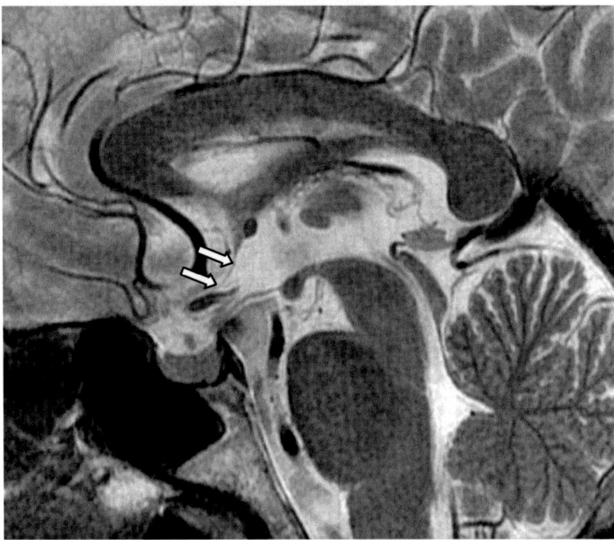

FIGURE 1-1 ■ Midline sagittal T2 MR image through the third ventricle. The thin membrane of the lamina terminalis (white arrows) corresponds to the anterior end of the embryonic neural tube.

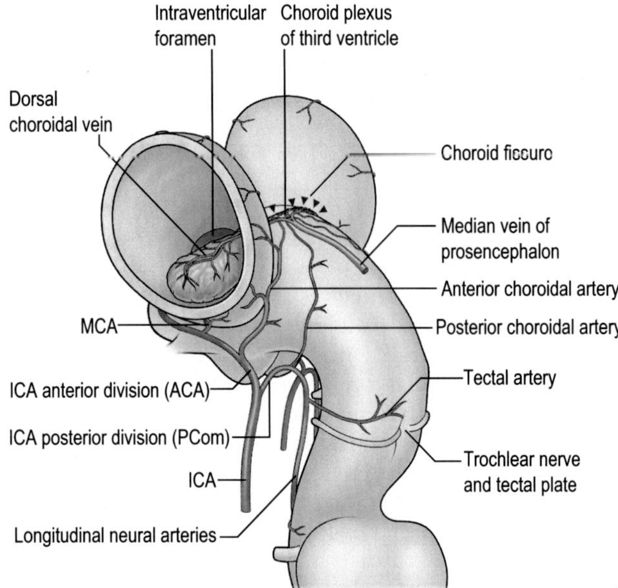

FIGURE 1-2 ■ Schematic of early embryo. The bulging telencephalic vesicles (here cut open to reveal the choroid plexus and interventricular foramen) represent the future cerebral hemispheres. Choroid fissure has appeared in the roof of the future third ventricle, forming the choroid plexus, which is proportionately much larger than in the adult. The choroid plexus is drained by the median prosencephalic vein, a forerunner of the vein of Galen.

terminologies (archicortex, paliocortex, archipallium, etc.) are obsolete and better avoided. The developing cerebral hemispheres are initially separate, with the first crossing fibres developing in the lamina terminalis to form the anterior commissure. Superior to this, formation of the corpus callosum begins, progressing posteriorly. The surface of the hemispheres from an initially smooth (lissencephalic) appearance becomes progressively convoluted. The mesenchymal soft tissues overlying the brain, deriving mainly from the neural crest, differentiate into skull, dura mater and enveloping the

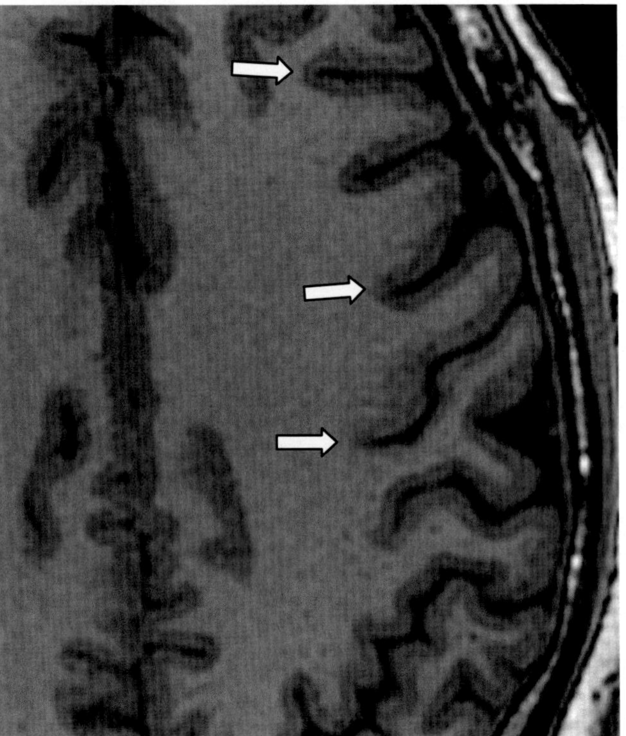

FIGURE 1-3 ■ T2 MR image demonstrates cortical thickness. Note that cortex is thicker over surface and sides of gyri, and thinnest in the depths of the sulci (arrows).

brain the vascular meninx primitiva. Cavitation within the meninx primitiva separates the pia mater from arachnoid mater, producing the subarachnoid space, and modification of the primordial vascular plexus produces the surface vessels of the brain.

Cerebral Cortex, Lobar Anatomy and Deep Grey Matter Structures

If we consider neuroradiology begins with the first radiograph of a skull taken in 1895,[3] we could imagine the disappointment of those pioneers as they realised that the brain was invisible to the 'new radiation'. Indeed most of the history of neuroradiology has involved the quest for an image of the brain. This was achieved with the first CT images in 1972. The cerebral hemispheres can now be examined in superlative detail by MRI at 1.5 and 3 T, and high-field systems are offering the beginnings of MR microscopy, to probe details of the cerebral cortex.

The cerebral cortex itself consists of arrays of neurons (estimated to number 100 billion, each one communicating synaptically with many adjacent neurons in a system of astonishing complexity) which on Nissl staining appear to be arranged in layers.[4,5] The cortex varies from 2 to 5 mm in thickness. Cortical thickness, though not its internal structure, is readily apparent on standard T1 IR and T2 sequences (Fig. 1-3).

Isocortex, as described above, has six layers, allocortex has three, with mesocortex in between, all layers being numbered from superficial to deep. Probably, equal numbers of glial cells are present in the cortex, interacting metabolically with neurons and synapses as well as with the rich network of cortical capillaries. Precise

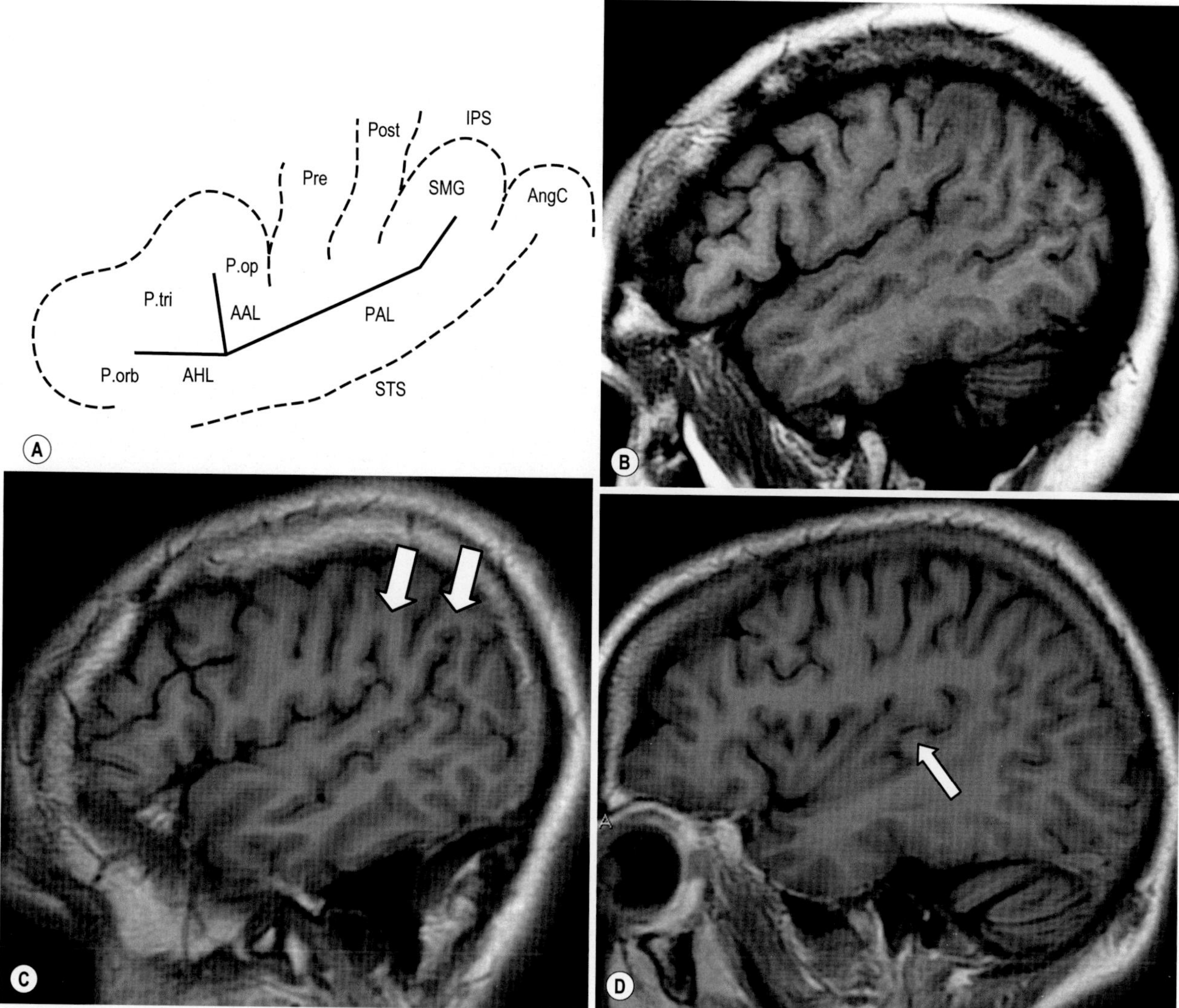

FIGURE 1-4 ■ **Sulcal and gyral relationships of the lateral hemisphere. Schematic and sagittal MR images.** (A) Schematic showing Sylvian fissure in bold. Adjacent sulci of frontal, parietal and temporal lobes represented by dashed lines. Note that the anterior ascending and horizontal limbs of the Sylvian fissure divide the M-shaped inferior frontal gyrus, below the inferior frontal sulcus, into three parts. Broca's area (motor speech) classically occupies the pars opercularis. Wernicke's area (receptive speech) is usually centred on the supramarginal gyrus. (B) The M-shape of the inferior frontal gyrus is well defined in this image. Low signal change in the supramarginal gyrus is evident in this patient with receptive dysphasia and an infarct of Wernicke's area. (C) The inverted horseshoe-shaped supramarginal and angular gyri are well shown in this image (arrows). (D) More medial parasagittal image demonstrates the triangular-shaped insular cortex. Note the consistent bulge of Heschl's gyrus (primary auditory cortex) arising from the superior surface of the temporal lobe (arrow). Abbreviations: PAL, posterior ascending limb; AAL, anterior ascending limb; AHL, anterior horizontal limb; P.op, pars opercularis; P.tri, pars triangularis; P.orb, pars orbitalis; Pre, precentral gyrus; Post, postcentral gyrus; IPS, intraparietal sulcus; SMG, supramarginal gyrus; AngG, angular gyrus; STS, superior temporal sulcus.

functions of glial cells are not clear-cut, but they are certainly not mere supporting cells.[6] The surface of the cortex is formed by a continuous layer of superficial astrocyte foot processes with associated basement membrane forming the glia limitans to which is applied the pia mater, with a potential subpial space intervening.

The cortical mantle over the surface of each hemisphere is folded into a series of elevated gyri separated by sulcal clefts. These form the basis of the separation into the lobes of the brain, which were originally named for the overlying skull bones. Gratiolet (in 1854) adopted this schema, adding precise boundaries which became widely adopted.[7] The lobar terminology represents a convenient though arbitrary system (which has varied over time and between authors) and is largely devoid of ontogenic significance. Six lobes in each hemisphere are often described: frontal, parietal, occipital, temporal, insula and limbic. With familiarity, patterns emerge from the initially bewildering array of brain convolutions allowing quite accurate identification of the major subdivisions.[8,9] The interhemispheric fissure and Sylvian (or lateral) fissure (Fig. 1-4) are immediately obvious.

The central sulcus is the other main landmark of the hemisphere separating the precentral gyrus (motor) from the postcentral gyrus (sensory) and can usually be confidently identified on axial and sagittal images (Fig. 1-5). From these landmarks other sulci and gyri can be sequentially identified.[8,10,11]

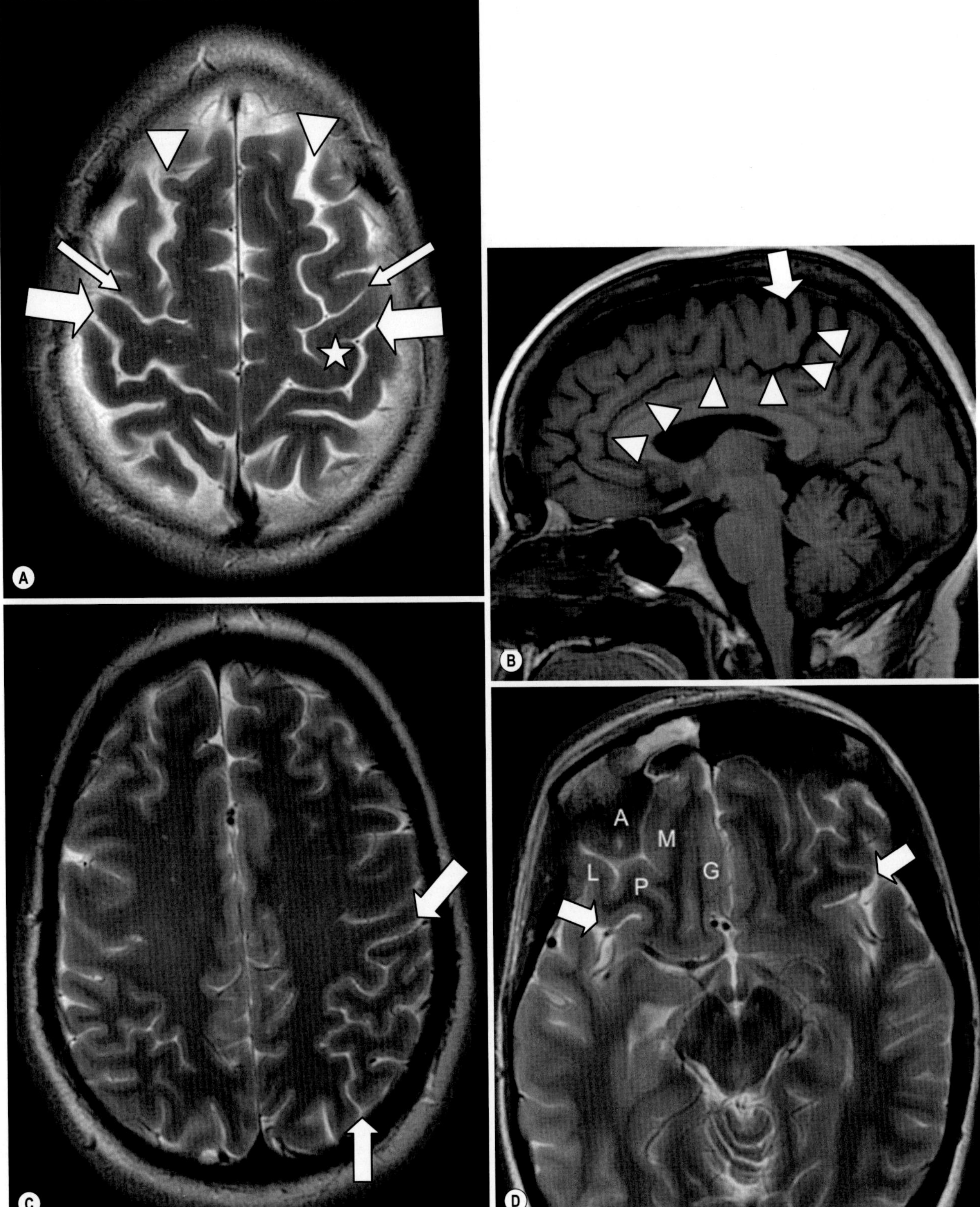

FIGURE 1-5 ■ (A) Axial T2 MR image near vertex. The superior frontal sulcus (arrowheads) is readily identified on most brains between the superior and middle frontal gyri. It typically meets the precentral sulcus (small arrows) almost at a right angle. Posterior to this lies the central sulcus. The bulge in the precentral gyrus (star) represents the hand motor area. (B) Sagittal T1 image. Paralleling the corpus callosum, the cingulate sulcus (arrowheads) as it approaches the splenium turns towards the brain surface. This extension, the pars marginalis of the cingulate sulcus, lies immediately posterior to the central sulcus (large arrow). (C) On axial images, the intraparietal sulcus (arrows) separates the superior parietal lobule (medially) from the inferior parietal lobule (laterally). Anteriorly, it merges with the postcentral sulcus. (D) More caudally, the frontobasal sulci are demonstrated. Note the H-shaped orbital sulci separating the anterior (A), posterior (P), medial (M) and lateral (L) orbital gyri. Gyrus rectus (G) is separated from the medial orbital gyrus by the olfactory sulcus. Arrows indicate the Sylvian fissure.

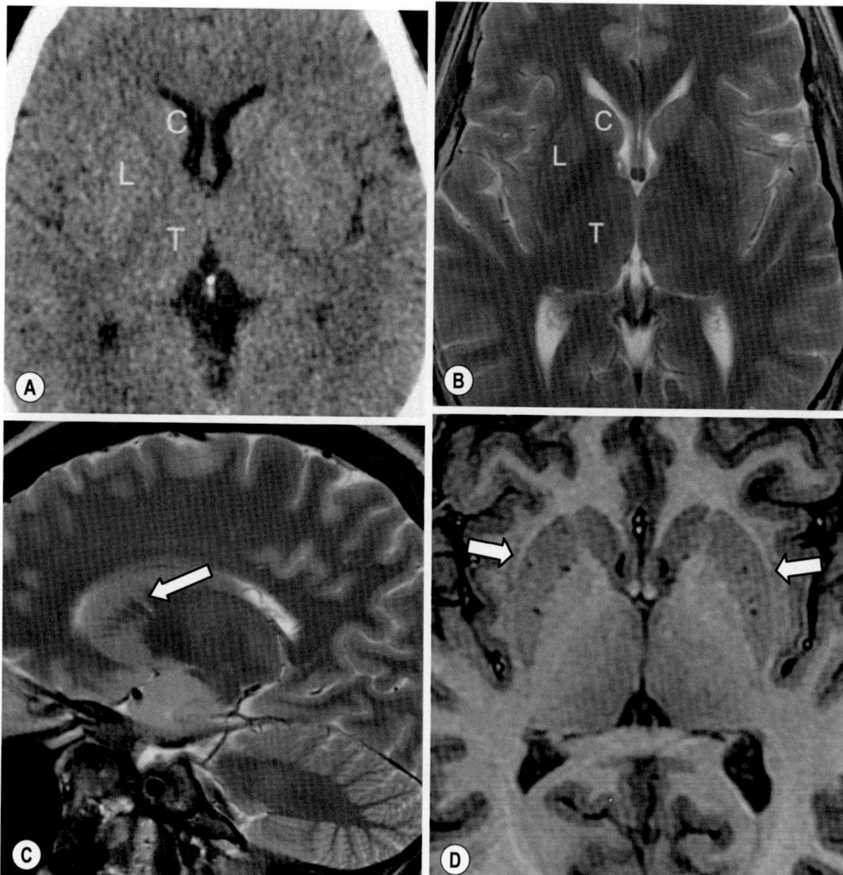

FIGURE 1-6 ■ (A, B) Standard axial CT and T2 MRI images through the basal ganglia and internal capsule. The caudate (C) and lentiform nuclei (L) and the thalami (T) are well demonstrated by CT and MRI together with the intervening V-shape of the internal capsule. (C) Parasagittal T2 image through the basal ganglia. Note the striated appearance of the grey matter bridges crossing the internal capsule, linking the caudate and lentiform nuclei (arrow). (D) T1 axial image shows the thin grey matter layer of the claustrum between the lentiform nucleus and the insula cortex, separating the white matter of the external capsule medially from the extreme capsule laterally.

The deep grey matter structures principally comprise the basal ganglia, amygdala and thalamus and are well demonstrated by CT and MRI (Fig. 1-6). The basal ganglia are part of the extrapyramidal system including the caudate nucleus, globus pallidus, putamen, nucleus accumbens and substantia nigra. The globus pallidus and caudate are linked across the intervening internal capsule by a series of grey matter bridges giving a striated appearance, the origin of the term corpus striatum for this region.

Beneath the internal capsule, these nuclei are linked by the nucleus accumbens. Physiological punctate calcification of the basal ganglia is commonly seen with ageing on CT images after the age of about 30 years.[12,13] Iron deposition is also encountered in the basal ganglia, increasing with age from the second decade (Fig. 1-7).[14] Similarly, calcification in the pineal gland is seen in about 40% of subjects by the age of 20 years (Fig. 1-8).[15]

The thalami are paired large nuclear masses forming most of the lateral walls of the third ventricle, above and behind the hypothalamus. They often are in contact across the ventricle at the massa intermedia. The posterior border, or pulvinar, bulges convexly into the quadrigeminal cistern and overlies the medial (visual) and lateral (olfactory) geniculate bodies.

White Matter Centre

The anatomy of the white matter of the brain has generally received little attention in the imaging literature, which is surprising given the ubiquity of white matter diseases. The medullary core of the brain is formed of bundles of axons, supporting glial cells and penetrating blood vessels. Its whitish colour derives from the fatty myelin sheaths contributed by oligodendrocytes (in the periphery myelin sheaths are formed by Schwann cells). The lipid content accounts for the low density of white matter on CT images and for the characteristic high signal on T1 and low signal on T2 MRI sequences. The white matter is less metabolically active than grey matter and consequently receives a much smaller proportion of the brain's blood supply. On axial anatomic or imaging sections the white matter core presents an oval aspect, Vieussens (eighteenth century) terming the component in each hemisphere, the centrum semiovale (Fig. 1-9).[16] Long after Schwann (1839) established the cell theory, anatomists considered the white matter to be an amorphous continuum, which paradoxically, in imaging terms it has remained until recently. Tractography with MRI diffusion tensor imaging (DTI) can now reveal white matter bundles and their pathways in the living brain. Some of the larger tracts are apparent even on standard sequences. It is conventional in neuroradiology to describe lesions as lying in the subcortical (U-fibres immediately below the cortex), deep (white matter core) or periventricular (thin band of white matter adjacent to the ependyma) white matter.

Axons entering or leaving the cortex can be classified into several types (Fig. 1-9). Thus subcortical U-fibres link one gyrus locally to adjacent gyri with a U-shaped band deep to the sixth layer of the cortex.

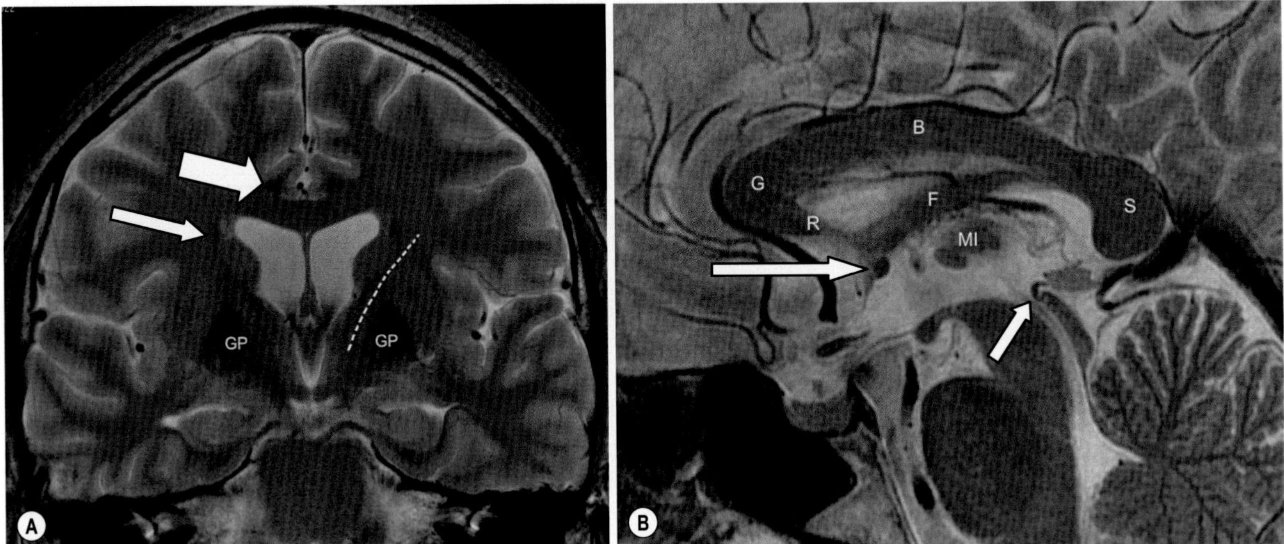

FIGURE 1-7 ■ (A) Coronal T2 MR image. Low signal bundles of the cingulum (arrow) within the cingulate gyrus and the superior longitudinal fasciculus (thin arrow). The internal capsules are well seen (dotted line) between the caudate and lentiform nuclei. Note low signal of iron deposition in the globus pallidus (GP) and the flow voids of CSF passing through the foramen of Monro. (B) Sagittal T2 MR image. The corpus callosum genu (G), rostrum (R), body (B) and splenium (S) are shown. Note the anterior commissure (long arrow) and posterior commissure (short arrow) forming the posterior border of the cerebral aqueduct. Also shown are the fornix (F) and the massa intermedia (MI), or thalamic adhesion, within the third ventricle.

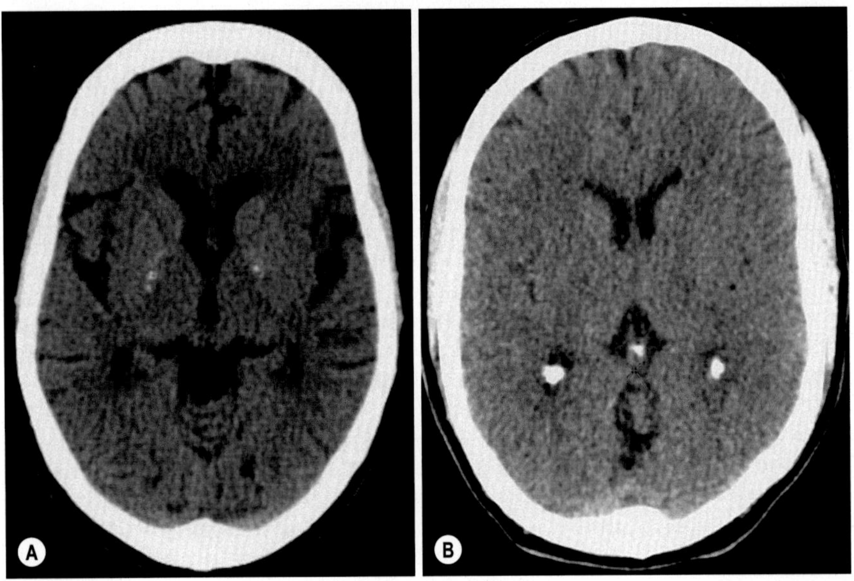

FIGURE 1-8 ■ **Axial CT images.** (A) Normal age-related calcification of the globus pallidus on each side. (B) Midline calcification of the pineal gland. Note the paired internal cerebral veins immediately anterior to the pineal calcification. Typical calcification is also present in the choroid plexuses in the trigones bilaterally.

Ascending/descending tracts carry sensory information to the thalamus and cortex, or project motor fibres via the internal capsule to traverse the brainstem. For example, the corona radiata and internal capsule bearing the descending corticospinal tract, corticocerebellar tracts traverse the cerebellar peduncles and the ascending spinothalamic tracts.

Association tracts link cortical areas in different lobes of the same hemisphere. The most prominent are the superior longitudinal fasciculus (SLF I, II and III) running in the white matter of the parietal lobe linking parieto-occipital and frontal lobes, the arcuate fasciculus, the extreme capsule, the fronto-occipital fasciculus (running with the subcallosal bundle of Muratoff, the combination being visible on standard T2 sequences MRI), the uncinate fasciculus linking anterior and mesial temporal structures with the frontobasal region, and the cingulum bundle, also visible on standard MRI (Fig. 1-7).

Commissural tracts are crossing fibres linking corresponding regions of opposite hemispheres, the largest of these being the corpus callosum, a mammalian innovation only absent in marsupials and monotremes. This dense bundle of fibres containing up to 190 million axons has a rostrum, genu, body and splenium. Anteriorly, its fibres fan out into the forceps minor and posteriorly from the larger splenium into the forceps major. Consisting of densely packed axons with relatively low metabolic requirements, it is less susceptible to ischaemic disease but is a typical site of demyelination, particularly on its ventricular surface. It also provides a common route of

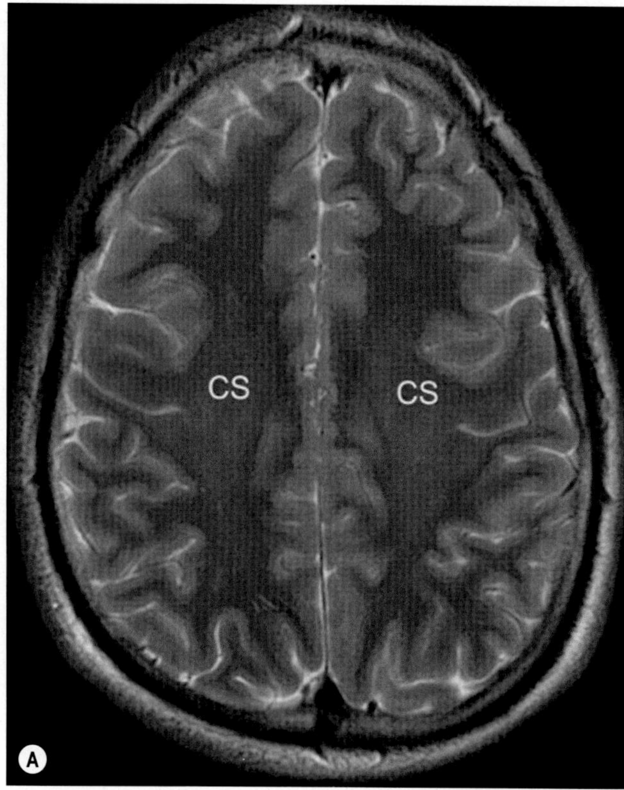

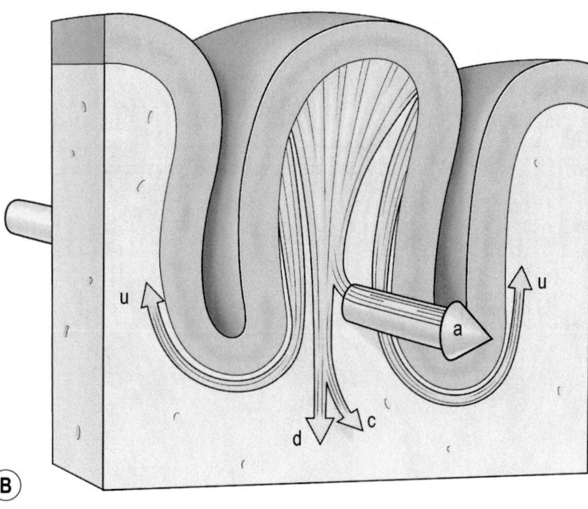

FIGURE 1-9 (A) Axial T2 MRI demonstrates the white matter core of the cerebral hemispheres, the centrum semiovale (CS). (B) Schematic demonstrating the several types of white matter tract: subcortical U-fibres (u), ascending/descending tracts (d), association tracts (a) and commissural tracts (c).

spread for aggressive neoplasms (butterfly glioma). The anterior commissure (AC), a dense bundle of axons, runs in the anterior wall of the third ventricle and is well demonstrated on sagittal and axial sections. The posterior commissure (PC), although more difficult to visualise directly on sagittal images, can be readily pinpointed since it is located at the point where the cerebral aqueduct opens into the third ventricle. The AC–PC line is a basic imaging plane for stereotaxic procedures and is thus easily drawn on sagittal images. There are several other smaller commissures, including the fornix (or hippocampal) commissure and the habenular commissure.

Limbic System, Hypothalamus and Pituitary Gland

Following the isocortical mantel over the hemisphere to its medial edges, the structures of the limbic system are encountered. These include the amygdala, hippocampus, parahippocampal gyrus, cingulate gyrus, subcallosal gyri and associated structures.

Limbic structures are associated with memory processing, emotional responses, fight-or-flight responses, aggression and sexual response: in summary, with activities contributing to preservation of the individual and the continuation of the species. These structures are demonstrated in detail by coronal and sagittal MRI. The limbic system is often rather misleadingly described as a phylogenetically ancient part of the brain: the hippocampus is unequivocally a mammalian innovation while the isocortex itself has equally ancient antecedents.

The core limbic structures are located in the medial temporal lobe readily amenable to high-resolution MRI.

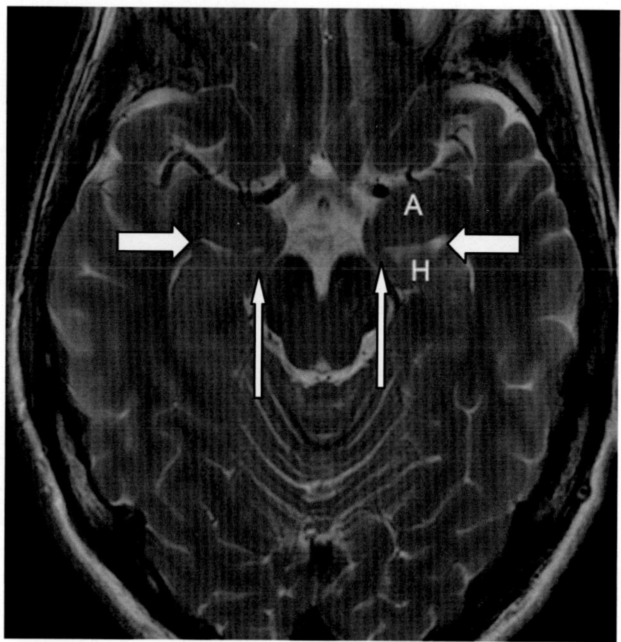

FIGURE 1-10 **Axial T2 MR image of mesial temporal structures.** The uncal recess of the temporal horn of the lateral ventricle turns medially, separating the amygdala (A) from the hippocampal head (H). The uncus lies medially (thin arrows).

The amydala is the most anterior structure, separated from the hippocampal head by the uncal recess of the temporal horn (Fig. 1-10). The medial lying uncus (hook) has anterior amygdaloid and posterior hippocampal components.

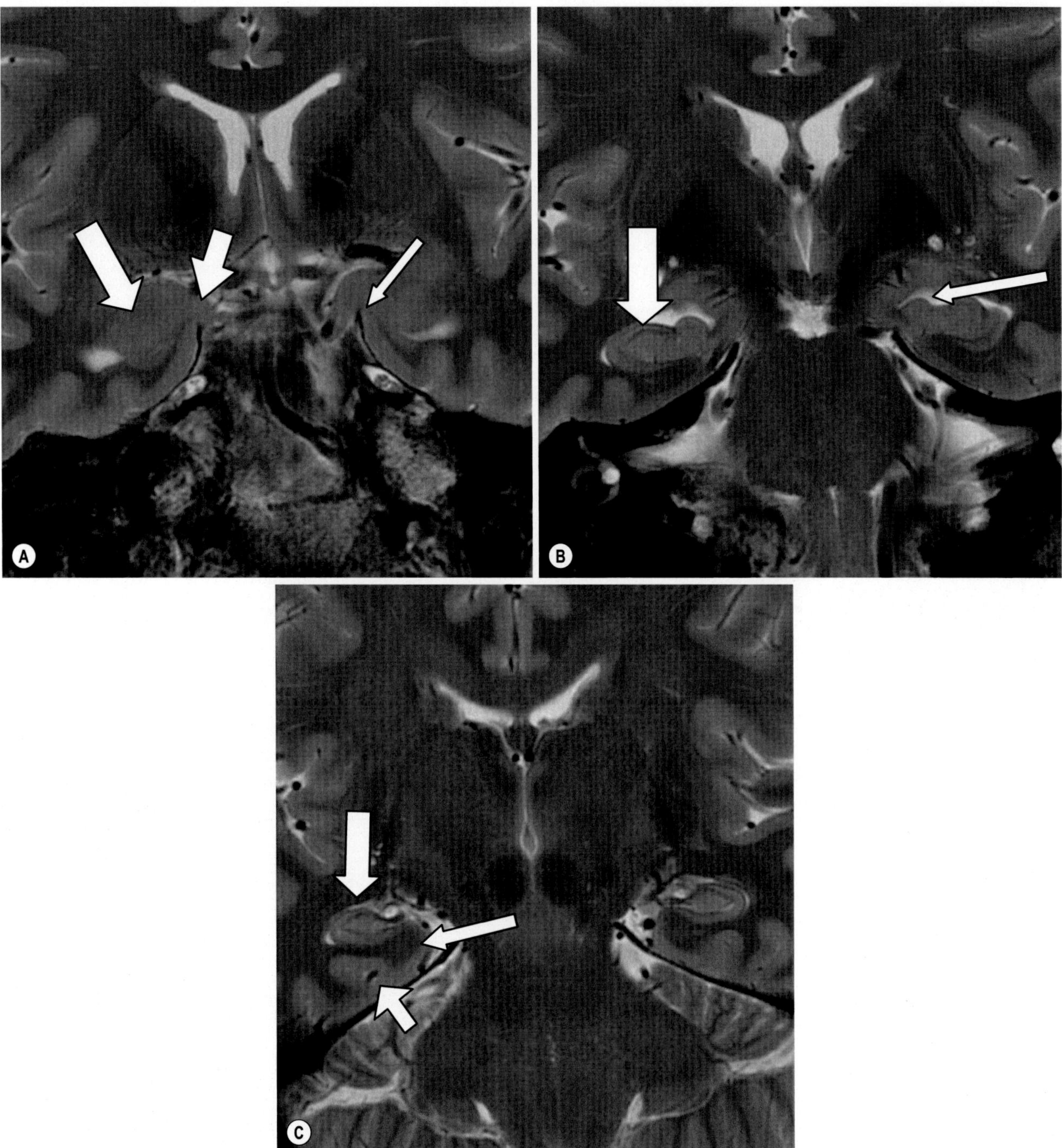

FIGURE 1-11 ■ Coronal T2 MR images from anterior to posterior, demonstrating the main limbic structures of the mesial temporal lobe. Compare with the structures on the schematic picture. (A) Amygdala (large arrow), uncus (short arrow), free margin of tentorium cerebelli (thin arrow). (B) Hippocampal head (large arrow), uncal recess of temporal horn separating posterior aspect of amygdala superiorly from hippocampal head inferiorly. (C) Body of hippocampus (large arrow), parahippocampal gyrus (long arrow), collateral sulcus (short arrow).

The hippocampal head, body and tail are well shown on coronal imaging, along with the parahippocampal gyrus (Fig. 1-11).

The white matter connections of the hippocampus via the fibria-fornix system are visualised on coronal and sagittal images. A thinned layer of hippocampal tissue, the indusium griseum, extends over the corpus callosum but is not visible on standard imaging.

The hypothalamus forms the floor of the third ventricle and its side walls anteriorly following an oblique line inferiorly from the foramen of Monro to the midbrain aqueduct. It consists of a group of nuclei serving a number of autonomic, appetite-related and regulatory functions for the body as well as controlling and producing hormonal output from the pituitary gland. The hypothalamus is intimately linked to other limbic structures and might be considered the output for the limbic system.

The pituitary infundibulum (or pituitary stalk), a hollow conical structure, extends inferiorly from the hypothalamus to the pituitary gland. The pituitary

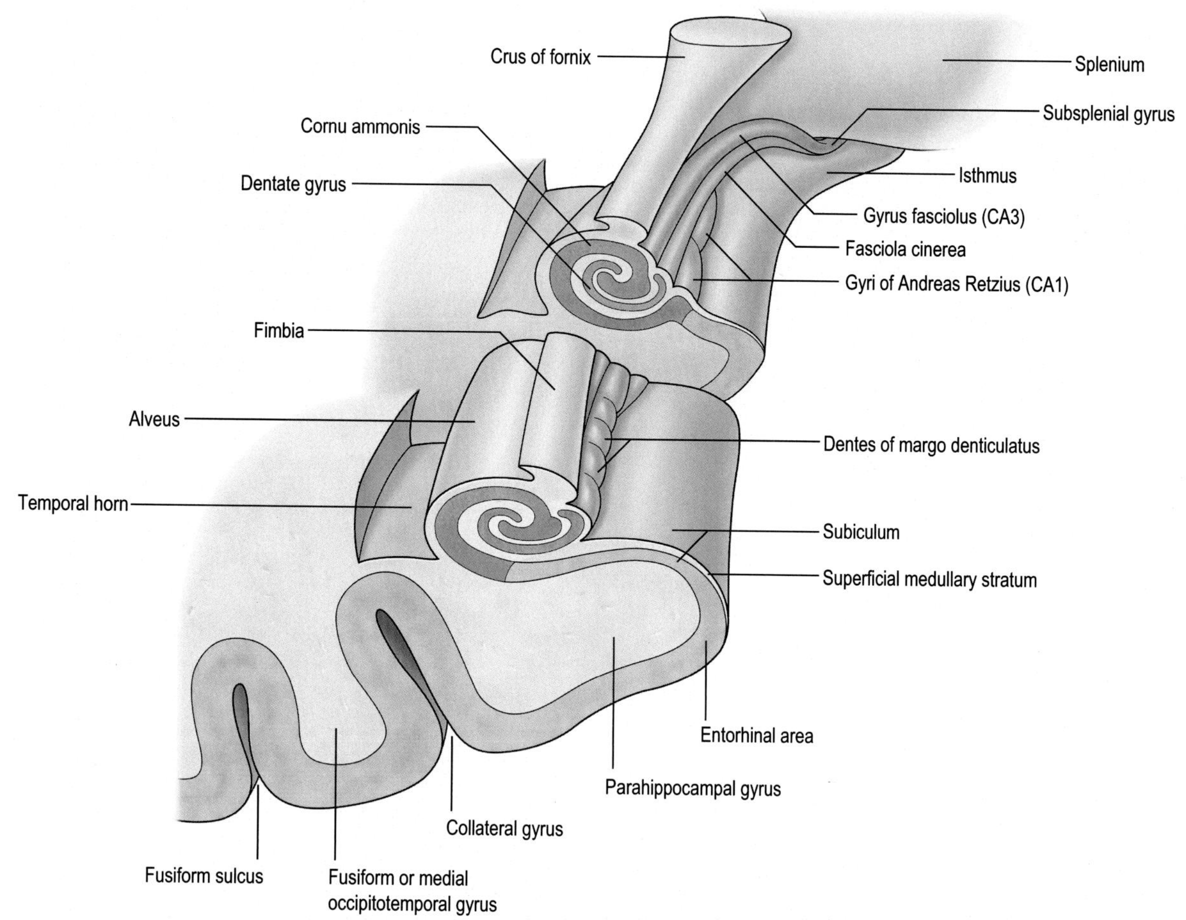

FIGURE 1-11, Continued ■ (D) Schematic illustration of hippocampal structures.

gland varies considerably in size, with sometimes only a thin rim of glandular tissue visible at the floor of the pituitary fossa. In young females, the gland may fill the fossa with a convex upper border. Anterior and posterior lobes can be distinguished on MRI, the posterior lobe often returning a high signal on T1-weighted images due to neurosecretory granules in the neurohypophysis. Both gland and stalk show strong contrast enhancement.

Ventricular System and Subarachnoid Space

The ventricular system, filled with cerebrospinal fluid, is the mature derivative of the cavity of the neural tube. Thus, the telencephalon contains the lateral ventricles; the diencephalon, the third ventricle; the midbrain, the cerebral aquaduct and the brainstem, the fourth venrticle (Fig. 1-12). The ventricles are lined by modified glial cells constituting the ependyma.

The lateral ventricles are divided into frontal horn, body, occipital (posterior) and temporal horns. The junction of the body, occipital and temporal horn is known as the trigone indented posteromedially by the calcar avis, the impression of the deep calcarine fissure. The sites of the original outpouchings of the telencephalic vesicles form the interventricular foramina of Monro linking the lateral ventricles with the anterosuperior aspect of the third ventricle. The third ventricle is a midline, slit-like cavity bordered laterally by the bulky grey matter of the thalami that frequently make contact with each other centrally as the massa intermedia. Antero-inferiorly and inferiorly lies the hypothalamus. A number of important structures are identified in the walls of the third ventricle on sagittal midline MRI slices (Figs. 1-7 and 1-13).

From the posteroinferior aspect of the third ventricle, the cerebral aqueduct (of Silvius) traverses the midbrain emerging into the rhomboid-shaped fourth ventricle (Fig. 1-14). The floor of the fourth ventricle is formed by the pons and medulla oblongata and it is roofed by the cerebellum, with its tented apex, the fastigium. There are two lateral apertures, the foramina of Luschka and a single posterior one, the foramen of Magendie allowing efflux of cerebrospinal fluid (CSF) into the subarachnoid space. At the inferior aspect of the fourth ventricle the embryonic continuation of the neural tube cavity into the central canal of the spinal cord is commonly obliterated in the adult.

As described above, the cavity of the ventricular system is invaginated, from the choroid fissure by the choroid plexus, a vascular membrane with pial and ependymal layers. Anterior and posterior choroidal arteries enter this membrane. Choroid plexus is present in both lateral ventricles and extends through the interventricular foramina into the third ventricle forming the roof. In the fourth ventricle the choroid plexus extends laterally into both foramina of Luschka, often projecting into the

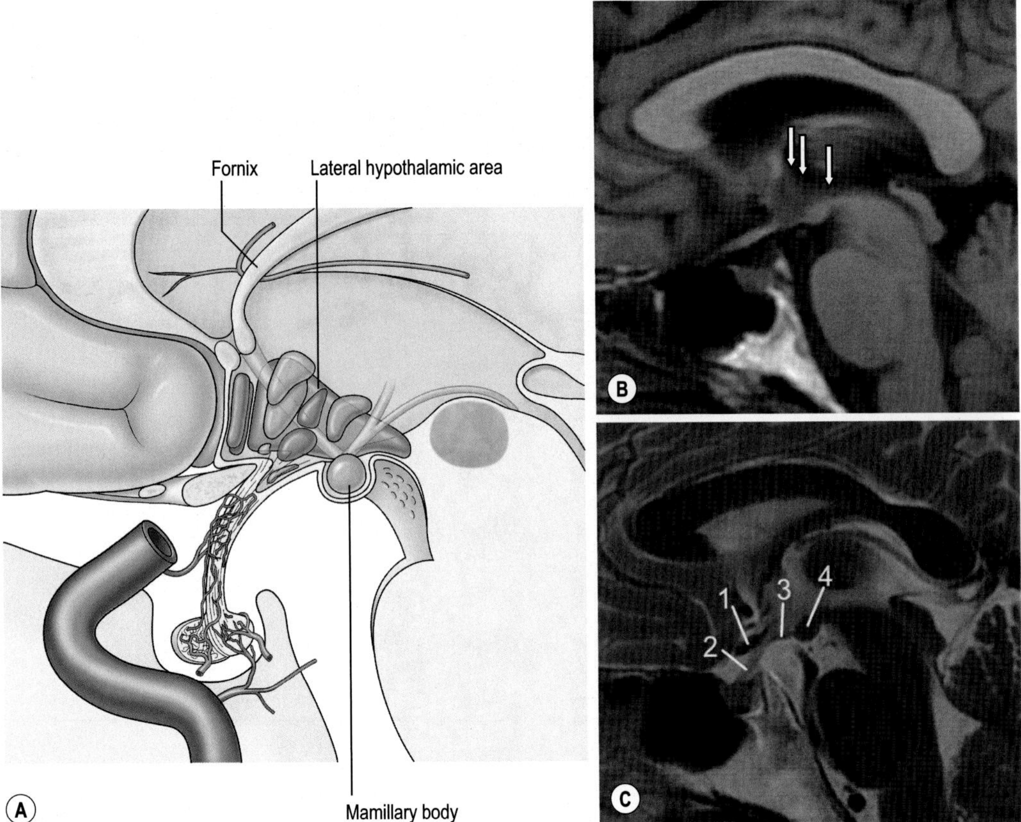

FIGURE 1-12 ■ (A) Schematic diagram depicting the nuclei of the hypothalamus in the lateral wall and floor of the third ventricle. Preoptic nuclei in red. Paraventricular and anterior nuclei in yellow. Medial and infundibular nuclei in blue. Posterior nucleus and mamillary body in orange. Blood supply to the pituitary gland is also shown with the superior and inferior hypophyseal arteries arising from the internal carotid artery. (B) Sagittal T1 image. Hypothalamic border (hypothalamic sulcus) is well seen in this example (arrows). (C) Sagittal T2 image demonstrates the structures in the floor of the third ventricle: Optic chiasm (1), pituitary infundibulum (2), tuber cinereum (3) and mamillary bodies (4).

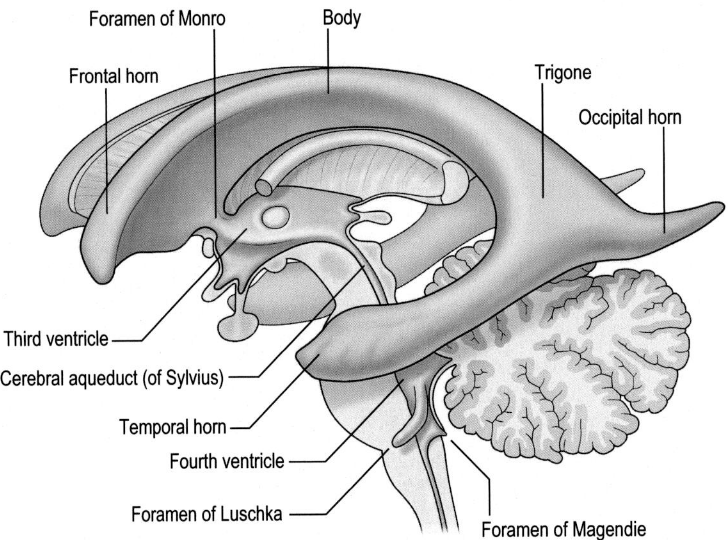

FIGURE 1-13 ■ **Schematic illustration of the components of the ventricular system.** Note the two anterior recesses (chiasmatic and infundibular) and the two posterior recesses (pineal and suprapineal) of the third ventricle.

subarachnoid space. Fourth ventricular choroid plexus is supplied by branches of the posterior inferior cerebellar artery.

CSF flows from the fourth ventricular foramina into the subarachnoid space (Fig. 1-15). Over the superior convexity of the brain, the subarachnoid space is thin. At the base conversely, because of irregularity of the inferior surface of the brain and skull, the spaces become widened in places which are known as subarachnoid cisterns, named for adjacent structures.

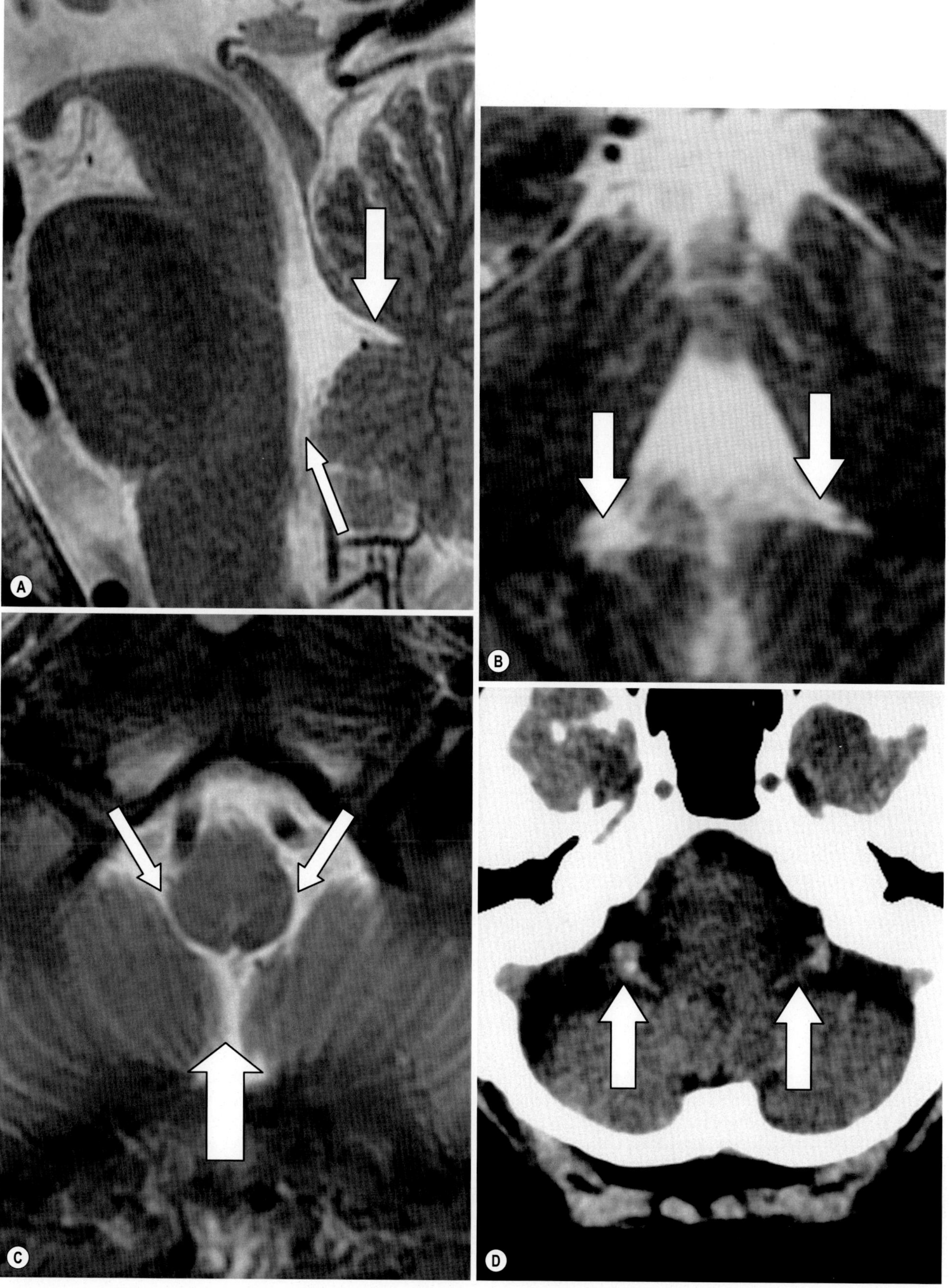

FIGURE 1-14 ■ (A) Sagittal T2 MR image. Flow void of CSF within the aqueduct is present. The tented apex of the fourth ventricle, the fastigium (large arrow) and the foramen of Magendie (small arrow) are well shown. (B) The rhomboid shape of the fourth ventricle is apparent in coronal images. The lateral recesses (arrows) funnel into the foramina of Luschka. (C) Axial MR image through the caudal fourth ventricle demonstrate the foramen of Magendie (large arrow) and foramina of Luschka (small arrows). (D) Axial CT. Tufts of choroid plexus typically project through the foramina of Luschka into the subarachnoid space and may be calcified (arrows).

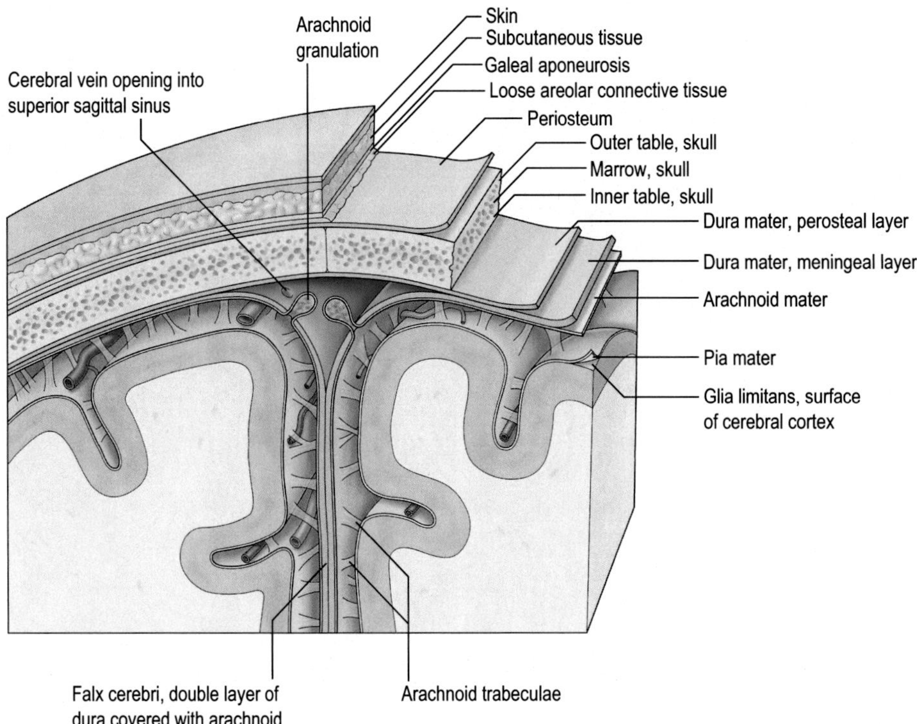

FIGURE 1-15 ■ Schematic showing the relationship of the subarachnoid space to the surrounding meninges.

CSF is produced in part from the choroid plexuses, and in part from transudation of fluid from brain capillaries into the ventricles at a rate of approximately 500 mL per day. The total volume of CSF in the ventricles, intracranial and spinal subarachnoid space is about 150 mL. Thus, total CSF volume is turned over several times a day. Previous concepts that the majority of CSF is reabsorbed into the dural venous sinuses at the arachnoid granulations no longer appear tenable.[17,18] Whether the granulations are involved at all in CSF reabsorption remains debatable and their major functions are unknown in adults as well as infants in whom they are not fully formed. The major routes of CSF reabsorption appear to be along the cranial nerve linings, large vessel adventitia and the cribriform plate into the lymphatic system, via the spinal, especially lumbar, epidural space as well as directly back into the capillaries and venules of the brain.

Cerebellum

The cerebellum occupies the bulk of the posterior fossa, lying posterior to the fourth ventricle and brainstem to which it is linked by the white matter tracts of the paired superior, middle and inferior cerebellar peduncles. It is separated from the occipital lobes by the dural fold of the tentorium cerebelli. The cerebellum displays much finer folding than the cerebral hemispheres, the folds being termed folia. There are two cerebellar hemispheres joined by a midline portion, the cerebellar vermis, which is divided into a number of lobules readily identified on sagittal MRI (Fig. 1-16). Cerebellar cortex overlies the cerebellar white matter. Within the white matter on each side are the cluster of paired deep cerebellar nuclei, the largest of which are the two dentate nuclei. The principal functions of the cerebellum involve the coordination of skilled voluntary movements and muscle tone, each cerebellar hemisphere serving this function for the same side of the body.

Brainstem

The brainstem is usually considered to include the midbrain, pons and medulla oblongata and extends from the posterior commissure at the opening into the third ventricle to the pyramidal decussation at the cervicomedullary junction. This may be divided into the hindbrain or rhombencephalon, comprising the medulla oblongata and pons (as well as the cerebellum which develops from them) and the mesencephalon or midbrain.

The midbrain (Fig. 1-17) consists of the anteriorly lying cerebral peduncles containing the descending and ascending tracts. These are separated by the grey matter nuclei of the substantia nigra from the midbrain tegmentum. The tegmentum extends posteriorly to the cerebral aqueduct (of Silvius). Posterior to the aqueduct lies the tectal (or quadrigeminal) plate with its superior and inferior colliculi. Cranial nerve IV arises here also, the only cranial nerve to arise from the dorsal surface of the brainstem. Grey matter structures within the midbrain include the substantia nigra and red nuclei, readily identified on MRI, as well as the upper cranial nerve nuclei. The medial forebrain bundle bringing limbic fibres from the septal area and hypothalamus ends in the reticular formation, a loose array of neurons, part of the limbic midbrain.

The pons (Fig. 1-17) comprises a bulbous convexity anteriorly, the basis pontis, containing masses of transversely oriented fibres which enter the large middle cerebellar peduncles on each side. Amongst these fibres are the dispersed bundles of the corticospinal tracts which

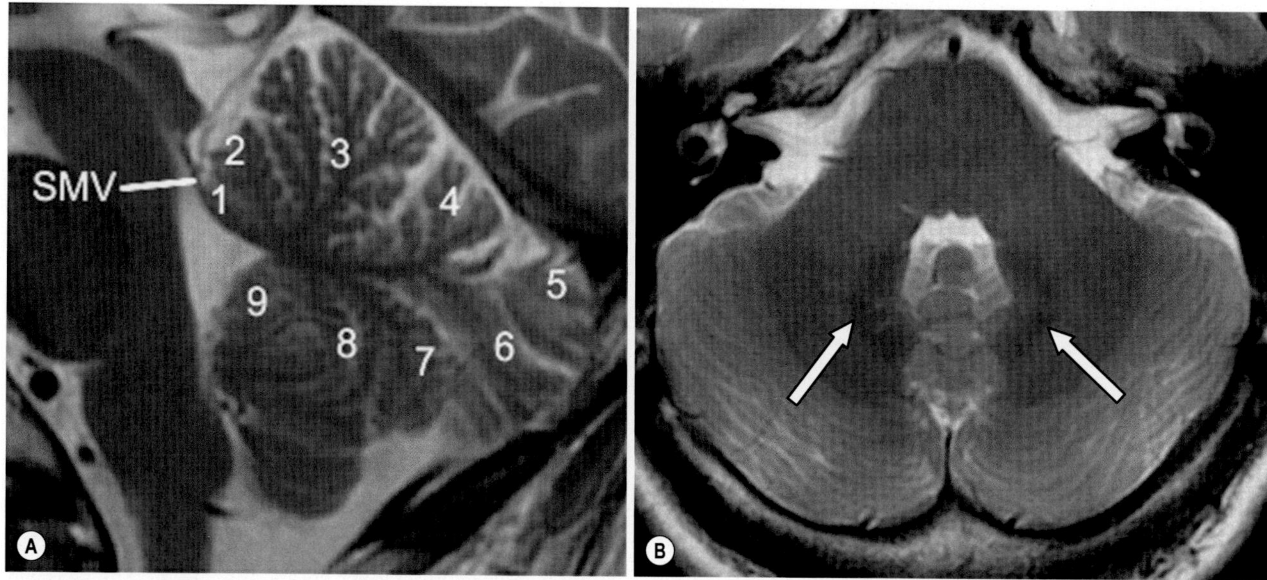

FIGURE 1-16 ■ **T2 MR images.** (A) Sagittal image of cerebellum. Lobules of vermis are demonstrated: lingula (1), central (2), culmen (3), declive (4), folium (5), tuber (6), pyramid (7), uvule (8) and nodule (9). The roof of the fourth ventricle is formed by the superior medullary velum (SMV). (B) Axial image at level of pons and internal auditory meatus. Iron deposition in the dentate nuclei gives low signal change (arrows).

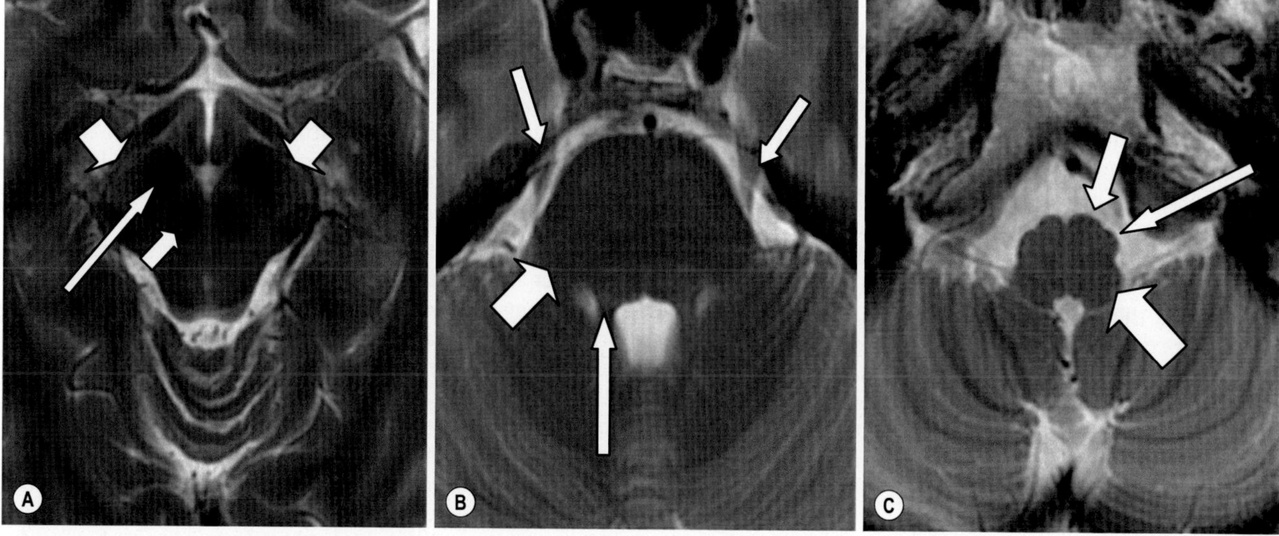

FIGURE 1-17 ■ **Axial T2 MR images through brainstem.** (A) Midbrain. Note the low signal indicating iron accumulation in the red nuclei (short arrow) and substantia nigra (long arrow). The cerebral peduncles contain the ascending and descending tracts from the cerebral hemispheres (broad arrows). (B) Pons. The trigeminal nerves can be seen running anteriorly into Meckel's cave (short arrows). The superior (long arrow) and middle cerebellar peduncles (broad arrow) are separated by CSF in the inferior extension of the ambient cistern. (C) Medulla oblongata. On each side three bulges are visible in the contour of the medulla: the pyramids (short arrow), olives (long arrow) and the inferior cerebellar peduncle (broad arrow).

separate as they leave the midbrain and reform as they enter the pyramids of the medulla. The posterior part of the pons, the pontine tegmentum, forms the floor of the upper part of the fourth ventricle, and contains cranial nerve nuclei (V, VI, VII, VIII).

The medulla oblongata (Fig. 1-17) consists of an inferior closed portion, with its central canal extending into the spinal cord, and a superior open portion related to the inferior portion of the fourth ventricle. The closed part of the medulla extends from the C1 spinal roots to the obex at the lower margin of the fourth ventricle. The ventral surface of the medulla is marked by two bulges on each side: medially lie the pyramids and laterally, the olives. The medulla transmits ascending sensory tracts posteriorly and descending motor tracts anteriorly both of which cross the midline, or decussate within the closed medulla (sensory decussation lying slightly higher). The lower cranial nerve nuclei lie within the medulla but are not visible with imaging. In cross-section the medulla oblongata is, however, well demonstrated on MRI.

Cerebral Vasculature

The internal carotid arteries (ICA) supply the anterior cerebral circulation while the vertebral forming the

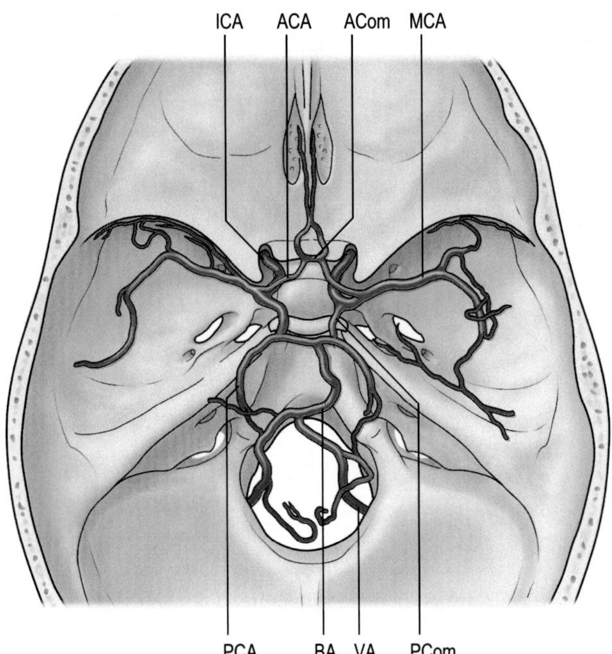

FIGURE 1-18 ■ CTA of a relatively symmetrical and complete circle of Willis. Anterior cerebral artery (ACA), anterior communicating artery (ACom), internal carotid artery (ICA), middle cerebral artery (MCA), posterior communicating artery (PCom), posterior cerebral artery (PCA), basilar artery (BA), vertebral artery (VA).

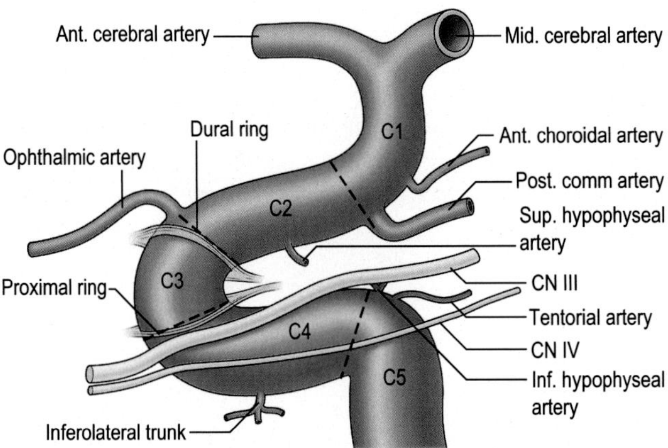

FIGURE 1-19 ■ Schematic illustration of the carotid syphon. The emergence of the ICA from the petrous bone into the cavernous sinus is shown inferiorly (not labelled) and the dural rings where it exits the cavernous sinus are shown proximal to the ophthalmic artery. The close relationship of the cranial nerves to the artery is indicated (CN V and VI are not shown). The segments of the ICA are numbered. Small branches of the ICA are shown and the close relationship of the origins of the posterior communicating and anterior choroidal arteries are apparent.

basilar artery supply the posterior circulation (Fig. 1-18), the two meeting at the circle of Willis. The external carotid arteries (ECA) supply most extracranial head and neck structures (except the orbits) and make an important contribution to the supply of the meninges. There are numerous anastomoses between the external carotid arteries and the anterior and posterior circulation.

The aortic arch gives rise to three main branches, brachiocephalic, left common carotid and left subclavian arteries. The common carotid arteries run within the carotid sheath, lateral to the vertebral column, and bifurcate usually at the fourth cervical vertebrae into external and internal carotid arteries.

Anterior Circulation

The internal carotid artery can be divided into a number of segments C1–C5. The cavernous segment (Fig. 1-19) gives branches to dura, pituitary gland and cranial nerves before its first major branch, the ophthalmic artery.[19] The tentorial and inferior hypophyseal vessels may arise as a meningohypophyseal trunk. The inferolateral trunk supplies adjacent cranial nerves and anastomoses with the ECA. After leaving the cavernous sinus, it pierces the dura and enters the subarachnoid space at the level of the anterior clinoid process (Fig. 1-20). The posterior communicating artery is of very variable size, sometimes occurring as a fetal-type posterior cerebral artery. The anterior choroidal artery supplies the posterior limb of internal capsule, cerebral peduncle and optic tract, medial temporal lobe and choroid plexus. The supraclinoid segment of the ICA divides into the anterior (ACA) and middle cerebral arteries (MCA).

The anterior cerebral artery[20,21] is divided into three anatomical segments: horizontal or precommunicating segment (A1), vertical or postcommunicating segment (A2) and distal ACA including cortical branches (A3). The A1 segment is joined to the contralateral A1 segment by the anterior communicating artery. The A1 segment gives rise to perforating branches, the medial lenticulostriate arteries. The recurrent artery of Heubner is the largest of the perforating branches doubling back on the parent artery, arising from the A1 or A2 segment. One or other A1 segment may be hypoplastic, or the A2 segments may fuse to give a midline azygous anterior cerebral artery. Cortical branches of the ACA supply the medial aspect of the cerebral hemisphere.

The middle cerebral artery[22] is divided into four anatomical segments: horizontal segment (M1), insular segment (M2), opercular segment (M3) and cortical branches (M4 segments). Medial and lateral lenticulostriate arteries are perforating branches that arise from the M1 segment supplying the basal ganglia and capsular regions. The M1 segment divides as a bifurcation or trifurcation. Cortical branches supply the lateral surface of the cerebral hemispheres.

Posterior Circulation

The vertebral arteries usually arise as the first branches of the subclavian arteries (V1), then entering the foramen transversarium of the sixth cervical vertebra. They run upwards through each vertebra (V2) before arching around the anterior arch and behind the lateral mass of the atlas (V3) to pierce the dura mater and enter the subarachnoid space at the level of the foramen magnum (V4), fusing with their fellow in front of the lower pons, to form the basilar artery (Fig. 1-21). The left vertebral artery is commonly larger. The vertebral arteries give muscular branches, which anastomose with the ascending pharyngeal and occipital arteries, posterior meningeal

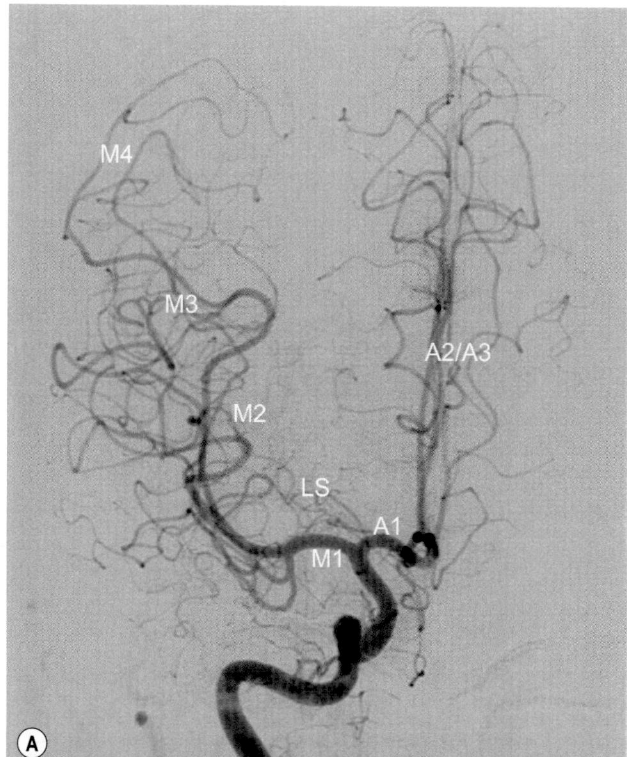

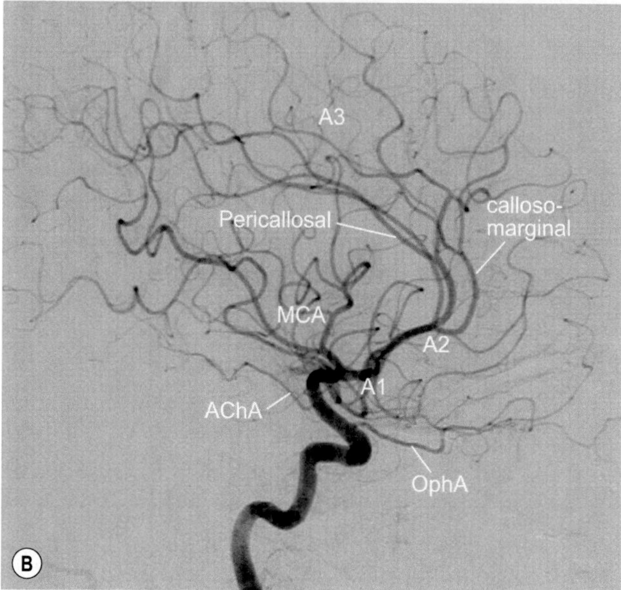

FIGURE 1-20 ■ Digital subtraction angiography (DSA) of the ICA. (A) AP view. (B) Lateral view. Segments of the MCA (M1–4), and ACA (A1–3) are visible. Anterior choroidal artery (AChA), ophthalmic artery (OphA), lenticulostriate arteries (LS).

branches, as well as supplying the cervical spinal cord. After entering the cranial cavity, each vertebral artery gives off a posterior inferior cerebellar artery (PICA) supplying the brainstem, inferior cerebellar hemisphere, vermis and the choroid plexus.

The basilar artery runs superiorly on the anterior surface of the pons giving off anterior inferior cerebellar (AICA), superior cerebellar (SCA) and posterior cerebral arteries on both sides as well as perforating branches. It terminates just above the tip of the dorsum sellae.[23]

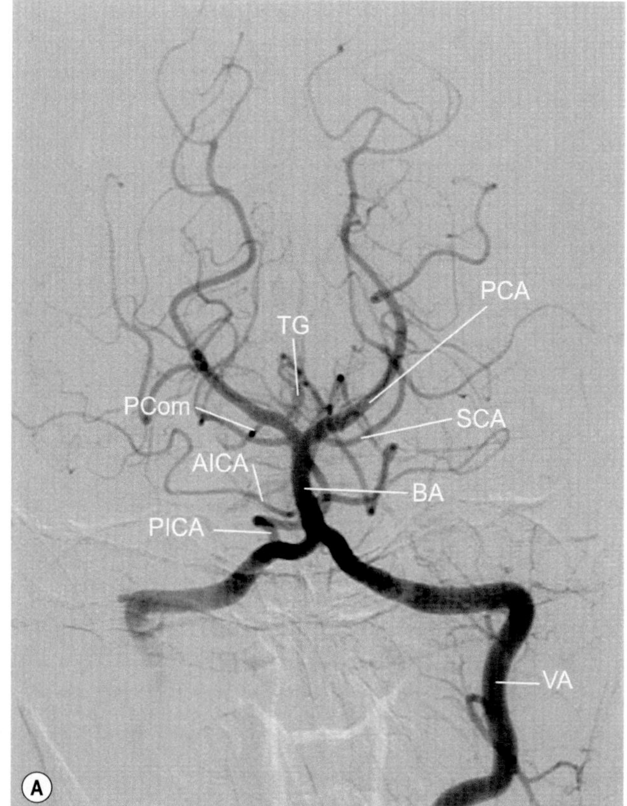

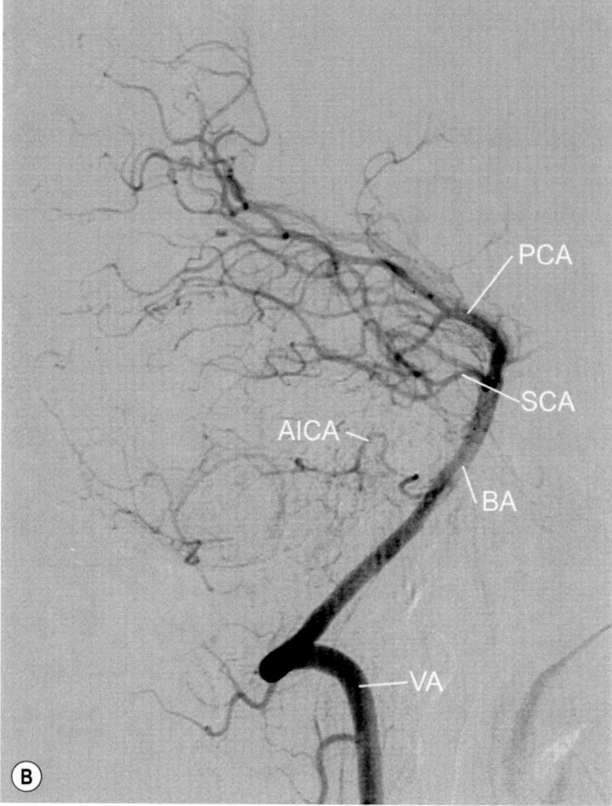

FIGURE 1-21 ■ DSA of the vertebrobasilar circulation. (A) AP and (B) lateral views. vertebral artery (VA), basilar artery (BA), posterior inferior cerebellar artery (PICA), anterior inferior cerebellar artery (AICA), superior cerebellar artery (SCA), posterior cerebral artery (PCA), posterior communicating artery (PCom), thalamogeniculate (TG) perforating arteries.

The AICAs enter the cerebellopontine angle, and supply the surrounding structures; their branches include the internal auditory arteries, to the nerves in the internal auditory meatus. The cerebellar branches anastomose with those of the PICA. The SCAs arise several millimetres below the posterior cerebral arteries from which they are separated by the tentorium cerebelli. They pass around the brainstem to fan out over the superior surface of the cerebellar hemispheres.

The posterior cerebral arteries are the terminal branches of the basilar artery, each of which has four segments. P1 (precommunicating) segment joins the posterior communicating artery to become the P2 (ambient) segment and then P3 (quadrigeminal) segment. The P4 segment is the terminal segment, and includes the occipital and inferior temporal branches. There is reciprocity in calibre of the precommunicating (P1) segments of the posterior cerebral arteries and the posterior communicating arteries: at one extreme is the so-called fetal origin of the posterior cerebral artery. Here, the P1 segments may be hypoplastic and even invisible on vertebral angiography. The posterior communicating arteries and P1 segments give off the thalamoperforating arteries and thalamogeniculate arteries, which enter the posterior perforated substance. Posterior choroidal arteries, medial and lateral arise from the P2 segment. Cortical branches arise from the P2 segment (anterior and posterior temporal arteries) and from the P4 segment, supplying a considerable portion of the inferior surface of the temporal lobe and the medial surface of the occipital lobe, including the visual cortex.

External Carotid Artery

The major branches of the external carotid artery are shown in Fig. 1-22; in general they are named simply for their territory of supply.

Anastomotic Pathways

There are three main categories of collateral supply to the brain: extracranial–intracranial anastomoses, the circle of Willis and leptomeningeal collaterals. The extracranial—intracranial collaterals are actual or potential anastomotic connections between branches of the external carotid artery and the internal carotid or vertebral arteries. These play a role in chronic cerebrovascular occlusive disease and their knowledge is of vital importance for interventional endovascular procedures.[24]

The circle of Willis[25] plays a critical role as a collateral supply in acute and chronic cerebrovascular occlusive disease. The circle of Willis is well demonstrated with axial projections of MR or CT angiograms. A complete circle of Willis is only found in about 40% of people and various segments of the circle may be sufficiently small or absent to be ineffective as a collateral channel. Common variations include absence or hypoplasia of one of the A1 segments and of one or both posterior communicating arteries. The fetal origin of the posterior cerebral artery from the internal carotid artery occurs in 20–30%.

There are other developmental connections between the anterior (carotid) and posterior (vertebrobasilar) circulation that may persist into adult life, the commonest, the trigeminal artery found in less than 1% of normal people (Fig. 1-23). The so-called otic artery is most likely fictitious.[26]

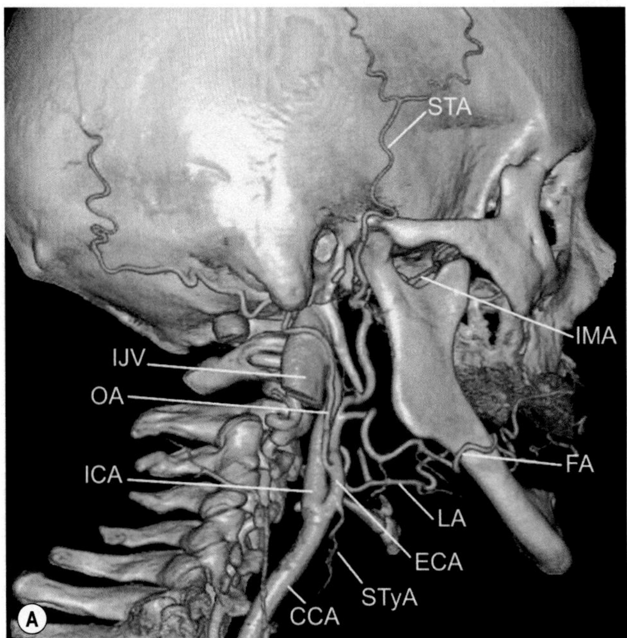

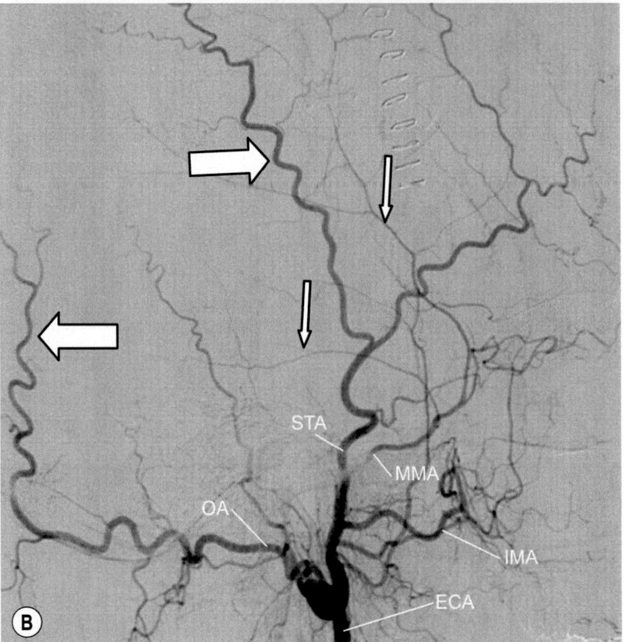

FIGURE 1-22 ■ (A) CTA image of external carotid arteries. Common carotid artery (CCA), internal carotid artery (ICA), external carotid artery (ECA), superficial thyroid artery (STyA), lingual artery (LA), facial artery (FA), occipital artery (OA), internal maxillary artery (IMA), superficial temporal artery (STA). The ascending pharyngeal artery arises at the CCA bifurcation following the course of the ICA but is not visible on this study. Internal jugular vein (IJV). (B) DSA of external carotid artery. The middle meningeal artery (MMA) is the first branch of the IMA. Note that the scalp branches have a 'corkscrewing' course (large arrows) readily distinguished from the meningeal branches, which have a much straighter course (small arrows).

Leptomeningeal (pial) collaterals are end-to-end anastomoses between distal branches of the intracerebral arteries that can provide collateral flow across vascular watershed zones. These are highly variable and are of

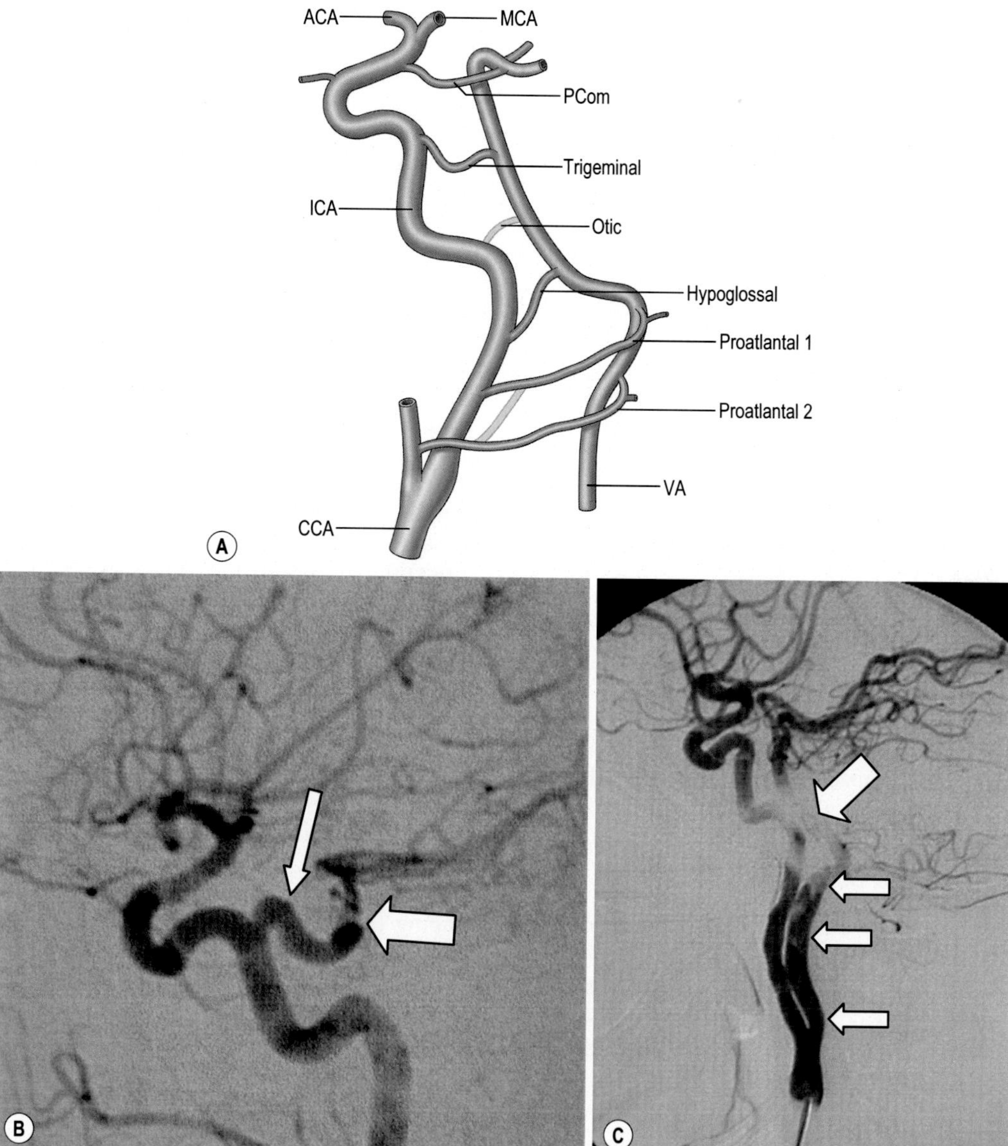

FIGURE 1-23 ■ (A) Schematic diagram showing the series of embryonic anastomoses between the anterior and posterior circulation which form and regress until the final one, the posterior communicating artery, is established. (B) DSA: the persistent trigeminal artery (small arrow) is most frequently encountered. (C) DSA: the persistent hypoglossal artery (small arrows) is extremely rare, arising from the ICA and traversing the hypoglossal canal to reach the basilar artery. Broad arrows in (A) and (B) indicate the basilar artery.

great importance in acute occlusion of intracerebral vessels.

Intracranial Veins

The dural sinuses run within the major dural septa: the superior sagittal sinus between the layers of the upper part of the falx cerebri and the inferior sagittal sinus in the lower border of the falx, running backwards to join the great vein of Galen.[27] The straight sinus is formed by the confluence of the vein of Galen and inferior sagittal sinus and runs downwards towards the torcular herophili. The transverse (or lateral) sinuses are often asymmetric in size; the right is usually the dominant one. They become the sigmoid sinuses as they turn downward to discharge into the internal jugular veins, which run in the lateral portion (the pars vascularis) of the jugular foramina.

The superior petrosal sinuses extend from the cavernous sinus to the sigmoid sinuses. The inferior petrosal sinuses connect the cavernous sinus to the jugular.

Cerebral veins consist of two groups: the deep, subependymal veins and the superficial cortical veins. The former are rather constant, while the latter are extremely variable. In the angiographic series, the cortical veins fill before the deep ones. The deep and superficial groups are in fact joined by fine medullary veins.

The septal veins course directly posteriorly on the septum pellucidum, to join the thalamostriate veins. They meet at the foramina of Monro, forming the venous angle, from which the internal cerebral veins run posteriorly on the roof of the third ventricle, near the midline. The confluence of internal cerebral and basal veins of Rosenthal gives rise to the midline great vein of Galen, which enters the straight sinus.

Most superficial cortical veins drain upwards and medially to the superior sagittal sinus. Veins in the inferior frontoparietal and temporal regions drain to the superficial middle cerebral vein, thence to the sphenoparietal sinus and cavernous sinus. Inferior parietal, posterior temporal and occipital veins drain directly to the transverse sinuses. Two large cortical veins running posterosuperiorly across the parietal lobe to the superior sagittal sinus and posteroinferiorly over the temporal lobe to the transverse sinus are the superior and inferior anastomotic veins (of Trolard and Labbé, respectively); it is uncommon for both to be well developed.

The anatomy of the posterior fossa veins is very variable. There are three principal drainage pathways: the vein of Galen, the superior petrosal sinus and direct tributaries into the transverse and straight sinuses.

TECHNIQUES FOR IMAGING THE BRAIN AND CEREBRAL VASCULATURE

Computed Tomography

In the acute neurological setting, speed and ready availability of computed tomography (CT) have led to it being the common first-line imaging choice. Recent advances in CT have positively impacted neuroimaging, offering lower dose and faster and higher resolution imaging.

Indications, Risks and Benefits

The radiologist should have a good understanding of the specific indications, risks and benefits of CT, as well as those of alternative imaging techniques.[28] There is a wide range of indications for CT of the brain, used either as a primary technique of investigation or as a secondary technique when MRI is unavailable, contraindicated or unsuccessful (Table 1-1).[29]

In the acute setting, CT offers rapid detection of surgically treatable conditions, such as haemorrhage, hydrocephalus, extra-axial collection or mass lesions, allowing quick treatment decisions. Acute head trauma is one of most frequent primary indications, with CT replacing skull radiography, allowing rapid detection of potentially life-threatening primary and secondary findings of intracranial trauma.[30,31] The speed and ease of CT is integral to its utility in acute stroke, allowing exclusion of intracranial haemorrhage, detection of early ischaemic changes and rapid progression to thrombolysis. The addition of CT angiography and perfusion allows assessment of vascular patency and changes in cerebral perfusion.[32] Computed tomography offers a first-line assessment of intracranial haemorrhage: when combined with CT angiography, most causative intracranial aneurysms and many vascular malformations can be identified.[33]

Beyond the brain, CT offers exquisite assessment of bone and is widely used to detect and characterise bony lesions or fractures of the calvarium, skull base or spine. Brain and cervical spine imaging can be easily combined, allowing detection of the third of patients with moderate to severe head injuries who also have cervical spine trauma.

As CT uses ionising radiation, it requires medical justification of the investigation and radiation dose, using low-dose techniques where possible to adhere to the ALARA (as low as reasonably achievable) principle. Imaging alternatives, commonly magnetic resonance imaging (MRI), should always be considered, especially where radiation dose is of higher concern, such as children.[34] Further, MRI may provide more detailed information on the underlying pathological process and therefore may be a more appropriate investigation.

TABLE 1-1 **Indications for CT of the Brain**

Primary Indications	Secondary Indications (when MRI Is unavailable or contraindicated, or if radiologist deems CT to be appropriate)
Acute head trauma	Diplopia
Suspected acute intracranial haemorrhage	Cranial nerve dysfunction
Vascular occlusive disease or vasculitis (including use of CT angiography and/or venography)	Seizures
Aneurysm evaluation	Apnoea
Detection or evaluation of calcification	Syncope
Immediate postoperative evaluation following surgical treatment of tumour, intracranial haemorrhage, or haemorrhagic lesions	Ataxia
Treated or untreated vascular lesions	Suspicion of neurodegenerative disease
Suspected shunt malfunctions, or shunt revisions	Developmental delay
Mental status change	Neuroendocrine dysfunction
Increased intracranial pressure	Encephalitis
Headache	Drug toxicity
Acute neurological deficits	Cortical dysplasia, and migration anomalies or other morphological brain abnormalities
Suspected intracranial infection	
Suspected hydrocephalus	
Congenital lesions (such as, but not limited to, craniosynostosis, macrocephaly and microcephaly)	
Evaluating psychiatric disorders	
Brain herniation	
Suspected mass or tumour	

However, MRI examination times are much longer and availability may still necessitate CT in the first instance.

Technique and Protocols

There continue to be rapid advances in CT technology, which have major implications for neuroimaging techniques and protocols. Knowledge of current technology and upcoming changes are vital for the practising radiologist.

Spiral CT has revolutionised CT and offers major advances for neuroimaging. Rapid, continuous imaging of the area of interest, by use of slip-ring technology, enables acquisition of a volume data set. Improvements in hardware, most notably, multidetector configuration, and software, have both improved speed, and spatial resolution in the *z*-axis, enabling the acquisition of isotropic data. The ability to cover whole organs in one tube rotation offers major advantages for assessment of both cerebral vasculature and perfusion.[35]

Data can be resampled according to need, and edited (e.g. skull removal), allowing the radiologist to highlight relevant data and optimise interpretation. Multiplanar reformatting (MPR) of data is useful in many situations in both brain and spine. Sagittal images provide good visualisation of the midline structures such as the craniocervical junction and pituitary fossa (Fig. 1-24), while coronal images improve assessment of structures in the axial plane, e.g. the superior aspects of the brain, floor of the middle cranial fossa. Slice thickness can be manipulated according to need and streak artefacts can be reduced from the skull, allowing better visualisation of the posterior fossa and sellar regions.

While volume rendering (VR) and multiple intensity projection (MIP) have particular utility for neurovascular imaging, VR can also be helpful for depicting complex fractures of calvarium, skull base or spine, allowing assessment of integrity and alignment. Single slice techniques, however, still offer an equivalent assessment of the brain in the axial plane and have the advantage that the gantry can be angled to avoid irradiation of the globes.[36]

Intravenous contrast is most commonly administered to further evaluate a known pathology with blood–brain barrier breakdown, such as tumour or abscess, or a suspected pathology within an area of observed abnormality: for example, vasogenic oedema. The addition of intrathecal contrast provides exquisite myelographic images, allowing detailed assessment of intracranial subarachnoid spaces: for example, in CSF leak (Fig. 1-25). For the spine, CT myelography offers an alternative to MRI in assessment of spinal cord or nerve root compression.

Viewing the Images

Ionising radiation produced by CT is absorbed to varying degrees by the body, reflecting the linear attenuation coefficient and electron density. Thus, a grey scale of variable densities (Hounsfield units) is produced, ranging from −1000 for air to +1000 for bone/calcification, with water as 0.

Contrast between structures is maximised by limiting the grey-scale spectrum to a central window level and width that focuses on the likely densities within. This narrows the viewing spectrum to benefit the grey-scale capabilities of the human eye, which are considerably less than a CT imaging device. For the brain, a window level set in the range of 35–50 and width of 70–150 provides a good baseline setting. Assessment using specific bone window settings, with a higher window level and width, e.g. 80–500/600–2000, is key not only for trauma patients but also for all patients and should be performed to detect bone lesions. A bony reconstruction algorithm and filter can enhance fine bony detail (Fig. 1-26). Variable window width and centre level settings are also helpful to accentuate contrast differences between oedematous and normal brain, for example in detection of acute stroke,[37] while letting structures outside the set window level be distinguished such as haemorrhage and calcification.

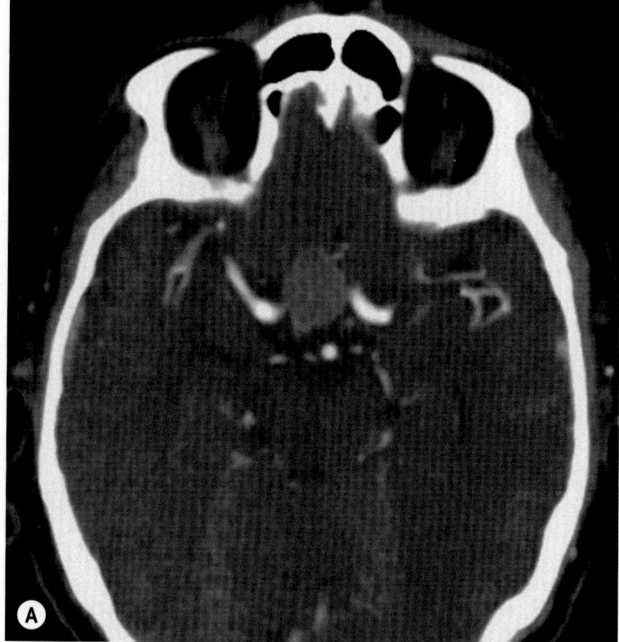

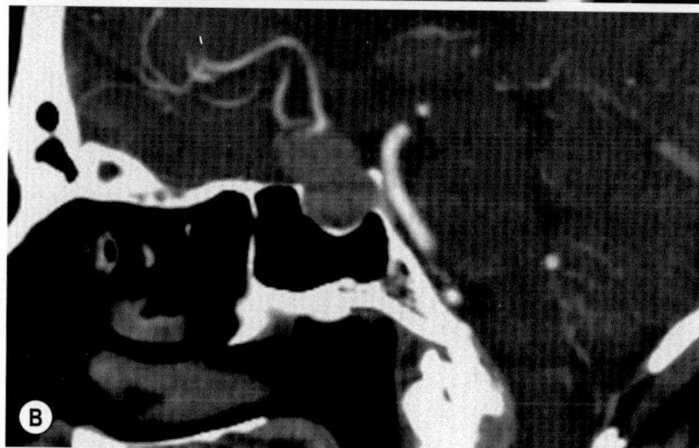

FIGURE 1-24 ■ (A) A 60-year-old man, with reducing vision. Spiral CT (dual bolus contrast) reveals an enhancing suprasellar mass. (B) Sagittal reformat provides a good assessment of midline structures and confirms this as a mixed sellar/suprasellar mass lesion. It was confirmed pathologically as a pituitary macroadenoma.

Slice thickness should be optimised according to personal preference and need. Thicker slices offer less noise,

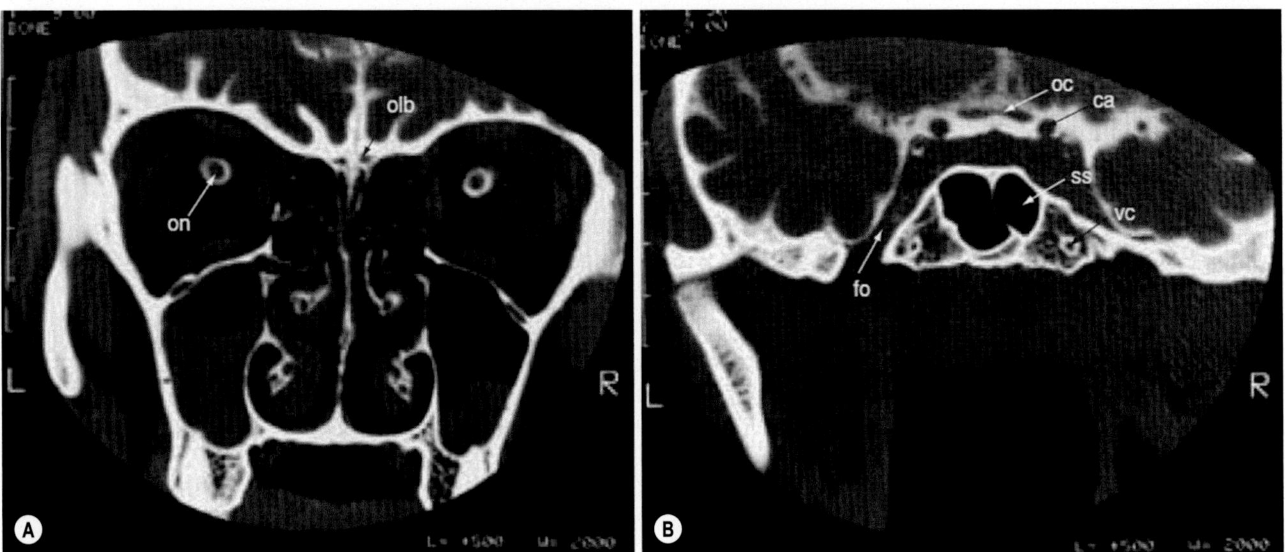

FIGURE 1-25 ■ Thin-section (1.5 mm) CT slices at the (A) level of the olfactory grooves and (B) foramen ovale. The intrathecal contrast outlines the subarachnoid space and extends into the optic nerve sheaths, outlining the optic nerves. ca = carotid artery, fo = foramen ovale, oc = optic chiasm, olb = olfactory bulb, on = optic nerve, ss = sphenoid sinus, vc = vidian canal.

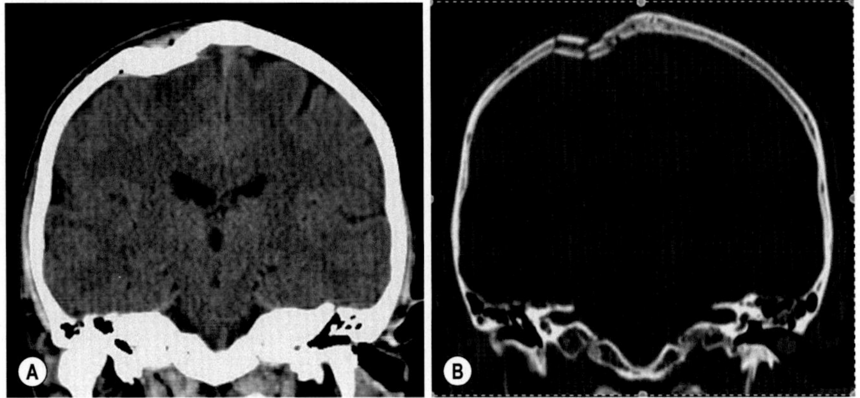

FIGURE 1-26 ■ (A) A 20-year-old man following blunt trauma. Coronal reformat of spiral CT, viewed on soft-tissue windows (window centre 35, width 70), shows a depressed right posterior skull fracture, with underlying parenchymal oedema. (B) Assessment of the comminuted fragments and displacement is optimised by use of a high-resolution bone algorithm and filter (window centre 800, width 2000).

while thinner slices reduce partial volume and artefacts, e.g. posterior fossa. Further viewing possibilities are also available where iterative data reconstructive techniques are used. This reconstructive technique reduces noise, and ultimately dose, producing a smoother appearance.[38] It can be blended with back-projection techniques, to produce best subjective viewing conditions (Fig. 1-27).

Magnetic Resonance Imaging

MRI is a key diagnostic technique for imaging of the neuraxis, allowing detailed assessment of the anatomy and pathological findings of the brain and spine.

Indications, Risks and Benefits

The choice of cross-sectional neuroimaging technique is dependent on a number of factors, including the clinical status of the patient, the speed of examination required and the suspected pathology. Some of the indications for MR of the brain are listed in Table 1-2.[39]

The full extent of involvement and the underlying pathological process are commonly easier to define using MRI. The superior soft-tissue contrast of MRI ensures that many pathological findings are detected earlier than CT. In many cases, this is due to the high inherent sensitivity of MRI to water, which is increased at an early stage in many parenchymal lesions. MRI also offers a high contrast for other compositions, such as fat and subacute haemorrhage, which show T1 shortening (Fig. 1-28). The technique can be used for follow-up of parenchymal haematoma, to confirm expected evolution and help exclude underlying tumour or vascular malformation.[40]

When clinical symptomatology points to the posterior fossa, MRI should be performed whenever possible. Both

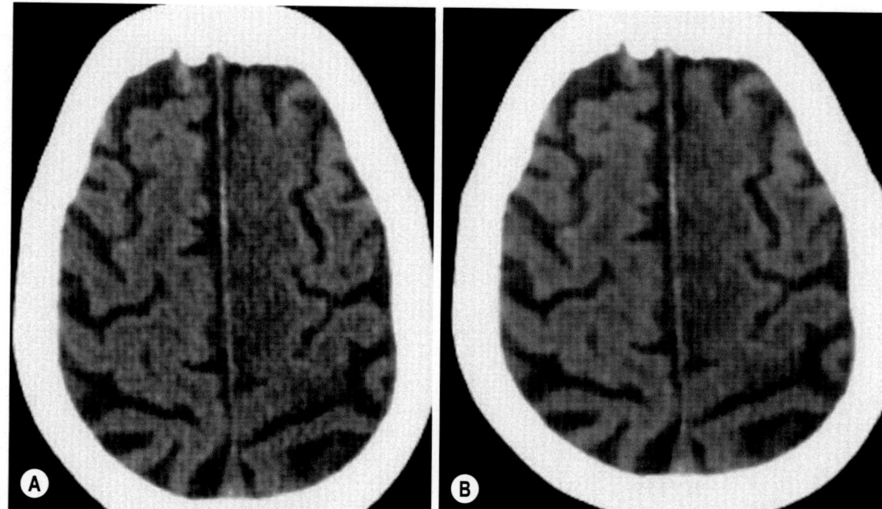

FIGURE 1-27 ■ **A 67-year-old woman with anterior cerebral artery infarct.** (A) Reduced-dose CT brain, reformatted using filtered back projection, shows a slightly noisy appearance. Low attenuation with sulcal effacement of the left paramedian frontal lobe present, in keeping with anterior cerebral infarction. (B) Same examination reconstructed by iterative reconstruction reduces image noise and has a much smoother appearance.

TABLE 1-2 **Indications for MRI of the Brain**

Primary Indications	Extended Indications
Seizures	Suspicion of acute intracranial haemorrhage or evaluation of chronic haemorrhage
Cranial nerve dysfunction	Neuroendocrine dysfunction
Diplopia	Functional imaging
Ataxia	Brain mapping
Acute and chronic neurological deficits	Blood flow and brain perfusion study
Suspicion of neurodegenerative disease	Image guidance for intervention or treatment planning
Primary and secondary neoplasm	Spectroscopy (including evaluation of brain tumour, infectious processes, brain development and/or degeneration, and ischaemic conditions)
Aneurysm	Volumetry
Cortical dysplasia and other morphological brain abnormalities	Morphometry
Vasculitis	Tractography
Encephalitis	Post-traumatic conditions
Brain maturation	
Headache	
Mental status change	
Hydrocephalus	
Ischaemic disease and infarction	
Suspected pituitary dysfunction	
Inflammation or infection of the brain or meninges, or their complications	
Postoperative evaluation	
Demyelination and dysmyelination disorders	
Vascular malformations	
Arterial or venous/dural sinus abnormalities	
Suspicion of non-accidental trauma	

brainstem and cerebellum are best depicted on MR, without the streak artefacts from the skull base that are common on CT. Further, MRI should be used as the primary investigation for assessment of spinal disease, including symptoms of spinal cord dysfunction or neural compression. It provides best assessment of the soft tissues of the spine, including the intervertebral discs, as well as valuable information on bone integrity, alignment and marrow composition. For patients in whom MR is not suitable, CT offers an alternative.

A safe MR examination necessitates that patients are interviewed and screened prior to the examination to exclude individuals who may be at risk or have contraindication to exposure to the MRI environment: for example, ferrometallic clips. Patients suffering from anxiety or claustrophobia may require sedation or anaesthesia. The examination is significantly longer than CT and is dependent on sequences used, which can be problematic for some patients. Under certain clinical conditions, very rapid acquisitions such as echo-planar imaging

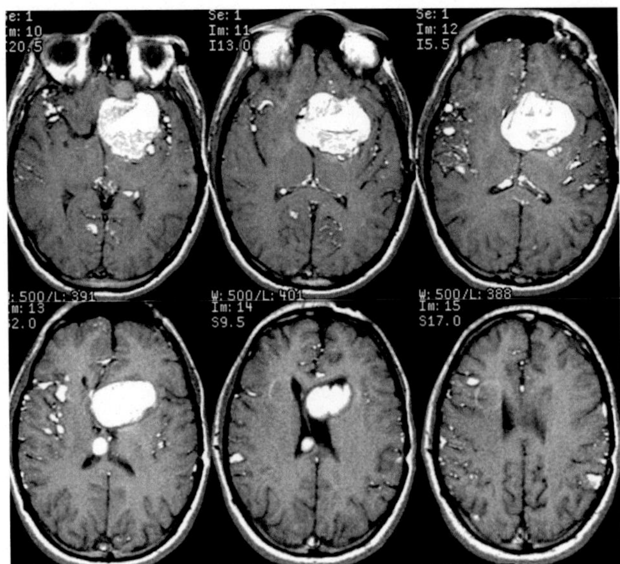

FIGURE 1-28 ■ A 25-year-old male patient with headaches. Axial T1-weighted MR images (unenhanced) reveal a T1 hyperintense mass lying to the left of the midline, with scattered globules of T1 hyperintensity within the subarachnoid spaces and ventricular system. Findings are in keeping with a ruptured dermoid, with spread of fat within cerebrospinal fluid.

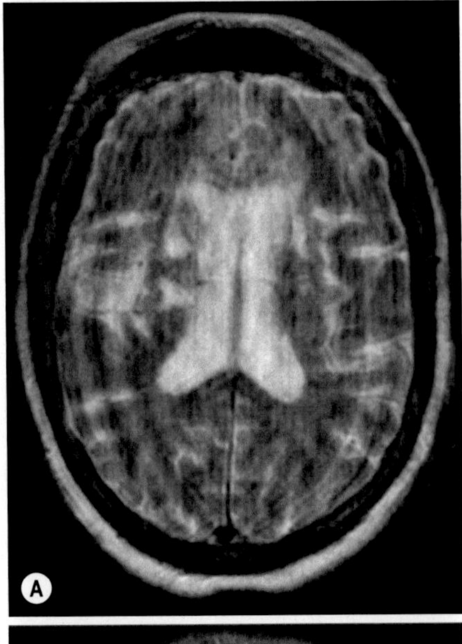

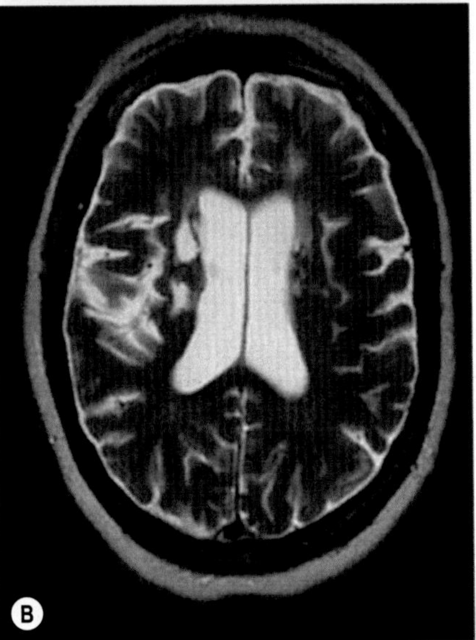

FIGURE 1-29 ■ A 78-year-old woman with multifocal chronic deep white matter infarcts. (A) Axial T2-weighted FSE MR image acquired using conventional sequence is severely degraded by motion artefact. (B) Axial T2-weighted FSE acquired with motion correction (PROPELLER) during the same examination shows correction of any patient motion and marked improvement in image quality.

or single-shot fast spin-echo imaging can be performed, although this necessitates lower-resolution techniques. Motion correction can be extremely helpful, particularly in the moving or confused patient (Fig. 1-29).[41]

Technique and Protocols

Most imaging of the neuraxis is performed using superconducting magnets of 1.5 T or higher. Use of 3 T MRI is becoming more widespread for structural and functional imaging, offering the advantage of either shorter imaging times, or higher resolution, which can offer benefit in subtle pathologies.[42] There are significant advantages of higher-field imaging for more specialised sequences, including MR angiography, MR spectroscopy and functional MRI, due to inherent higher signal to noise. Ultra-high magnetic fields, up to 7 T, will likely become more available in the future, offering further advantages in these areas.[43]

Advances in coil technology have lead to widespread use of multichannel coils, speeding up imaging time by use of parallel imaging. Combined coils, such as brain and spine, have now become commonplace, removing the necessity to change coil during an examination of the brain and spine.

A wide variety of pulse sequences are available for MR imaging of the neuraxis, constantly evolving with advancing techniques. The exact protocol used depends on both the clinical question and the available hard and software. Most imaging examinations of the brain or spine use a multi-contrast approach, incorporating at least both T1-weighted and T2-weighted imaging, which can be acquired using a number of different techniques. T2-weighted FLAIR sequences are commonly added, due to their high sensitivity to lesion detection, with particular utility in cortical and periventricular regions, where suppression of cerebrospinal fluid enhances lesion detection.

Images should be optimised using variable image parameters, including TE, TR, flip angle. Slice thickness, spatial resolution, signal-to-noise ratio, acquisition time and contrast are all interrelated and should be carefully controlled. A maximum slice thickness of 5 mm with a 2.5-mm gap should be used in the brain, but thinner slices often offer benefit and, when obtained with a 3D technique, offer the option of multiplanar reconstruction. Such T1 volume studies are commonplace, but there is now increasing availability of volume T2-weighted sequences. T2*-weighted imaging, using a gradient-echo sequence, or susceptibility-weighted imaging (SWI), is

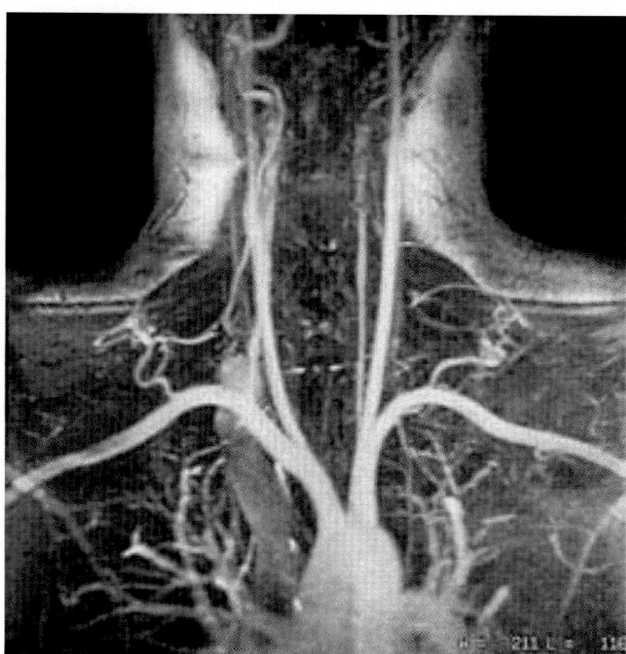

FIGURE 1-30 ■ Contrast-enhanced MRA of aortic arch. A 3D gradient-echo sequence has been acquired during the first pass of an intravenously injected gadolinium bolus. It shows the origins of the great vessels.

important for detection of acute or chronic haemorrhage or calcification and has a significant impact on the detection of cerebral microhaemorrhages, the clinical importance of which is being increasingly recognised.[44]

Intravenous administration of gadolinium can be used to assess the integrity of the blood–brain barrier. Care should be made with the choice of agent, especially where patients have renal dysfunction, in order to limit the risk of nephrogenic systemic fibrosis.[45]

Contrast medium administration is useful in a wide range of indications: for example, in the assessment of tumours or infection. It can be useful to detect acute demyelinating plaques, where enhancement is indicative of improved response disease-modifying treatments.[46] MR angiography or venography of the neurovascular circulation can be performed using intravenous contrast, either targeted to a specific vascular phase or using a time-resolved technique, to assess the vasculature (Fig. 1-30). Alternatively, unenhanced techniques, commonly time-of-flight or phase contrast can be used.

Diffusion-Weighted Imaging

Diffusion-weighted imaging is key to include as part of an acute stroke protocol for detection of cytotoxic oedema, but also has a wider utility: for example, in encephalitis, abscess, brain tumours and metabolic conditions.[47] This technique exploits the presence of random motion (Brownian motion) of water molecules to produce image contrast.[48] A pair of diffusion sensitising gradients around the 180 refocusing RF pulse of a T2-weighted sequence assess whether molecular motion has occurred. Mobile molecules acquire phase shifts, which prevent their complete rephasing and result in signal loss, proportional to the degree of motion. The degree of phase shift and signal loss depends also on the strength and duration of the diffusion sensitising gradient, which is expressed by the '*b*-value': 1000 s mm^{-2} is commonly used in stroke imaging. The apparent diffusion coefficient (ADC) can be calculated and provides a quantitative assessment of water movement in tissue.

A further feature of diffusion in the brain is its directional dependence, or anisotropy. This is particularly prominent in compacted white matter tracts, and least evident in grey matter. DTI explores anisotropy in a variety of directions on a pixel-by-pixel basis. This technique has utility in assessment of white matter structure and lesions thereof, such as diffuse axonal injury.[49]

MR Perfusion Imaging

Perfusion imaging can be performed for a variety of indications, such as stroke or tumour. T2*-weighted techniques exploit the magnetic susceptibility effects within the brain tissue during the first pass of an intravenously injected gadolinium-based contrast agent, causing a transient signal drop on temporal imaging.[50] The sequential changes in signal intensity, plotted as a time–signal intensity curve, allow generation of the relative cerebral blood volume (rCBV), proportional to the area under the curve. Other measurements that can be derived are time to peak and mean transit time (MTT) of the gadolinium bolus. Using tracer kinetics, the relative cerebral blood flow can be estimated by dividing the rCBV by the MTT.

The technique, however, at present is only semiquantitative and cannot provide absolute values. An emerging non-contrast technique, arterial spin labelling, does not require exogenous contrast medium and has the advantage of providing absolute values of perfusion parameters.[51] Alternatively, T1-weighted perfusion imaging can assess accumulation and distribution of gadolinium. Pharmacokinetic modelling can be used to gain data on contrast leakage, including permeability, which can provide useful functional information: for example, in neuro-oncology.[52]

Magnetic Resonance Spectroscopy

Magnetic resonance spectroscopy (MRS) allows investigation of biochemical changes in brain pathologies, by detection of metabolites on ^{1}H-MRS peaks.[53] A change in the resonance intensity of these marker compounds may reflect loss or damage to a specific cell type. The acquisition of long echo time data allows the detection of *N*-acetylaspartate (NAA), creatine (Cr/PCr) and choline (Cho) in normal brain, and lactate in areas of abnormality. The methyl resonance of NAA produces a large sharp peak at 2.01 ppm and acts as a neuronal marker, as it is almost exclusively found in neurons in the human brain. The creatine peak (3.03 ppm) arises from both phosphocreatine- and creatine-containing substances in the cell and choline (3.22 ppm) is thought to arise from choline-containing substances in the cell membrane. The acquisition of short echo time data detects further resonances from additional metabolites, such as *myo*-inositol, glutamate and glutamine.

Current clinical uses in neuroimaging include assessment of brain tumours, stroke, metabolic conditions and demyelination.

Functional MRI

Functional MRI (fMRI) can be used to study cortical activation. It measures a tiny increase in signal intensity on T2*-weighted acquisitions in the relevant cortex during neuronal activation.[54] During cortical activation there is an increase in rCBF and thus an increase in oxygen delivery to the activated brain, which exceeds the local oxygen metabolic requirement. There is a net increase in oxyhaemoglobin concentration in the venules and veins in the vicinity of the activated brain, which results in a tiny increase in MR signal, the so-called *b*lood *o*xygenation *l*evel-*d*ependent or, BOLD effect. The magnitude of this MR signal change is tiny and quantitative comparison must be made between the MR signal during the resting state and the activation state during multiple repetitions in order to detect activation.

Although fMRI is being increasingly used for brain mapping, it does have clinical applications, such as identification of eloquent cortex, prior to surgery in patients with structural lesions.[55]

Nuclear Medicine

Single-Photon Emission Computed Tomography

Single-photon emission computed tomography (SPECT) images are formed from detection of gamma rays emitted during radionuclide decay. Gamma rays or photons are detected by a gamma camera, which, if rotated about the patient's head, allows reconstruction of tomographic slices of distribution of activity in that part of the patient.

Clinical applications of SPECT include dementia, cerebrovascular disease, epilepsy, encephalitis and head injury.[56] Radionuclide imaging of the brain requires radiopharmaceuticals that cross the blood–brain barrier. SPECT may be used to produce images of rCBF using a variety of radiopharmaceuticals: e.g. ^{99m}Tc-hexamethylpropyleneamine oxime (HMPAO) (Fig. 1-31). SPECT can also be used to image uptake at neurotransmitter receptors using various radiopharmaceuticals, usually labelled with ^{123}I. Many different SPECT radiopharmaceuticals are taken up into intracranial tumours: for example, ^{201}Tl.

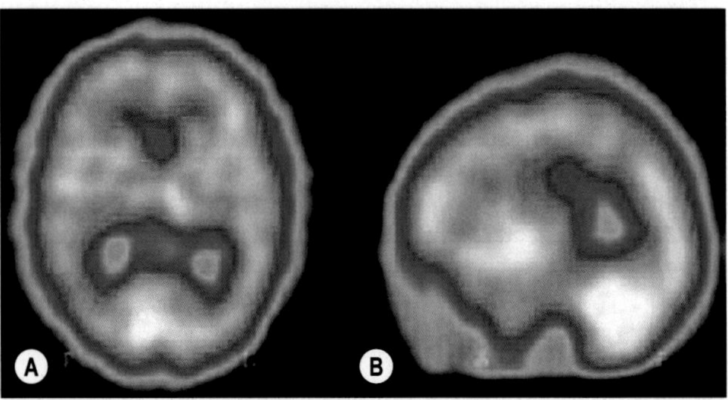

FIGURE 1-31 ■ **SPECT**. Normal ^{99m}Tc-HMPAO SPECT of the brain, axial (A) and sagittal (B) images.

SPECT is available in most nuclear medicine departments, is relatively inexpensive and has good patient acceptability, although it has inherently poorer resolution than PET.

Positron Emission Tomography

Positron emission tomography (PET), like SPECT, produces tomographic images.[56] Positron-emitting radioisotopes decay by emission of positrons, which combine with an adjacent electron in an annihilation reaction with the emission of two high-energy gamma rays in opposing directions. Detection of these simultaneously emitted photons allows calculation of their site of origin and, therefore, a map of radiopharmaceutical distribution in the patient. PET can be used to study different physiological processes in the brain.

A cyclotron is required to generate positron-emitting isotopes that can be made from a variety of biologically interesting compounds. Physiological parameters can be derived: for example, cerebral glucose uptake, using^{1,8} fluorodeoxyglucose (FDG); oxygen metabolism, using $^{15}O_2$ or ^{11}CO; and rCBF, using $H_2{}^{15}O$. A number of radiopharmaceuticals are available for PET receptor imaging. FDG, [^{11}C]-methionine and [^{18}F]-α-methyltyrosine are used for tumour imaging.

The disadvantages of PET compared with SPECT are its limited availability and high cost due to the necessity of a cyclotron close to the PET unit.

VASCULAR IMAGING TECHNIQUES

Imaging techniques for the assessment of intra- and extracranial vessels have evolved over recent decades with traditional digital subtraction angiography (DSA) no longer the universal reference standard. Following introduction of new CT and MR applications, the role of DSA is increasingly restricted to the endovascular treatment of diseases as well as for the diagnosis of certain pathological conditions such as small dural or pial AV fistulas or head and neck pathologies. This section discusses the techniques of vascular imaging (invasive and non-invasive). Doppler ultrasound is covered elsewhere.

Conventional Catheter Digital Subtraction Angiography

General principles and basic arteriographic techniques are described elsewhere. Most diagnostic cerebral angiography is performed under local anaesthesia. Using the standard Seldinger technique, the transfemoral route is almost exclusively used for catheterisation of the cerebral vessels. There has been a move towards using 4Fr catheters, often with multipurpose or vertebral curves, with Sidewinder curves reserved for difficult access.

A complete diagnostic study may involve catheterisation of six vessels. Internal and external carotid runs are necessary to exclude or verify the presence of dural or pial AV fistulas. And separate catheterisation of the two vertebral arteries may be needed. Angiographic runs usually start with the internal carotid artery. Contrast medium can be injected manually or by pump injector. For 3D DSA, an automatic pump injection (20 mL of contrast medium at a rate of 5 mL s^{-1}) is needed for smaller-calibre 4Fr catheters.

A biplane angiography unit is of major advantage in neuroangiography. It allows simultaneous acquisition of two projections (such as AP and lateral or two oblique views) during a single injection, reducing the number of contrast medium injections.

Routine cerebral angiography is carried out with a frame rate of two or three images per second, while for the investigation of teriovenous malformations (AVMs) a frame rate of six images per second is usually preferred. Flat detector (FD)-equipped angiography machines have become the norm for neuroangiographic imaging. With this equipment, it is possible to obtain not only high-quality 3D vascular volumes (3D rotational angiography) but also CT-like images (FD-CT) of brain parenchyma that allow detection of intraparenchymal and subarachnoid haemorrhages. This technological breakthrough also allows for removal of the bony structures and offers high-resolution 3D images of the cerebral vessels. As a result, planning of endovascular treatment of aneurysms or AVMs is much easier, even in difficult anatomical locations, such as the carotid siphon[57] (Fig. 1-32). The ability to obtain CT images of the brain also reduces the need to transfer patients from the angiography suite to a CT facility, should complications occur.

Nowadays, the indications for diagnostic DSA have been dramatically reduced. In departments where CTA is routinely used, cerebral angiography is used to resolve discrepancies between two non-invasive methods and as an integral part of endovascular interventional procedures.

DSA is still required in most patients with subarachnoid haemorrhage and negative CTA, in order to exclude a small dural or pial fistula. In cases of intraparenchymal haematoma, DSA is part of the diagnostic work-up, in order to exclude or to reveal the presence and angioarchitecure of a brain AVM. DSA is now less commonly required in carotid artery disease to confirm a significant stenosis suspected on non-invasive imaging, or to reveal intracranial haemodynamic changes, due to severe stenosis. Preoperative angiography is sometimes performed in glomus jugulare tumours and meningiomas to assess tumour vascularity, and is frequently combined with preoperative embolisation in very vascular tumours.

The principal modern use of intra-arterial angiography is related to therapeutic interventions, such as brain aneurysm or AVM embolisation, or in the context of intra-arterial treatment of acute stroke.[58] Follow-up DSA after aneurysm and AVM treatment remains widely used. Ongoing improvements in magnetic resonance angiography (MRA) technology are likely to further reduce indications for DSA, but patients with non-MRI compatible implants will continue to need catheter angiography.

There are very few absolute contraindications to cerebral angiography. A well-documented history of

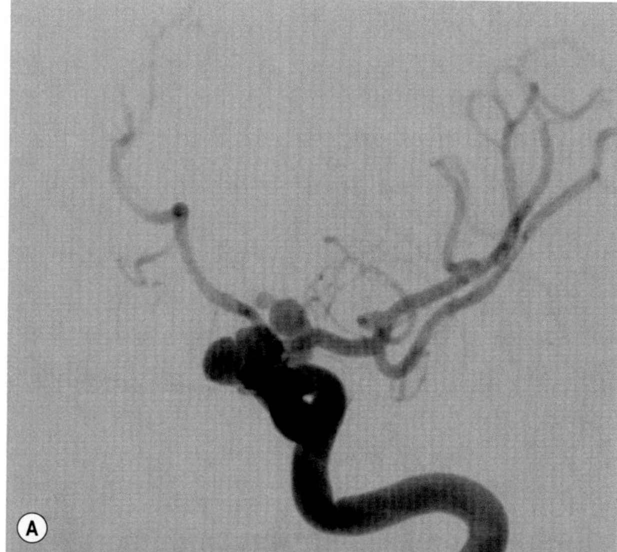

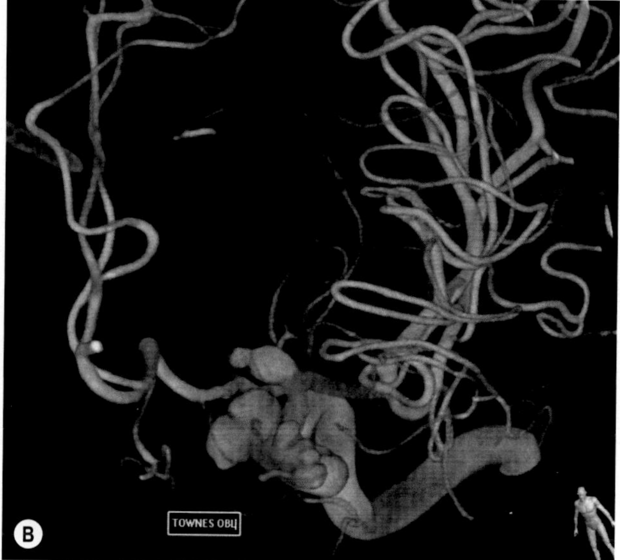

FIGURE 1-32 ■ (A) Standard 2D DSA image showing multiple aneurysms of the carotid syphon and ICA termination. (B) A 3D image can be rotated into any projection to display the aneurysms more clearly, assisting in planning the endovascular approach.

untoward reactions to contrast media is probably the most important contraindication. Severe renal failure is a relative contraindication, because haemodialysis can follow the DSA. Treatment with anticoagulant drugs does not contraindicate arteriography, provided the prothrombin level is within the normal therapeutic range.

Local and general complications of arteriography are discussed elsewhere. Specific risks of catheterisation of the aortic arch or cervical arteries include cerebral thromboembolism and damage to the arteries by the catheter or guidewire, which include spasm, thrombosis and dissection. Older patients with severe atherosclerotic disease should be treated with extreme caution, during catheterisation, because of the higher possibility of thromboembolic complications.[59] Reported risks of cerebral angiography in studies published over the past 15 years are reported to vary from 0.3 to 1.5%.[60,61]

Computed Tomography Angiography (CTA)

Selective imaging of blood vessels with CT has become possible with the introduction of helical CT systems. Over the past decade, the use of multidetector CT angiography has revolutionised the demonstration of intra- and extracranial vessels. Even more recently, dual-energy CT has increased diagnostic capabilities of tomography.[62]

Modern multidetector CT units are able to cover an area from the aortic arch up to the circle of Willis or the entire intracranial circulation from the skull base to the vertex with a single data acquisition. Timing of data acquisition in relation to the administration of contrast medium is critical for maximum arterial opacification. All modern CT systems provide an automated bolus detection system. This is more satisfactory because it adjusts for individual variations in circulation time.

For the cervical arteries, the reference axial image for the smart prep should be at the level of aortic arch, while for the intracranial angiogram, it may be placed at a level cranial to the carotid bifurcation (C4-C5 vertebrae). Typical volumes of 100–120 mL of contrast medium are given at a rate of 3–4 mL s^{-1}.

The quality of CT angiograms depends heavily on postprocessing of the image data. Separation of vessels running close to bone (near the skull base and cranial vault) may be difficult. These difficulties can be at least partially resolved by using thick-section multiplanar reformats (which can be angled in such a way to exclude bone) and by interactive viewing of the source data. With newer technology of dual-energy systems, accurate highlighting of bone structures on CTA data sets is very easy. The highlighted pixels can be removed by a single click, removing the bony structures. The dual-energy approach reliably isolates even complex vasculature, for example, at the base of the skull where CTAs are difficult to interpret,[63] and plaque characterisation in carotid stenosis is more reliable.

In neurovascular angiography, the immediate availability and fast examination time in MDCT have proven highly beneficial in the non-invasive investigation of supra-aortic extracranial and intracranial vessels for the vast majority of pathologies. In most centres where MDCT is available, CTA is the first and often the only examination needed for diagnosis. In the setting of possible thrombectomy, in acute stroke, CTA is usual in the diagnostic algorithm.[64]

Studies have shown that CTA is an excellent tool for the detection of intracranial aneurysms in cases of subarachnoidal haemorrhage. CTA has been used successfully for the evaluation of carotid artery stenosis, cervical artery dissection and intracranial vascular stenosis.[65–67] It has also been suggested that it could be the only diagnostic test in patients with perimesencephalic subarachnoid haemorrhage, although this remains controversial.[68]

CTA is also used to examine the cerebral venous system (CT venography) for suspected superficial or deep cerebral venous system thrombosis.

CTA has certain advantages over MRA: it can be used in claustrophobic patients and patients with cardiac pacemakers, or other implants that preclude MR data acquisition. It is also quicker and more easily performed than MRA. Its disadvantages are the use of ionising radiation and iodinated contrast media.

Magnetic Resonance Angiography

The basic principles of MRI are discussed elsewhere. MRA relies on inflow of unsaturated spin (time-of-flight (TOF) MRA) or the accumulation of phase shifts proportional to the flow velocity (phase contrast MRA). MRA may be used in conjunction with gadolinium-based contrast media (contrast-enhanced (CE) MRA). Both TOF and phase contrast techniques can be performed with a 2D or 3D data acquisition.

MRA is useful for the evaluation of extracranial atherosclerotic disease, as well as for the detection of intracranial arterial or venous pathology. For the cervical vessel disease, a systematic review and meta-analysis showed that MRA is highly accurate for the diagnosis of high-grade ICA stenoses and occlusion with both TOF and CE techniques, CE MRA is highly accurate for distinguishing occlusions from high-grade stenoses, whereas both CE MRA and especially TOF MRA appear to be poor diagnostic tools for moderate ICA stenosis.[69] For imaging of the intracerebral vessels, 3D TOF MRA is the technique of choice, with a single-slab 3D TOF acquisition being adequate for imaging the circle of Willis. Data are usually displayed as maximum intensity projections, but inspection of the source data should always be performed to resolve difficult cases, to confirm the suspicion of an artefact or to clarify possible false-positive results.

Over recent years major advances in MRA techniques allowed for the measurement of arterial blood flow in various cerebrovascular conditions (quantitative MRA (QMRA)), detection of aneurysms (3D TOF MRA), assessment of intracranial stenosis and, to a limited extent, AVMs.

MRA is, however, still usually not the first-choice examination in everyday practice, especially for the evaluation of SAH or intracerebral hematomas. It is, however, widely used for the follow-up of aneurysms after endovascular treatment (Fig. 1-33).

Phase contrast MRA is based on the detection of phase shifts generated by a flow-encoding gradient. Although generally inferior to 3D MRA, it is more sensitive for detection of slow flow (with the appropriate velocity encoding) and can therefore be used for imaging cerebral veins. It does not suffer from T1-contamination artefact and it can provide information about the direction of blood flow.

The administration of a gadolinium-based contrast medium has been shown to have some benefit in conjunction with intracranial 3D TOF MRA for conditions such as AVMs and intracranial stenosis, while, more recently, contrast-enhanced, time-resolved 4D MRA has shown promising results for the pretreatment assessment of AVMs.[70]

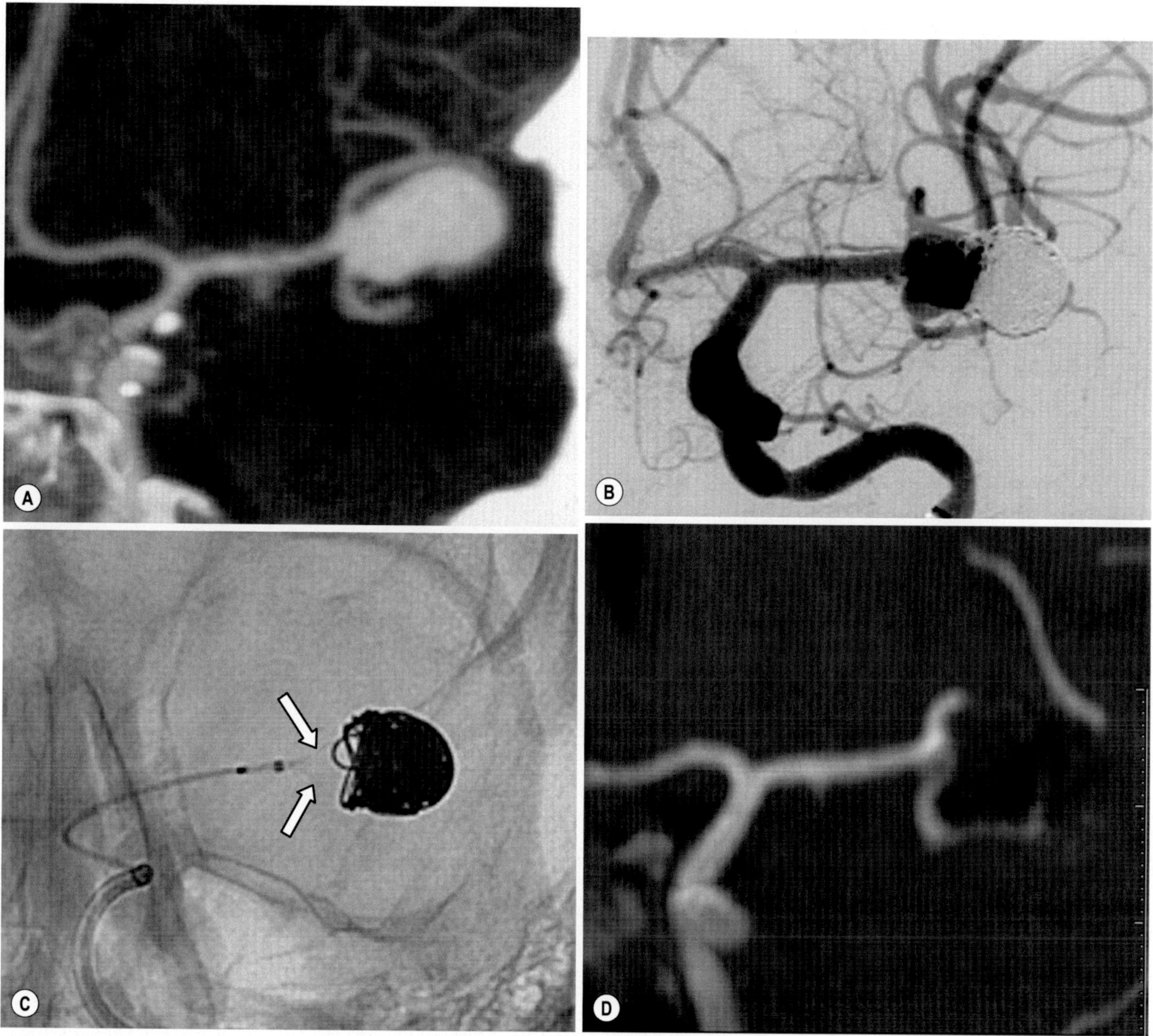

FIGURE 1-33 ■ **Patient with ruptured left MCA aneurysm.** (A) CTA shows wide-neck aneurysm. (B) Initially treated by coiling. Loose packing at aneurysm neck led to compaction and refilling of the aneurysm. (C) Re-treatment with intrasaccular flow diverter (WEB device) (arrows). (D) A 6-month follow-up MRA shows complete occlusion of aneurysm, and demonstrates the normal convexity of the recess of the WEB device.

TRAUMA TO THE SKULL AND BRAIN

HEAD INJURY

Head injuries are either open (penetrating) or closed (non-penetrating), the latter being by far the more common in civilian practice. The main indication for imaging is suspected intracranial haemorrhage where prompt neurosurgical evacuation may modify outcome. Because it shows haemorrhage particularly well, CT generally is recommended in preference to MRI for this purpose. Furthermore CT is more widely available on a 24-h basis and is easier to perform following major trauma. Thus there are clear recommendations from the Royal College of Radiologists[71] and the National Institute of Clinical Excellence (NICE)[72,73] about the indications for and appropriate timing of CT following trauma. During the subsequent clinical course, imaging may be required to assess neurological deterioration or other complications, or perhaps failure to improve, and later to make a final assessment of overall damage for long-term prognosis. For many of these less acute indications, MRI may be preferred. Despite the numerous published guidelines for imaging of the head and cervical spine in trauma, they are only guidelines and many individual brain injury units have their own variations. The principles behind these, however, are simply the application of common sense on a case-by-case basis.

Skull Fractures

Detection of fractures of the cranial vault by plain radiography of the skull is now appreciated to be less useful in assessing the probability of intracranial haemorrhage

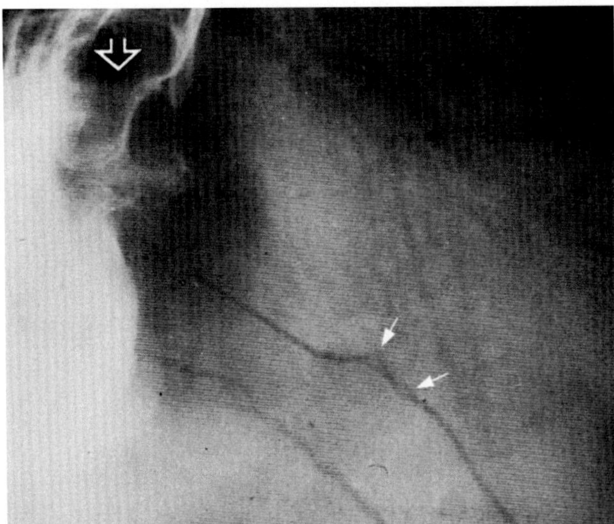

FIGURE 1-34 ■ Bilateral vault fracture, with fluid level in sphenoid sinus (open arrow). Two fracture lines are seen; the more anterior (upper on this radiograph) is better defined and is therefore on the side nearer the radiographic plate. Apparent islands of bone within (small arrows) are typical of an acute fracture. This radiograph has been obtained with the patient in the supine brow up position.

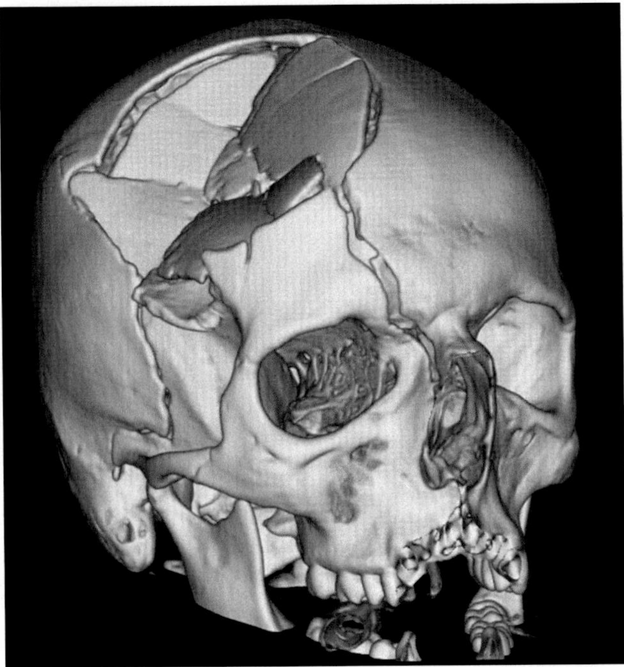

FIGURE 1-35 ■ **Stellate comminuted depressed fracture produced by a direct blow.** CT volume rendered image.

than had been previously suggested. Clinical assessment appears to be a better guide and this, in turn, guides the need for CT. Thus the role of skull radiography has greatly diminished. In any event simple linear fractures are often of little consequence in themselves. Like fractures elsewhere, these may be simple or comminuted. They sometimes branch, and must be distinguished from vascular markings (Fig. 1-34), including the groove in the squamous temporal bone caused by a deep temporal artery.[74] Acute fractures are usually straighter, more angulated, more radiolucent and do not have corticated margins. A fracture passing through a sinus or air cell is effectively compound, and of much greater potential significance than a simple fracture. A compound fracture is one in which the cranial cavity is in real or potential communication with the exterior. Depressed fractures (Fig. 1-35) are usually comminuted and often compound; bone fragments embedded in brain substance often are removed or relocated to reduce the risk of post-traumatic epilepsy. Acuteness of the fracture may be determined by demonstrating overlying scalp swelling on CT. Fractures of the skull base are important because of bleeding or leakage of CSF; air and fluid within the sphenoid sinus may indicate that the leptomeninges have been torn. CT is extremely helpful in assessing fractures of the skull base, including the petrous bone, where it may also reveal ossicular dislocation, a treatable cause of traumatic hearing loss. Growing fractures (leptomeningeal cysts) usually occur after severe head injuries early in life.[74] The dura mater underlying a linear fracture is torn, often with laceration of the underlying brain. Exposure of the remodelling bone to pulsation of the CSF results in progressive widening of the fracture line over weeks or months.

Traumatic Haemorrhage

Trauma may cause bleeding into the scalp, between the cranial vault and the dura mater (extradural—but also termed epidural), between the dura and arachnoid mater (subdural), or into the subarachnoid space, brain or ventricular system. The aim of imaging in the acute stage is to identify patients with intracranial bleeding requiring surgery; they represent less than 1% of patients with well-documented head injury. CT is the imaging procedure of choice, rather than MRI, as haematomas are about the most readily recognisable abnormality on plain CT.

Extradural Haemorrhage

The **acute extradural (or epidural) haematoma** is a relatively stereotyped lesion (Figs. 1-36 and 1-37). Because the dura mater tends to adhere to the skull, the haematoma is seen on CT sections as a biconvex dense area immediately beneath the skull vault, convex towards both the brain and the vault. The temporoparietal convexity is the most common site, in which lesions are easily detected on axial sections. The haematoma often lies beneath a fracture of the squamous part of the temporal bone. They tend not to cross cranial sutures. Areas of low density within them may indicate continuing bleeding (Fig. 1-37), and add further urgency to the assessment. Frontal, vertical and posterior cranial fossa collections (Fig. 1-38) can be difficult to diagnose; coronal images may be required. Even then, shallow extradural haematomas may be overlooked, especially when adjacent to contused or haemorrhagic brain. Wide-window CT images may help distinguish the intermediate density of the clot from bone and underlying brain. The underlying brain is displaced, but often appears intrinsically normal. MRI can be helpful on occasions (Fig. 1-39).

Subdural Haemorrhage

Subdural bleeding is often, but not always, associated with damage to the brain, and arises from rupture of veins

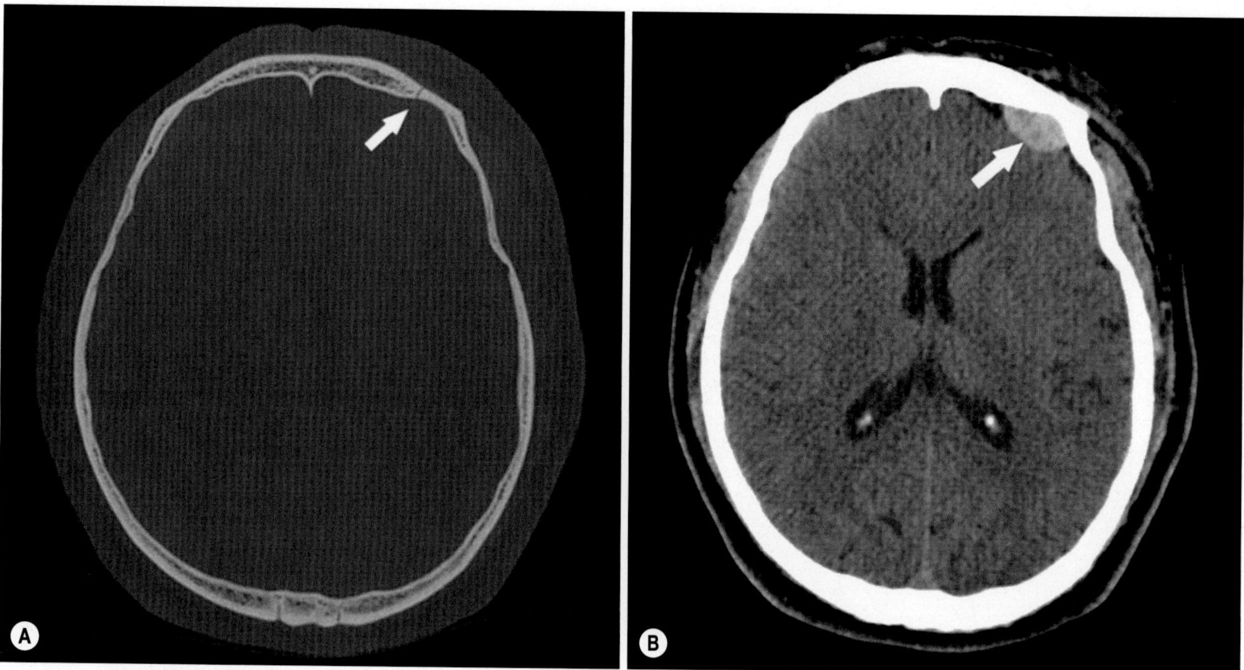

FIGURE 1-36 ■ (A, B) CT: axial 'brain and bone windows' from equivalent levels demonstrate an undisplaced fracture of the left frontal bone (A, arrow), with a small extradural haematoma overlying the adjacent frontal lobe (B, arrow). Soft-tissue contusion overlying the fracture site is also noted.

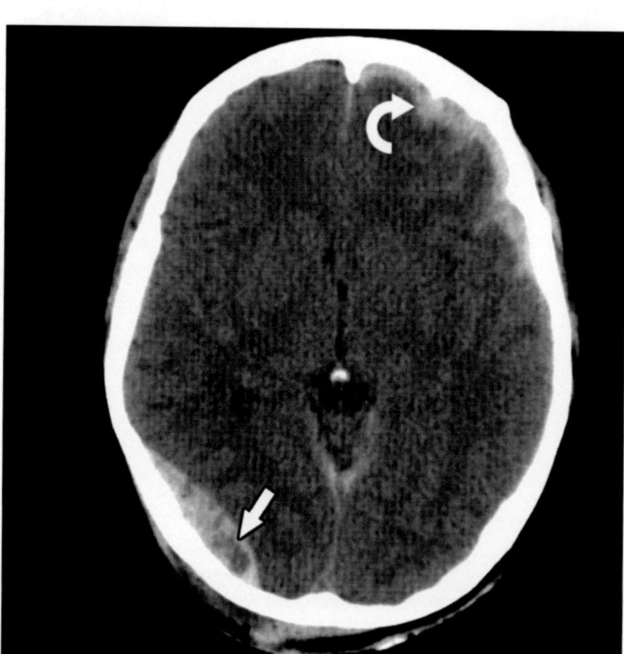

FIGURE 1-37 ■ **Trauma.** CT: a biconvex extradural haematoma overlies the right parieto-occiptal region. Note the central low attenuation (arrow) within the haematoma, indicative of active haemorrhage. A crescent of fresh subdural blood is also seen overlying the left frontal and temporal lobes (curved arrow).

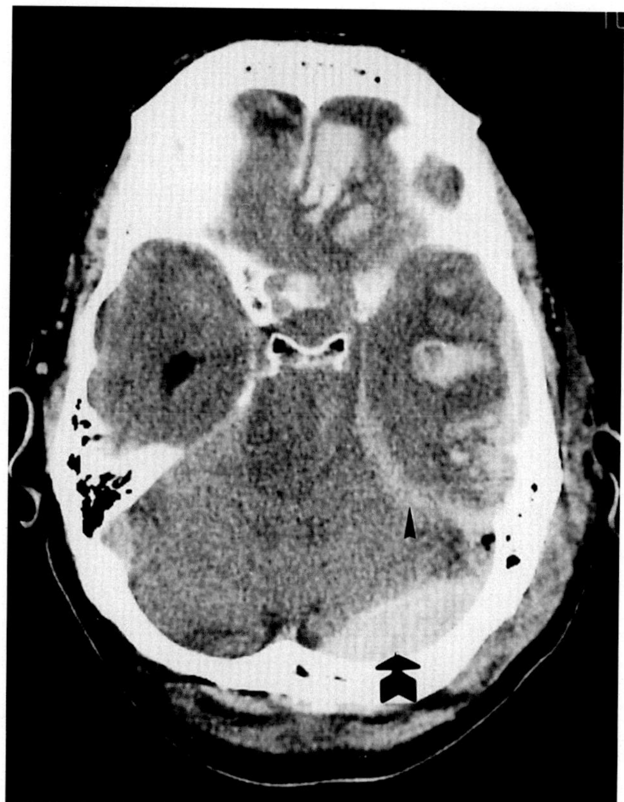

FIGURE 1-38 ■ **Trauma.** CT: A biconvex density of blood over the left cerebellar hemisphere indicates an extradural haematoma (thick arrow). A crescent of fresh subdural blood spreads over the left temporal lobe and tracks along the tentorium in a comma-shaped fashion (arrowhead); this feature differentiates it from an extradural. Typical sites of haemorrhagic contusions are also seen; gyrus recti and temporal lobe.

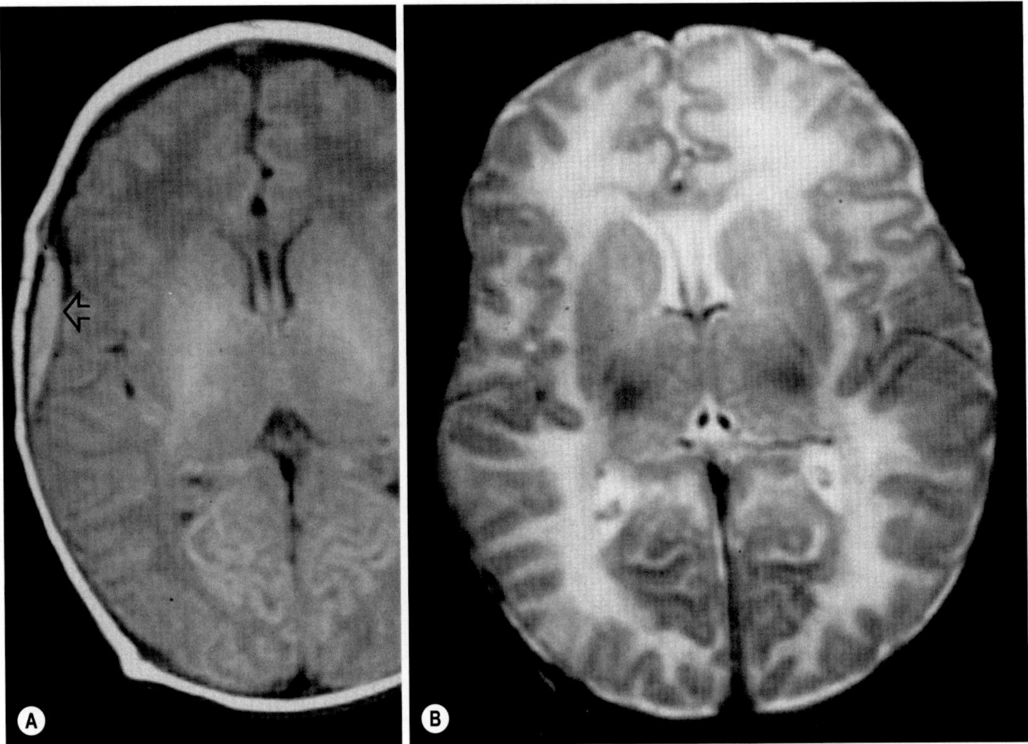

FIGURE 1-39 ■ **Acute extradural haematoma.** MRI in a neonate with traumatic delivery. (A) Axial T_1-weighted image (750/16). Slightly hyperintense epidural collection (arrow) in the right temporal region. (B) Axial T_2-weighted image (3000/120), epidural collection is hypointense and is invisible except for deformation of the underlying cortex. This is the MR signature of deoxyhaemoglobin.

which cross the subdural space; vault fractures are much less commonly present in patients with subdural haematomas than extradural bleeds.

Subdural haematomas are seen most commonly over the cerebral convexities, under the temporal and occipital lobes, or along the falx cerebri. They lie in the virtual space between the dura and arachnoid maters and may be extensive. This is because the blood within them, while under less pressure, is less restricted and tends to spread out over the surface of the brain; bleeding may even extend over an entire cerebral hemisphere. They may follow minor head injuries, and sometimes seem to develop spontaneously, especially in the elderly and in patients with haematological abnormalities. In such situations they are often diagnosed during the investigation of persistent headache, or perhaps transient but repetitive focal neurological deficits. Large ones requiring operative evacuation are usually associated with a reduced conscious state of the patient.

On axial CT and MRI, the cerebral surface typically is concave (Fig. 1-40), but on coronal images may appear more convex. Acute lesions are usually hyperdense on CT, but mixed density is also common. They become progressively less dense over time, and typically end up of similar density to CSF within a few weeks or months. During this evolution there is often a period when the attenuation of the haematoma is similar to that of cerebral tissue; the resulting 'isodense subdural' haemotoma[75] can be difficult to identify (Fig. 1-41) and is a well-recognised pitfall on CT which continues to cause problems.[76] MRI is better at making this diagnosis when these

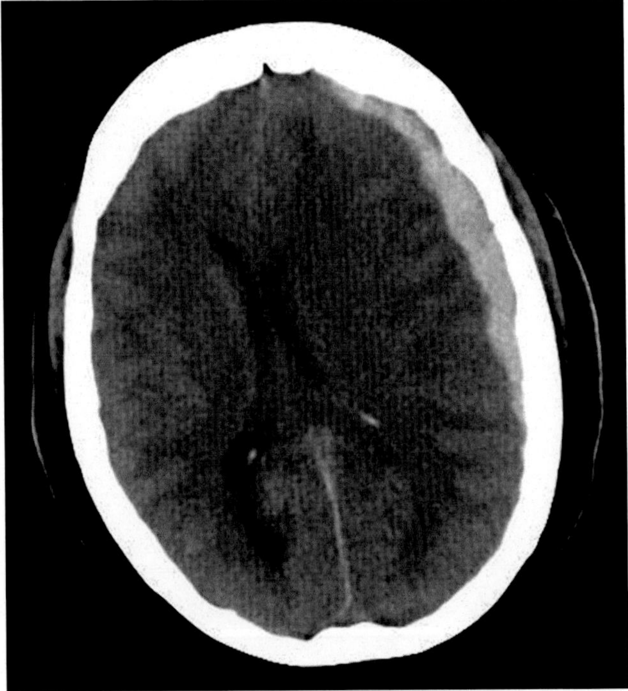

FIGURE 1-40 ■ **Acute subdural haematoma.** CT: Heterogeneous density of irregular shape occupies extra-axial space overlying the left cerebral convexity. There is quite severe mass effect exhibited by effacement of convexity sulci, narrowing of the left-sided ventricular system and midline shift. (Courtesy of Dr Dan Scoffings.)

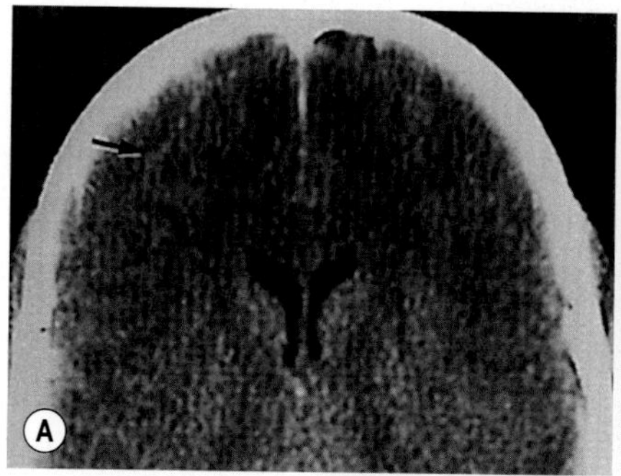
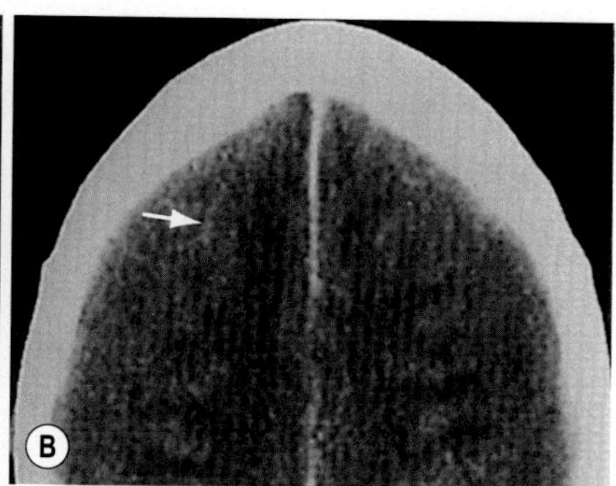

FIGURE 1-41 ■ **Bilateral isodense subdural haematomas on contrast-enhanced CT.** The ventricles (A) are slit-like and displaced medially, giving a 'rabbit's ears' appearance. A higher section (B) indicates that the normal grey–white interface lies too near the midline; the cortex appears abnormally thick. On close inspection, both sections show cortical vessels (arrows) displaced away from the cranial vault.

lesions are of some long-standing. Most resolve spontaneously with time, but some persist, sometimes for years. Occasionally these lesions enlarge progressively at a variable, but usually slow, rate and eventually may require evacuation. The high morbidity of these lesions, particularly in the aged, is due in large part to the associated swelling, contusion or laceration of the underlying brain. It is often evident that midline displacement is greater than would be accounted for by the mass of the haematoma alone. Dilatation of the contralateral ventricle is a bad prognostic sign.

The interhemispheric subdural haematoma extends along the falx cerebri and may spread onto the tentorium, giving a characteristic comma shape on axial CT sections (see Fig. 1-38).

Coronal CT sections may be useful in distinguishing supra- and infra-tentorial bleeding. Sub- or extradural collections low in the posterior cranial fossa, which may be life-threatening, may be overlooked, and the presence of unexplained hydrocephalus after acute head injury should prompt thorough examination of that region (see Fig. 1-42).

The CT attenuation of the blood in a subacute subdural haematoma slowly decreases: as a rule of thumb, it remains denser than the brain for 1 week, and is less dense after 3 weeks (Fig. 1-43). There is thus an interim period of up to 2 weeks when it may be 'isodense' with brain (see Fig. 1-41). Not all isodense haematomas are subacute: an acute bleed can be isodense in a very anaemic patient, and if there is continued leakage of venous blood, a chronic haematoma may not be of low density. Indirect signs may then be crucial: midline shift, with compression of the ipsilateral ventricle; contralateral ventricular enlargement; effacement of cerebral sulci; and medial displacement of the junction between the white and grey matter ('buckling'). Some of these signs may be absent if there are bilateral collections; the frontal horns may then lie closer together than normal, giving a 'rabbit's ear' configuration (see Fig. 1-41). Intravenous contrast medium, by highlighting the vessels on the surface of the brain, may remove any doubts about the extracerebral location of the lesion. The increasing use of MRI for nonacute problems should help overcome this diagnostic problem in the future.

Chronic subdural collections are usually biconvex. Their density is less than that of brain, approaching that of CSF. Fluid–fluid levels may be seen between denser blood elements in the more dependent portions and serous fluid above, particularly if haemorrhage has been repeated. The membrane on their deep surface frequently shows contrast enhancement.

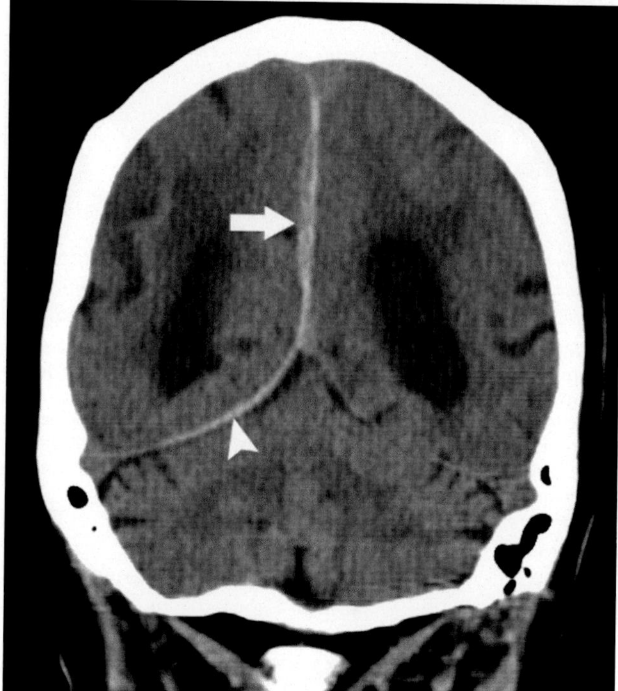

FIGURE 1-42 ■ CT: Coronal reformatted image demonstrates a subtle parafalcine subdural haematoma (arrow) with layering over the tentorium cerebelli (arrowhead). Reformatted coronal images are useful for identifying the latter, which may be difficult to identify on axial images.

PRIMARY CEREBRAL DAMAGE IN CLOSED HEAD INJURY

This is commonly associated with intracerebral haemorrhage, usually small and multifocal. An important feature is that the haemorrhages tend to enlarge and become more conspicuous over the initial few days after injury. Primary cerebral damage may be described as either superficial or deep. Interestingly, these patterns of injury usually are mutually exclusive. Deep damage generally is considered to occur more commonly in high speed accidents and to have a worse prognosis, but exceptions are encountered quite frequently, and as in all forms of head

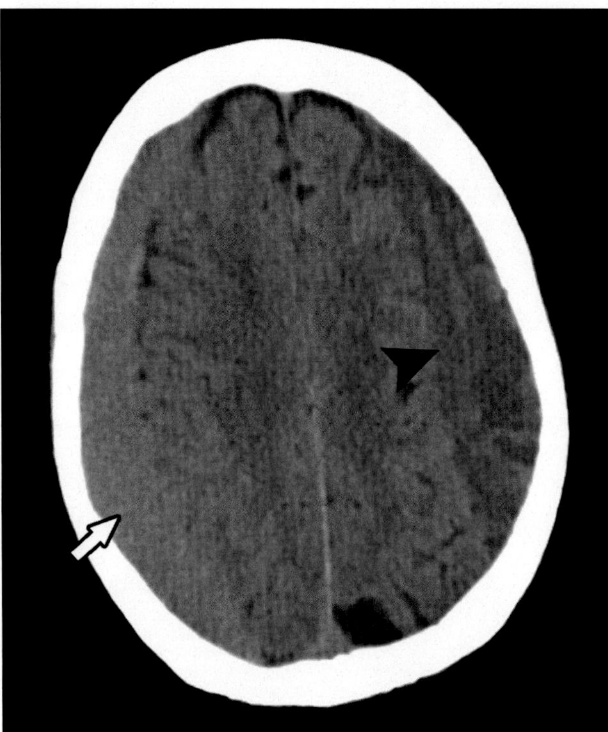

FIGURE 1-43 ■ **Bilateral subacute haematomas.** CT: The subdural haematoma overlying the right cerebral convexity is isodense to brain parenchyma (arrow), and results in mass effect with effacement of the adjacent cortical sulci. The subdural collection overlying the left convexity (arrowhead) is of lower attenuation than brain parenchyma but denser than CSF, and is therefore older than that on the right side.

injury, prognosis must be guarded in the initial few months following the injury.

Superficial Primary Cerebral Damage

This consists of cerebral contusions (see Fig. 1-38) and cortical lacerations. The underlying white matter also usually is damaged to a variable extent. The lesions usually are quite extensive, and typically involve the inferior parts of the frontal lobes and the anterior parts of the temporal lobes, but they can be found elsewhere. The mechanism is rotation of the brain with respect to the skull, especially the sphenoid ridges and the anterior cranial fossa. The term contrecoup contusion often is used because commonly this type of cerebral damage lies diametrically opposite the site of impact, as defined by skull fracture or scalp haematoma (Fig. 1-44). However, the cause is rotation, not linear acceleration of the brain. On CT, contusion appears as superficial low density areas with mild to moderate mass effect, which tends to increase a little in the initial days and subsequently contracts into a region of focal atrophy and sometimes cavitation. Multiple, usually small hyperdense haemorrhages are often present within the low density areas in the early stages. On MRI, they appear as mixed signal lesions, later contracting to regions of persistent mainly cortical cerebral damage. MRI is not much more sensitive in assessing the extent of contusions than CT.

Deep Primary Cerebral Damage

This pattern of injury is considerably less common. The mechanism here is differential rates of rotational acceleration within brain substance itself, producing shearing forces which damage axons and microvasculature. The injury is microscopic and may not be detected at all by

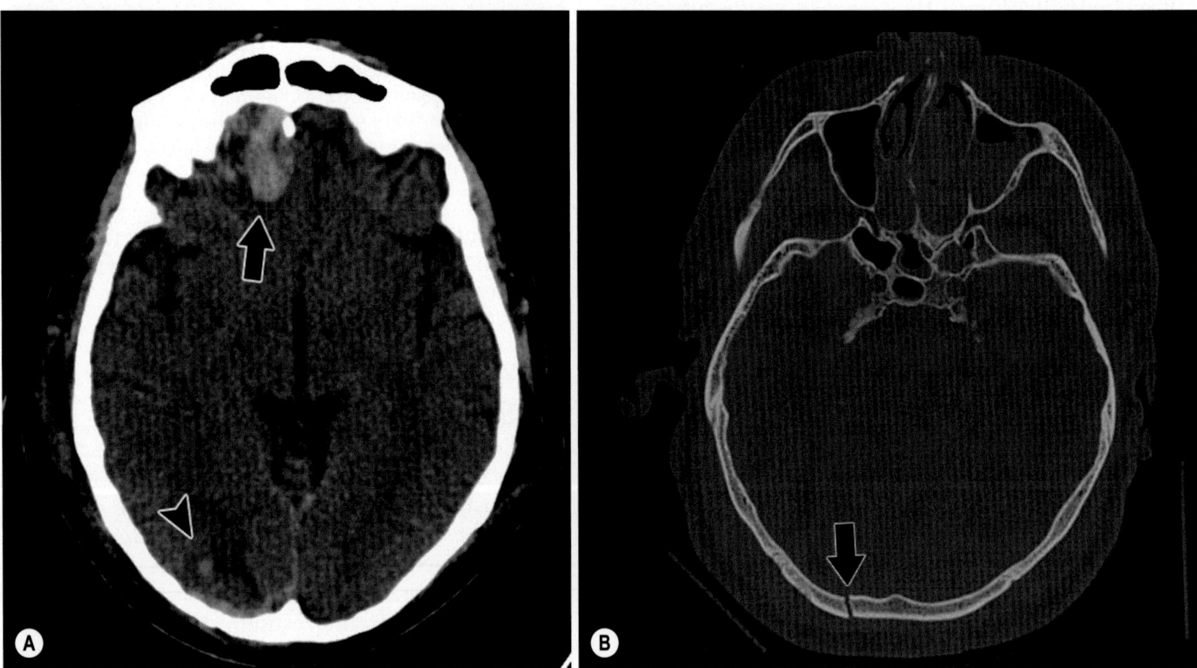

FIGURE 1-44 ■ **Contrecoup injury.** (A) Haemorrhagic 'contrecoup' contusion is demonstrated within the anterior right frontal lobe (arrow). A 'coup' contusion of the occipital lobe resulting from the direct impact is also seen (arrowhead), adjacent to a fracture of the right occipital bone (B, arrow).

CT or MRI, unless diffuse atrophy subsequently develops in the brain. Its presence is most often recognised on imaging by the presence of so-called marker lesions. These probably represent small areas of microvascular damage with haemorrhage or infarction, but they are a reliable guide to the presence of diffuse axonal injury, though not to its extent. They are small multifocal lesions, and tend to occur in more or less characteristic sites: high parasagittal cerebral white matter, corona radiata, posterior corpus collosum and subcortical white matter almost anywhere. They usually are not visible on CT unless haemorrhagic; many more may be on MRI, whether haemorrhagic or not. Susceptibility-weighted MRI (T_2 'star' acquisitions) often shows still more lesions, even long after the event, as small dark patches of haemosiderin (Fig. 1-45). Characteristically the surrounding brain appears normal. Quantitative diffusion tensor imaging has been considered to demonstrate the axonal damage in a few reported cases, but only when it has been exceptionally severe.

When the vascular component of the shearing injury is severe there may be larger haemorrhages in the basal ganglia and elsewhere, a pattern sometimes termed diffuse axonal injury of the brain.

Primary Brainstem Injuries

These usually only occur with deep cerebral damage. The most common is a haemorrhagic lesion in the dorsolateral midbrain. Another is the pontomedullary rent, usually not compatible with life and therefore rarely seen on imaging.

OTHER TYPES OF INTRACRANIAL HAEMORRHAGE AFTER CLOSED HEAD INJURY

Subarachnoid Haemorrhage

Head injury is probably the most common cause overall of subarachnoid haemorrhage. It commonly accompanies superficial cerebral damage, but may be minor and inconspicuous and is usually not recognised radiologically or clinically.

Intraventricular Haemorrhage

When isolated, intraventricular haemorrhage usually seems to be the result of tears in the attachments of the septum pellucidum to the corpus callosum.

Isolated Large Intracerebral Haemorrhage

Although rare, intracerebral haemorrhage is encountered from time to time and is often a source of diagnostic confusion. Cerebral angiography may show a false aneurysm.

SECONDARY CEREBRAL DAMAGE WITH CLOSED HEAD INJURY

This results mainly from the effects of raised intracranial pressure, local pressure cones and fluctuations in systemic

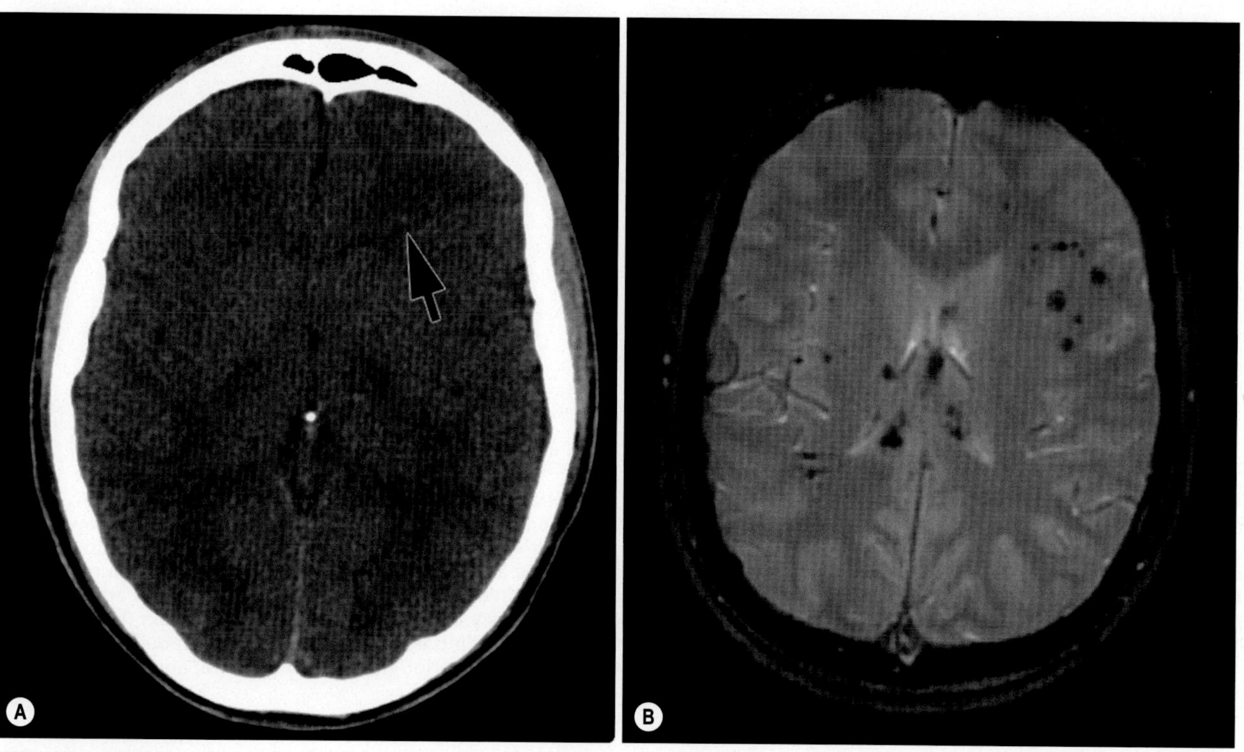

FIGURE 1-45 ■ **Diffuse axonal injury.** On unenhanced CT imaging (A) a subtle focus of high attenuation is present at the grey–white matter interface (arrow). (B) Axial T_2*-weighted MR image (660/25) at the equivalent level demonstrates numerous further foci of haemorrhage not seen on CT, manifesting as multiple hypointense punctate foci within the subcortical and deep white matter of both hemispheres and within the corpus callosum.

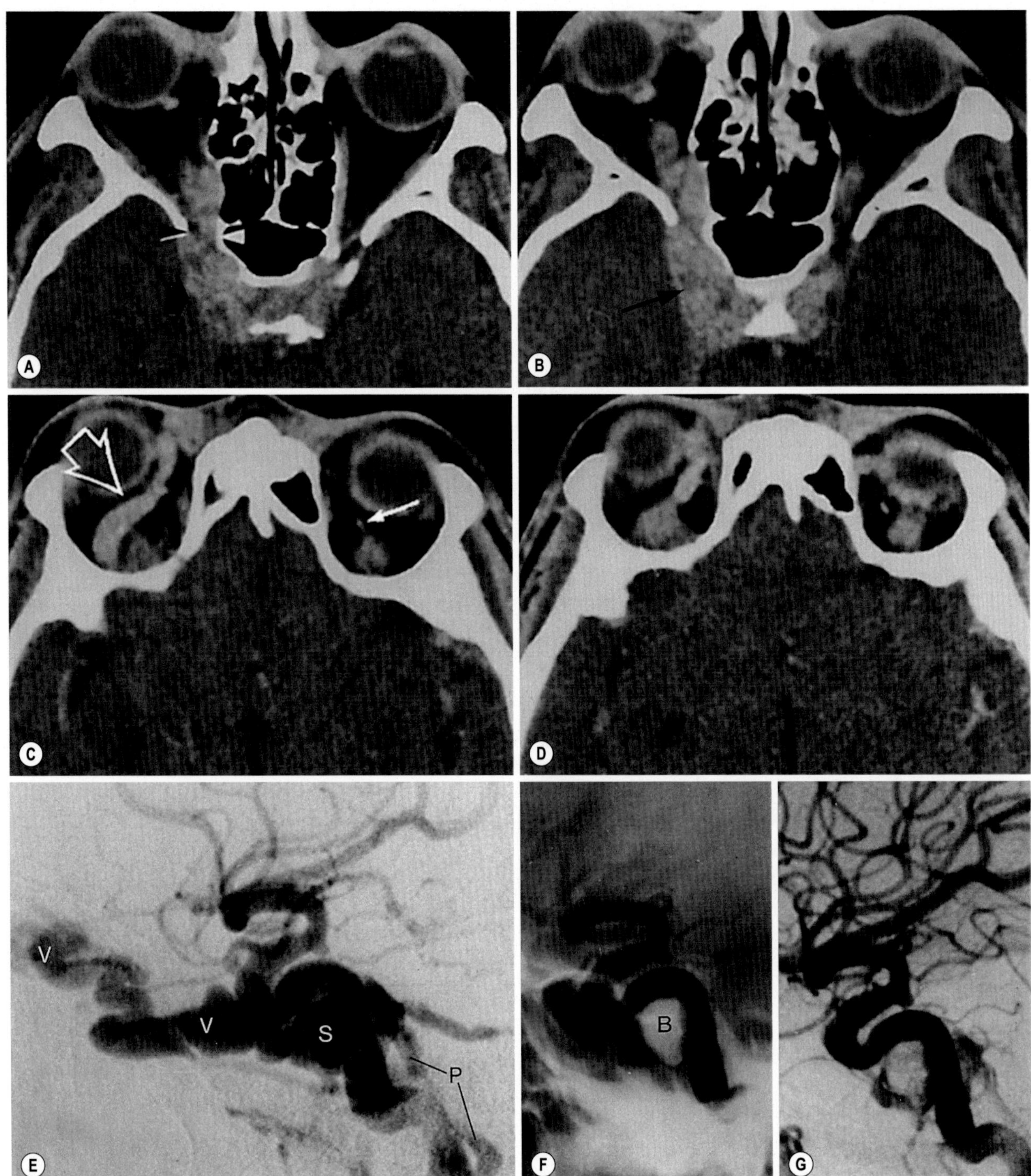

FIGURE 1-46 ■ **Post-traumatic caroticocavernous fistula.** (A–D) Axial contrast-enhanced CT: the right cavernous sinus (A, arrow) is enlarged, and a large enhancing mass runs forwards into the orbit through a widened superior orbital fissure (A, arrowheads). A sigmoid structure (C, open arrow) in the upper part of the right orbit represents the greatly dilated superior ophthalmic vein (cf. normal left side in C, small white arrow). Some of the extraocular muscles are thicker than on the left, and there is marked right proptosis. (E) Intra-arterial DSA, lateral projection, arterial phase, following injection into the right internal carotid artery. Contrast medium floods into the cavernous sinus (S), and drains anteriorly into a grossly dilated superior ophthalmic vein (V); there is also shunting posteriorly and via the inferior petrosal sinus (P). Intracranial arterial filling is poor. (F, G) After therapeutic detachment of a balloon (B) in the cavernous sinus (F, lateral projection), shunting particularly anteriorly, is greatly reduced, and intracranial filling much improved (G).

blood pressure and blood oxygen saturation. A common serious problem in the initial 2 or 3 d after a major head injury is diffuse cerebral swelling due to an increase in the cerebral blood volume, appropriately referred to as hyperaemic brain swelling, and less appropriately as brain oedema. It is a potent cause of raised intracranial pressure in this period and may trigger drastic neurosurgical decompression by wide craniectomies. The appearance of brain substance on CT and MRI is not affected, so it is not directly recognisable by imaging alone.

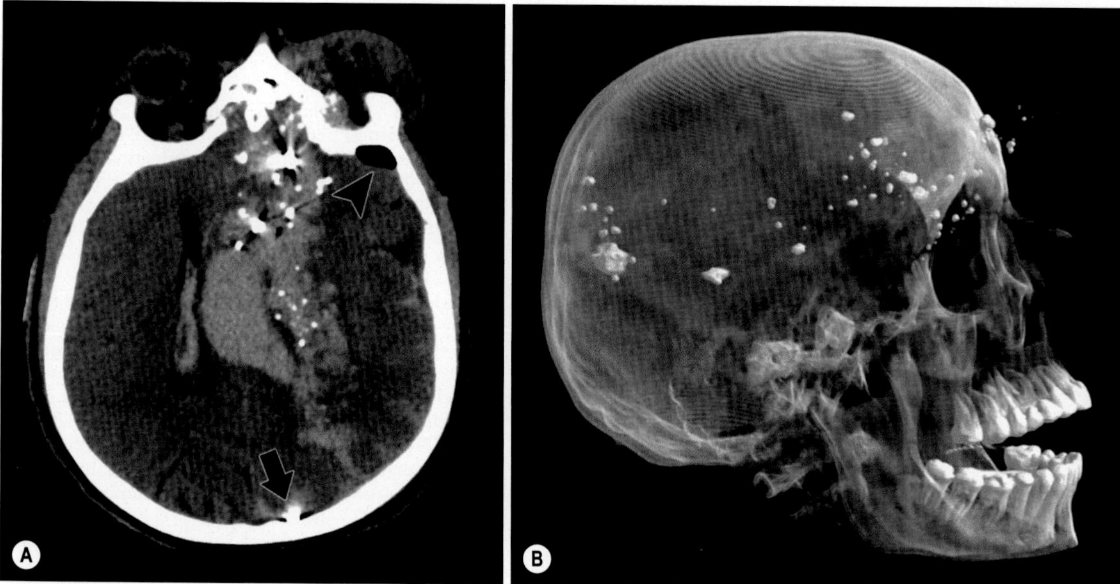

FIGURE 1-47 ■ **Gunshot injury.** (A) Axial CT: The site of projectile penetration is through the left frontal sinus and has resulted in extensive intraparenchymal haematoma with extension into the lateral ventricles, in addition to pneumocephalus (arrowhead). Multiple metallic density projectile fragments lie along the projectile tract, the larger fragments resulting in streak artefact. Note the large fragment adjacent to the occipital bone, with no exit site (arrow). (B) A partially transparent volume-rendered image is useful for identifying the relative position of the numerous projectile fragments.

Secondary cerebral damage consists of infarctions and brainstem haemorrhage. Infarcts most commonly occur in the cortical distributions of one or both posterior cerebral arteries, and haemorrhages are most often found in the ventral mid-brain and upper ponds. Both probably, but certainly the latter, are due to pressure cones across the tentorial incisura.

OTHER COMPLICATIONS WITH CLOSED HEAD INJURIES

Hydrocephalus requiring shunting is an uncommon complication and generally is of a communicating type.

CSF fistulae are associated with skull base fractures and may present with otorrhoea or rhinorhhoea. Most heal within 10 d or so, but a small number may persist or become intermittent, and eventually require surgical repair. Detailed imaging may be necessary to identify the site of the leak.[77] CSF leaks are associated with intracranial air, which may be extradural if the meninges are intact, or if they are torn, subarachnoid or intraventricular. These are often referred to as aerocoeles or pneumocephalus.

Cranial nerve palsies are usually associated with skull base fractures and are immediate and permanent. Delayed cranial nerve palsies also may occur in the absence of fracture and may be reversible. Virtually any nerve or branch that traverses the skull base can be involved.

An arteriovenous fistula may be an immediate or a delayed complication (Fig. 1-46). The most common occurs between the internal carotid artery and the cavernous sinus,[78] and is termed a direct carotid cavernous fistula. These usually are torrential, and may require urgent endovascular treatment to preserve vision, sometimes at a time when the overall outcome is in the balance. Alternatively they may be chronic and the patient may present with an alarming engorged exophthalmos.

Penetrating Head Injuries

Although uncommon, such injuries are increasing in frequency in civilian practice. Appearances on imaging vary with the penetrating agent and the trajectory of the cerebral penetration. Intracerebral haemorrhage usually dominates the appearances on imaging (Fig. 1-47). Direct vascular injury is more common than in closed head injury, resulting in larger haemorrhages and more frequent false aneurysms.

REFERENCES

1. O'Rahilly R, Muller F. The Embryonic Human Brain, an Atlas of Developmental Stages. 3rd ed. Hoboken, NJ: Wiley-Liss; 2006. pp. 31–92.
2. Lasjaunias P, Berenstein A, ter Brugge K. Surgical Neuroangiography. 2nd ed. vol 1 Clinical Vascular Anatomy and Variations. Berlin: Springer-Verlag; 2001. pp. 480–96.
3. Thomas AMK, Banerjee AK. The History of Radiology. Oxford: Oxford University Press; 2013.
4. Swanson LW. Brain Architecture: Understanding the Basic Plan. 2nd ed. Oxford: Oxford University Press; 2012.
5. Nieuwenhuys R, Voogd J, van Huijzen C. The Human Central Nervous System. 4th ed. Berlin: Springer-Verlag; 2008. pp. 491–510.
6. Temburni MK, Jacb MH. New functions for glia in the brain. Proc Natl Acad Sci USA 2001;98:3631–2.
7. Yousry T. The cerebral lobes and their boundaries. Int J Neuroradiol 1998;4:342–8.
8. Naidich TP, Brightbill TC. Systems for localizing fronto-parietal gyri and sulci on axial CT and MRI. Int J Neuroradiol 1996;2: 313–38.
9. Chen CY, Zimmerman RA, Parrish B, et al. MR of the cerebral operculum: topographic identification and measurement of interopercular distances in healthy infants and children. Am J Neuroradiol 1995;16:1677–87.

10. Kido DK, LeMay M, Levinson AW, Benson WE. Computed tomographic localization of the precentral gyrus. Radiology 1980;135:373–7.
11. Naidich TP, Brightbill TC. The intraparietal sulcus: a landmark for localization of pathology on axial CT scans. Int J Neuroradiol 1995;1:3–16.
12. Cohen CR, Duchesneau PM, Weinstein MA. Calcification of the basal ganglia as visualized by computed tomography. Radiology 1980;134:97–9.
13. Sarwar M, Ford K. Rapid development of basal ganglia calcification. Am J Neuroradiol 1981;2:103–4.
14. Drayer BP, Burger P, Darwin R, et al. Magnetic resonance imaging of brain iron. Am J Neuroradiol 1986;7:373–80.
15. Zimmerman RA, Bilaniuk L. Age-related incidence of pineal calcification detected by computed tomography. Radiology 1982;142:659–62.
16. Clarke E, O'Malley CD. The Human Brain and Spinal Cord: A Historical Study Illustrated by Writings from Antiquity to the Twentieth Century. 2nd ed. San Francisco: Norman Publishing; 1996. pp. 585–7.
17. Greitz D, Greitz T, Hindmarsh T. A new view on the CSF-circulation with the potential for pharmacological treatment of childhood hydrocephalus. Acta Paediatr 1997;86:125–32.
18. Koh L, Zakharov A, Johnston M. Integration of the subarachnoid space and lymphatics: is it time to embrace a new concept of cerebrospinal fluid absorption? Cerebrospinal Fluid Res 2005;2:6.
19. Willinsky R, Lasjaunias P, Berenstein A. Intracavernous branches of the internal carotid artery: comprehensive review of their variations. Surg Radiol Anat 1987;9:201–15.
20. Perlmutter D, Rhoton AL. Microsurgical anatomy of the anterior cerebral-anterior communicating-recurrent artery complex. J Neurosurg 1976;45:259–72.
21. Perlmutter D, Rhoton AL. Microsurgical anatomy of the distal anterior cerebral artery. J Neurosurg 1978;49:204–28.
22. Gibo H, Carver C, Rhoton AL, et al. Microsurgical anatomy of the middle cerebral artery. J Neurosurg 1981;54:151–69.
23. Campos C, Churojana A, Rodesch G, et al. Basilar tip aneurysms and basilar tip anatomy. Intervent Neuroradiol 1998;4:121–5.
24. Lasjaunias P, Berenstein A, ter Brugge KG. Surgical Neuroangiography. 2nd ed. vol 1: Clinical Vascular Anatomy and Variations. Berlin: Springer-Verlag; 2001. pp. 165–478.
25. Wolpert SM. The circle of Willis. Am J Neuroradiol 1997;18:1033–4.
26. Bhattacharya JJ, Lamin S, Thammaroj J. Otic or mythic? Am J Neurordiol 2004;25:160–2.
27. Cure JK, van Tussel P, Smith MT. Normal variant anatomy of the dural venous sinuses. Semin Ultrasound CT MR 1994;15:499–519.
28. Making the Best Use of Clinical Radiology. IRefer Guidelines. Royal College of Radiologists, UK. Version 7.0.1. 2012.
29. ACR-ASNR Practice Guideline for the Performance and Interpretation of Computed Tomography (CT) of the Brain. American College of Radiology/American Society of Neuroradiology. Resolution 12. Revised 2010.
30. Head injury: Triage, assessment, investigation and early management of head injury in infants, children and adults. National Institute for Health and Clinical Excellence (NICE) Clinical Guideline 56. 2007.
31. Early Management of Patients with a Head injury. Scottish Intercollegiate Guidelines Network (SIGN) Guideline no. 110. May 2009.
32. Lui YW, Tang ER, Allmendinger AM, et al. Evaluation of CT perfusion in the setting of cerebral ischemia: patterns and pitfalls. Am J Neuroradiol 2010;31:1552–63.
33. Fischbein NJ, Wijman CAC. Nontraumatic intracranial hemorrhage. Neuroimaging Clin N Am 2010;20:469–92.
34. Pearce MS, Salotti JA, Little MP, et al. Radiation exposure from CT scans in childhood and subsequent risk of leukaemia and brain tumours: a retrospective cohort study. Lancet 2012;380:499–505.
35. Orrison WW, Snyder KV, Hopkins LN, et al. Whole-brain dynamic CT angiography and perfusion imaging. Clin Radiol 2011;66:566–74.
36. Reichelt A, Zeckey C, Hildebrand F, et al. Imaging of the brain in polytraumatized patients comparing 64-row spiral CT with incremental (sequential) CT. Eur J Radiol 2012;81:789–93.
37. Lev MH, Farkas J, Gemmete JJ, et al. Acute stroke: improved nonenhanced CT detection—benefits of soft-copy interpretation by using variable window width and center level settings. Radiology 1999;213:150–5.
38. Rapalino OO, Kamalian SS, Kamalian SS, et al. Cranial CT with adaptive statistical iterative reconstruction: improved image quality with concomitant radiation dose reduction. Am J Neuroradiol 2012;33:609–15.
39. ACR-ASNR Practice Guideline for the performance and interpretation of magnetic resonance imaging (MRI) of the brain. American College of Radiology/American Society of Neuroradiology. Resolution 21. Revised 2008.
40. Barkovich AJ, Atlas SW. Magnetic resonance imaging of intracranial hemorrhage. Radiol Clin North Am 1988;26:801–20.
41. Forbes KP, Pipe JG, Karis JP, et al. Brain imaging in the unsedated pediatric patient: comparison of periodically rotated overlapping parallel lines with enhanced reconstruction and single-shot fast spin-echo sequences. Am J Neuroradiol 2003;24:794–8.
42. Stobo DB, Lindsay RS, Connell JM, et al. Initial experience of 3 Tesla versus conventional field strength magnetic resonance imaging of small functioning pituitary tumours. Clin Endocrinol (Oxf) 2011;75:673–7.
43. van der Kolk AG, Hendrikse J, Luijten PR. Ultrahigh-field magnetic resonance imaging: the clinical potential for anatomy, pathogenesis, diagnosis, and treatment planning in brain disease. Neuroimaging Clin N Am 2012;22:343–62, xii.
44. Charidimou A, Krishnan A, Werring DJ, Jäger HR. Cerebral microbleeds: a guide to detection and clinical relevance in different disease settings. Neuroradiology 2013;5:655–74.
45. Medicines, Healthcare products Regulatory Agency. Drug Safety Update. Available at <http://www.mhra.gov.uk/Safetyinformation/DrugSafetyUpdate/CON087741>.
46. Filippi M, Rocca MA. MR imaging of multiple sclerosis. Radiology 2011;259:659–81.
47. da Cruz LCH Jr, editor. Clinical Applications of Diffusion Imaging of the Brain. London: Elsevier; 2011.
48. Yang E, Nucifora PG, Melhem ER. Diffusion MR imaging: basic principles. Neuroimaging Clin N Am 2011;21:1–25, vii.
49. Shenton ME, Hamoda HM, Schneiderman JS, et al. A review of magnetic resonance imaging and diffusion tensor imaging findings in mild traumatic brain injury. Brain Imaging Behav 2012;6:137–92.
50. Copen WA, Schaefer PW, Wu O. MR perfusion imaging in acute ischemic stroke. Neuroimaging Clin N Am 2011;21:259–83.
51. Duyn JH, van Gelderen P, Talagala L, et al. Technological advances in MRI measurement of brain perfusion. J Magn Reson Imaging 2005;22:751–3.
52. Lacerda S, Law M. Magnetic resonance perfusion and permeability imaging in brain tumors. Neuroimaging Clin N Am 2009;19:527–57.
53. Barker PB, Bizzi A, De Stefano N, et al. Clinical MR Spectroscopy. Cambridge, UK: Cambridge University Press; 2009.
54. Stroman PW. Essentials of Functional MRI. Boca Rotan, FL: CRC Press; 2011.
55. Pillai JJ. The evolution of clinical functional imaging during the past 2 decades and its current impact on neurosurgical planning. Am J Neuroradiol 2010;31:219–25.
56. Van Heertum RL, Tikofsky RS, Ichise M. Functional Cerebral SPECT and PET Imaging. Lippincott Williams & Wilkins; 2013.
57. Anxionnat R, Bracard S, Ducrocq X, et al. Intracranial aneurysms: clinical value of 3D digital subtraction angiography in the therapeutic decision and endovascular treatment. Radiology 2001;218:799–808.
58. Adams HP Jr, del Zoppo G, Alberts MJ, et al. Guidelines for the early management of adults with ischemic stroke. Stroke 2007;38:1655–711.
59. Fifi JT, Meyers PM, Lavine SD, et al. Complications of modern diagnostic cerebral angiography in an academic medical center. J Vasc Interv Radiol 2009;20:442–7.
60. Dawkins AA, Evans AL, Wattam J, et al. Complications of cerebral angiography: A prospective analysis of 2,924 consecutive procedures. Neuroradiology 2007;49:753–9.
61. Willinsky RA, Taylor SM, TerBrugge K, et al. Neurologic complications of cerebral angiography: prospective analysis of 2,899 procedures and review of the literature. Radiology 2003;227:522–8.

62. Fleischmann D, Boas FE. Computed tomography—old ideas and new technology. Eur Radiol 2011;21:510–7.
63. Morhard D, Fink C, Graser A, et al. Cervical and cranial computed tomographic angiography with automated bone removal: dual energy computed tomography versus standard computed tomography. Invest Radiol 2009;44:293–7.
64. Latchaw RE, Alberts MJ, Lev MH, et al. Recommendations for imaging of acute ischemic stroke: a scientific statement from the American Heart Association. Stroke 2009;40:3646–78.
65. Luo Z, Wang D, Sun X, et al. Comparison of the accuracy of subtraction CT angiography performed on 320-detector row volume CT with conventional CT angiography for diagnosis of intracranial aneurysms. Eur J Radiol 2012;81:118–22.
66. Brown DL, Hoffman SN, Jacobs TL, et al. CT angiography is cost-effective for confirmation of internal carotid artery occlusions. J Neuroimaging 2008;18:355–9.
67. Teasdale E, Zampakis P, Santosh C, Razvi S. Multidetector computed tomography angiography: Application in vertebral artery dissection. Ann Indian Acad Neurol 2011;14:35–41.
68. Ruigrok YM, Rinkel GJ, Buskens E, et al. Perimesencephalic hemorrhage and CT angiography: A decision analysis. Stroke 2000; 31:2976–83.
69. Debrey SM, Yu H, Lynch JK, et al. Diagnostic accuracy of magnetic resonance angiography for internal carotid artery disease: a systematic review and meta-analysis. Stroke 2008;39: 2237–48.
70. Hadizadeh DR, Kukuk GM, Steck DT, et al. Noninvasive evaluation of cerebral arteriovenous malformations by 4D-MRA for preoperative planning and postoperative follow-up in 56 patients: comparison with DSA and intraoperative findings. Am J Neuroradiol 2012;33:1095–101.
71. Royal College of Radiologists. Making the Best Use of a Department of Clinical Radiology: Guidelines for Doctors. London: RCR; 2007.
72. National Institute for Clinical Excellence. Head Injury: Guidelines. London: NICE; 2003. Available at <http://www.nice.org.uk/guidance/CG4/guidance/pdf/English/download.dspx>.
73. Mayor S. NICE recommends greater use of CT imaging for head injuries. BMJ 2003;326:1414.
74. Du Boulay GH. Principles of X-Ray Diagnosis of the Skull. London: Butterworth; 1980.
75. Naidich TP, Moran CJ, Pudlowski RM, Naidich JB. CT diagnosis of isodense subdural hematoma. Adv Neurol 1979;22:73–105.
76. Boviatsis EJ, Kouyialis AT, Sakas DE. Misdiagnosis of bilateral isodense chronic subdural haematomas. Hosp Med 2003;64: 374–5.
77. Avdin K, Guven K, Sencer S, et al. MRI cisternography with gadolinium-containing contrast medium: its role, advantages and limitations in the investigation of rhinorrhoea. Neuroradiology 2004;46:75–80.
78. Peeters FLM, Kroger R. Dural and direct cavernous sinus fistulas. Am J Roentgenol 1979;132:599–606.

CHAPTER 2

Benign and Malignant Intracranial Tumours in Adults

Ruchi Kabra • Caroline Micallef • H. Rolf Jäger

CHAPTER OUTLINE

RADIOLOGICAL INVESTIGATIONS IN INTRACRANIAL TUMOURS

Plain radiographic findings in brain tumours are of historical interest and may show signs of raised intracranial pressure (such as erosion of the lamina dura of the dorsum sellae, or a 'J-shaped' sella), tumour calcification or enlargement of middle meningeal artery grooves in meningiomas.

Magnetic resonance imaging (MRI) is the preferred investigation for patients with suspected intracranial tumours. It provides a better soft-tissue differentiation and tumour delineation than CT and advanced MR imaging techniques, such as diffusion-weighted (DWI) and perfusion-weighted (PWI) imaging and MR spectroscopy (MRS), allow the assessment of physiological and metabolic processes.

Intra-arterial angiography for brain tumours is now mostly performed in conjunction with preoperative or palliative tumour embolisations.

COMPUTED TOMOGRAPHY

Most clinically symptomatic brain tumours are detectable on CT, by virtue of mass effect and/or altered attenuation. Intra-axial tumours are usually of low attenuation on non-enhanced CT images. Primary intracranial lymphoma is usually iso- to slightly hyperdense to the brain parenchyma. High attenuation areas within a tumour indicate tumour calcification or recent intratumoural haemorrhage. Tumours frequently exhibiting these two features are listed in Table 2-1.

Bone-window settings can reveal bone erosion or hyperostosis, associated with extra-axial tumours.

Contrast enhancement improves the visualisation of strongly enhancing mass lesions such as meningiomas, schwannomas, metastases and certain types of glial tumours.

CT perfusion has emerged as a technique to assess the relative cerebral blood volume (rCBV) and permeability changes in brain tumours.[1] The newer 320-detector row CT system provides full brain coverage.[2] CT perfusion has the advantage of a direct relationship between the CT attenuation coefficient and contrast material concentration in tissue.

MAGNETIC RESONANCE IMAGING

Structural MRI

The MRI protocol for structural tumour imaging should include T2-weighted, fluid-attenuated recovery

TABLE 2-1 **Commonly Calcified and Haemorrhagic Lesions**

Commonly Calcified Lesions	Commonly Haemorrhagic Lesions
Oligodendrogliomas (90%)	GBM (grade 4 glioma)
Choroid plexus tumours	Oligodendroglioma
Ependymoma	Metastases
Central neurocytoma	– Melanoma
Meningioma	– Lung
Craniopharyngioma	– Breast
Teratoma	
Chordoma	

(FLAIR) sequence and T1-weighted images before and after injection of a gadolinium-based contrast medium.

Most tumours appear hypointense on T1 and hyperintense on T2 and FLAIR images. The latter provide a particularly good contrast between normal brain tissue and glial tumours and show signal loss in cystic tumour components.[3] Highly cellular tumours such as lymphomas and primitive neuroectodermal tumours have decreased water content and therefore appear relatively hypointense on T2 images. Intratumoural haemorrhage or calcification is also hypointense on T2 images and becomes more conspicuous on T2* or susceptibility-weighted images (SWI) where magnetic susceptibility effects are stronger. Hyperintensities on T1 images can be due to haemorrhage, calcification, melanin (in metastatic melanomas) or fat.

Enhancement with gadolinium is seen in vascular extra-axial tumours such as meningiomas, and in intra-axial tumours which disrupt the blood–brain barrier. This is generally a feature of high-grade intra-axial tumours, but can also be present in certain low-grade tumours, such as pilocytic astrocytomas and WHO grade II oligodendrogliomas. The visibility of contrast enhancement on MR can be improved by doubling or tripling the gadolinium dose,[4] or by using high relaxivity gadolinium compounds.[5] Post-contrast FLAIR sequences are useful to assess leptomeningeal disease.

MR images may be acquired in an intraoperative setting where an MR imaging facility is available in an operating theatre environment. With tumours, in particular, images may be acquired during surgery, thus guiding the extent of lesion resection in near real time while preserving eloquent regions of the brain.

Advanced Physiological and Molecular Imaging Methods

DWI, PWI, MRS, functional MRI (fMRI) and positron emission tomography (PET) provide additional information about brain tumours which can be useful in specific clinical settings.

MR Perfusion Imaging

There are three main methods of PWI:

1. Dynamic susceptibility-weighted contrast-enhanced (DSC) imaging exploits the susceptibility effects of gadolinium, which, because of its paramagnetic properties, causes a transient signal loss on T2*-weighted images during the passage of a gadolinium bolus.
2. Dynamic contrast-enhanced (DCE) imaging measures the increase of signal intensity on a series of T1-weighted images following gadolinium administration.
3. Arterial spin labelling (ASL) uses magnetically labelled blood as endogenous tracer to assess blood flow and does not require an injection of a contrast medium.

DSC is currently the most widely used perfusion technique in brain tumours. rCBV measurements derived from DSC correlate closely with angiographic and histological markers of tumour vascularity and the expression of vascular endothelial growth factor (VGEF).[6] It provides an indirect measure of tumour neovascularity and high-grade glial tumours tend to have higher rCBV values than low-grade tumours.[7] Leakiness of contrast agent into the extravascular space due to disruption of the blood–brain barrier can lead to inaccuracies of the rCBV calculations in DSC PWI, especially in high-grade tumours. Several mathematical models have been developed to correct for this problem which can also be minimised by administering an extra gadolinium dose prior to DSC PWI ('preloading dose').[8]

In DCE PWI, T1-weighted images are acquired beyond the duration of the first pass of the gadolinium bolus, typically for about 5 min. The shape of the time–signal intensity curve is influenced by tissue perfusion, vascular permeability and the extravascular-extracellular space. Several mathematical models can be used to quantify contrast leakage into the extravascular space as a measure of microvascular permeability. The most frequently used parameter is the transfer coefficient K^{trans} which is influenced by endothelial permeability, vascular surface area and flow. DCE images can also be analysed using a model-free approach by looking at the slope of the time–signal intensity curve.[9]

ASL uses labelling of endogenous hydrogen to measure cerebral blood flow (rCBF).[10] As hydrogen is freely diffusible and crosses the blood–brain barrier immediately, it is not possible to measure tissue blood volume in the same way as with DSC PWI where the tracer (gadolinium) stays (or is assumed to stay) predominantly in the intravascular compartment. Studies of brain tumours have demonstrated, however, a good correlation between rCBF measurements obtained with ASL and rCBV measurements derived from DSC PWI[11] and the clinical use of ASL techniques in neuro-oncology is likely to increase.

MR Diffusion Imaging

DWI measures Brownian motion of water molecules within tissue. The apparent diffusion coefficient (ADC)

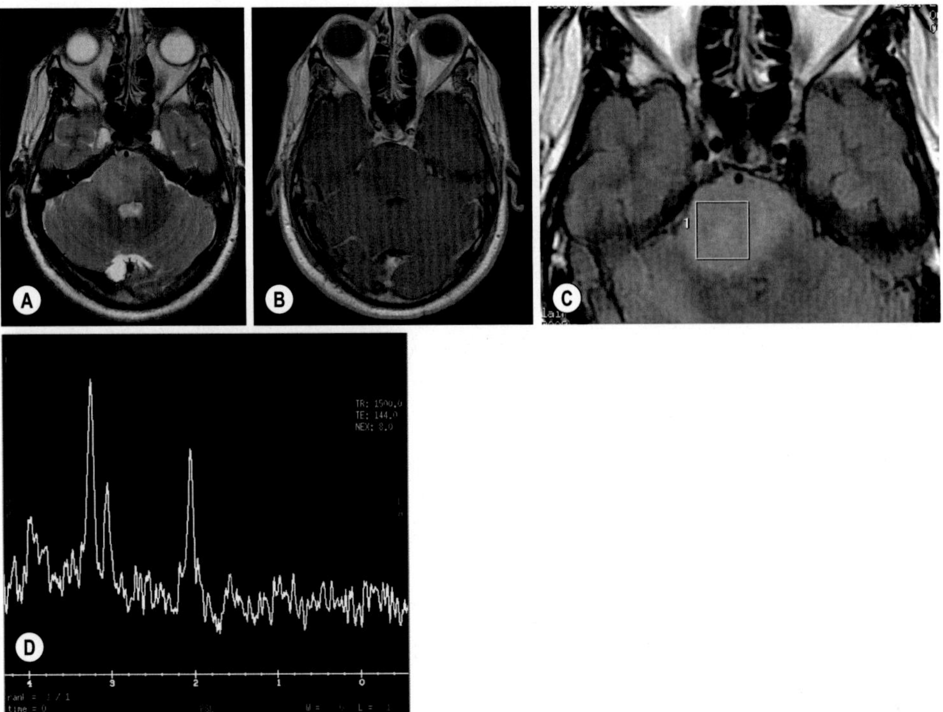

FIGURE 2-1 ■ **Proton magnetic resonance spectroscopy.** Single voxel magnetic resonance spectroscopy. Diffusely infiltrative brain stem glioma which is hyperintense on T2WI (A) and hypointense on contrast-enhanced T1WI (B). A magnified FLAIR image (C) demonstrates placement of the spectroscopy voxel within the tumour. The spectrum (D) demonstrates that the choline peak (3.22 ppm) is elevated and much higher than the creatine peak (3.03 ppm) and the *N*-acetylaspartate peak (2.01 ppm). (CHO = choline, PCr/Cr = creatine, NAA = *N*-acetylaspartate)

describes the overall water diffusibility in tissue and is an indicator of disruption of tissue microstructure, cellular density and matrix composition in tumours. ADC measurements correlate inversely with the histological cell count of gliomas[12] and positively with the presence of hydrophilic substances in the tumour matrix.[13]

There is increasing evidence that DWI using multiple (low and high) *b* values is helpful in brain tumours.[14]

Diffusion tensor imaging (DTI) provides additional information about the direction of water diffusion.[15] The tendency of water to move in some directions more than others is called anisotropy and can be quantified using parameters such as fractional anisotropy (FA). Compact white matter tracts show normally a high degree of anisotropy that can be lost if they are infiltrated by tumour cells which destroy the ultrastructural boundaries formed by myelin sheaths.

Post-processing of DTI allows the depiction of important white matter tracts and their connections (tractography), which can be displayed in direction-encoded colour images. Tractography is useful in the preoperative assessment of brain tumours and helps to differentiate between displacement and infiltration of white matter tracts.[16]

MR Spectroscopy

MRS analyses the biochemistry of a brain tumour and provides semiquantitative information about major metabolites.[17,18] A common pattern in brain tumours is a decrease in *N*-acetylaspartate (NAA), a neuron-specific marker, and creatine (Cr), and an increase in choline (Cho), lactate (Lac) and lipids (L) (Fig. 2-1). The concentration of Cho is a reflection of the turnover of cell membranes (due to accelerated synthesis and destruction) and is more elevated in regions with a high neoplastic activity. Lactate (Lac) is the end product of non-oxidative glycolysis and a marker of hypoxia in tumour tissue. This is of interest, as tumour hypoxia is now recognised as a major promoter of tumour angiogenesis and invasion. Lac is probably associated with viable but hypoxic tissue, whereas mobile lipids is thought to reflect tissue necrosis with breakdown of cell membranes.

The choice of echo time (TE) is an important technical consideration for performing MRS. It can be short (20–40 ms), intermediate (135–144 ms) or long (270–288 ms). MRS with a short TE has the advantage of demonstrating additional metabolites which may improve tumour characterisation, such as *myo*-inositol, glutamate/glutamine (Glx) and lipids, but is hampered by baseline distortion and artefactual NAA peaks. Intermediate echo times have a better defined baseline and quantification of NAA and Cho is more accurate and reproducible. Long echo times lead to a decrease of signal to noise.

MRS is presently a sensitive but not very specific technique. Single voxel spectroscopy provides good-quality spectra but is prone to sampling errors. Chemical shift imaging (CSI) is technically more demanding but provides 2D or 3D spectra and larger area coverage. With 3T MRI systems it is now possible to obtain a 16 × 16 × 16 array of spectra with a voxel size of 1 cm^3 in 5–10 min.[19]

fMRI

Blood oxygen level-dependent (BOLD) imaging detects changes in regional cerebral blood flow during various forms of brain activity. Paradigms using motor tasks, language and speech productions and memory are able to show activation of relevant cortical areas. The main use of fMRI in tumour imaging is the preoperative localisation of eloquent cortical regions which may have been displaced, distorted or compressed by the tumour[18] and identifying any evidence of functional reorganisation. This can improve the safety of surgery and allow for a more radical resection. The BOLD effect is an **indirect** measure of neuronal activity that may be influenced by numerous physiological factors as well as the MR relaxation properties of soft tissue such that activation within a tumour may reflect angiogenesis rather than eloquent function and susceptibility effects from blood products, for instance, may mask areas of brain activation. Other important caveats include the inability of discriminating between indispensable and expandable brain regions and accurate assessment of the distance between a lesion and an area of functional activity. To this effect, other non-BOLD techniques such as arterial spin labelling (ASL) are being developed and may reduce these pitfalls in the futures.

When possible an indicated fMRI should be combined with MR tractrography in order to minimise intraoperative injury to white matter tracts connected to eloquent cortical areas (Fig. 2-2).

Positron-Emission Tomography (PET)

The most widely used PET tracer in oncological imaging is fluorodeoxyglucose [^{18}F] (FDG), which provides a measure of glucose metabolism that correlates closely with the proliferative activity of tumours. Its limitation in neuro-oncoly is the high physiological baseline glucose metabolism of the brain., which may result in a poor lesion to background contrast. New PET radiopharmaceuticals, for brain tumour imaging[20] include amino acid analogues such as [^{11}C]methionine (MET) and [^{18}F]fluoroethyl-L-tyrosine (FET), nucleoside analalogues such as [^{18}F]fluorothymidine (FLT) and hypoxia markers such as [^{18}F]fluoromisonidazole (F-MISO). Radioactively labelled choline, [^{11}C]choline (CHO) or [^{18}F]choline, can be used to assess membrane cell turnover and 68Ga-DOTATOC shows a high uptake in meningiomas.[21]

PET imaging is currently mostly used in combination with computed tomography (PET/CT), but the availability of PET/MRI systems is likely to increase in future, allowing simultaneous acquisition and registration of high-resolution MR sequences and molecular information from PET.

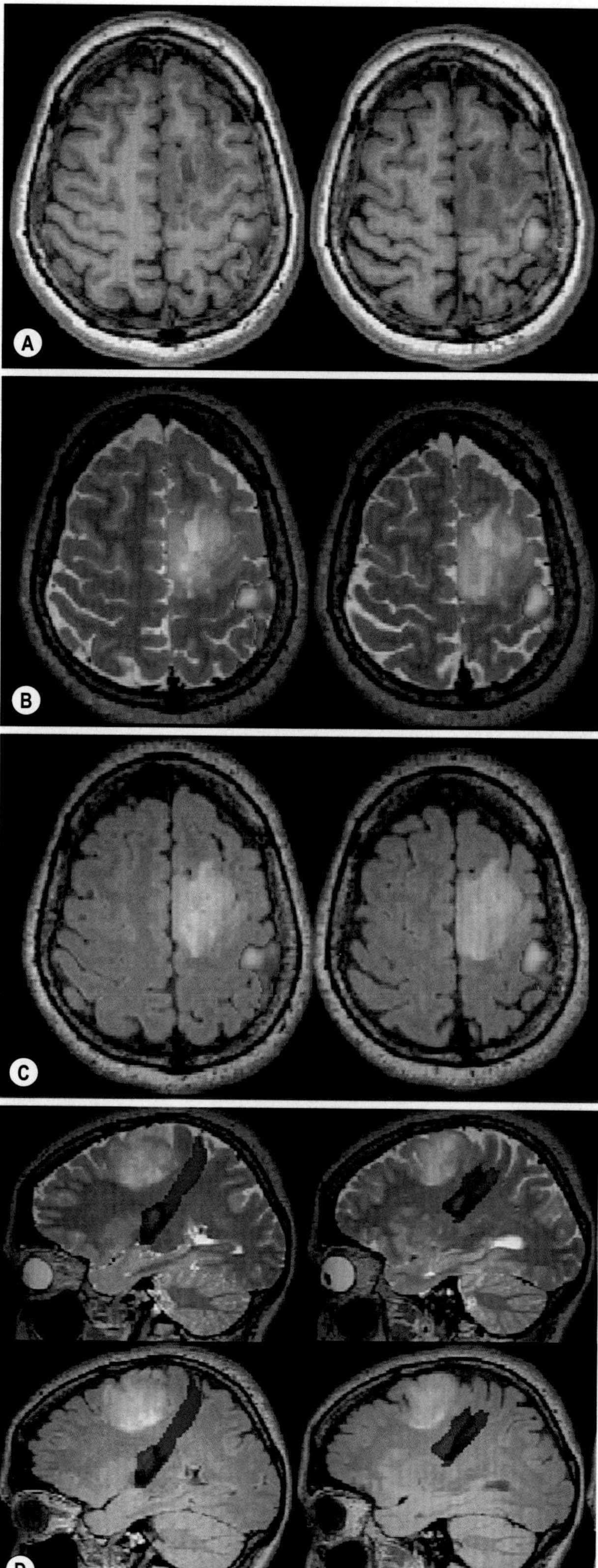

FIGURE 2-2 ■ **fMRI in a patient with a frontal low-grade glioma.** The fMRI of right-hand movement shows activation in the left pre- and post-central gyri, posterolateral to the tumour which appears hypointense on TW1 (A), and hyperintense on T2WI (B) and FLAIR images (C). Sagittal images of DTI (D) show non-invaded corticospinal tracts posterior to the tumour (right hand in red and, right foot in blue).

CLASSIFICATION OF INTRACRANIAL TUMOURS

There are several ways of classifying brain tumours: primary versus secondary intra-axial (arising from the brain parenchyma) versus extra-axial (arising from tissues covering the brian, such as the dura), and various regional classifications (supratentorial, infratentorial, intraventricular, pineal region and sellar region tumours).

The World Health Organisation (WHO) classification of intracranial tumours is a universally accepted histological classification of brain tumours. It was extensively revised in 1993 with the incorporation of immunohistochemistry into diagnostic pathology and updated in 2000, when genetic profiles were added, stratifying neoplasms by their overall biological potential.[22,23] The latest revision is from 2007 with the introduction of eight new entities and three new variants to the previous classification.[24] The WHO classification no longer relies on standard pathological features alone but includes information from immunochemistry and molecular tumour profiling. An outline of this classification is given in Table 2-2.

Intra-axial tumours, which conform largely to the tissue types 1, 4, 5 and 9, will be discussed first, followed by extra-axial tumours corresponding to the tissue types 2, 3, 6, 7 and 8.

TABLE 2-2 **Abbreviated WHO Classification of Brain Tumours**

1	**Tumours of Neuroepithelial Tissue**
1.1	Astrocytic tumours
1.2	Oligodendroglial tumours
1.3	Oligoastrocytic tumours
1.4	Ependymal tumours
1.5	Choroid plexus tumours
1.6	Other neuroepithelial tumours
1.7	Neuronal and mixed neuronal-glial tumours
1.8	Pineal region tumours
1.9	Embryonal tumours
2	**Tumours of Cranial and Paraspinal Nerves**
2.1	Schwannoma
2.2	Neurofibroma
3	**Tumours of the Meninges**
3.1	Meningioma
3.2	Mesenchymal tumours
3.3	Haemangioblastoma
4	**Lymphoma and Haematopoietic Tumours**
5	**Germ Cell Tumours**
5.1	Germinoma
5.2	Teratoma
5.3	Choriocarcinoma
5.4	Other germ cell tumours
6	**Cysts and Tumour-Like Conditions**
6.1	Rathke's cleft cyst
6.2	Epidermoid cyst
6.3	Dermoid cyst
6.4	Colloid cyst
7	**Tumours of the Sellar Region**
7.1	Pituitary adenoma
7.2	Craniopharyngioma
7.3	Others
8	**Local Extension from Regional Tumours**
9	**Metastases**

INTRA-AXIAL TUMOURS

NEUROEPITHELIAL TUMOURS

Neuroepithelial tumours account for 50–60% of all primary brain tumours and represent a broad spectrum of neoplasms arising from or sharing morphological properties of neuroepithelial cells. They include glial neoplasms, choroid plexus tumours, tumours with predominant neuronal phenotype (ganglioglioma, dysembryoplastic neuroepithelial tumour and neurocytoma), pineal tumours and embryonal tumours (neuroectodermal tumours, medulloblastoma).

Gliomas

Gliomas are the commonest neuroepithelial tumours and may originate from astrocytic or oligodendrocytic cell lines. Assessment of the DNA profile and gene expression in tumours plays an increasing role in the characterisation of gliomas and has prognostic implications.[25]

Presently the most relevant molecular and gene abnormalities are isocitrate dehydrogenase (IDH1 or IDH2) mutation, 1p and 19q chromosomal translocation, methylation status of the DNA repair gene 0-6-methylguanine-DNA-methyltransferase (MGMT) and overexpression of the epidermal growth factor receptor (EGFR).

Astrocytic Tumours

Astrocytomas account for approximately 75% of glial neoplasms and range from the benign pilocytic astrocytomas (WHO grade I) to glioblastoma (WHO grade IV), the most malignant astrocytic tumour, and show a distinct age distribution: pilocytic astrocytomas (WHO grade 1) occur mainly in children and young adults; infiltrative low-grade astrocytomas (WHO grade II) are most frequent in the third decade of life; anaplastic astrocytomas (WHO grade III) have a peak incidence around 40 years; and glioblastoma (WHO grade IV) usually occurs after 40 years.

Pilocytic astrocytomas are non-invasive, well-circumscribed, potentially resectable neoplasms which are classified as WHO grade I. They have a low proliferative potential, do not show any IDH mutations and have a predilection for the posterior fossa (Fig. 2-3) and optic nerve/chiasm in children and young adults. Cerebral pilocytic astrocytomas are much less common and usually seen in an older age group (Fig. 2-4). Pilocytic astrocytomas have usually a cystic component and show enhancement, which can be nodular or ring-like. Infratentorial pilocytic astrocytomas in adults are frequently mistaken for haemangioblastomas, which have a similar appearance and represent the commonest primary intra-axial tumour below the tentorium cerebelli in adults, associated in about 20% with von Hippel–Lindau disease. There is evidence that DSC perfusion imaging may help distinguish between the two, as haemangioblastomas have a considerably higher rCBV than pilocytic astrocytomas.[26]

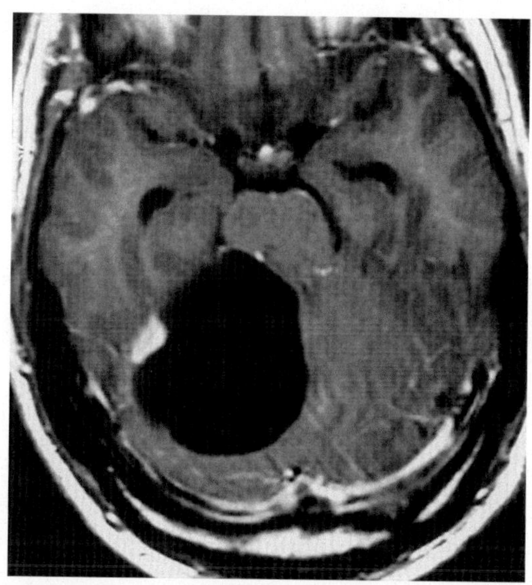

FIGURE 2-3 ■ Cerebellar pilocytic astrocytoma. Axial T1W post-gadolinium MRI. There is a cystic lesion in the cerebellum with a small, enhancing mural nodule but otherwise non-enhancing cyst wall. The fourth ventricle is compressed, causing hydrocephalus (note enlargement of the temporal horns). The differential diagnosis of this lesion is a cerebellar haemangioblastoma.

Diffuse astrocytomas (WHO grade II) are infiltrating low-grade tumours which occur typically in the cerebral hemispheres of young adults, involving cortex and white matter with less well-defined borders than pilocytic astrocytomas. WHO grade II astrocytomas have a low mitotic activity but show a propensity to progress to a higher histological grade, usually within 3–10 years. They frequently show IDH1 and IDH2 mutations, which have a favourable impact on overall survival.[27] WHO grade II astrocytomas appear iso- or hypodense on CT and show areas of calcification in up to 20%. MRI is better in defining the extent of the low-grade gliomas (Fig. 2-5). They are hyperintense on T2 images and FLAIR images and hypo/isointense on T1 images and show no contrast enhancement as opposed to pilocytic (WHO grade I) and anaplastic (WHO grade III) astrocytomas.

Anaplastic astrocytomas (WHO grade III) are high-grade gliomas with an increased mitotic activity and raised immunohistochemical proliferation indices. The majority of anaplastic astrocytomas show contrast enhancement but up to a third may be non-enhancing.[28] Infiltration of the peritumoural tissues is more extensive than in grade II lesions.[29,30]

Pleomorphic xanthoastrocytoma (PXA) is a rare, relatively benign low-grade tumour arising near the surface of the brain, with a predilection for the temporal lobe, and presents usually with epilepsy in children and young adults. The tumour is usually well circumscribed, may enhance strongly and has a cystic component in over 50%. Despite its fat content, it is T1 hypointense and T2 hyperintense on MRI. It can occasionally transform to a more aggressive anaplastic WHO grade III tumour.

Glioblastoma (WHO grade IV) has the worst prognosis but is unfortunately also the commonest primary intracranial neoplasm in adults,[31] showing poorly differentiated, often highly pleomorphic glial tumour cells with florid microvascular proliferation and necrosis. About 90% of glioblastomas arise de novo (primary glioblastoma) and 10% are from malignant transformation of

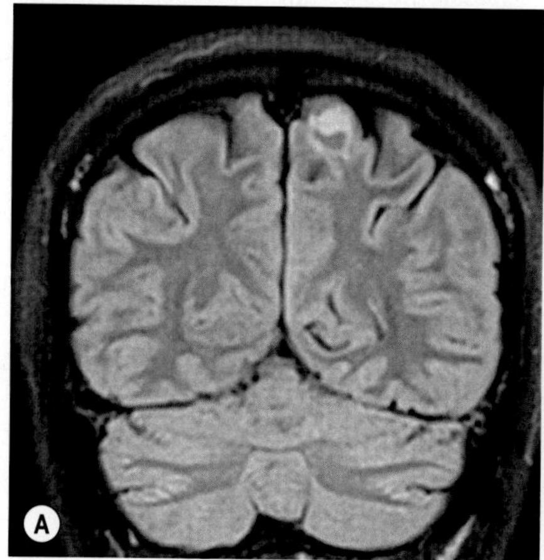

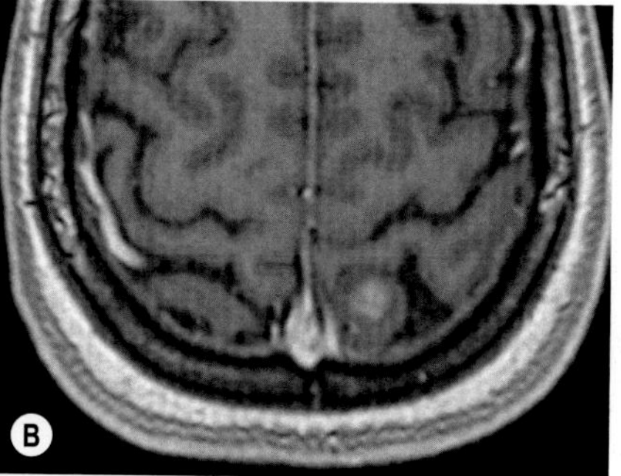

FIGURE 2-4 ■ Cerebral pilocytic astrocytoma in a young adult female patient presenting with epilepsy. FLAIR image (A) shows a well-defined, partially solid (hyperintense) and partially cystic (hypointense) lesion involving the left parietal cortex. The contrast-enhanced T1WI (B) shows uniform enhancement of the solid component.

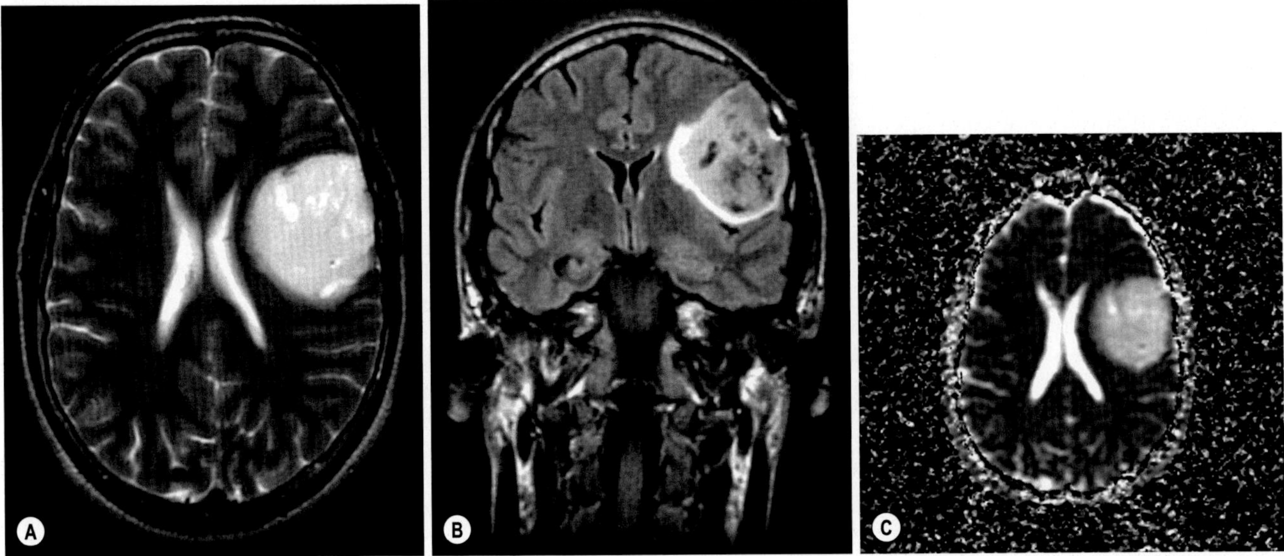

FIGURE 2-5 ■ Low-grade glioma (WHO grade II astrocytoma). Axial T2W (A), FLAIR (B) images showing a left frontal hyperintense mass lesion with well-defined borders and small cystic areas. On the ADC map (C) the glioma is easily identified as an area of increased diffusivity compared to normal brain parenchyma.

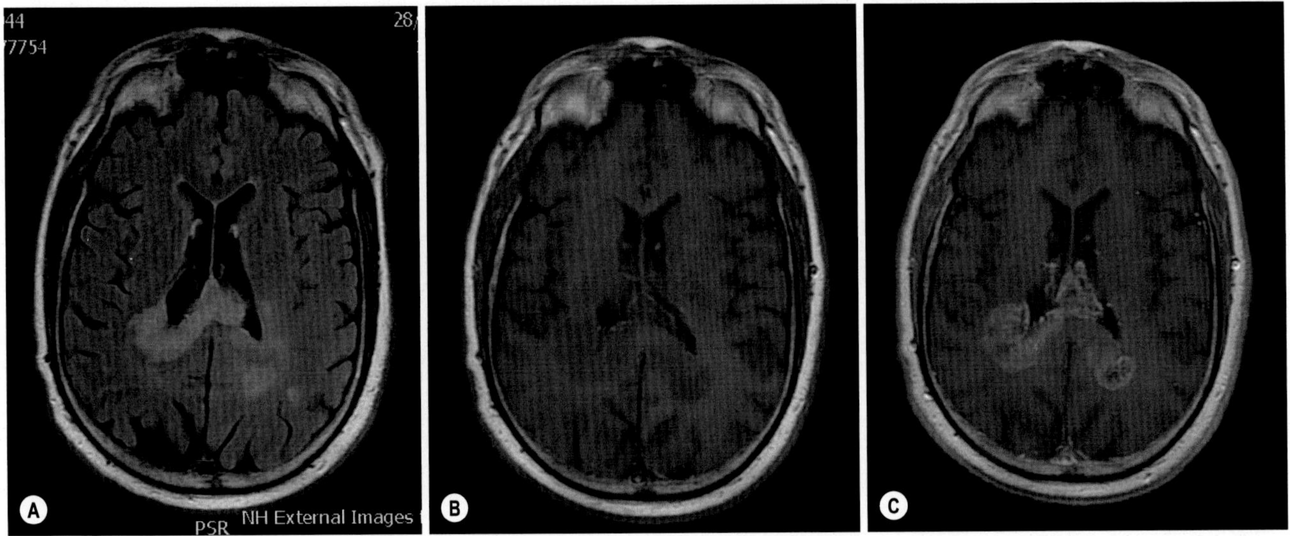

FIGURE 2-6 ■ Glioblastoma. A 55-year-old patient with a 'butterfly' glioblastoma. The tumour appears hyperintense on FLAIR images (A) and infiltrates and thickens the splenium of the corpus callosum and surrounds the trigones of both lateral ventricles. On the pre-contrast T1WI images (B) the glioblastoma appears hypointense and the post-contrast T1WI (C) shows widespread inhomogeneous enhancement of the tumour.

lower-grade astrocytomas (secondary glioblastoma). The two groups have different genetic characteristics: primary glioblastomas, which occurs in a slightly older age group, show EGFR overexpression and secondary glioblastomas show IDH mutations like the lower-grade gliomas from which they arise. Methylation of the DNA repair gene MGMT is associated with a better response to temozolomide and better prognosis in glioblastomas.

The MRI appearances of glioblastomas are heterogeneous, showing a mixture of solid tumour portions, central necrosis and surrounding oedema. The solid portion is usually T1 hypo and T2/FLAIR hyperintense but to a lesser degree than the areas of central necrosis and surrounding oedema, which have signal intensities similar to CSF on T2 images. The oedema is usually infiltrated by strands of tumour cells, which cannot be detected on standard MR images. The solid portion of the glioblastomas may show complete or partial or enhancement with contrast (Fig. 2-6). The extent of enhancement of the solid tumour seems to correspond to different molecular profiles and appears to have an influence on patient survival.[32,33]

The standard treatment for glioblastoma (GBM) consists of surgery (with a variable extent of resection depending on tumour location and the patient's clinical status), followed by a combination of radiotherapy and chemotherapy with temozolomide. Second-line treatment includes anti-angiogenesis drugs and other experimental drugs. The assessment of tumour response and progression in GBM had traditionally been based on measurements of enhancing tumour portions known as Macdonald criteria.[34] With the advent of combined chemoradiation as standard therapy and antiangiogentic drugs as second-line treatment, new phenomena such a pseudoprogression and pseudoresponse have to be taken into account and have made an assessment solely based on assessment of enhancing tumour portion unreliable.[35,36] The Response Assessment in Neuro-Oncology (RANO) Working Group has therefore published recommendations for updated response criteria for high-grade gliomas.[37]

Pseudoprogression is due to an inflammatory reaction, which results in a temporary increase of contrast enhancement and oedema, usually within 12 weeks of chemoradiation, and subsides subsequently without additional treatment (Fig. 2-7). Pseudoprogression is more frequently observed in patients with methylation of the DNA repair gene MGMT, and is associated with a better prognosis (longer overall survival). There are certain histological similarities between the inflammatory response in pseudoprogression and classical radiation necrosis

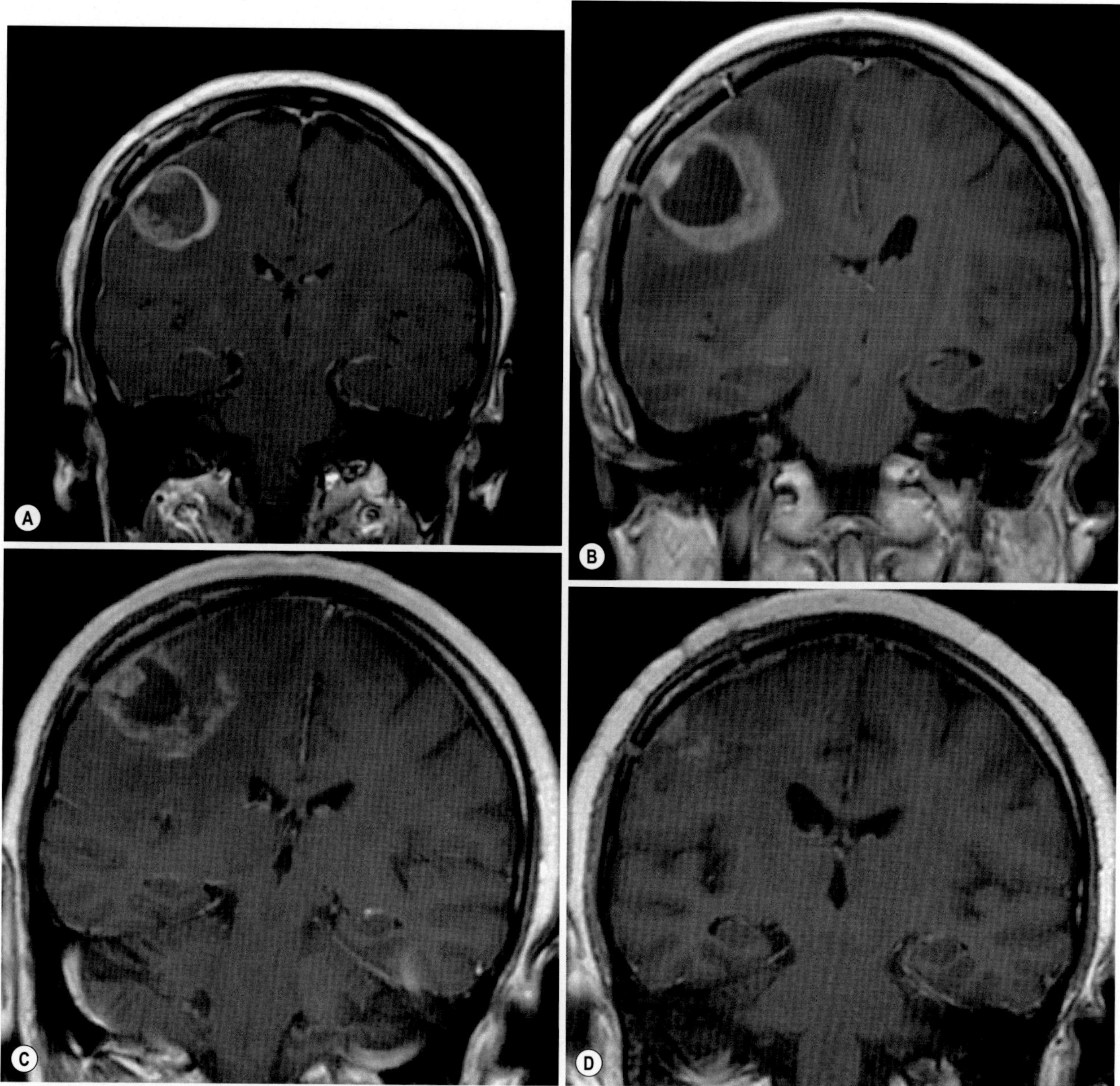

FIGURE 2-7 ■ **Pseudoprogression.** Series of contrast-enhanced T1WI in a patient with glioblastoma before (A) and at 6 weeks (B), 16 weeks (C) and 6 months (D) after treatment with temozolomide and radiotherapy. The baseline images (A) show an irregular ring-enhancing mass lesion. Six weeks following combined chemoradiation (B) there is an increase of enhancement and associated oedema. Both the enhancement and oedema decrease subsequently (C, D) without altering the treatment, leaving a small amount of residual enhancement at the site of the tumour after 6 months (D). The time course of these appearances is typical for 'pseudoprogression', an inflammatory response to chemoradiation associated with a favourable outcome.

which is a delayed complication of radiation treatment occurring 6–12 months after treatment. Advanced MR imaging such as DSC and DCE perfusion imaging shows promise in differentiating theses two conditions from true tumour progression.

Pseudoresponse is characterised by a decrease of enhancement and oedema following the administration of antiangiogenic drugs without improved survival.[37,38] In pseudoresponse the tumour progresses by infiltrative patterns without neoangiogenesis, resulting in an increase of non-enhancing T2/FLAIR hyperintense tumour portions (Fig. 2-8).

Antiangiogenic treatment can also be associated with non-enhancing areas of markedly decreased ADC, which appears to correspond to an atypical gelatinous necrotic tissue rather than tumour and are associated with improved outcome.[39]

Oligodendrogliomas account for 10–15% of all gliomas and occur predominantly in adults. They are diffusely infiltrating neoplasms, which are found almost exclusively in the cerebral hemispheres, most commonly in the frontal lobes, and typically involving subcortical white matter and cortex (Fig. 2-9). The WHO classification distinguishes between WHO grade II (well-differentiated low-grade) and WHO grade III (anaplastic high-grade) oligodendrogliomas. The former are slowly-growing tumours with rounded homogeneous nuclei; the latter have increased tumour cell density, mitotic activity,

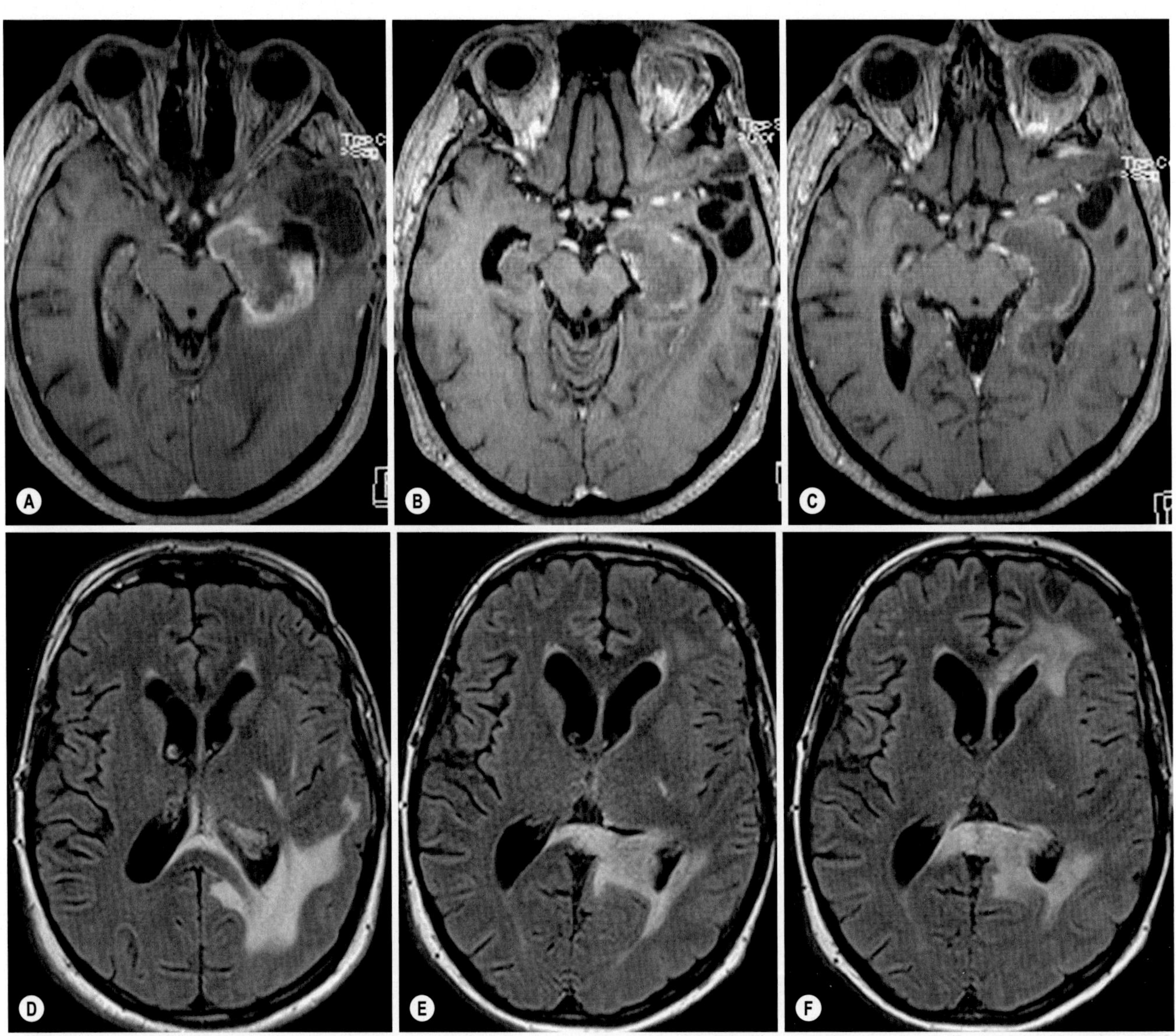

FIGURE 2-8 ■ **Pseudoresponse.** Series of contrast-enhanced T1WI (A–C) and FLAIR images (D–F) in a patient with glioblastoma receiving anti-VGEF therapy as second-line treatment. The baseline images show an enhancing tumour component in the left temporal lobe and a non-enhancing FLAIR hyperintense component in the left peritrigonal region extending into the splenium of the corpus callosum (D). Six weeks after anti-angiogenesis treatment there is marked decrease of enhancement (B) and some resolution of oedema in the left peritrigonal region (E); there is, however, thickening and increased signal intensity of the splenium of the corpus callosum consistent with increasing amount of tumour infiltration. Sixteen weeks post-treatment the enhancement remains minimal (C) but there has been a further increase in the non-enhancing infiltrative tumour in the splenium of the corpus callosum and also around the frontal horn of the left lateral ventricle (F). These appearances are typical for 'pseudoresponse'.

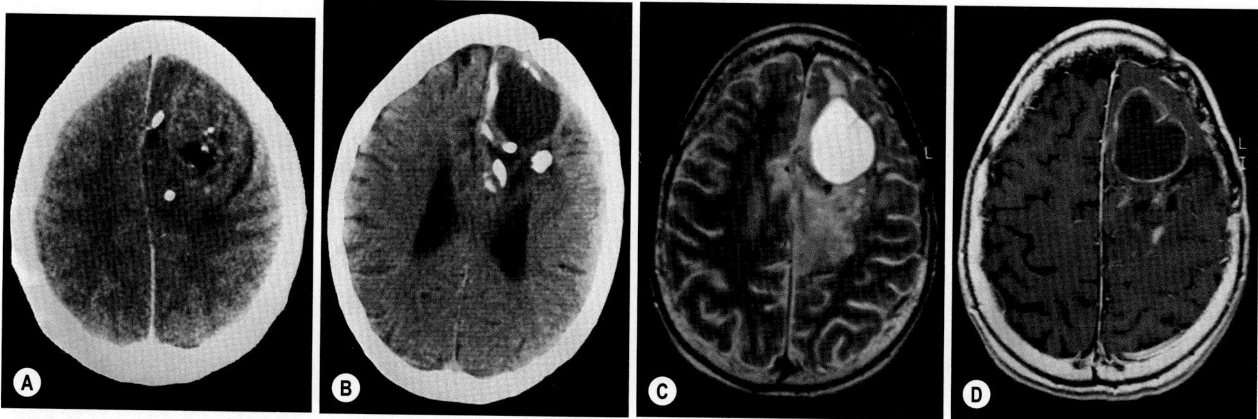

FIGURE 2-9 ■ **WHO grade II oligodendroglioma.** CT after IV contrast medium (A) shows a large left frontal tumour that involves the cortex. It is predominantly solid with irregular enhancement, but there are also cysts and coarse calcification. Follow-up after 2 years with CT (B), T2W MRI (C) and T1W post-contrast MRI (D) shows more extensive cyst formation and calcification than on the first image. The calcification is much less apparent on MRI and appears as non-specific low signal areas. Posterior infiltration of the tumour is, however, best seen on MRI (C). Note that the patient had undergone a left frontal craniotomy after the first CT.

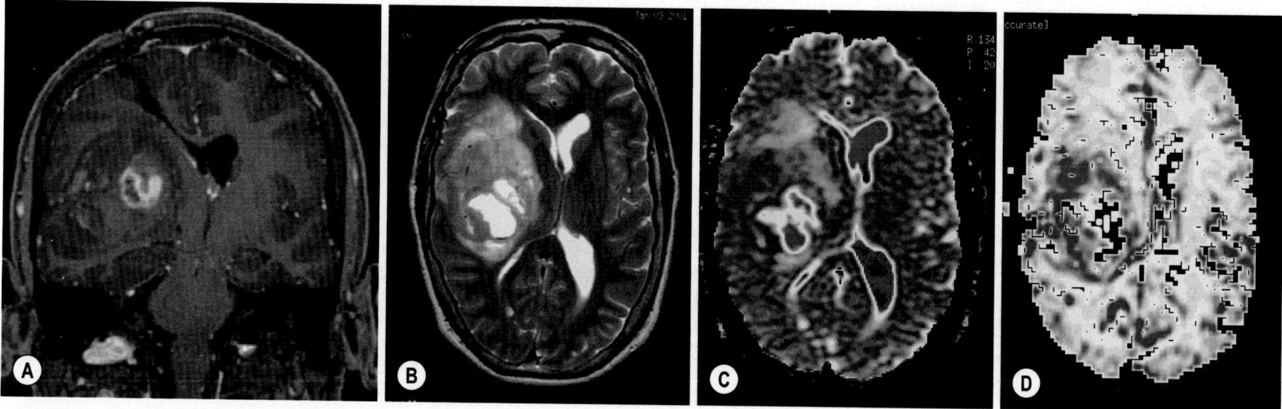

FIGURE 2-10 ■ **Grade III oligodendroglioma.** Post-contrast T1WI (A), T2WI (B), ADC map of diffusion-weighted MRI (C) and rCBV of perfusion-weighted MRI (D) of a WHO grade III oligodendroglioma. There is patchy enhancement within the tumour (A). The T2WI (B) show a central hyperintense cystic area surrounded by more hypointense solid tumour components which have a decreased ADC corresponding to the dark blue areas in (C) and increased rCBV, corresponding to the dark red areas in (D).

microvascular proliferation and necrosis. Both low- and high-grade oligodendral tumours express proangiogenic mitogens and may contain regions of increased vascular density with finely branching capillaries that have a 'chicken wire' appearance. This contributes to their appearance on contrast-enhanced MRI and MRP. Up to 90% of oligodendrogliomas contain visible calcification on CT, which can be central, peripheral or ribbon-like (Fig. 2-9).[40] On MRI, intratumoural calcification appears typically T2 hypo- and T1 hyperintense and causes marked signal loss on T2* or SWI images. Intratumoural haemorrhage, which occurs uncommonly in oligodendrogliomas, may have a similar appearance. Contrast enhancement is variable and often heterogeneous. Unlike in astrocytomas, contrast enhancement is not a reliable indicator of tumour grade it oligodendrogliomas: it occurs in about 20% of WHO grade II tumours and in over 70% of WHO grade III oligodendrogliomas.[41] Low-grade oligodendrogliomas may also have an elevated rCBV on PWI.[42]

Allelic loss on the chromosomes 1p and 19q is present in 80% of oligodendrogliomas and is associated with better response to chemotherapy. Oligodendrogliomas with 1p/19q loss appear to have a significantly higher rCBV than those with intact 1p and 19q[43] (Fig. 2-10). Conventional MR images may provide a further clue to the oligodendroglioma genotype: tumours with intact 1p/19q show more homogeneous signal on T1- and T2-weighted (T1W, T2W) images and have sharper borders than the tumours with chromosome deletions.[44,45]

MRS of low-grade tumours with oligodendral elements shows increased levels of *myo*-inositol/glycine as well as glutamine and glutamate.[17]

The Role of Advanced Physiological MR Imaging in Glial Tumours

The use of PWI, DWI and MRS as an adjunct to structural imaging can improve the prediction of the histological tumour type and grade, tumour infiltration of surrounding tissue, treatment response and patient survival. These techniques are also helpful for differentiating treatment-related complications from tumour progression. Low-grade (WHO grade II) oligodendrogliomas tend to have higher rCBV values and lower ADC values than WHO grade II astrocytomas.[46] This can be explained by increased vascular density and higher cellular density in low-grade oligodendrogliomas and differences in tumour matrix composition.

Several studies have shown the use of PWI to distinguish low-grade from high-grade glial tumours. The formation of new blood vessel (angiogenesis) represents an important aspect of tumour progression and growth in glial tumours, and is reflected in the much higher rCBV values of WHO grade III and IV tumours compared to WHO grade II tumours. PWI significantly increases the sensitivity and positive predictive value of conventional MR imaging in glioma grading with a sensitivity of 95% for distinguishing low-grade from high-grade gliomas when an rCBV threshold of 1.75 is used.[47]

Combining minimum ADC with maximum rCBV measurements further improves the accuracy of glioma grading, particularly the distinction between WHO grade II and III tumours.[48] For oligodendrogliomas ADC values were better than rCBV values in distinguishing between WHO grade II and III tumours.[41]

DWI appears also useful to identify the MGMT promotor methylation status in glioblastomas. Tumours with methylated MGMT, which have a better prognosis, demonstrated a significantly higher minimum ADC.[49]

In MRS, glial tumours are characterised by an increase in Cho and decrease in NAA, which can be expressed in a choline to NAA index (CNI). Low-grade tumours have generally a lower CNI than high-grade tumours; WHO grade IV tumours show additionally an increase in lipid and lactate as markers of hypoxia and necrosis.[19]

Infiltration of peritumoural regions in gliomas can also be assessed with physiology-based MR techniques.[16,19] The peritumoural regions of high-grade gliomas show a more marked decrease in ADC, fractional anisotropy and NAA and increase in CBV compared to low-grade tumours. This is a reflection of the more invasive nature of these tumours, which destroy ultrastructural boundaries with a consequent decrease in ADC and FA; and replace normal brain tissue, resulting in a drop of NAA. Metastases, on the other hand, are surrounded by 'pure' vasogenic oedema, which contains no infiltrating tumour cells. The peritumoural regions in metastases show therefore no increase in rCBV or decrease in FA.

Physiological and molecular MR imaging have also a role in predicting patient survival and treatment response.

Measurements on baseline rCBV in gliomas are strongly predictive of patient outcome[50] and have proved to be a better predictor of time to progression than histological grading.[51] Diffusion tensor imaging can be used to grade the invasiveness of glioblastoma, which correlates with progression-free survival.[52]

Response to radiation and/or chemotherapy may be evident on PWI, DWI and MRS before any significant tumour volume changes occur.[19] Indicators of a good response to therapy are an early decrease of rCBV and an early increase of ADC.[53,54] Treatment with antiangiogenic agents usually results in a rapid decrease of permeability (K^{trans}) and rCBV.

Treatment complications can also be assessed with PWI, DWI and MRS. The role of these methods in distinguishing radiation necrosis from tumour recurrence is well established,[9,55,56] and there is increasing evidence that these techniques are also helpful in the diagnosis of pseudoprogression.[36,57,58]

Radiation necrosis is a late complication of radiotherapy or gamma knife surgery, and can present as an enhancing mass lesion, difficult to distinguish from recurrent tumour on conventional imaging.[56] FDG-PET, PWI and DWI may help to distinguish between radiation necrosis and tumour recurrence (Fig. 2-11).[56,59] In radiation necrosis the enhancing lesion has a low glucose metabolism (FDG uptake) and low rCBV, both of which tend to be high in tumour recurrence. On DCE perfusion imaging, recurrent tumours show a much higher maximum slope of enhancement than radiation necrosis.[9] ADC measurements of the enhancing components in recurrent tumour are significantly lower than in radiation necrosis, mirroring the higher cellular density in recurrent neoplasms.

In addition to the above indications, PWI, DWI and MRS may in future be increasingly used in the context of stereotactic tumour biopsies and help to direct tissue sampling towards areas with maximal angiogenesis, cellular density and metabolic activity.

Tumours of Predominantly Neuronal Cell Origin

These include gangliocytomas, gangliogliomas, dysembryoplastic neuroepithelial tumours (DNET) and central neurocytomas. The latter is discussed later in the chapter in the section 'Intraventricular Tumours'.

Gangliogliomas and Gangliocytomas

These are slow-growing tumours with a low malignant potential, which occur preferentially in young adults and in the temporal lobe presenting with epilepsy. Gangliogliomas contain a mixture of neural and glial elements with neoplastic large ganglion cells; gangliocytomas have only neuronal elements. CT and MRI show peripherally located mixed solid/cystic lesions which commonly calcify. Enhancement can be variable and is often peripheral (Fig. 2-12).

Dysembryoplastic neuroepithelial tumours (DNETs) are highly polymorphic tumours that arise during embryogenesis. They are preferentially located in the supratentorial cortex and frequently manifest through intractable complex partial seizures. DNETs appear variable on imaging but are usually hypodense on CT and T1 hypointense and T2 hyperintense on MRI (Fig. 2-13). Small intratumoural cysts may be present and cause a 'bubbly' appearance. Calcification is seen in about 25% and they enhance in 20–40% of cases. Thinning of the overlying bone is present in approximately half of the cases, reflecting the extremely slow growth of these tumours which allows bone remodelling to occur.[60]

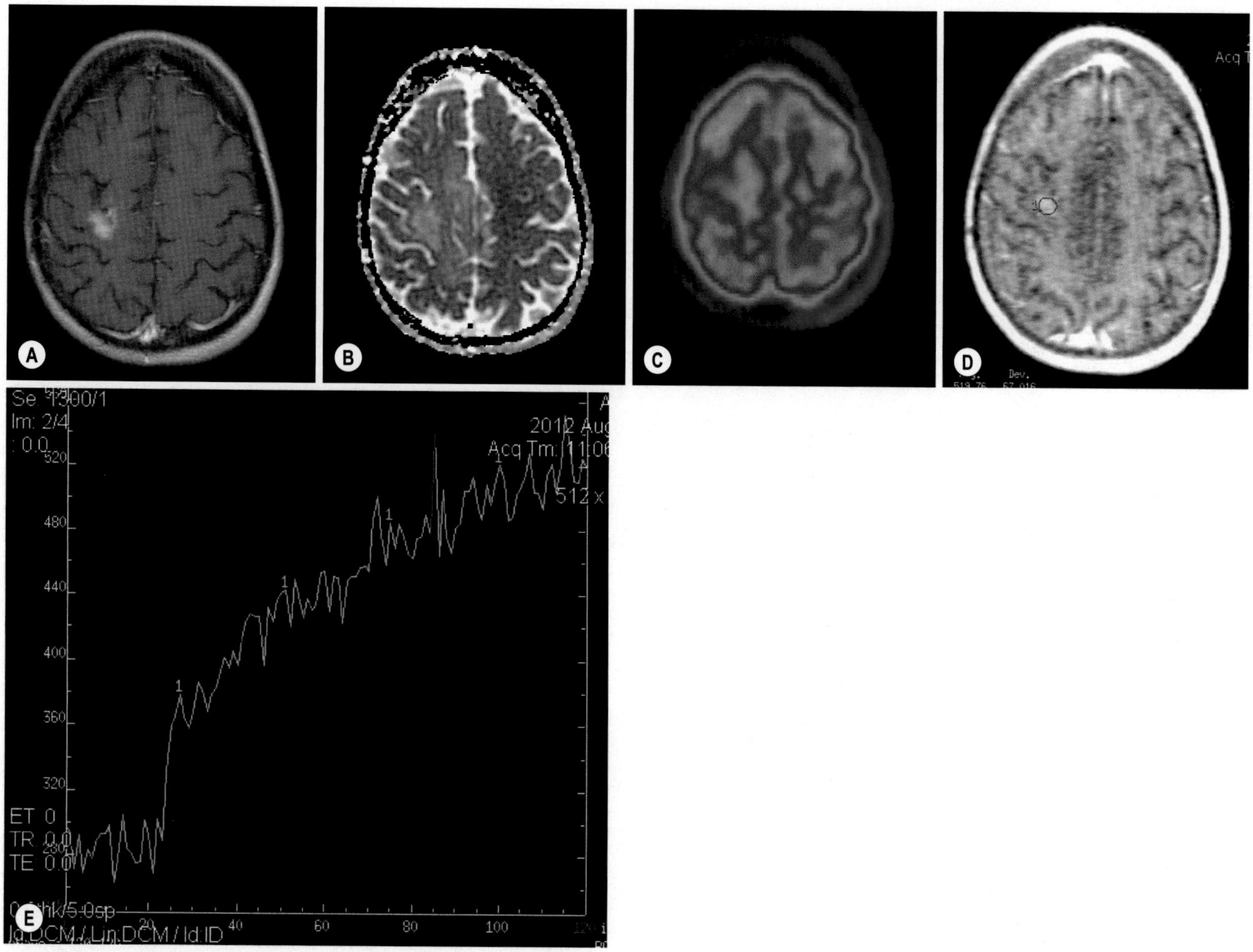

FIGURE 2-11 ■ **Radiation necrosis.** Contrast-enhanced T1WI (A), ADC map (B), FDG-PET (C) and DCE perfusion imaging (D, E) in a patient with radiation necrosis following radiotherapy for a high-grade glioma. On the contrast-enhanced T1WI (A) there is an enhancing area which is indistinguishable from tumour recurrence. The corresponding region shows an increased ADC (B) and decreased glucose metabolism on the FDG-PET (C). A ROI placed over this area on DCE perfusion images (D) demonstrates a slow rise of signal intensity without washout (E). All the findings in (B–E) are typical for radiation necrosis and not for tumour recurrence.

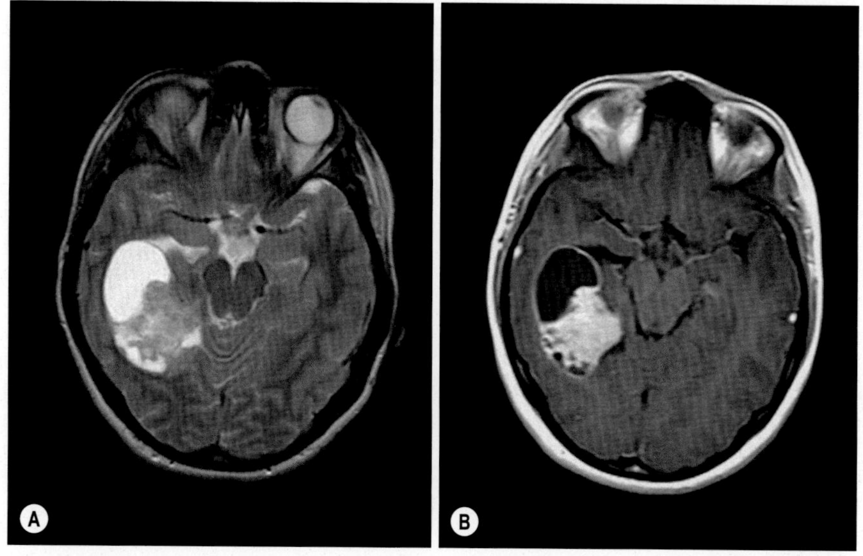

FIGURE 2-12 ■ **Ganglioglioma (WHO grade I).** T2WI (A) and post-contrast T1WI (B) of a WHO grade I ganglioglioma showing a well-defined, non-infiltrating tumour with a cystic component anteriorly and markedly enhancing solid component posteriorly. There is also enhancement of the cyst wall.

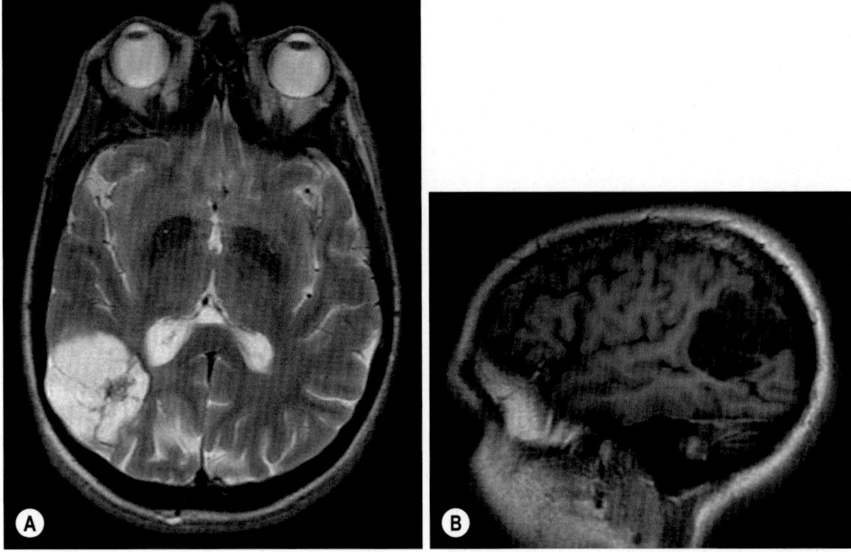

FIGURE 2-13 ■ **Dysembryoplastic neuroepithelial tumour (DNET).** An axial T2WI (A) and a sagittal T1WI (B) showing a T1-hypointesne and T2-hyperintense cortically based tumour with a 'bubbly' appearance. Thinning and remodelling of the overlying bone is also demonstrated.

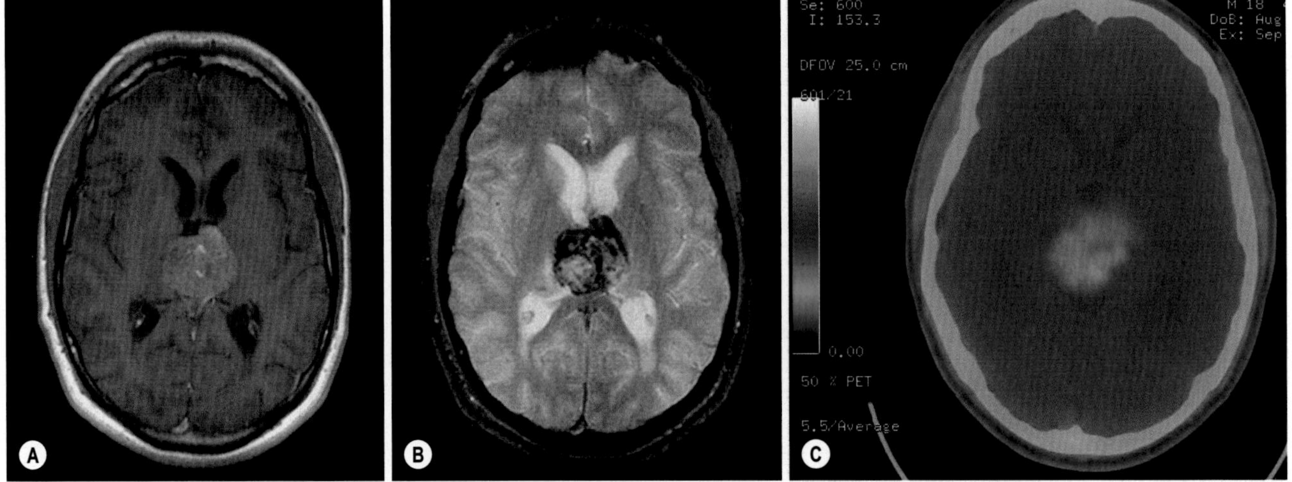

FIGURE 2-14 ■ **Pineal tumour.** Pineal germ cell tumour in an 18-year-old male patient presenting with Parinaud's syndrome. Contrast-enhanced T1WI (A) shows an enhancing pineal region tumour compressing the third ventricle, which contains areas of susceptibility artefact (signal dropout) on T2*WI (B) and avid tracer uptake on a choline PET (C).

Pineal Region Tumours

Pineal region tumours account for approximately 1% of intracranial tumours in adults, whereas they represent 10% of all paediatric brain tumours. They present either with obstructive hydrocephalus secondary to aqueduct compression or with problems with eye movements and accommodation, caused by compression of the underlying tectal plate. More than half of all pineal region tumours are of germ cell origin (germinoma, teratoma, yolk sac tumours and choriocarcinoma).[61] The diagnosis of a germ cell tumour is often made by the presence of marker proteins (such as α-fetoprotein or chorionic gonadotrophin) in the cerebrospinal fluid.

Germinomas account for the majority of pineal region tumours and occur primarily in young men. They are usually rounded, and often iso- or hyperdense on CT and grey matter isointense on standard MRI. They show marked, homogeneous contrast enhancement and virtually never calcify. They tend to displace physiological calcification within the pineal gland. Germinomas may be multifocal (the second commonest site being the hypothalamic region associated with diabetes insipidus which usually occurs only late in suprasellar astrocytomas) or show diffuse subependymal and subarachnoid spread, best appreciated on contrast-enhanced T1 images.[62] They show restricted diffusion on DWI due to dense cellularity with high choline and reduced NAA and MRS.

Teratomas appear more lobulated and inhomogeneous on CT and MRI, reflecting fat content and calcification. The margins of these tumours are often irregular and enhancement is usually inhomogeneous (Fig. 2-14).

The remaining pineal region tumours are mainly of pineal cell (pineoblastomas, pineocytomas) or glial origin (astrocytomas). Pineocytomas are largely histologically benign tumours, usually occurring in young adults, that lack specific imaging features although they tend to enhance and, by contrast with germinomas, contain physiological pineal calcification centrally within the mass. Pineoblastomas occur in children and belong to the group of primitive neuroectodermal tumours (PNETs). They behave like cerebellar medulloblastomas, with frequent seeding via the CSF. They tend to be of low signal intensity on T2 images and can appear bright on DWI. Benign pineal cysts are common and must be differentiated from pineal tumours. They are smooth and well defined and can exhibit rim enhancement. Their signal on T1, proton density-weighted and FLAIR images may be higher than CSF due to their protein content. They do not, however, cause hydrocephalus or a midbrain syndrome.

Embryonal Neuroepithelial Neoplasms

The revised WHO classification (2007) lists the following embryonal neuroepithelial neoplasms: medulloblastomas and its variants, primitive neuroectodermal tumour (PNET) and atypical teratoid/rhabdoid tumour (ATRT). Medulloblastomas are the commonest posterior fossa tumour in children and arise classically from the super medullary velum at the roof of the fourth ventricle (Fig. 2-15). Gene expression profiling has identified for distinct molecular subgroups of medulloblastomas with different clinical outcomes. PNETs are extracerebellar and have a poorer prognosis than medulloblastomas, as have ATRTs, which occur nearly always in children below 5 years of age.

Imaging features of the embryonal neuroepithelial neoplasms reflect their high cellular density and they appear hyperdense on CT, hyperintense on DWI and of intermediate-to-low density on T2 images.

They enhance with IV contrast medium and have a propensity for dissemination in the subarachnoid space with leptomeningeal deposits. Staging of these tumours requires therefore a contrast–enhanced MRI of the entire neuroaxis.[30]

LYMPHOMAS

Lymphoma of the CNS can be primary (PCNSL) or secondary in patients with systemic lymphoma. Secondary CNS lymphoma is more common and occurs usually with non-Hodgkin's lymphomas, Hodgkin's lymphomas having a very low risk of CNS involvement.

Immunocompromised patients have an increased risk of developing PCNSL, but the incidence in the HIV-infected population has markedly decreased since the widespread introduction of antiretroviral therapy. In contradistinction, there has been an increased incidence of PCNSL in the immunocompetent population.

Primary CNS lymphoma (PCNSL) invariably involves the brain parenchyma, whereas secondary CNS lymphoma affects the leptomeninges in two-thirds and the brain parenchyma in one-third of cases.[63]

PCNSL appears as a single (less frequently multiple) lobulated enhancing mass, often abutting an ependymal or meningeal surface Enhancement is usually uniform in immunocompetent patients and irregular or ring-like in immunocompromised patients. The high cellular density and nucleus-to-cytoplasm ratio make PCNSL appear hyperdense on CT (Fig. 2-16) and hypointense on T2 images. The ADC of PCNSL is lower than in gliomas[64] or toxoplasmosis,[65] which is an important differential diagnosis in immunocompromised patients. PCNSL grows in an angiocentric fashion around existing blood vessels without extensive new vessel formation. PCNSL show findings on PWI which differentiates them from high-grade gliomas. They tend to have a much lower rCBV than high-grade gliomas and characteristically show a high percentage signal recovery, overshooting the baseline on the time–signal intensity curves of DSC studies.[66]

A characteristic clinical feature of PCNSL is a rapid resolution of the tumour following administration of steroids and/or radiotherapy

Secondary CNS lymphoma can cause enhancement of the leptomeninges, subependyma, dura, cranial nerves and superficial cerebral lesions.[63] Lymphoma has a high glucose metabolism on FDG-PET, which can be more apparent than contrast enhancement (Fig. 2-17).

METASTASES

The primary neoplasms that most commonly metastasise to the brain are carcinoma of the lung, breast and malignant melanoma. Generally, metastases appear as multiple rounded lesions with a tendency to seed peripherally in the cerebral substance, at the grey/white matter junction. They can, however, occur anywhere in the cerebrum, brainstem or cerebellum, and can also spread to the meninges. Metastases are characterised by oedema in the surrounding white matter which is often disproportionate to the size of the tumour itself. On T2 images, the neoplastic nodule may blend with the surrounding oedema, giving a picture of widespread vasogenic oedema and obscuring the diagnosis. Most metastases enhance strongly with IV contrast medium, either uniformly, or ring-like if the metastasis has outgrown its blood supply. Most metastases from lung and breast are similar in density to normal brain parenchyma on CT, but some types are spontaneously dense, particularly deposits from malignant melanoma.[67]

Haemorrhage occurs in about 10% of metastases, resulting in high signal on T1 images and high or low signal on T2 images. Similar signal characteristics can also occur in non-haemorrhagic metastases from melanoma, due to the paramagnetic properties of melanin (Fig. 2-18). Small metastases and those that are not made

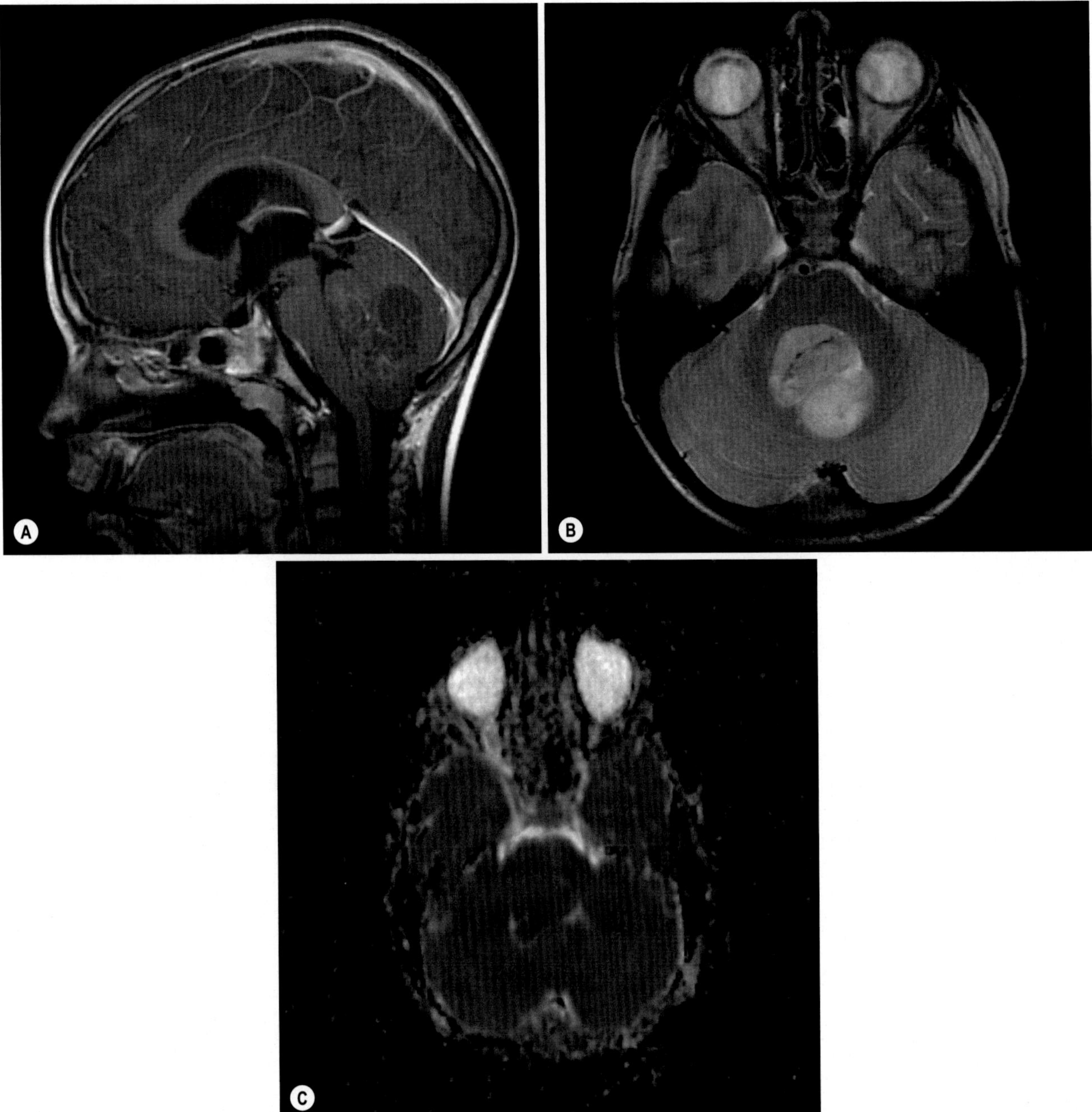

FIGURE 2-15 ■ **Medulloblastoma.** Sagittal gadolinium-enhanced T1W (A), axial T2W images (B) and ADC map (C) demonstrate a heterogeneously enhancing mass posterior to the fourth ventricle, which is obliterated. The increased cellularity of this tumour is reflected by its relative hypointensity on the ADC map. (Courtesy of Dr R. Gunny.)

conspicuous by surrounding oedema are often only detected on contrast-enhanced studies. Increasing the contrast dose or relaxivity of gadolinium compounds can improve the sensitivity for detection of metastases on MRI.[5]

Advanced MR imaging methods can also contribute towards the diagnosis and differential diagnosis of metastases. DWI may help to predict the histology of metastases. Well-differentiated adenocarcinoma metastases are hypointense on trace-weighted DWI, whereas small cell and neuroendocrine metastases are hyperintense, due to their higher cellularity.[68,69] On standard MRI it may occasionally be difficult to distinguish a single metastasis from a glioma. PWI and MRS of the peritumoural rather than intratumoural region were shown to be useful in differentiating the two, as mentioned above.

DWI is helpful to differentiate cystic metastasis from cerebral abscesses (Fig. 2-19).[69] The latter contain more viscous fluid and pus and show a more marked restriction of water diffusion than necrotic tumours. Abscesses appear therefore bright on trace-weighted DWI and dark on ADC maps (Fig. 2-20).

INTRAVENTRICULAR TUMOURS

Approximately a tenth of all primary intra-axial brain tumours involve the ventricular system. The precise anatomical location of the tumour within the ventricles often provides an important clue to the nature of the lesion. Common intraventricular tumours and cysts and their sites of predilection are summarised in Table 2-3. Intraventricular tumours arising from neuroepithelial tissue (ependymomas, central neurocytoma and choroid plexus tumours) are discussed first.

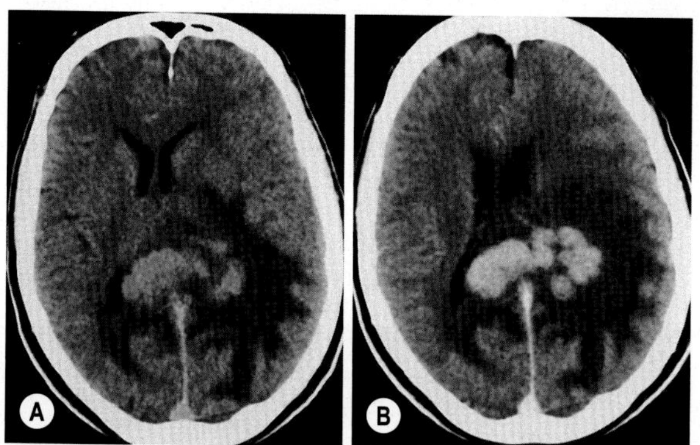

FIGURE 2-16 ■ **Primary cerebral lymphoma.** CT before (A) and after IV contrast medium (B). An irregular mass that is hyperdense to grey matter expands the splenium of the corpus callosum and extends into the left hemisphere. It is surrounded by extensive white matter oedema and enhances avidly with contrast.

Ependymoma

Ependymomas arise from neoplastic transformation of the ependyma and account for about 5% of adult primary brain tumours, being twice as frequent in children. Ependymomas are usually intraventricular, although extraventricular rests of ependymal cells may give rise to hemisphere tumours. Supratentorial tumours occur in young adults and fourth ventricular ependymomas (Fig. 2-21), which frequently extend through the foramina of Magendie and Luschka, and have two age peaks, at 5 and 35 years of age. They are well-demarcated lobulated mass lesions which show calcification on CT in over 50% and are of mixed signal intensity on MRI (predominantly hyperintense on T2 and iso- to hypointense on T1 images). MRI may demonstrate small cysts but calcification is less conspicuous than on CT. Enhancement is mild to moderate and often heterogeneous.

TABLE 2-3 **Intraventricular Lesions**

Tumour	Typical Site
Colloid cyst	Foramen of Monro/third ventricle
Meningioma	Trigone of lateral ventricle
Choroid	Fourth ventricle
Ependymoma	Lateral ventricle (more common in children) and fourth ventricle
Neurocytoma	Lateral ventricles (involving septum pellucidum)
Metastases	Lateral ventricles, ependyma and choroid plexus

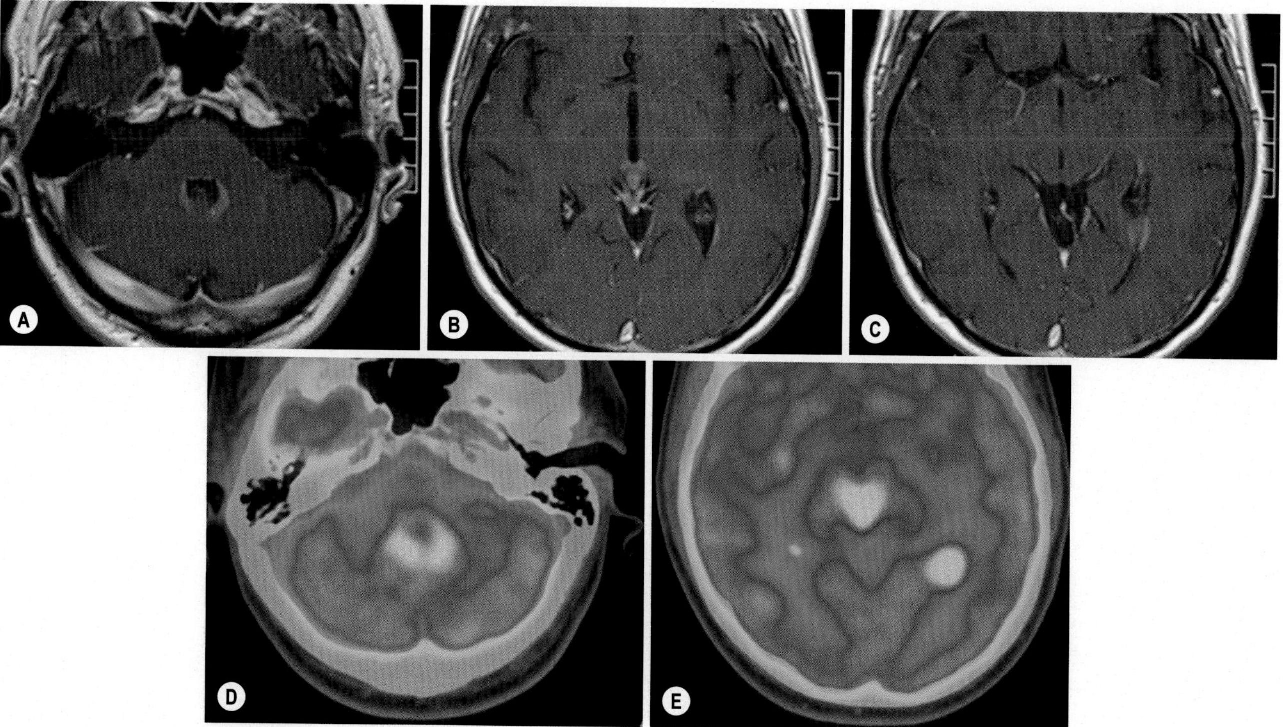

FIGURE 2-17 ■ **Secondary cerebral lymphoma.** Contrast-enhanced T1WI (A–C) and FDG-PET/CT (D, E) in a patient with secondary CNS (B-cell) lymphoma showing focal thickening and enhancement of the ependyma lining the fourth ventricle (A), the third ventricle posteriorly and left occipital horn (B) and atrium of the left lateral ventricle (C). These lesions are more conspicuous on the FDG-PET which show avid tracer uptake (D, E).

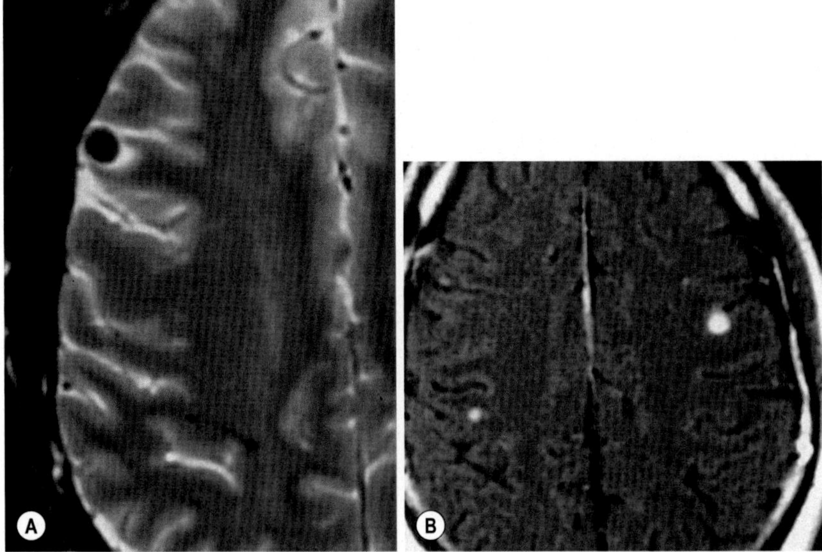

FIGURE 2-18 ■ Metastases. (A) Melanoma (MRI): axial T2W (2000/80). There are at least three foci of signal hypointensity in the right hemisphere, the largest in the right posterior frontal cortex and the others deeper in the subcortical parietal region. This T2 shortening is attributable to melanin. (B) Axial post-contrast T1W with magnetisation transfer (650/16). At a slightly different level, this post-contrast study discloses at least four rounded hyperintense metastatic deposits, all in the cortex or subcortical regions.

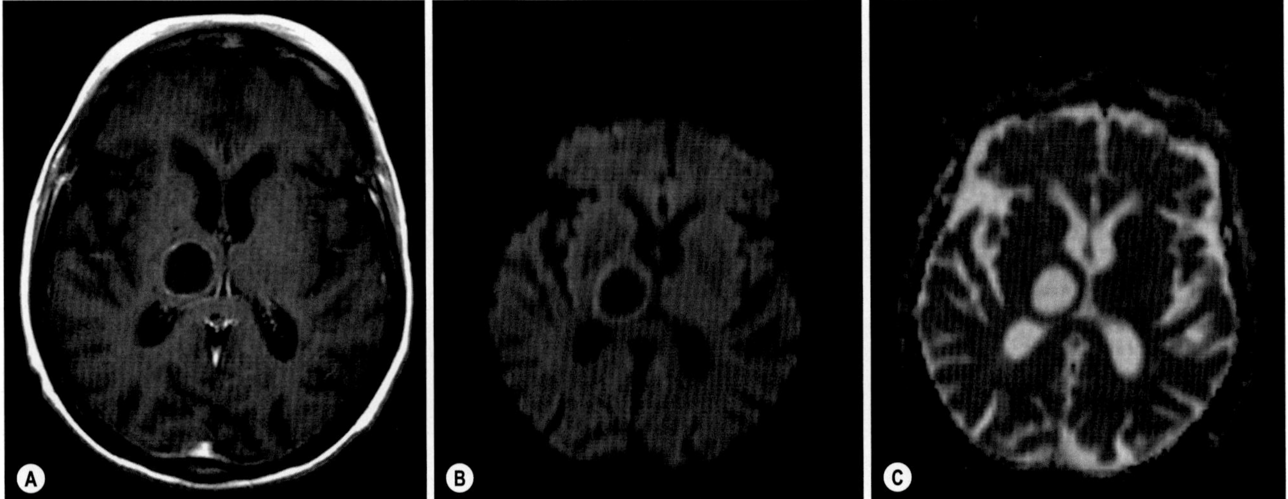

FIGURE 2-19 ■ Cystic metastasis from CA breast. Axial T1W post-contrast image (A) demonstrates a peripherally enhancing, centrally necrotic lesion in the right thalamus. The lesion appears dark on the trace-weighted DW image (B) and bright on the ADC map (C), which is consistent with a relatively unrestricted diffusion in the centre of the mass.

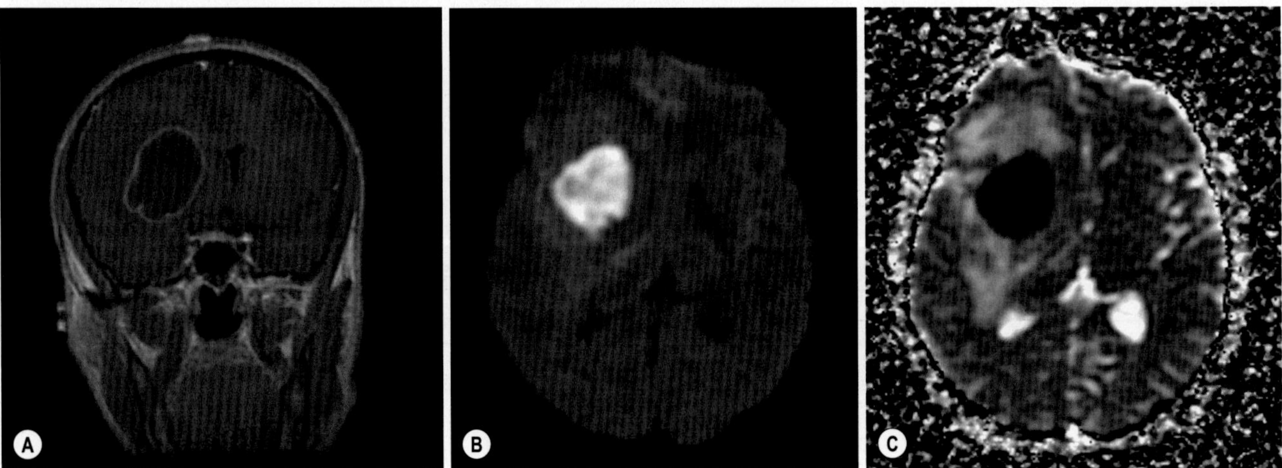

FIGURE 2-20 ■ Brain abscess.

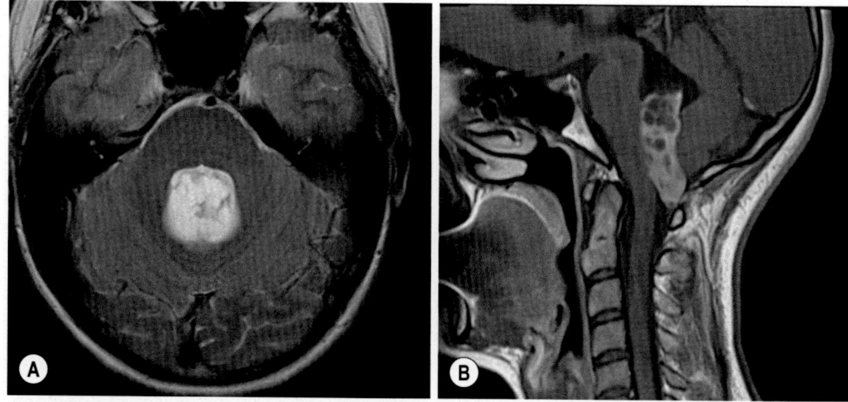

FIGURE 2-21 ■ Ependymoma of the fourth ventricle. (A) The axial T2WI demonstrates a relatively well-circumscribed hyperintense partially solid and cystic mass expanding the fourth ventricle. (B) Sagittal post-contrast T1WI shows a heterogeneously enhancing mass expanding the inferior part of the fourth ventricle and extending through the foramen of Magendie. There is dilatation of the ventricular system in keeping with obstructive hydrocephalus.

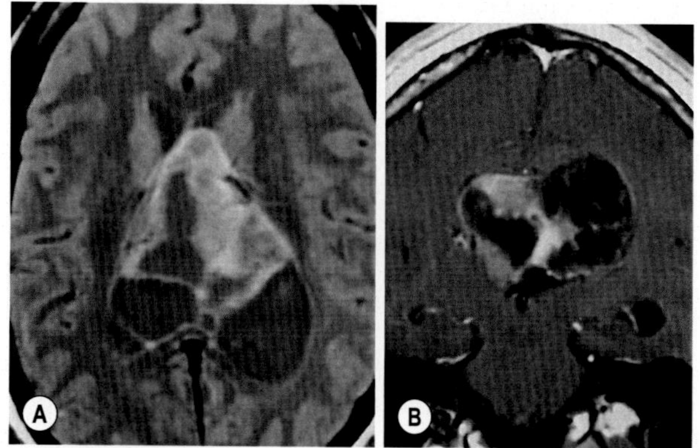

FIGURE 2-22 ■ Central neurocytoma. Axial proton density (A) and coronal T1W post-gadolinium (B) MRI. A partly cystic, multi-septated, enhancing mass, which is related to the septum pellucidum, fills the bodies of both lateral ventricles and causes hydrocephalus with dilatation of the left temporal horn.

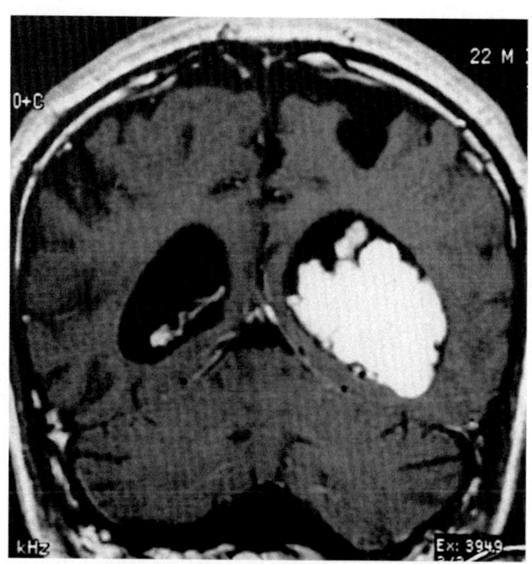

FIGURE 2-23 ■ Choroid plexus papilloma. Coronal T1W post-gadolinium MRI. There is a lobulated, strongly enhancing tumour in the trigone of the left lateral ventricle. Both lateral ventricles are dilated due to hydrocephalus associated with this tumour.

Central Neurocytoma

Central neurocytomas are slow-growing intraventricular tumours of purely neuronal origin.[70] They may rarely arise outside the ventricular system. Before the advent of immunohistological methods they were frequently misdiagnosed as subependymal oligodendrogliomas. These relatively benign tumours occur predominantly in the second and third decades of life, and represent probably the commonest lateral ventricular masses in this age group. They typically arise from the septum pellucidum and occupy the frontal horns and bodies of the lateral ventricles, and sometimes extend through the foramen of Monro. CT frequently shows calcification and small cysts. MRI shows a heterogeneously enhancing mixed-signal intensity mass containing septated cysts, susceptibility artefact from calcification and grey-matter-isointense nodules (Fig. 2-22). Obstructive hydrocephalus is common.

Choroid Plexus Tumours

Choroid plexus papillomas are WHO grade I tumours and much more common than the more aggressive atypical choroid papillomas (WHO grade II), which show a higher mitotic count, or choroid plexus carcinomas (WHO grade III). The location and incidence of choroid plexus papillomas vary with age. They are relatively more common in childhood (3% of primary brain tumours), presenting as a 'cauliflower-like' mass in the trigone of the lateral ventricle (Fig. 2-23). In adults, papillomas are less common, and occur predominantly in the fourth ventricle. CT shows an iso- to hyperdense mass with punctate calcification and homogeneous enhancement. On MRI the papillomas appear as lobulated, intraventricular masses of heterogeneous, predominantly intermediate signal intensity on both T1 and T2 images, with intense contrast enhancement. Angiography, which is rarely indicated, shows a highly vascular mass supplied predominantly by the anterior and posterior choroidal arteries. Choroid plexus

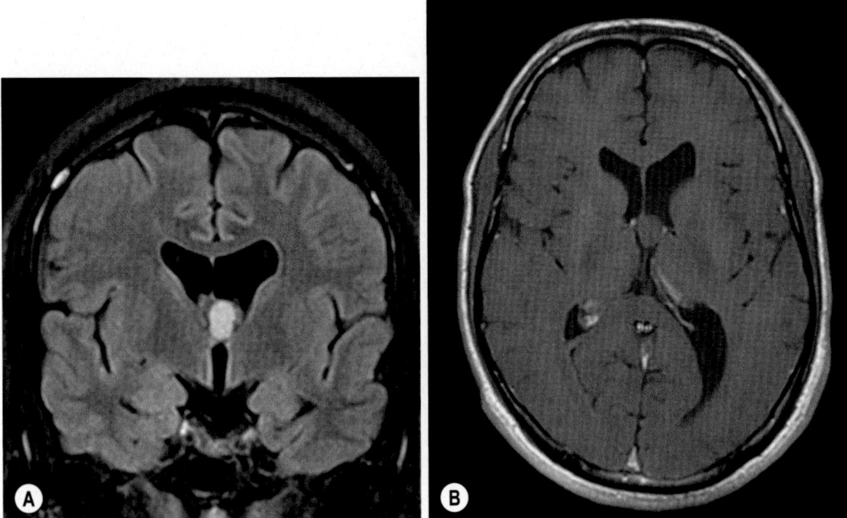

FIGURE 2-24 ■ **Colloid cyst.** FLAIR image (A) shows a well-circumscribed mass at the foramen on Monro, which is homogeneously hyperintense due to proteinaceous cyst content. It does not enhance and appears isointense on post-contrast T1WI (B). There is mild dilation of the left lateral ventricle.

carcinomas are rare, highly malignant tumours that invade the adjacent brain parenchyma to a greater degree than papillomas.

Colloid Cyst

This occurs exclusively at the paraphysis, which lies in the posterior lip of the foramen of Monro, between the third and lateral ventricles. They tend to cause hydrocephalus, by intermittently or continuously obstructing the outflow of cerebrospinal fluid from the lateral ventricles and are smooth, spherical lesions, which are characteristically hyperdense on unenhanced CT imaging. Their MR appearance varies depending on the cyst content (calcium, cholesterol, haemosiderin); some can have similar a signal to CSF, but most are of high signal on T2 and T1 FLAIR images (Fig. 2-24).

Meningioma

This is the commonest cause of a mass in the trigone of the lateral ventricle after the first decade of life. The CT and MRI appearances are similar to those of extraventricular meningiomas (see below): a well-defined, globular lesion which is usually hyperdense on CT and may give similar signal to cerebral cortex on T1 and T2 images. They usually show marked contrast enhancement on CT and MRI.

EXTRA-AXIAL TUMOURS

Primary extra-axial neoplasms arise from the meningothelial arachnoidal cells (meningiomas), mesenchymal pericytes (haemangiopericytoma) or cranial nerves (schwannomas, neurofibromas) and include developmental cysts or tumour-like lesions (epidermoid and dermoid cysts). Metastatic involvement of the meninges and tumours in specific regions (around the sella turcica and skull base) are discussed separately. Overall, meningiomas represent the commonest non-glial intracranial neoplasm, accounting for approximately 20% of all primary intracranial tumours. Multiple meningiomas and cranial nerve tumours are found in neurofibromatosis type 2. Extra-axial lesions occur much more frequently in adults than in children and account for the majority of primary infratentorial tumours in adults, with three lesions sharing a predilection for the cerebellopontine region: vestibular schwannoma, meningioma and epidermoid cysts.

When analysing an extra-axial lesion, it is important to pay attention to associated bone changes: meningiomas tend to induce a hyperostotic bone reaction, whereas epidermoid cysts and schwannomas tend to cause bone thinning resulting in enlargement of, for example, the middle cranial fossa or internal auditory meatus. Other features distinguishing extra- from intra-axial mass lesions are 'buckling' and medial displacement of the grey–white matter interface, a CSF cleft separating the base of the mass from adjacent brain, and a broad base along a dural or calvarial surface.[71]

MENINGIOMAS

Meningiomas originate from arachnoid cell rests, related to arachnoid granulations of the dura mater, and may assume a spherical, well-circumscribed shape or be flat, infiltrating ('en plaque') lesions.[72]

There are several histological types of meningioma, including meningothelial, fibrous/fibroblastic, transitional and psammomatous tumours. The WHO

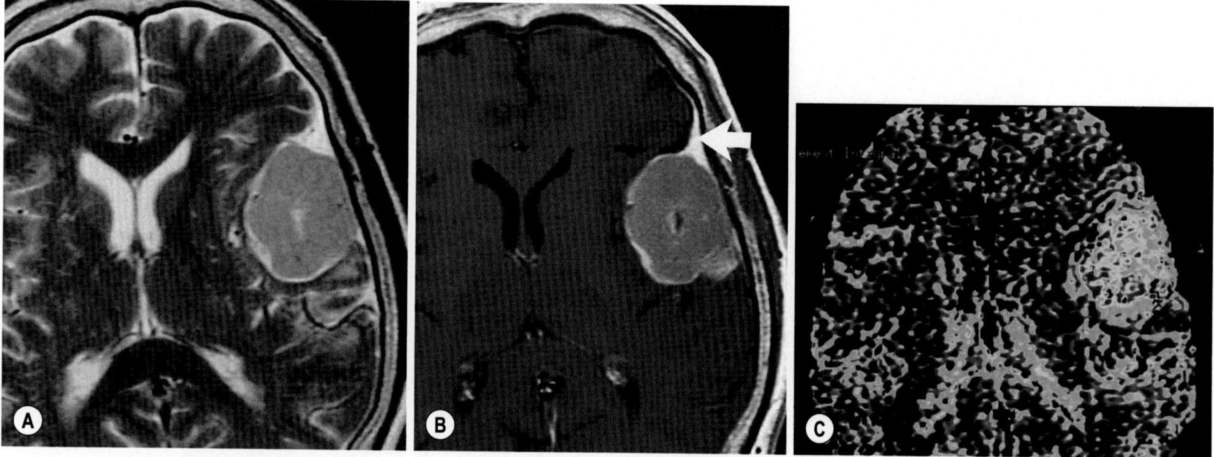

FIGURE 2-25 ■ Meningioma with perfusion-weighted imaging. Axial T2W (A), gadolinium-enhanced T1W (B) and perfusion-weighted (C) MRI. A grey matter isointense mass deeply indents the left cerebral convexity (A). Its broad dural base, the surrounding displaced cerebral sulci and the small pial vessel between the tumour and the brain surface (arrowhead) are all features of an extra-axial lesion. The tumour enhances and there is a 'dural tail' (arrow) (B), which is a frequent radiological finding in meningioma, but is not pathognomonic (see Fig. 2-30). Perfusion-weighted MRI (C): a colour map of the relative cerebral blood volume (rCBV) shows increased blood volume of the tumour compared with normal cortex and white matter, confirming its highly vascular nature.

classification for brain tumours distinguishes three types of meningiomas.[24]

The majority of meningiomas are typical (WHO grade I) meningiomas and have a good prognosis, with a low recurrence rate following surgical resection. Diagnosis of a grade II (atypical) meningioma is based on evidence of a high mitotic index, various patterns of disordered growth or brain invasion (although this is not formally a pathological criterion, it corresponds prognostically to WHO grade II). Grade III (anaplastic) meningiomas demonstrate excessive mitotic activity and have a sarcoma-, carcinoma- or melanoma-like appearance under light microscopy.[73]

Of meningiomas, 90% are supratentorial, arising, in decreasing order of frequency, from the parasagittal region, cerebral convexities, sphenoid ridge and olfactory groove. Infratentorial meningiomas are most frequently located on the posterior surface of the petrous bones and clivus and can mimic vestibular schwannomas. Bone sclerosis is in favour of meningioma and enlargement of the internal auditory meatus is much more common in schwannomas.

Many meningiomas are incidentally discovered on CT or MRI performed for other indications. CT is well suited to demonstrate effects on adjacent bone such as hyperostosis associated with benign meningiomas or bone destruction associated with atypical meningiomas. Sixty per cent of meningiomas are spontaneously hyperdense and up to 20% contain calcification[74] and enhancement is usually intense and uniform.

On MRI, meningiomas appear frequently isointense to cerebral cortex on both T1 and T2 images and may be difficult to detect without IV contrast medium. Meningiomas can have 'capping cysts' of similar MRI signal intensity to CSF. As on CT, meningiomas enhance vividly and homogeneously, except for the uncommon cystic and very densely calcified tumours, which may produce foci of low signal within the mass. There may also be a linear, contrast-enhancing 'dural tail' extending from the tumour along the dura mater. The 'dural tail' sign, once thought to be pathognomonic for meningioma (Fig. 2-25), can also be seen with other tumours such as schwannoma or metastasis.

Vasogenic oedema is not infrequently associated with meningiomas. The extent of the vasogenic oedema does not correlate with the size of the meningioma and, as with metastases, even small lesions can cause quite extensive oedema. The presence of intra-axial oedema, however, is thought to correspond to an increased likelihood of recurrence.[75]

Meningiomas abutting the superior sagittal or transverse sinuses can compress or invade these venous structures. The distinction between compression and occlusion is important for preoperative planning, and can be made by MRA or CTA.

Physiological MR imaging methods may also of help in the diagnosis and prognostication of meningiomas using non-invasive methods.

MRS may show an alanine peak, which is characteristic for a meningioma but is seen in less than 50% of cases. However, no MRS data have been clinically correlated to patient outcomes.[76]

DWI has been used to investigate the differences between typical and atypical meningiomas with conflicting results. A decrease in ADC values of benign meningiomas at follow-up was thought to raise suspicion of transformation to a higher grade[77] following initial reports of significantly lower ADC values in non-typical meningiomas.[78] However, a more recent study did not show any significant correlation between ADC values and meningioma histology.[79]

Meningiomas have usually a markedly elevated rCBV on PWI, which can be used to differentiate them from dural metastases, which tend to have a lower rCBV.

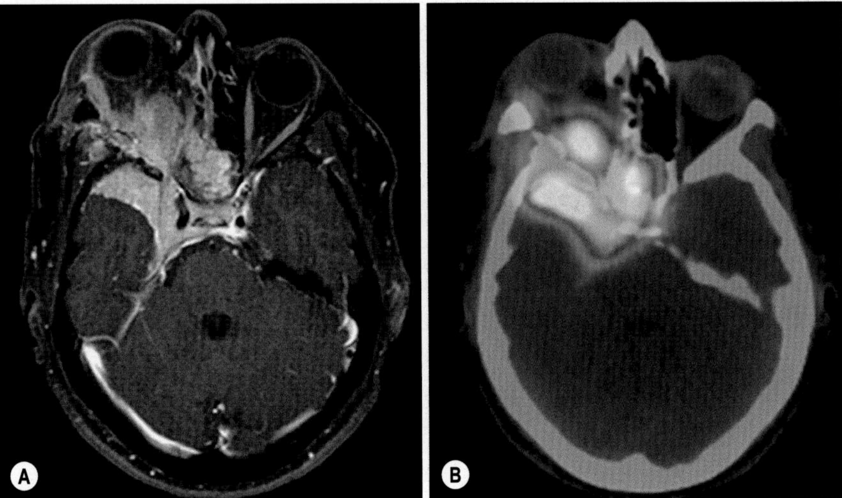

FIGURE 2-26 ■ **Meningioma.** Post-contrast T1W1 (A) demonstrates an avidly enhancing extra-axial mass centred on the right planum sphenoidale and extending to the petrous apex, cavernous sinus, orbital apex and also involving the right optic nerve sheath and intraconal structures, as well as the sphenoid and ethmoid sinuses. On PET imaging (B) there is avid ^{68}Ga-DOTATOC uptake, which is a somatostatin analogue, due to the high density of somatostatin receptors in meningiomas.

Furthermore, the CBV of peritumoural odema has been found to be higher when surrounding malignant meningiomas[80] (Fig 2-25).

On PET imaging meningiomas show a high uptake of ^{68}Ga-DOTATOC (Fig. 2-26), which can be useful for differentiating meningiomas from other similarly looking tumours and to distinguish residual/recurrent tumour from postoperative enhancement or to improve radiotherapy planning in skull base meningiomas.[21]

Angiography is now mostly performed in the context of preoperative embolisation to minimise intraoperative blood loss. The cardinal angiographic findings are supplied from meningeal vessels and a dense, homogeneous, persistent blush. Parasitisation of cortical vessels by tumours over the cerebral convexity or of branches of the ophthalmic artery by subfrontal masses is not rare.

With preoperative embolisation now being frequently performed, it is important to be aware of the post-embolisation MRI appearances of meningiomas which typically include a decrease in enhancement and reduced perfusion of the devascularised segment of the meningiomas.[81]

Haemangiopericytomas enter into the differential diagnosis for meningiomas. Features suggestive of a haemangiopericytoma rather than meningioma are a lobulated (rather than spherical) dural-based mass, absence of calcification and hyperostosis and multiple areas of flow void on MRI, reflecting the high vascularity of these tumours.[82]

CRANIAL NERVE SHEATH TUMOURS

Cranial nerve sheath tumours, originating from cranial nerves, account for 6–8% of primary intracranial tumours. Most are benign neoplasms arising from Schwann cells ('schwannomas') of the nerve sheaths. Schwannomas arise eccentrically from the sheath and compress the parent nerve rather than invading it. All cranial nerves except I (olfactory) and II (optic), which are white matter tracts of the cerebrum, have nerve sheaths, but schwannomas usually grow on the sensory nerves, most frequently from the superior vestibular division of the vestibulocochlear nerve (often inaccurately called 'acoustic neuroma') and, with decreasing frequency, from the trigeminal, glossopharyngeal and lower cranial nerves. Pure motor cranial nerves rarely form schwannomas. Multiple cranial nerve schwannomas are found in neurofibromatosis type 2 and bilateral vestibular schwannomas are pathognomonic of this condition. Neurofibromas are benign tumours, composed of fibroblasts, reticulin and a mucoid matrix in addition to Schwann cells. Cranial nerve tumours are T1 iso/hypointense and T2 hyperintense, and larger lesions often contain areas of cystic degeneration. Cranial nerve tumours almost invariably show marked enhancement with IV contrast, which is solid in two-thirds and ring-like or heterogeneous in one-third of cases.

Vestibular schwannomas account for over 80% of cerebellopontine lesions. They smoothly erode the posterior edge of the porus acusticus, widening the internal auditory meatus (IAM) and often present as an oval component within the cerebellopontine angle cistern, giving rise to the 'ice-cream cone' appearance.[83] CT has been largely replaced by MRI for imaging tumours of the cerebellopontine angle with a sensitivity approaching 100% and a very high specificity.[84] Thin-section T2 imaging with sequences such as CISS/DRIVE/C-FIESTA resolve the 7th and 8th nerves in detail (Fig. 2-27). Tumours as small as 4 mm causing focal nerve thickening can be detected, and MRI is often used for screening patients with asymmetrical sensorineural hearing loss.[85] If the findings are equivocal, gadolinium-enhanced images refute or confirm the suspicion of a tumour.

T2* W or SWI images demonstrate microhaemorrhages in most vestibular schwannomas, which is a useful differentiating feature from meningiomas.[86]

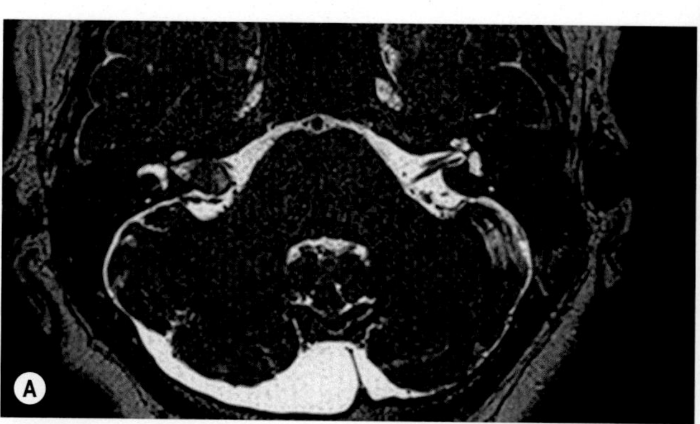
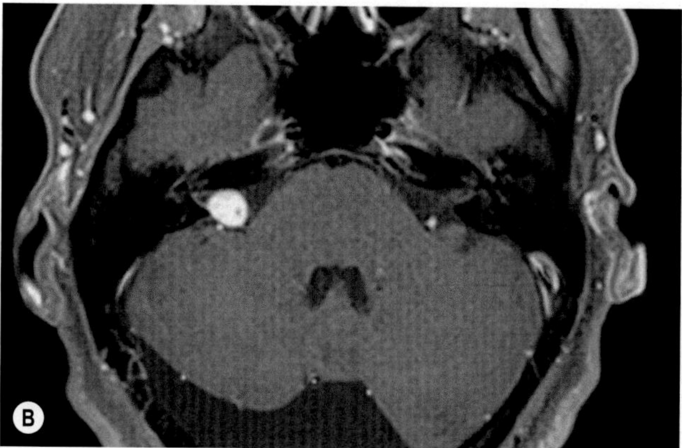

FIGURE 2-27 ■ Vestibular schwannoma. (A) Thin-section T2W CISS imaging shows a vestibular schwannoma with a small cystic component medially, expanding the right internal auditory meatus. (B) Post-contrast T1WI demonstrates marked enhancement of the tumour.

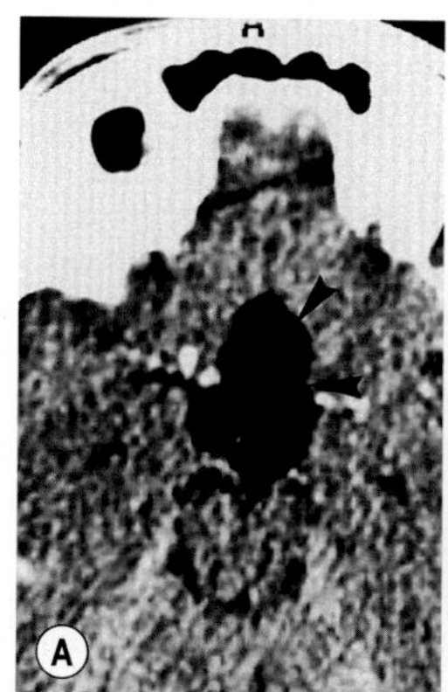
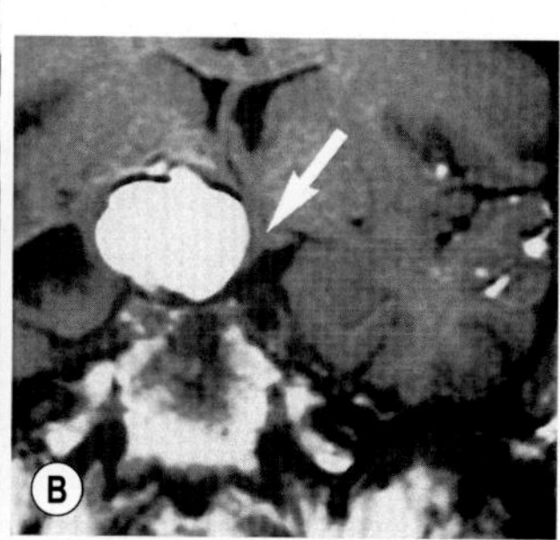

FIGURE 2-28 ■ Suprasellar dermoid tumours. CT (A). There is a midline, fat density tumour (arrowheads) occupying the suprasellar region. (B) Coronal T1W MRI of a different patient with a ruptured dermoid tumour. There is a lobulated high signal mass in the chiasmatic cistern, compressing and displacing the optic chiasm to the left (arrow). Fat globules, which have spilled into the subarachnoid space, are seen as high signal foci in the left Sylvian fissure. The patient has had previous surgery via a right temporal approach, causing right temporal atrophy and enlargement of the right temporal horn.

Vestibular schwannomas appear usually isointense to normal brain parenchyma on DWI, and have raised ADC values. Meningiomas can have similar appearances on DWI[87] but PWI demonstrates significantly lower rCBV measurements in vestibular schwannomas than in meningiomas.[88]

EPIDERMOID AND DERMOID TUMOURS

Epidermoid and dermoid cysts, or 'pearly tumours',[89] result from inclusion of ectodermal epithelial tissue or cutaneous ectoderm, respectively, during the closure of the neural tube.

Intracranial dermoids account for 0.04 to 0.6% of all intracranial tumours and are usually located along the midline. Dermoids contain all skin elements, including fat, and appear therefore of very low density on CT and of high signal intensity on T1 images (Fig. 2-28). They may rupture and release their contents into the subarachnoid space, which is demonstrated as fatty globules within the basal cisterns or ventricles. Dermoid cysts often remain asymptomatic, but can present with aseptic meningitis in the event of rupture.[90]

Epidermoid cysts represent approximately 0.2 to 1.8% of all intracranial tumours and can be central (chiasmatic and quadrigeminal plate cisterns) or eccentric (cerebellopontine angle, middle cranial fossa, Sylvian fissure). Although present at birth, these lesions grow slowly by accumulating desquamated epithelium and conform to the shape of the portion of the subarachnoid space they occupy, sometimes invaginating into the brain parenchyma. On CT, epidermoid cysts generally appear as well-circumscribed, lobulated, non-enhancing, homogeneously hypodense lesions (of similar density to CSF). There is typically no surrounding oedema.[91] On MRI, epidermoid cysts have a signal intensity close to that of CSF on T1, T2 and FLAIR images which can make them difficult to distinguish from other cystic lesions[92] such as arachnoid cysts (Fig. 2-29). The latter often have better defined margins and cause bone thinning. DWI is the most helpful MRI sequence for making the diagnosis of epidermoid tumours. They appear bright on DWI, as opposed to arachnoid cysts, which appear dark, like CSF.

MENINGEAL METASTASES

Meningeal metastases may involve the pachymeninges (dura mater), leptomeninges (arachnoid and pia mater) or both. Contrast-enhanced MRI is much more sensitive than contrast-enhanced CT for detection of metastatic meningeal involvement. Carcinomatosis of the dura mater, common in carcinoma of the breast, manifests itself as focal curvilinear or diffuse contrast enhancement closely applied to the inner table of the skull, which does not follow the convolutions of the gyri. Focal segmental lesions may be difficult to distinguish from en plaque meningioma (Fig. 2-30). Leptomeningeal carcinomatosis produces linear or finely nodular contrast enhancement of the surface of the brain, extending into the sulci and following the convolutions of the brain. It may be

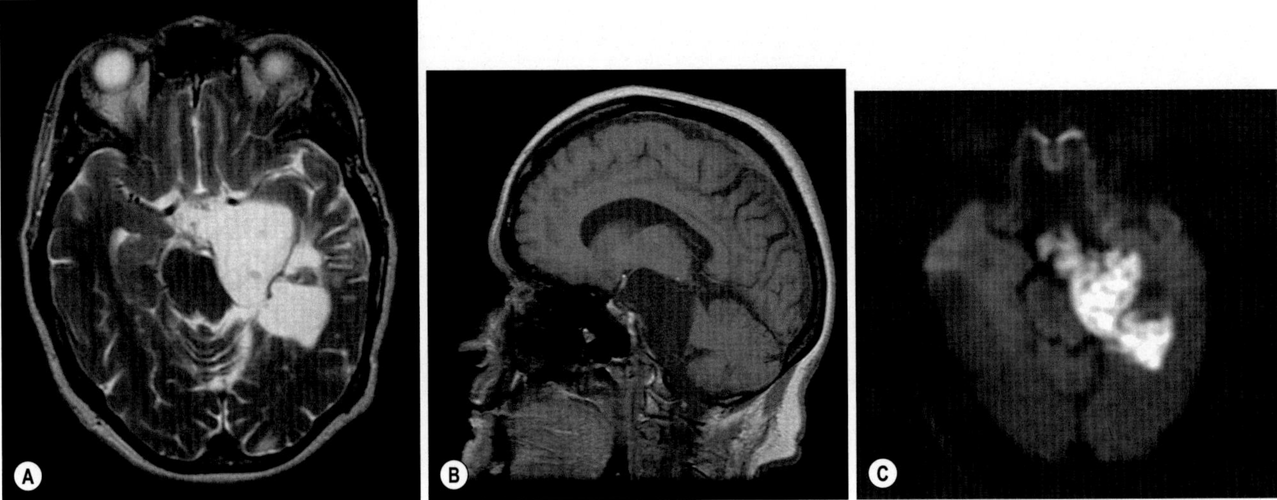

FIGURE 2-29 ■ Epidermoid tumour. Axial T2W image (A) and sagittal gadolinium-enhanced T1W image (B) show a large non-enhancing lesion of similar signal intensity to CSF, which occupies the chiasmatic and ambient cisterns, and distorts the medial aspect of the left temporal lobe. On the trace-weighted DW image (C), the lesion appears markedly hyperintense, indicating restricted diffusion.

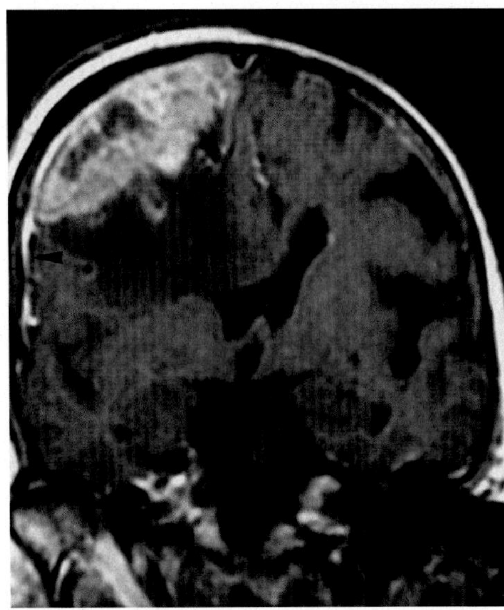

FIGURE 2-30 ■ Dural metastasis from carcinoma of the breast. Coronal T1W post-contrast MRI. There is a heterogeneously enhancing mass with an irregular surface that arises from the dura over the right cerebral convexity. It displaces the underlying brain and causes considerable low signal oedema within it. There is a 'dural tail' extending away from the tumour (arrowhead).

indistinguishable from infective meningitis or sarcoidosis. Leptomeningeal disease is commonly seen in leukaemia, lymphoma and breast or lung cancer.

SKULL BASE TUMOURS

Tumours of the skull base include a large pathological spectrum, such as metastases, myeloma/plasmacytoma, meningioma, caudally extending pituitary adenomas, direct extension of nasopharyngeal malignancies as well as tumours and inflammatory lesions arising in the paranasal sinuses. Two specific lesions of the central and posterior skull base are discussed below: chordomas and glomus jugulare tumours.

Chordomas

Chordomas originate from malignant transformation of notochordal cells and their most frequent location in the skull base is the spheno-occipital synchrondrosis of the clivus, followed by the basiocciput and petrous apex: tumours away from the midline are considerably less common. Chordomas are locally invasive and uncommonly metastasise. They present usually with pain and lower cranial nerve palsies. Both MRI and CT are usually performed to assess intracranial chordomas.[93] Bone destruction and calcification are well demonstrated on CT with bone window settings and the tumour is hyperattenuating in relation to the adjacent neural axis. MRI demonstrates a mass which is of intermediate-to-low signal intensity on T1 images and of very high signal intensity on T2 images, frequently containing septae of low signal which gives a characteristic 'soap-bubble' appearance[83] (Fig. 2-31). The solid components show variable, but often marked, contrast enhancement. Fat-suppressed T1W spin-echo sequences are particularly helpful for demonstrating the extent of the tumour and distinguishing pathological enhancement from the high signal of adjacent clival fat. Partial encasement or displacement of the intracranial vessels is common but arterial narrowing or stenoses are rare. Both MR and CT angiography can readily assess the relationship of the tumour to the surrounding vessels and hence aid in surgical planning.

The differential diagnosis includes chondrosarcoma, metastasis and nasopharyngeal carcinoma.

Glomus Jugulare Tumours

Glomus jugulare tumours (chemodectomas) arise from paraganglion cells, the precursors of the chemo- and

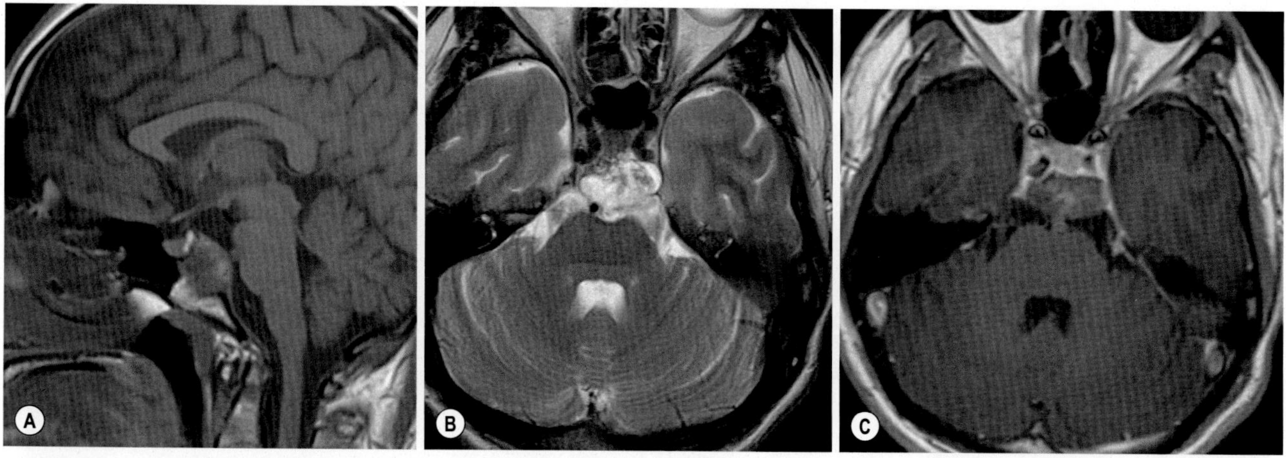

FIGURE 2-31 ■ **Chordoma.** Sagittal T1W image (A) shows a mass arising from the clivus. The mass has partially replaced the normal hyperintense bone marrow and destroyed the cortex posteriorly. On axial T2WI (B) the mass is predominantly hyperintense with with septae of low signal, giving a 'soap-bubble' appearance. Contrast-enhanced T1WI (C) shows patchy enhancement of the tumour.

baroreceptors of great vessels. The most common site is the jugular bulb and their presentation is with pulsatile tinnitus, deafness, vertigo and lower cranial nerve palsies. The tumour causes enlargement of the pars vasorum of the jugular foramen, and any associated bone destruction is well demonstrated on CT (Fig. 2-32). Glomus jugulare tumours enhance intensely on CT and MRI due to their extreme vascularity. On MRI, they appear hyperintense on T2 images and tend to contain areas of flow void corresponding to dilated vessels. These tumours frequently obstruct the internal jugular vein, which may show signal changes indicative of thrombosis.[94]

PITUITARY REGION TUMOURS

Imaging of the pituitary gland and sellar/parasellar region requires high-resolution images, as the pituitary gland is of small volume and in close proximity to many important structures.[95] The differential diagnosis for sellar and parasellar masses is large and, in addition to pituitary tumours, non-neoplastic lesions such as arachnoid cysts or giant aneurysms (Fig. 2-33) must be considered.

Pituitary Adenomas

Pituitary adenomas are the most common neoplasms in the sellar region and comprise 10 to 15% of all intracranial neoplasms. They are classified as microadenomas (diameter < 1 cm) and macroadenomas (> 1 cm) and become symptomatic either because of their endocrine activity (microadenomas and functioning macroadenomas) or by the mass effect they exert (non-functioning macroadenomas) on adjacent structures such as the optic nerves and chiasm, which leads to visual symptoms.

Non-functioning microadenomas are not uncommon and can be found incidentally on MRI studies performed for other reasons.

MRI is the investigation of choice for the detection of microadenomas. Two methods are typically employed, sometimes in conjunction. The first is a standard spin-echo (SE) T1 pre- and post-contrast imaging in the coronal and sagittal plane using a high-resolution technique (3-mm thin slices with small intervals). Fat-saturated T1 images should be performed after administration of IV contrast medium to eliminate high signal from fat in the clivus and clinoid processes, which could be mistaken for enhancement. The second method utilises the different potential enhancement characteristics of adenomas versus normal pituitary tissue by performing dynamic pituitary MRI, which involves the acquisition of a series of rapid images with a time interval of approximately 10–15 s following contrast.[96] A newer imaging technique employs spoiled gradient recalled (SPGR) acquisition in the steady state sequence which gives 1-mm-thin sections and excellent soft-tissue contrast. However, it has the disadvantage of a lower signal-to-noise ratio than SE sequences.[97]

Functioning microadenomas can produce prolactin (prolactinomas), ACTH (in Cushing's disease) or growth hormone (eosinophilic microadenomas). Prolactinomas are the most common functioning microadenomas and tend to arise laterally within the anterior lobe of the pituitary gland. They may depress the floor of the sella turcica or expand one side of the gland, causing a subtle upwardly convex bulge and contralateral displacement of the infundibulum. Microadenomas are best shown on contrast-enhanced images and usually enhance later and/or to a lesser degree than normal pituitary tissue (Fig. 2-34).

The primary treatment of prolactin-secreting microadenomas is medical and the role of imaging in cases of hyperprolactinaemia is therefore mainly to exclude a macroadenoma. Precise localisation of the microadenoma is, however, important in ACTH and thyroid-stimulating hormone (TSH)-producing adenomas, which are treated surgically. In cases where MRI is inconclusive, inferior petrosal and/or cavernous sinus venous sampling may be necessary to lateralise an adenoma in pituitary-driven Cushing's disease. Sensitivity and specificity of more than

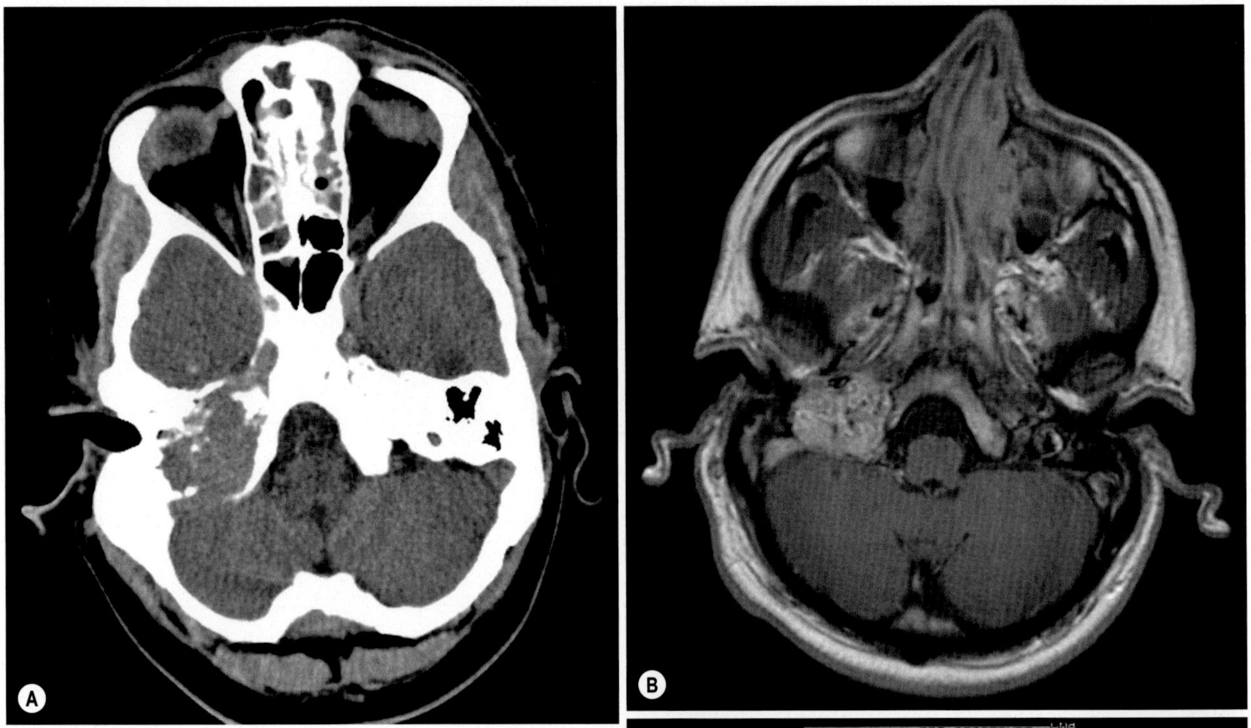

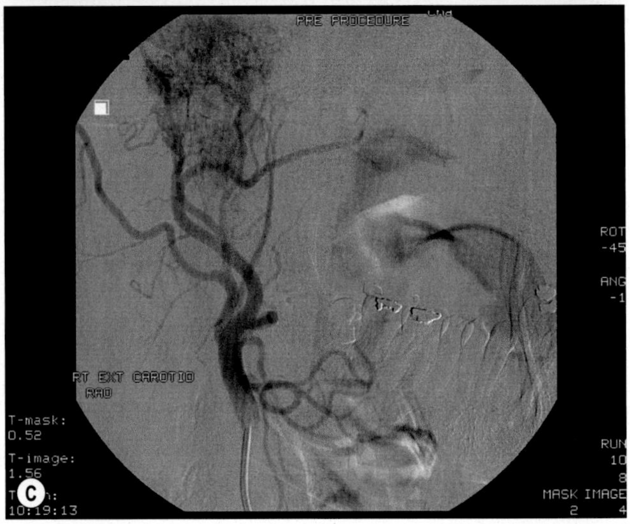

FIGURE 2-32 ■ **Glomus jugulare tumour.** An axial CT (A) demonstrates expansion of the right jugular foramen and bone destruction in the adjacent petrous bone by a mass that is markedly enhancing on an axial T1W post-contrast image (B). The mass contains areas of flow voids, corresponding to the dilated tumour vessels seen on the right external carotid artery angiogram (C). (Courtesy of Dr. M. Adams.)

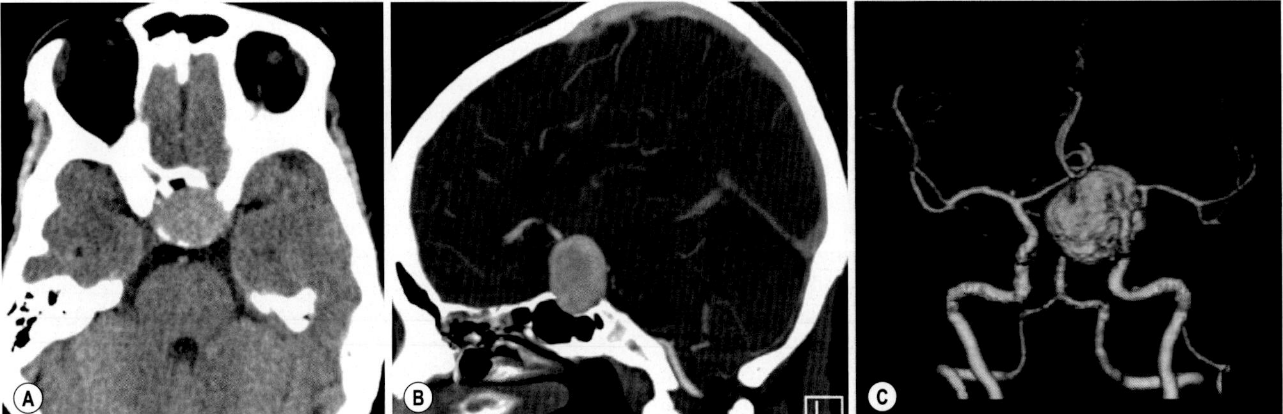

FIGURE 2-33 ■ **Aneurysm.** Axial-unenhanced CT (A) shows a homogeneous, intermediate-density mass expanding the sella turcica. Sagittal MPR images of the CTA angiogram (B) demonstrate this lesion to be highly vascular (B) and volume-rendered reconstructions (C) of the CTA confirm a left cavernous ICA aneurysm. A 'do not biopsy' lesion!

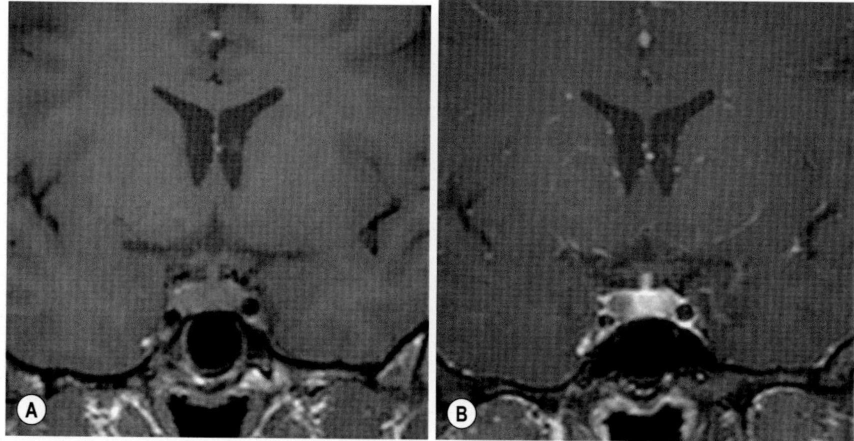

FIGURE 2-34 ■ **Pituitary microadenoma.** Pre-contrast T1WI (A) demonstrates asymmetrical enlargement of the anterior lobe of the pituitary gland on the right. Post-contrast T1WI (B) shows a right-sided microadenoma (<10 mm) abutting the cavernous sinus. It enhances to a much lesser degree than normal pituitary tissue, which makes it easily discernible.

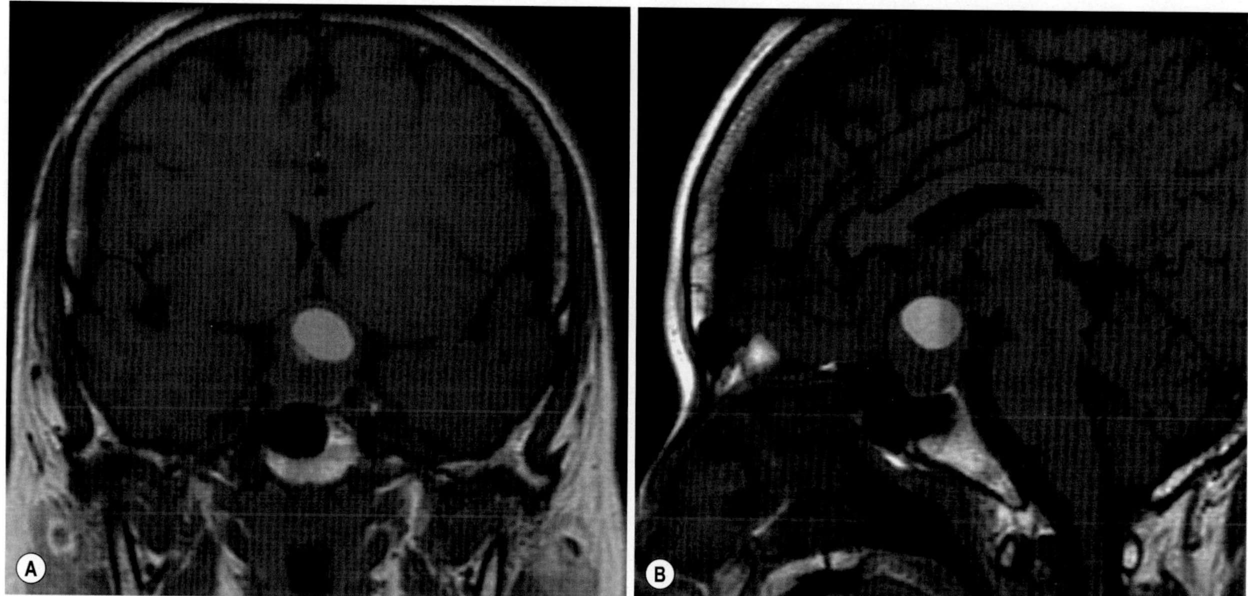

FIGURE 2-35 ■ **Pituitary apoplexy due to haemorrhage into a pituitary macroadenoma.** Coronal (A) and sagittal (B) T1W images demonstrate a hyperintense area at the superior aspect of the tumour that contains a fluid level and is consistent with a recent intratumoural haemorrhage. The optic chiasm is stretched across the apex of the mass.

90% is reported in detection of these lesions, but lesion localisation is not as high when compared with MRI.[98] Eosinophilic microadenomas can cause enlargement of the sella along with other features of acromegaly.

Macroadenomas balloon the pituitary fossa and can have a suprasellar component or extend inferiorly into the sphenoid sinus and clivus. Suprasellar extension leads first to elevation, then to compression of the optic chiasm and intracranial optic nerves, and large tumours may compress brain parenchyma, often in the region of the hypothalamus. Most macroadenomas are isointense with brain parenchyma on unenhanced T1W images and hyperdense on CT. Administration of IV contrast may show uniform or heterogeneous enhancement and facilitates the detection of cavernous sinus invasion, which is often a poor prognostic sign.[99] Enhancement and thickening of the dura (forming a 'dural tail') is frequently seen with large macroadenomas and is a helpful sign of an aggressive lesion, believed to be caused by venous congestion due to compression or invasion of the adjacent cavernous sinus.[100] Macroademomas may contain cystic or haemorrhagic components. Acute haemorrhage into a pituitary macroademona can lead to rapid expansion of the gland, resulting in acute compression of the optic chiasm (pituitary apoplexy). Haemorrhage appears hyperintense on non-enhanced T1W images and, in the acute stage, hyperdense on CT (Fig. 2-35).

Craniopharyngiomas

Craniopharyngiomas are suprasellar tumours which occur most frequently in childhood, but may arise in adult life, and have a second peak of incidence at about the 6th decade. Symptoms are due to compression of the optic chiasm or to raised ICP secondary to obstruction of the foramen of Monro.

They arise from epithelial remnants of Rathke's pouch, from which the anterior pituitary develops, and can be cystic, solid or mixed cystic/solid (Fig. 2-36). Craniopharyngiomas tend not to expand the pituitary fossa unless they become very large which is a differentiating feature from pituitary macroadenomas.

The two main pathological subtypes are the adamantinomatous and squamous-papillary varieties, which vary in age at presentation, tumour location and imaging characteristics.[92] The adamantinomatous type, more common in children, is more likely to have large T1 hyperintense cystic components, whereas the squamous-papillary type, more frequent in adults, is more likely to be predominantly solid and associated cysts return low signal on T1W images, similar to CSF.

The solid components of craniopharyngiomas show intense contrast enhancement and may be partially calcified.

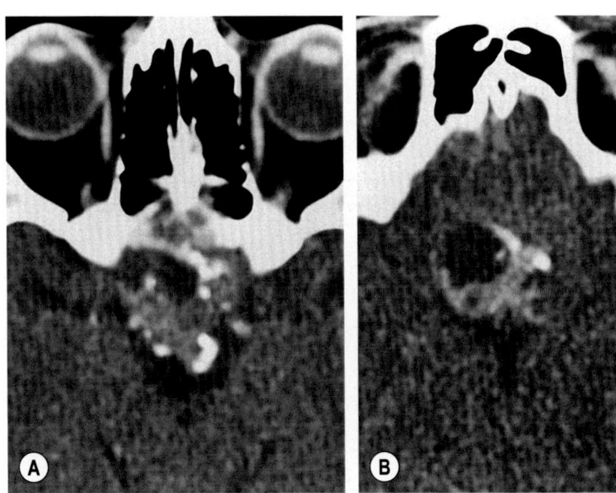

FIGURE 2-36 ■ **Craniopharyngioma.** CT following IV contrast medium. There is a partly calcified, partly cystic lesion in the suprasellar region. There is inhomogeneous enhancement of the solid tumour components.

Rathke's Cleft Cysts

Symptomatic Rathke's cleft cysts are less common than craniopharyngiomas and usually lie within the pituitary gland, but can also be found adjacent to the infundibulum, above the sella. On MRI, they appear frequently as T1 hyperintense cysts, reflecting the proteinaceous nature of the cyst fluid, but may also exhibit similar signal characteristics to CSF. In contradistinction to craniopharyngiomas, Rathke's cysts usually demonstrate thin and uniform walls which infrequently enhance following IV contrast.[101]

Other Sellar Region Tumours

Parasellar meningiomas can arise from the dura mater of the cavernous sinus or the tuberculum, dorsum or diaphragma sellae. Clinical presentation is with cranial nerve palsies or visual symptoms. Parasellar meningiomas are strongly enhancing masses which expand the cavernous sinus and frequently encase and narrow the cavernous portion of the internal carotid arteries. Suprasellar meningiomas often show a forward extension along the dura mater of the anterior cranial fossa and are associated with dilatation ('blistering') of the sphenoid sinus. Intracranial extension of optic nerve sheath meningiomas characteristically involves the planum sphenoidale.

Optic nerve gliomas are astrocytic tumours that occur in childhood and may involve the optic nerves, optic chiasm and optic tracts (Fig. 2-37). These tumours can be associated with NF1 but chiasmic tumours are more frequently seen in patients who do not have NF1.[102]

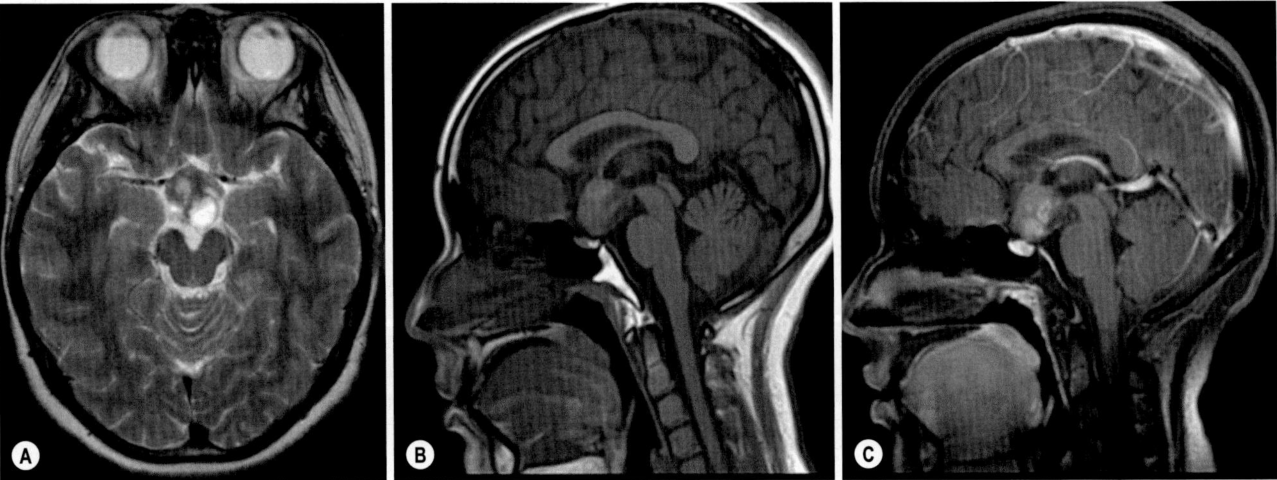

FIGURE 2-37 ■ **Intracranial optic nerve glioma.** T2WI (A), non-enhanced T1WI (B) and post-contrast T1WI (C) in a patient with an optic nerve glioma showing a mass centred on the optic chiasm with a cystic component posteriorly and solid T2 isointense (A) and T1 isointense (B) components that show heterogeneous enhancement (C). A normal enhancing pituitary gland is seen inferior to the mass (C).

Metastases, particularly from breast carcinoma, can cause thickening of the pituitary stalk and can present with diabetes insipidus. Similar appearances may be seen in histiocytosis and sarcoidosis.

REFERENCES

1. Hoeffner EG, Case I, Jain R, et al. Cerebral perfusion CT: technique and clinical applications. Radiology 2004;231:632–44.
2. Klingebiel R, Siebert E, Diekmann S, et al. 4-D Imaging in cerebrovascular disorders by using 320-slice CT: feasibility and preliminary clinical experience. Acad Radiol 2009;16(2): 123–9.
3. Bynevelt M, Britton J, Seymour H, et al. FLAIR imaging in the follow-up of low-grade gliomas: time to dispense with the dual-echo? Neuroradiology 2001;43:129–33.
4. Yuh W, Maley J. Contrast dosage in the neuroimaging of brain tumors. Principles and indications. Magn Reson Imaging Clin N Am 1999;6:113–24.
5. Essig M, Anzalone N, Combs SE, et al. MR imaging of neoplastic central nervous system lesions: review and recommendations for current practice. Am J Neuroradiol 2012;33(5):803–17.
6. Sugahara T, Koroghi Y, Kochi M, et al. Correlation of MR imaging-determined cerebral blood maps with histologic and angiographic determination of vascularity of gliomas. Am J Roentgenol 1998;171:1479–86.
7. Sugahara T, Korogi Y, Kochi M, et al. Perfusion-sensitive MR imaging of gliomas: comparison between gradient-echo and spin-echo echo-planar imaging techniques. Am J Neuroradiol 2001; 22:1306–15.
8. Paulson ES, Schmainda KM. Comparison of dynamic susceptibility-weighted contrast-enhanced MR methods: recommendations for measuring relative cerebral blood volume in brain tumors. Radiology 2008;249(2):601–13.
9. Narang J, Jain R, Arbab AS, et al. Differentiating treatment-induced necrosis from recurrent/progressive brain tumor using nnonmodel-based semiquantitative indices derived from dynamic contrast-enhanced T1-weighted MR perfusion. Neuro Oncol 2011;13(9):1037–46.
10. Petersen ET, Zimine I, Ho YC, Golay X. Non-invasive measurement of perfusion: a critical review of arterial spin labelling techniques. Br J Radiol 2006;79(944):688–701.
11. Järnum H, Steffensen EG, Knutsson L, et al. Perfusion MRI of brain tumours: a comparative study of pseudo-continuous arterial spin labelling and dynamic susceptibility contrast imaging. Neuroradiology 2010;52(4):307–17.
12. Sugahara T, Korogi Y, Kochi M, et al. Usefulness of diffusion-weighted MRI with echo-planar technique in the evaluation of cellularity in gliomas. J Magn Reson Imaging 1999;9:53–60.
13. Sadeghi N, Camby I, Goldman S, et al. Effect of hydrophilic components of the extracellular matrix on quantifiable diffusion-weighted imaging of human gliomas: preliminary results of correlating apparent diffusion coefficient values and hyaluronan expression level. Am J Roentgenol 2003;181:235–41.
14. Bai X, Zhang Y, Liu Y, et al. Grading of supratentorial astrocytic tumors by using the difference of ADC value. Neuroradiology 2011;53(7):533–9.
15. Le Bihan D, Mangin JF, Poupon C, et al. Diffusion tensor imaging: concepts and applications. J Magn Reson Imaging 2001;13:534–46.
16. Price SJ, Tozer DJ, Gillard JH. Methodology of diffusion-weighted, diffusion tensor and magnetisation transfer imaging. Br J Radiol 2011;84(Spec No 2):S121–6.
17. Law M. MR spectroscopy of brain tumors. Top Magn Reson Imaging 2004;15:291–313.
18. Vlieger EJ, Majoie CB, Leenstra S, Den Heeten GJ. Functional magnetic resonance imaging for neurosurgical planning in neurooncology. Eur Radiol 2004;14:1143–53.
19. Nelson SJ. Assessment of therapeutic response and treatment planning for brain tumors using metabolic and physiological MRI. NMR Biomed 2011;24(6):734–49.
20. Gulyás B, Halldin C. New PET radiopharmaceuticals beyond FDG for brain tumor imaging. Q J Nucl Med Mol Imaging 2012;56(2):173–90.
21. Graf R, Nyuyki F, Steffen IG, et al. Contribution of 68Ga-DOTATOC PET/CT to target volume delineation of skull base meningiomas treated with stereotactic radiation therapy. Int J Radiat Oncol Biol Phys 2013;85(1):68–73.
22. Kleihues P, Burger P, Scheithaur B. The new WHO classification of brain tumours. Brain Pathol 1993;3:255–68.
23. Kleihues P, Louis DN, Scheithauer BW, et al. The WHO classification of tumors of the nervous system. J Neuropathol Exp Neurol 2002;61:215–25; discussion 226–9.
24. Louis DN, Ohgaki H, Wiestler OD, et al. The 2007 WHO classification of tumours of the central nervous system. Acta Neuropathol 2007;114(2):97–109. Erratum: Acta Neuropathol 114(5):547.
25. Theeler BJ, Yung WK, Fuller GN, De Groot JF. Moving toward molecular classification of diffuse gliomas in adults. Neurology 2012; 2012;79(18):1917–26.
26. Kumar VA, Knopp EA, Zagzag D. Magnetic resonance dynamic susceptibility-weighted contrast-enhanced perfusion imaging in the diagnosis of posterior fossa hemangioblastomas and pilocytic astrocytomas: initial results. J Comput Assist Tomogr 2010;34(6): 825–9.
27. Leu S, von Felten S, Frank S, et al. IDH/MGMT-driven molecular classification of low-grade glioma is a strong predictor for long-term survival. Neuro Oncol 2013;15(4):469–79.
28. Upadhyay N, Waldman AD. Conventional MRI evaluation of gliomas. Br J Radiol 2011;84(Spec No 2):S107–11.
29. Wilms G, Demaerel P, Sunaert S. Intra-axial brain tumours. Eur Radiol 2005;15:468–84.
30. Young RJ, Knopp EA. Brain MRI: tumor evaluation. J Magn Reson Imaging 2006;24:709–24.
31. Nelson SJ, Cha S. Imaging glioblastoma multiforme. Cancer J 2003;9:134–45.
32. Pope WB, Chen JH, Dong J, et al. Relationship between gene expression and enhancement in glioblastoma multiforme: exploratory DNA microarray analysis. Radiology 2008;249(1):268–77.
33. Cirillo M, Esposito F, Tedeschi G, et al. Widespread microstructural white matter involvement in amyotrophic lateral sclerosis: a whole-brain DTI study. Am J Neuroradiol 2012;33(6): 1102–8.
34. Macdonald DR, Cascino TL, Schold SC Jr, Cairncross JG. Response criteria for phase II studies of supratentorial malignant glioma. J Clin Oncol 1990;8(7):1277–80.
35. Kong DS, Kim ST, Kim EH, et al. Diagnostic dilemma of pseudoprogression in the treatment of newly diagnosed glioblastomas: the role of assessing relative cerebral blood flow volume and oxygen-6-methylguanine-DNA methyltransferase promoter methylation status. Am J Neuroradiol 2011;32(2):382–7.
36. Hygino da Cruz LC Jr, Rodriguez I, Domingues RC, et al. Pseudoprogression and pseudoresponse: imaging challenges in the assessment of posttreatment glioma. Am J Neuroradiol 2011; 32(11):1978–85.
37. Wen PY, Macdonald DR, Reardon DA, et al. Updated response assessment criteria for high-grade gliomas: response assessment in neuro-oncology working group. J Clin Oncol 2010;28(11): 1963–72.
38. Hygino da Cruz LC, Rodriguez I, Domingues RC, et al. Pseudoprogression and Pseudoresponse: Imaging Challenges in the Assessment of Posttreatment Glioma. Am J Neuroradiol 2011; 32:1978–85.
39. Mong S, Ellingson BM, Nghiemphu PL, et al. Persistent diffusion-restricted lesions in bevacizumab-treated malignant gliomas are associated with improved survival compared with matched controls. Am J Neuroradiol 2012;33(9):1763–70.
40. Ricci P. Imaging of adult brain tumors. Neuroimaging Clin N Am 1999;9:651–69.
41. Khalid L, Carone M, Dumrongpisutikul N, et al. Imaging characteristics of oligodendrogliomas that predict grade. Am J Neuroradiol 2012;33(5):852–7.
42. Cha S, Tihan T, Crawford F, et al. Differentiation of low-grade oligodendrogliomas from low-grade astrocytomas by using quantitative blood-volume measurements derived from dynamic susceptibility contrast-enhanced MR imaging. Am J Neuroradiol 2005;26:266–73.
43. Jenkinson MD, Smith TS, Joyce KA, et al. Cerebral blood volume, genotype and chemosensitivity in oligodendroglial tumours. Neuroradiology 2006;48:703–13.

44. Jenkinson MD, du Plessis DG, Smith TS, et al. Histological growth patterns and genotype in oligodendroglial tumours: correlation with MRI features. Brain 2006;129:1884–91.
45. Kim JW, Park CK, Park SH, et al. Relationship between radiological characteristics and combined 1p and 19q deletion in World Health Organization grade III oligodendroglial tumours. J Neurol Neurosurg Psychiatry 2011;82(2):224–7.
46. Tozer DJ, Jäger HR, Danchaivijitr N, et al. Apparent diffusion coefficient histograms may predict low-grade glioma subtype. NMR Biomed 2007;20(1):49–57.
47. Law M, Yang S, Wang H, et al. Glioma grading: sensitivity, specificity, and predictive values of perfusion MR imaging and proton MR spectroscopic imaging compared with conventional MR imaging. Am J Neuroradiol 2003;24(10):1989–98.
48. Hilario A, Ramos A, Perez-Nuñez A, et al. The added value of apparent diffusion coefficient to cerebral blood volume in the preoperative grading of diffuse gliomas. Am J Neuroradiol 2012;33(4):701–7.
49. Romano A, Calabria LF, Tavanti F, et al. Apparent diffusion coefficient obtained by magnetic resonance imaging as a prognostic marker in glioblastomas: correlation with MGMT promoter methylation status. Eur Radiol 2013;23(2):513–20.
50. Brasil Caseiras G, Ciccarelli O, Altmann DR, et al. Low-grade gliomas: six-month tumor growth predicts patient outcome better than admission tumor volume, relative cerebral blood volume, and apparent diffusion coefficient. Radiology 2009;253(2):505–12.
51. Law M, Young RJ, Babb JS, et al. Gliomas: predicting time to progression or survival with cerebral blood volume measurements at dynamic susceptibility-weighted contrast-enhanced perfusion MR imaging. Radiology 2008;247(2):490–8.
52. Mohsen LA, Shi V, Jena R, et al. Diffusion tensor invasive phenotypes can predict progression-free survival in glioblastomas. Br J Neurosurg 2013 [Epub ahead of print].
53. Galbán CJ, Chenevert TL, Meyer CR, et al. The parametric response map is an imaging biomarker for early cancer treatment outcome. Nat Med 2009;15(5):572–6.
54. Galbán CJ, Chenevert TL, Meyer CR, et al. Prospective analysis of parametric response map-derived MRI biomarkers: identification of early and distinct glioma response patterns not predicted by standard radiographic assessment. Clin Cancer Res 2011; 17(14):4751–60.
55. Barajas RF Jr, Chang JS, Segal MR, et al. Differentiation of recurrent glioblastoma multiforme from radiation necrosis after external beam radiation therapy with dynamic susceptibility-weighted contrast-enhanced perfusion MR imaging. Radiology 2009; 253(2):486–96.
56. Shah R, Vattoth S, Jacob R, et al. Radiation necrosis in the brain: imaging features and differentiation from tumor recurrence. Radiographics 2012;32(5):1343–59.
57. Fatterpekar GM, Galheigo D, Narayana A, et al. Treatment-related change versus tumor recurrence in high-grade gliomas: a diagnostic conundrum–use of dynamic susceptibility contrast-enhanced (DSC) perfusion MRI. Am J Roentgenol 2012;198(1): 19–26.
58. Baek HJ, Kim HS, Kim N, et al. Percent change of perfusion skewness and kurtosis: a potential imaging biomarker for early treatment response in patients with newly diagnosed glioblastomas. Radiology 2012;264(3):834–43.
59. Fatterpekar GM, Galheigo D, Narayana A, et al. Treatment-Related Change Versus Tumor Recurrence in High-Grade Gliomas: A Diagnostic Conundrum—Use of Dynamic Susceptibility Contrast-Enhanced (DSC) Perfusion MRI. Am J Roentgenol 2012;198(1):19–26.
60. Stanescu Cosson R, Varlet P, Beuvon F, et al. Dysembryoplastic neuroepithelial tumors: CT, MR findings and imaging follow-up: a study of 53 cases. J Neuroradiol 2001;28:230–40.
61. Tien RD, Barkovich AJ, Edwards MS. MR imaging of pineal tumors. Am J Roentgenol 1990;155:143–51.
62. Sumida M, Uozumi T, Kiya K, et al. MRI of intracranial germ cell tumours. Neuroradiology 1995;37:32–7.
63. Haldorsen IS, Espeland A, Larsson EM. Central nervous system lymphoma: characteristic findings on traditional and advanced imaging. Am J Neuroradiol 2011;32(6):984–92.
64. Guo AC, Cummings TJ, Dash RC, Provenzale JM. Lymphomas and high-grade astrocytomas: comparison of water diffusibility and histologic characteristics. Radiology 2002;224:177–83.
65. Camacho DL, Smith JK, Castillo M. Differentiation of toxoplasmosis and lymphoma in AIDS patients by using apparent diffusion coefficients. Am J Neuroradiol 2003;24:633–7.
66. Mangla R, Kolar B, Zhu T, et al. Percentage signal recovery derived from MR dynamic susceptibility contrast imaging is useful to differentiate common enhancing malignant lesions of the brain. Am J Neuroradiol 2011;32(6):1004–10.
67. Young RJ, Sills AK, Brem S, Knopp EA. Neuroimaging of metastatic brain disease. Neurosurgery 2005;57:S10–23; discusssion S11–14.
68. Hayashida Y, Hirai T, Morishita S, et al. Diffusion-weighted imaging of metastatic brain tumors: comparison with histologic type and tumor cellularity. Am J Neuroradiol 2006;27:1419–25.
69. Guzman R, Barth A, Lovblad KO, et al. Use of diffusion-weighted magnetic resonance imaging in differentiating purulent brain processes from cystic brain tumors. J Neurosurg 2002;97: 1101–7.
70. Zhang D, Wen L, Henning TD, et al. Central neurocytoma: clinical, pathological and neuroradiological findings. Clin Radiol 2006;61:348–57.
71. Chiang IC, Kuo YT, Lu CY, et al. Distinction between high-grade gliomas and solitary metastases using peritumoral 3-T magnetic resonance spectroscopy, diffusion, and perfusion imagings. Neuroradiology 2004;46:619–27.
72. Drevelegas A. Extra-axial brain tumors. Eur Radiol 2005;15: 453–67.
73. Weber DC, Lovblad KO, Rogers L. New pathology classification, imagery techniques and prospective trials for meningiomas: the future looks bright. Curr Opin Neurol 2010;23(6):563–70.
74. Saloner D, Uzelac A, Hetts S, et al. Modern meningioma imaging techniques. J Neurooncol 2010;99(3):333–40.
75. Simis A, Pires de Aguiar PH, Leite CC, et al. Peritumoral brain edema in benign meningiomas: correlation with clinical, radiologic, and surgical factors and possible role on recurrence. Surg Neurol 2008;70(5):471–7; discussion 477.
76. Sibtain NA, Howe FA, Saunders DE. The clinical value of proton magnetic resonance spectroscopy in adult brain tumours. Clin Radiol 2007;62(2):109–19.
77. Hakyemez B, Yildirim N, Gokalp G, et al. The contribution of diffusion-weighted MR imaging to distinguishing typical from atypical meningiomas. Neuroradiology 2006;48(8):513–20.
78. Filippi CG, Edgar MA, Ulug AM, et al. Appearance of meningiomas on diffusion-weighted images: correlating diffusion constants with histopathologic findings. Am J Neuroradiol 2001;22: 65–72.
79. Santelli L, Ramondo G, Della Puppa A, et al. Diffusion-weighted imaging does not predict histological grading in meningiomas. Acta Neurochir (Wien) 2010;152(8):1315–19; discussion 1319.
80. Zhang H, Rödiger LA, Shen T, et al. Perfusion MR imaging for differentiation of benign and malignant meningiomas. Neuroradiology 2008;50(6):525–30.
81. Carli DF, Sluzewski M, Beute GN, van Rooij WJ. Complications of particle embolization of meningiomas: frequency, risk factors, and outcome. Am J Neuroradiol 2010;31(1):152–4.
82. Chiechi MV, Smirniotopoulos JG, Mena H. Intracranial hemangiopericytomas: MR and CT features. Am J Neuroradiol 1996; 17:1365–71.
83. Bonneville F, Savatovsky J, Chiras J. Imaging of cerebellopontine angle lesions: an update. Part 1: enhancing extra-axial lesions. Eur Radiol 2007;17(10):2472–82.
84. Sriskandan N, Connor SE. The role of radiology in the diagnosis and management of vestibular schwannoma. Clin Radiol 2011; 66(4):357–65.
85. Newton JR, Shakeel M, Flatman S, et al. Magnetic resonance imaging screening in acoustic neuroma. Am J Otolaryngol 2010;31(4):217–20.
86. Thamburaj K, Radhakrishnan VV, Thomas B, et al. Intratumoral microhemorrhages on T2*-weighted gradient-echo imaging helps differentiate vestibular schwannoma from meningioma. Am J Neuroradiol 2008;29(3):552–7.
87. Yamasaki F, Kurisu K, Satoh K, et al. Apparent diffusion coefficient of human brain tumors at MR imaging. Radiology 2005; 235(3):985–91.
88. Hakyemez B, Erdogan C, Bolca N, et al. Evaluation of different cerebral mass lesions by perfusion-weighted MR imaging. J Magn Reson Imaging 2006;24(4):817–24.

89. Osborn AG, Preece MT. Intracranial cysts: radiologic-pathologic correlation and imaging approach. Radiology 2006;239(3):650–64.
90. Orakcioglu B, Halatsch ME, Fortunati M, et al. Intracranial dermoid cysts: variations of radiological and clinical features. Acta Neurochir (Wien) 2008;150(12):1227–34.
91. Nagasawa D, Yew A, Safaee M, et al. Clinical characteristics and diagnostic imaging of epidermoid tumors. J Clin Neurosci 2011;18(9):1158–62.
92. Zada G, Lin N, Ojerholm E, et al. Craniopharyngioma and other cystic epithelial lesions of the sellar region: a review of clinical, imaging, and histopathological relationships. Neurosurg Focus 2010;28(4):E4.
93. Erdem E, Angtuaco EC, Van Hemert R, et al. Comprehensive review of intracranial chordoma. Radiographics 2003;23(4):995–1009.
94. Mafee MF, Raofi B, Kumar A, Muscato C. Glomus faciale, glomus jugulare, glomus tympanicum, glomus vagale, carotid body tumors, and simulating lesions. Role of MR imaging. Radiol Clin North Am 2000;38(5):1059–76.
95. Rennert J, Doerfler A. Imaging of sellar and parasellar lesions. Clin Neurol Neurosurg 2007;109(2):111–24.
96. Ouyang T, Rothfus WE, Ng JM, Challinor SM. Imaging of the pituitary. Radiol Clin North Am 2011;49(3):549–71, vii.
97. Patronas N, Bulakbasi N, Stratakis CA, et al. Spoiled gradient recalled acquisition in the steady state technique is superior to conventional postcontrast spin echo technique for magnetic resonance imaging detection of adrenocorticotropin-secreting pituitary tumors. J Clin Endocrinol Metab 2003;88(4):1565–9.
98. Liu C, Lo JC, Dowd CF, et al. Cavernous and inferior petrosal sinus sampling in the evaluation of ACTH-dependent Cushing's syndrome. Clin Endocrinol (Oxf) 2004;61(4):478–86.
99. Cottier J, Destrieux C, Brunereau L, et al. Cavernous sinus invasion by pituitary adenoma: MR imaging. Radiology 2000;215:463–9.
100. Rumboldt Z. Pituitary adenomas. Top Magn Reson Imaging 2005;16(4):277–88.
101. Huang BY, Castillo M. Nonadenomatous tumors of the pituitary and sella turcica. Top Magn Reson Imaging 2005;16(4):289–99.
102. Kornreich L, Blaser S, Schwarz M, et al. Optic pathway glioma: correlation of imaging findings with the presence of neurofibromatosis. Am J Neuroradiol 2001;22:1963–9.

CHAPTER 3

NEUROVASCULAR DISEASES

Amrish Mehta • Brynmor P. Jones

STROKE

Stroke is the third leading cause of death in Western populations and is the largest single cause of adult disability. It has a tremendous medical, social and economic impact. Over 130,000 cases develop in the UK every year. The annual cost to the NHS, UK families, businesses and public sector exceeds £7 billion.[1]

'Stroke' is an imprecise term used to describe the sudden onset of a persistent neurological deficit caused by partial or complete blockage (ischaemic stroke) or rupture of a cerebral blood vessel (haemorrhage). Ischaemic stroke, which constitutes the great majority of cases (~ 85%),[2] will be discussed in this section. An account of intracranial haemorrhage will follow in the next section.

A transient ischaemic attack (TIA) by definition resolves within 24 h. This includes amaurosis fugax, a transient loss of vision in one eye. The risk of stroke following a TIA is higher than previously thought, maybe up to 8% in the first week and 12% within a month,[3] and even more in those awaiting endarterectomy for a symptomatic carotid stenosis.[4] Indeed, up to 44% of clinical TIAs have recently been shown to actually represent small completed brain infarcts on imaging,[5] and in this situation, the risk of a persistent neurological deficit from a subsequent event is further increased.[6]

Whilst still essential for the exclusion of non-ischaemic causes of the fixed deficit and to identify surgical remedial lesions, imaging is now pivotal in modern acute stroke management and the strategies to recanalise the occluded artery.

Pathophysiology

Normal cerebral blood flow (CBF) is 50–55 mL/100 g brain tissue/min. Cerebral autoregulation responds to a fall in cerebral perfusion pressure (CPP) with vasodilatation and recruitment of collateral vessels, thus increasing cerebral blood volume (CBV) and reducing resistance, in order to maintain CBF. The average time a blood cell remains with a particular volume of tissue rises due to vasodilatation and collateral flow, resulting in a prolonged mean transit time (MTT) and thereby allowing improved oxygen delivery. After the vessels are fully dilated the autoregulatory system cannot properly respond to any further reduction in CPP and therefore CBF starts to decline. Oxygen extraction goes up to compensate, but once this is maximal any further fall in CBF causes cellular dysfunction. The loss of normal neuronal electrical function occurs when CBF falls to 15–20 mL/100 g/min. This may, however, be reversible, depending on the severity and duration of the ischaemia, such that irreversible infarction is likely to occur within minutes if the CBF <10, but moderate ischaemia (10–20) may be reversible for a few hours. At levels of CBF <10, hypoxaemia leads to failure of the ATP-driven cell integrity systems (glutamate, NMDA, Na^+/K^+), resulting in cell depolarisation and influx of Na^+ and water. Cellular swelling and cell death occurs (cytotoxic oedema). In time, structural breakdown of the blood–brain barrier occurs due to ischaemic damage to capillary endothelium. Leakage of intravascular fluid and protein into the extracellular space and later net influx of water to the infarcted area cause vasogenic oedema.[7–9] It is important to note that CBV generally remains preserved in infarction, unless there is a profound reduction in CPP, where it has been postulated that microvascular collapse due to inability of the vessels to remain patent may eventually result in a reduction in CBV.[10]

Following recanalisation of the occluded vessel, either spontaneously (33% within 48 h)[11] or following treatment, the ischaemic region becomes reperfused. This will occur with both viable and non-viable tissue.[12] Indeed, a state of 'post-ischaemic hyperperfusion' ensues where persistently vasodilated vessels result in an elevated CBV.[13] CBF is also elevated.

The Penumbra Model

Following a thromboembolic cerebral arterial occlusion, the decline in regional CBF in the affected brain parenchyma is not uniform. The accepted model, validated in animals and humans, is centred upon an infarct core with very low CBF and cell depolarisation. A peripheral zone—the penumbra—has moderately diminished CBF, resulting in loss of electrical function but preserved cell integrity. The duration of ischaemia in the penumbra is critical, and strategies to recanalise the vessel and restore normal CBF are likely to convey the greatest benefit here. Failure or, more crucially, a delay in achieving this, however, may lead to progression to infarction, especially as this tissue is poorly autoregulated and more vulnerable. Surrounding the penumbra is a zone of benign oligaemia. Here CBF is only mildly impaired and tissue is likely to survive.

Stroke Classification

The most commonly used classification system of ischaemic stroke (TOAST)[14] discriminates between large vessel thromboembolic, cardioembolic, small vessel and 'other' aetiologies. Precise allocation into these subtypes is sometimes difficult and strokes are not infrequently undetermined. A few points to consider are:

- Deep white matter infarcts are typically small vessel in nature but can result from emboli originating from large vessel atheroma or from a cardiac source.
- Middle cerebral artery (MCA) territory infarcts can arise from emboli from the heart or carotid artery, or from in situ thrombosis in the middle cerebral artery.
- Small peripheral infarcts in a vascular territory are usually embolic but the source is not always clear (i.e. cardiac vs carotid vs MCA) (Fig. 3-1).
- Peripheral infarcts involving multiple vascular territories must be from a proximal source and most likely the heart.
- The basilar artery supplies the posterior cerebral arteries (PCAs) unless the posterior communicating artery(s) is/are large, in which case emboli from the carotid circulation may enter their territory. Brainstem infarcts are commonly result from occlusion of short perforating vessels. A combination of infratentorial, thalamic and occipital infarcts suggests an occlusion of distal basilar artery, or 'top of the basilar' syndrome (Fig. 3-2).[15]

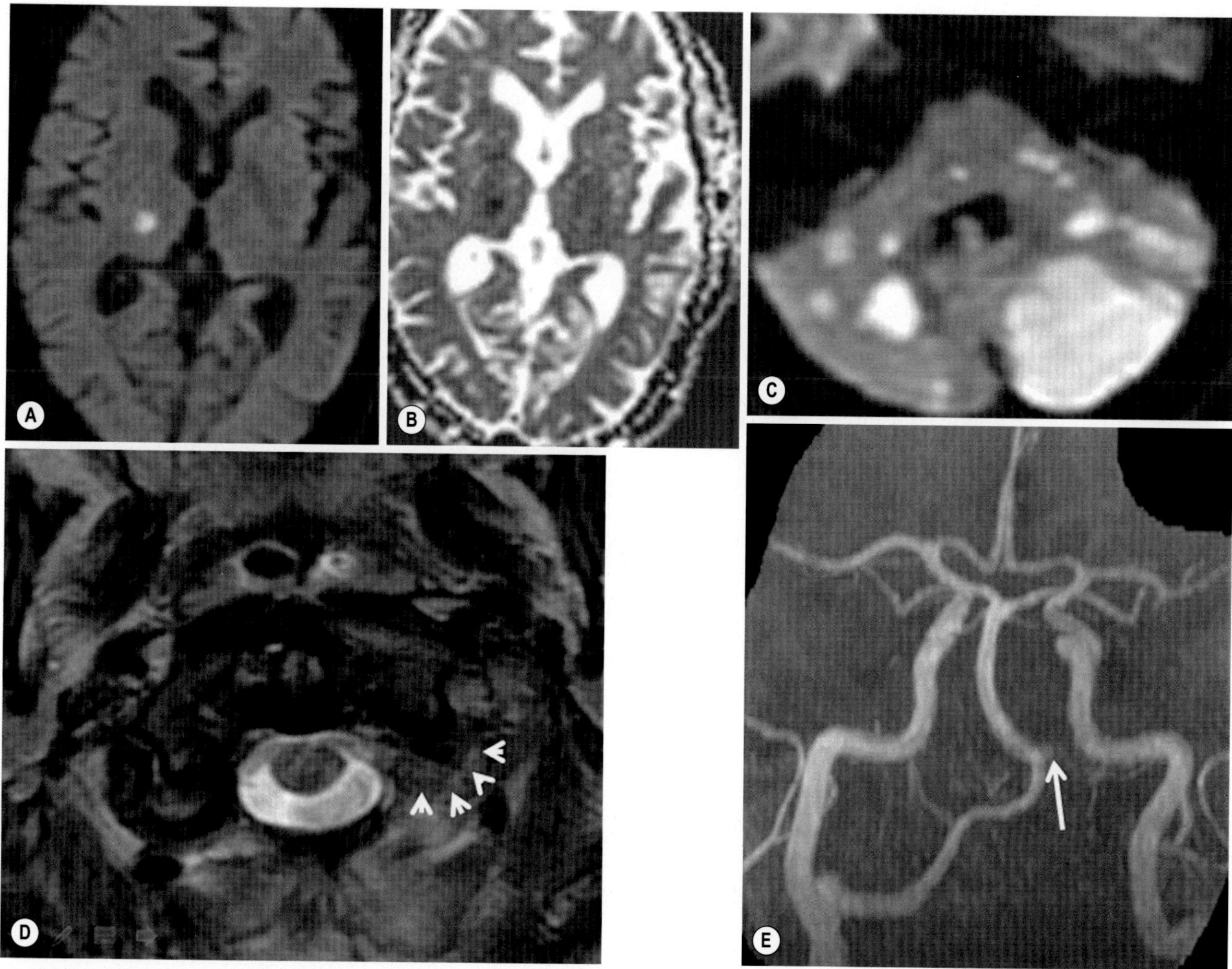

FIGURE 3-1 ■ There are multiple embolic posterior circulation infarcts in the right thalamus (hyperintense on DWI, A, and hypointense on ADC, B), and both cerebellar hemispheres (C). Note the absence of the normal flow-related signal void in the left vertebral artery at the skull base (D, white arrowheads) and absence of flow in the left vertebral artery on the TOF MRA (E, white arrow).

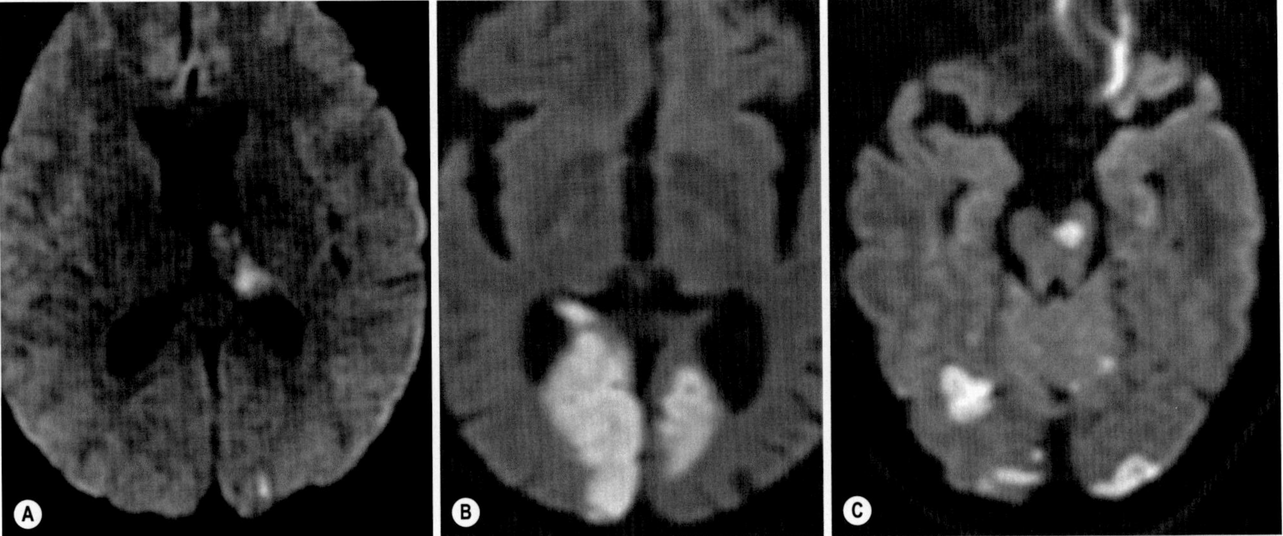

FIGURE 3-2 ■ **Basilar tip syndrome.** Multiple bilateral acute PCA territory infarcts depicted by hyperintensity on DWI are demonstrated in the left thalamus (A), both occipital lobes (B) consistent with impairment of flow at the basilar tip. In a different patient (C), there are multiple acute embolic infarcts in the posterior cerebral and superior cerebellar artery territories.

Causes

Large Vessel Thromboembolic Stroke (40%)

- Most commonly duc to thrombus at the site of atherosclerotic plaque or embolisation more distally (artery-to-artery).
- Sites: carotid bifurcation > intracranial internal carotid artery (ICA) > proximal MCA (> anterior cerebral artery (ACA)); vertebral artery origins > distal vertebral (VA) > basilar artery.
- Also vasculopathy (e.g. large vessel vasculitis, dysplasia such as fibromuscular dysplasia (FMD)), dissection.
- Haematological causes: deficiency of protein C/S/ antithrombin III; polycythaemia; pregnancy, oral contraceptives; paraneoplasia.

Cardioembolic Stroke (15–30%)

- Intracardiac thrombus: myocardial infarct, enlarged left atrial appendage, aneurysm, arrhythmia (especially paroxysmal atrial fibrillation (AF)); valvular disease—endocarditis, prosthetic valves, inadequate anticoagulation; right-to-left shunts.
- Cardiac tumours.

Small Vessel or Lacunar Stroke (15–30%)

- Small infarcts (<1.5 cm) in deep perforator territories; typically
  - Lenticulostriate perforators from M1 segment of MCA with infarcts in the lentiform nuclei, internal capsules and corona radiate.
  - Thalamic branches from posterior choroidal perforators from basilar tip, proximal PCAs and posterior communicating arteries cause infarcts in the thalami and posterior internal capsules.
  - Perforators from the basilar artery and its major branches resulting in brainstem infarcts.
- Small vessel pathology: hypertension/diabetes, etc. = ischaemic microangiopathy.
- Also vasculitis/ drugs/ radiation.
- Rarely Susac's syndrome/intravascular lymphoma/CADASIL (cerebral autosomal dominant arteriopathy with subcortical infarcts and leucoencephalopathy).

Borderzone Infarction

Also known as watershed ischaemia, this occurs at the boundaries of the major vessel territories—superficially between the leptomeningeal collaterals of the MCA and ACA which also extend into the corona radiata deep to the superior frontal sulcus, and those of the MCA and PCA. In the deep white matter of the inferior corona radiata and external capsules lies the deep borderzone between the cortical branches and deep M1 perforators of the MCA (Fig. 3-3).

Postulated mechanisms include local (e.g. carotid stenosis) and global (e.g. cardiac insufficiency) hypoperfusion, but embolic infarcts at these sites can also occur.

Borderzone ischaemia in the posterior fossa is uncommon but usually occurs between the superior cerebellar artery (SCA) and posterior inferior cerebellar artery (PICA) territories, and occasionally between the SCA, PICA and anterior inferior cerebellar artery (AICA) territories.

Global Hypoxic–Ischaemic Injury

Inadequate oxygen supply to the entire brain can be the consequence of severe hypotension or impaired blood oxygenation. Global hypoperfusion can result in watershed infarcts as described above, but profound hypoxia

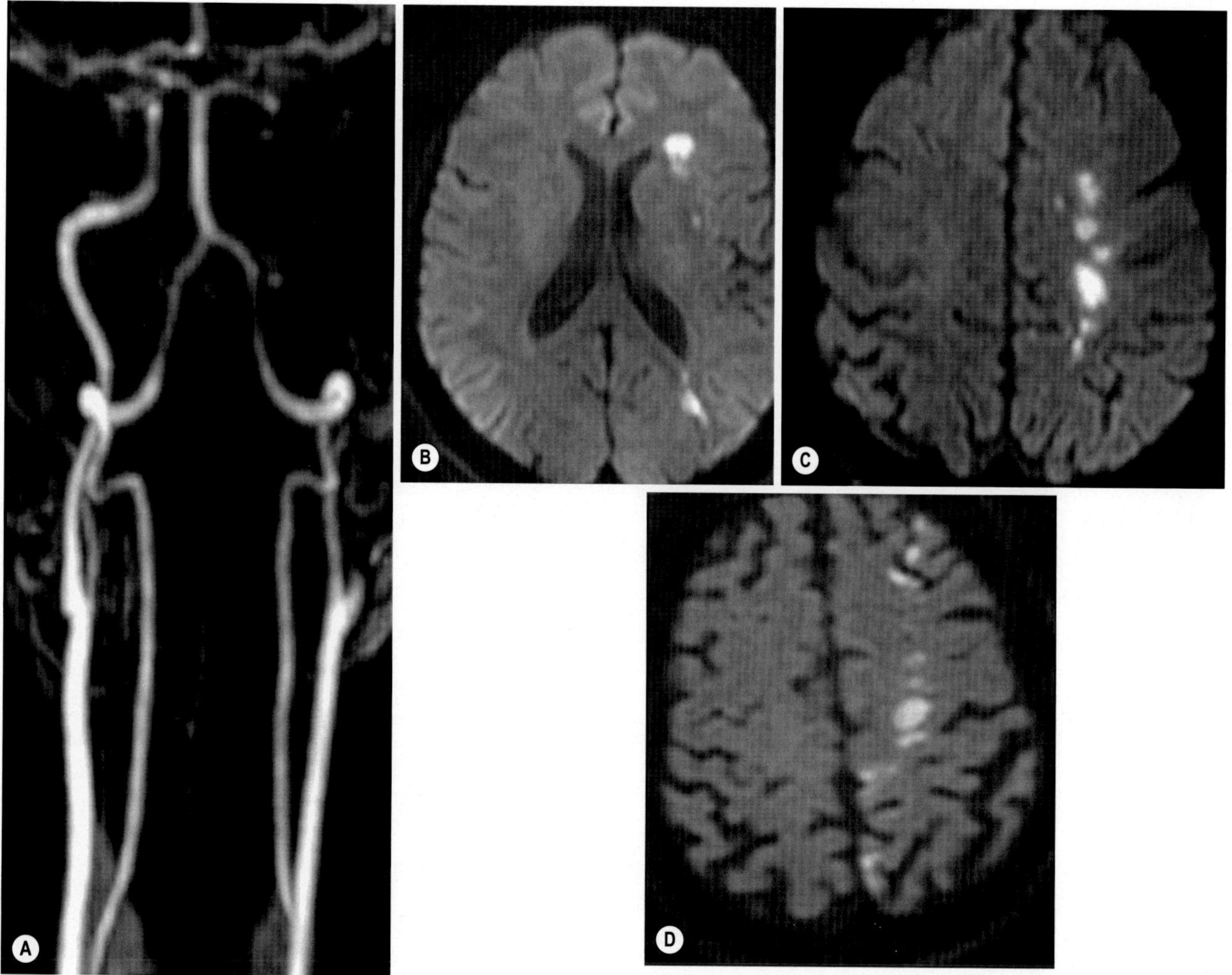

FIGURE 3-3 ■ **Borderzone ischaemia.** There is severe impairment of flow or occlusion in the left ICA from just after its origin (A). This is associated with acute infarcts on DWI in a typical distribution in the left frontal and parietal lobes (B–D), between the MCA and ACA, and MCA and PCA territories. These are presumed to be secondary to hypoperfusion in the left ICA territory. A linear distribution deep to the superior frontal sulcus is very suggestive of ACA–MCA borderzone ischaemia (C, D).

can also cause symmetric ischaemia in the basal ganglia, thalami and hippocampal formations. Anoxia due to defective blood oxygenation such as in carbon monoxide poisoning tends to cause infarcts in sensitive regions, typically, as in this case within the globus pallidus (Fig. 3-4).

Imaging Strategies and Goals in Acute Stroke

Standard Imaging

Brain imaging must be incorporated into the management paradigm of acute stroke. Currently, the only licensed therapy for vessel recanalisation in the acute period involves the administration of intravenous thrombolytic agents—mainly tissue plasminogen activator (tPA). This was derived from key studies (NINDS, ECASS-3 and SITS-MOST)[16–18] which demonstrated significant improvements in the degree of disability at 3 months in patients with ischaemic stroke treated with iv tPA provided they were within 4.5 h of onset, had sustained infarcts of less than one-third of the MCA territory and were less than 80 years old. Traditionally, imaging has been directed at these criteria, employing non-enhanced cranial computed tomography (NECT). Within the past 3 years in the UK following government-initiated restructuring of metropolitan stroke services and considerable investment, thrombolysis rates have risen dramatically from <1% to around 15% in most major hyperacute stroke units (HASUs)—with improvements in outcomes already becoming apparent.[19] In most of these centres, NECT continues to form the mainstay of acute stroke imaging.

Objectives of NECT in Acute Stroke

- To exclude haemorrhage and allow administration of aspirin therapy[20]
- To exclude an alternative cause of the fixed neurological deficit. Around 30% of patients presenting with a stroke-like episode have a non-vascular cause[21]

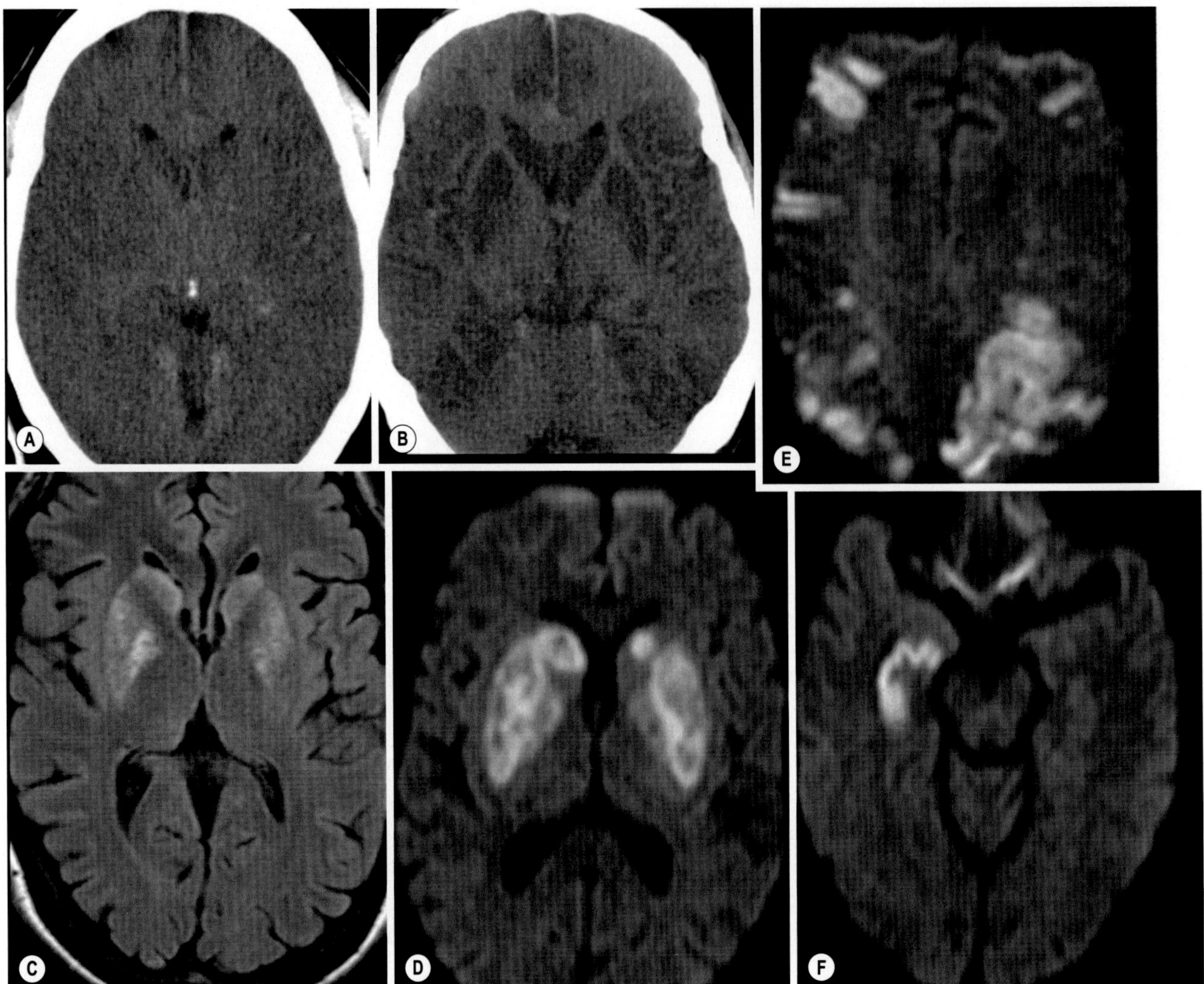

FIGURE 3-4 ■ **Global hypoxic—ischaemic insult.** The cranial imaging manifestations of global hypoperfusion or hypo-oxygenation typically vary according to their severity and age of the patient. In adults, the most common patterns are shown. On plain CT, bilateral symmetric grey matter hypodensity involving the basal ganglia, thalami and cerebral cortex is typical, acutely with cerebral swelling (A). When profound, the normal grey–white matter relationship is reversed (B). Signal change and restricted diffusion is demonstrated in the affected areas on MRI. Again, this is bilateral and symmetric. The basal ganglia are involved on FLAIR (C) and DWI (D), whilst the frontal and parietal lobes are infarcted in (E). Note that the hippocampal formations are also sensitive to global insults (F).

- To exclude infarcts > 1/3 MCA territory
- To establish that the infarct corroborates the clinical timeline and does not obviously appear subacute
- In cases of suspected posterior circulation stroke, to attempt to identify an obviously thrombosed basilar artery

Hyperacute Infarct Imaging Signs

A dense artery is the earliest detectable change on computed tomography (CT). As it is caused by fresh thrombus occluding the vessel it can be seen at the onset of the ictus. Thrombus may rapidly disperse, so this sign is not always present. When found in the proximal MCA or terminal ICA, it correlates with large infarcts and very poor outcomes[22] although it has a better prognosis if limited to an MCA branch within the sylvian fissure (the sylvian fissure 'dot' sign) (Fig. 3-5).[23] MCA calcification can mimic this sign but is often bilateral. The basilar artery may also appear dense in the case of posterior circulation infarcts, particularly the 'top of basilar' syndrome. The early parenchymal signs on CT are reduced grey matter density and brain swelling, manifest as effacement of sulci (Fig. 3-6). These changes are traditionally thought to reflect cytotoxic oedema, which reduces the Hounsfield number of grey matter so it is indistinguishable from adjacent white matter. In early MCA infarcts this causes a reduction in clarity of the margins of the lentiform nucleus and cortex, particularly in the insula. Hypodensity on early CT examinations affecting more than 50% of the MCA territory is associated with a high mortality rate,[24] and intravenous thrombolysis is contraindicated when more than one-third of the MCA territory is involved. However, infarct size evaluation is notoriously difficult in the acute

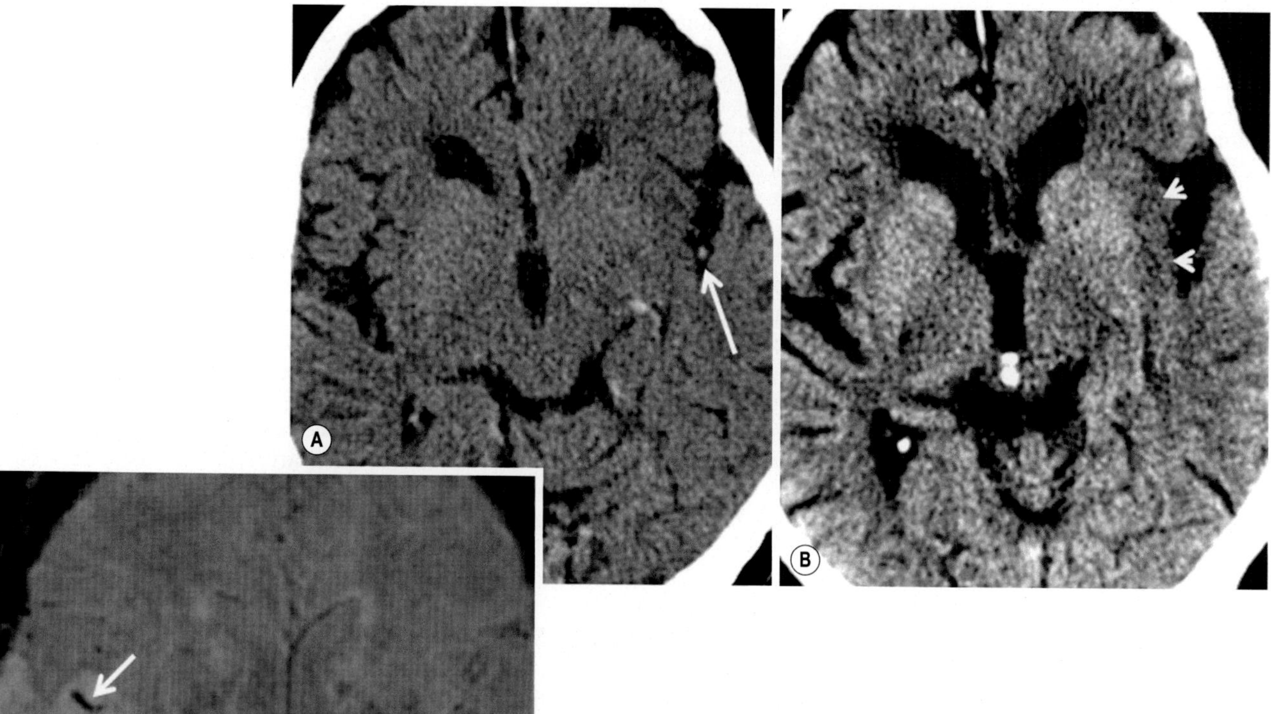

FIGURE 3-5 ■ **Sylvian 'dot' sign.** (A) There is thrombus within an M2 division of the left MCA—shown as a hyperdense dot in the left sylvian fissure (white arrow). This caused by an acute left MCA territory infarct involving the left insula with loss of conspicuity of the cortex. This is made more conspicuous by adjusting the window settings to W = 35, L = 35: the 'stroke' window (B, white arrowheads). Thrombus within a right M2 branch of a different patient is shown here as marked linear hypointensity ('blooming') on the SWI sequence (C, white arrows). This is caused by exaggerated sensitivity to susceptibility artefact afforded by SWI—in this case from deoxyhaemoglobin in acute thrombus.

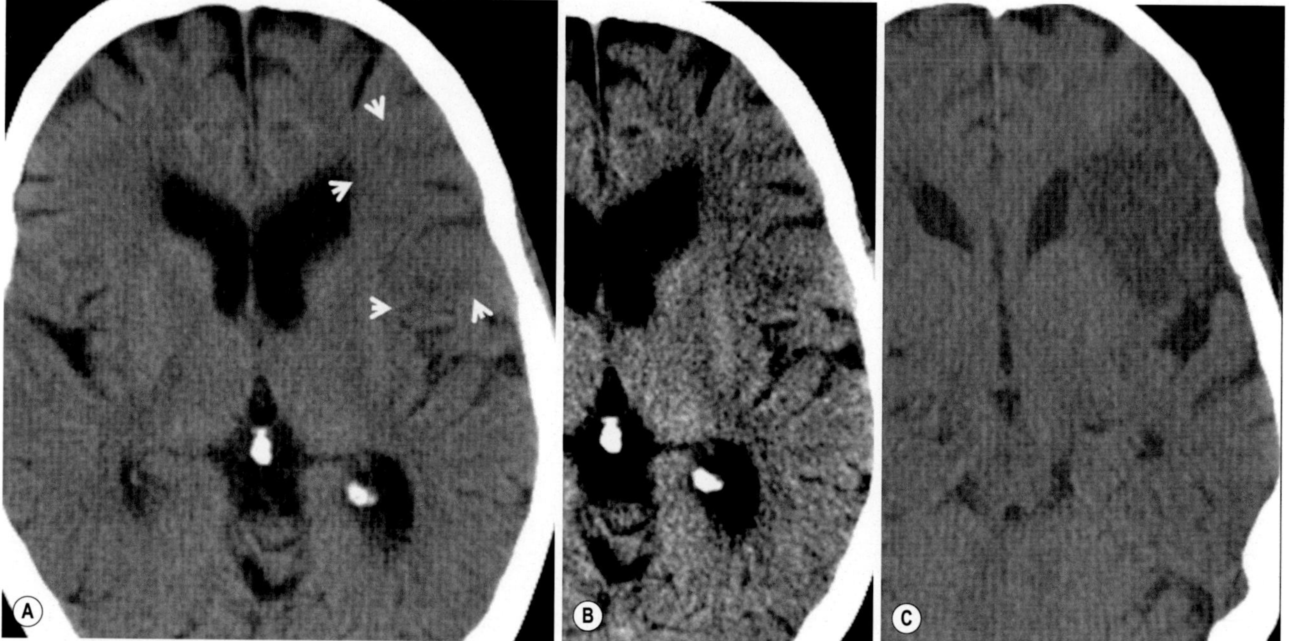

FIGURE 3-6 ■ **Evolution of infarct on CT.** In the hyperacute phase, there is subtle parenchymal swelling with sulcal effacement, and very mild cortical low attenuation with loss of grey–white matter differentiation (A, white arrowheads). This is more conspicuous when window settings are adjusted to 35/35 (B). Subacutely, there is well-demarcated and conspicuous wedge-shaped parenchymal low attenuation, with sulcal effacement (C).

phase, due to the lack of convincing parenchymal changes in 50–60% of NECT within 2 h. The sensitivity of CT for infarcts has been reported to be only 30% at 3 h[25] and 60% at 24 h. These difficulties have led to the development of the Alberta Stroke Program Early CT Score (ASPECTS).[26] ASPECTS can be used to predict outcome and risk of post-thrombolysis haemorrhage. It correlates well with diffusion weighted imaging (DWI) findings at presentation[27] and facilitates more accurate interpretation of emergency CT by nonexperts.[28] Even in patients not suitable for thrombolysis it seems intuitive that a methodical approach such as ASPECTS is likely to increase accuracy and reliability of CT interpretation, at least for supratentorial events (Fig. 3-7). The sensitivity to subtle grey matter low attenuation is enhanced using the 'stroke window' setting when reviewing images (window width = 35/window level = 35).

ASPECTS Infarct Size Scoring System

- Two NECT axial slices are examined (a, level of basal ganglia and internal capsule; b, bodies of the lateral ventricles)
- Ten regions are identified (four deep and six cortical)
- Starting with a score of 10, 1 point is deducted for each of these areas that is involved.
- If the score is <7, the infarct is considered >1/3 of an MCA territory

The key advantages of NECT are that it is very rapid, accessible, simple and safe. Speed is essential as the therapeutic window is closing all the time.

On magnetic resonance imaging (MRI), thrombus may cause loss of a normal arterial flow void. However, arterial high signal may be seen in a patent vessel on

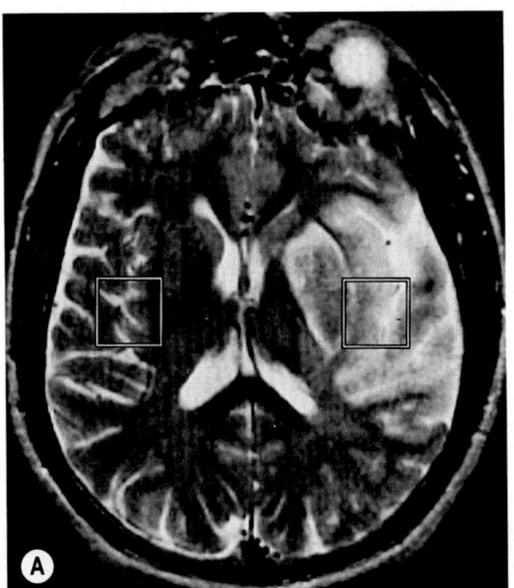

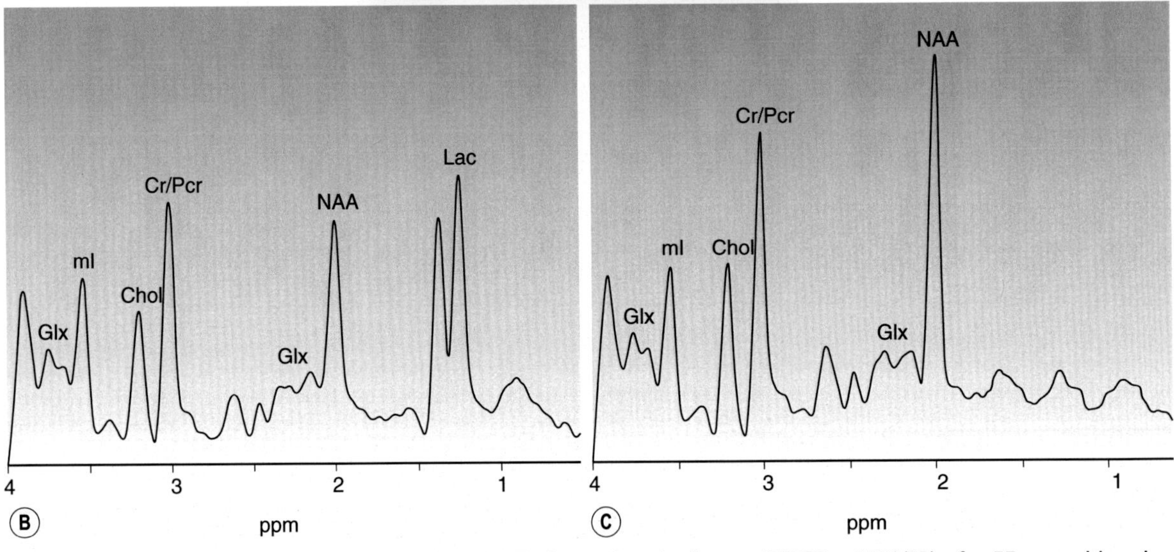

FIGURE 3-7 ■ MR spectroscopy in acute stroke. (A) Axial T2-fast spin-echo image (TR/TE = 3500/95) of a 55-year-old male stroke patient at 14 h from stroke onset, to show the positions of voxels within the infarct and contralateral hemisphere. (B) Proton spectrum (TR 2000/TE 30 ms) acquired at time of presentation on a 1.5 T MR system. The total creatine (3.03 p.p.m.) and choline (3.22 p.p.m.) are reduced, the NAA peak (2.01 p.p.m.) is almost absent and there is a large lactate doublet at 1.33 p.p.m. compared to the contralateral hemisphere. (C) Normal spectrum acquired from the contralateral hemisphere. Resonance peaks are lactate (Lac), N-acetyl aspartate (NAA), creatine (Cr/Pcr), myoinositol (ml), and glutamate and glutamine (Glx).

fluid-attenuated inversion recovery (FLAIR) MRI due to altered flow, a useful qualitative sign of reduced perfusion when the parenchyma usually still appears normal.[29] Intravascular enhancement due to sluggish flow in affected vessels—probably veins—may be seen on contrast-enhanced CT and MRI acutely.[30] Parenchymal MRI changes include cortical swelling and T1/T2 prolongation, more obvious on T2 sequences, particularly FLAIR. Parenchymal hyperintensity is often absent or very subtle in infarcts prior to 3 h,[31,32] suggesting that early parenchymal low density on CT may be due to abnormal perfusion (reduced CBV) rather than oedema.[33] Furthermore, brain swelling on CT without accompanying low density does not always progress to infarction. Such cases may also be due to abnormal perfusion, but a compensatory increase in CBV rather than a reduction.[34] Thus, whilst it is generally accepted that swelling with obvious low density on CT is an indication of infarction, perhaps subtle low density or swelling without low density are sometimes signs of compromised perfusion that may be reversible, particularly the latter. Diffusion-weighted imaging (DWI) has a pre-eminent role in acute stroke imaging due to its extremely high sensitivity and specificity,[35] with parenchymal hyperintensity as early as 5 min following the onset of infarction. DWI should be interpreted in conjunction with an apparent diffusion coefficient (ADC) map, which is derived from the DWI data and in the clinical environment is displayed as a grey scale 'image' for ease of use. 'Restricted diffusion' in acute infarcts returns high signal on DWI and appears dark on the ADC map (Figs. 3-8 and 3-9). Whilst DWI hyperintense areas (with appropriate ADC hypointensity) are considered to and almost always do represent areas of irreversible ischaemia, recently investigators have reported that following early recanalisation with either intravenous agents or mechanical embolectomy, DWI-positive areas may not progress to infarction. This phenomenon does not occur commonly and the proportion of the overall insult which appears to reverse is relatively small. Moreover, the effect is reduced in tissue with more profoundly reduced ADC. Nevertheless it does suggest that DWI-defined early ischemic injury physiologically represents the combination of irreversible ischemic core and a small potentially reversible surrounding area (Fig. 3-10).[36–38]

Whilst NECT has a much higher sensitivity than spin-echo MRI for the detection of acute haemorrhage, T2*-weighted gradient-echo imaging (GRE) has equivalent or superior sensitivity compared with CT.[39–41] The sensitivity for detection of deoxygenated haemoglobin—the key moiety in acute haemorrhage—is further enhanced with the susceptibility-weighted imaging (SWI) sequence.[42]

Advanced Imaging

The availability of neuroradiological expertise, multislice CT technology and improved access to MRI in some, typically neuroscience, units allows the delivery of advanced imaging techniques. These include 'penumbral imaging' which attempts to establish the relationship of the irreversible core infarct with any potentially salvageable but ischaemic penumbra; angiographic imaging to identify the site of vascular compromise and additional techniques such as permeability imaging and SWI. In the setting of hyperacute stroke, the challenge is to deliver this information rapidly.

Objectives of Penumbral Imaging

- To more accurately delineate the size of the core infarct
- To establish whether a penumbra of salvageable tissue is present

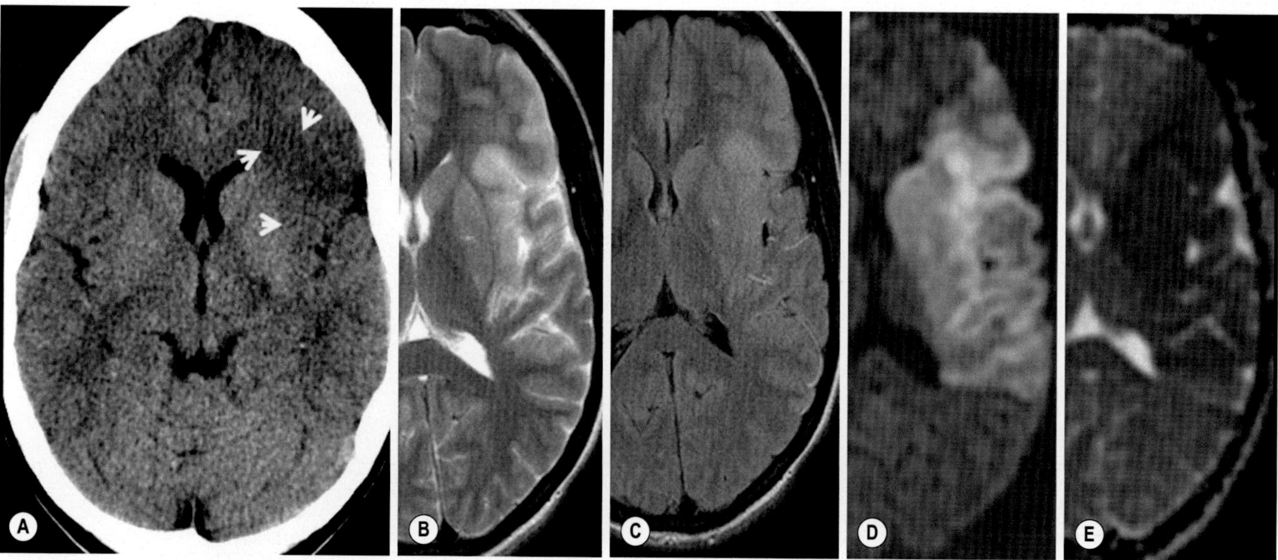

FIGURE 3-8 ■ An acute left MCA territory infarct presenting 7 h after onset is visible on CT (A) as low attenuation in the left frontal operculum and left insula. At this stage, not only is the infarct shown as T2 hyperintensity and gyral swelling but also more extensive involvement of the left MCA territory is identified on T2-weighted and FLAIR imaging (B, C). However, the full extent of involvement—including the basal ganglia—is only clearly demonstrated on DWI (D) as hyperintensity and on the corresponding ADC map (E) as hypointensity.

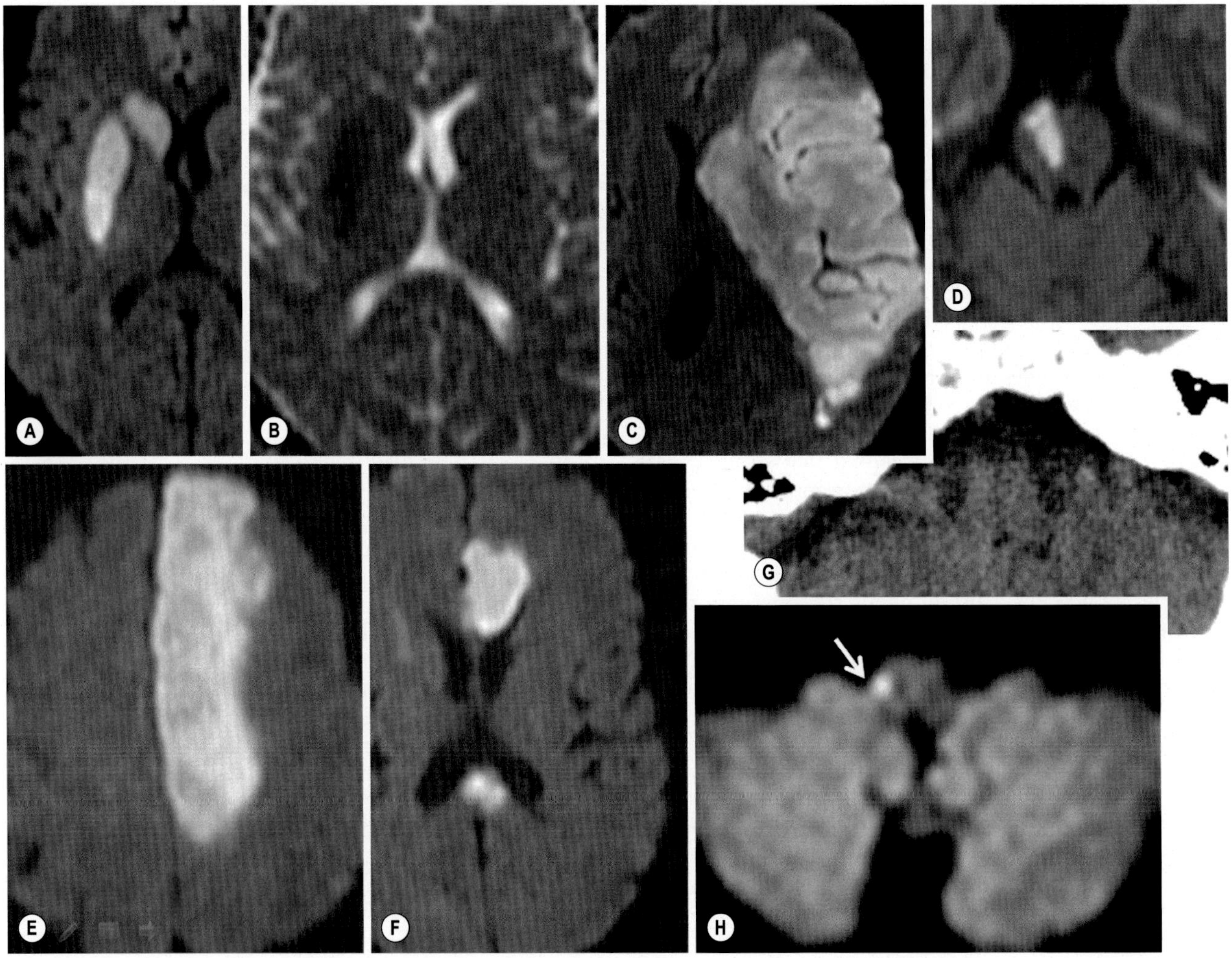

FIGURE 3-9 ■ **Acute territorial infarcts on DWI.** Acute right-sided striatal infarct with hyperintensity on DWI (A) and hypointensity on ADC (B). Other acute infarcts involving the entire left MCA (C) and left ACA (E, F) territories. Note the involvement of the left side of the genu and splenium of the corpus callosum in (F). However, the splenium is often supplied by the PCA. (D) A typical perforator infarct in the pons involving the anteromedial aspect of the basis pontis. A small right PICA territory infarct involving the posterolateral aspect of the right side of the medulla is shown on DWI (H, white arrow), but is inconspicuous on CT (G).

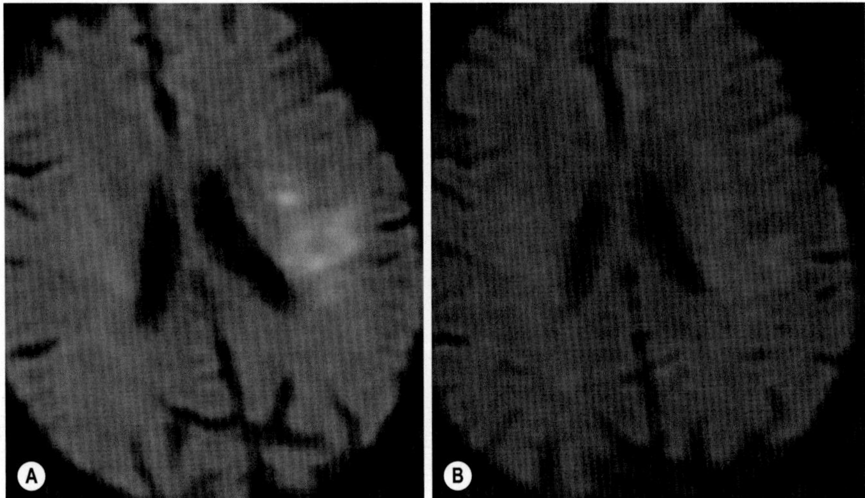

FIGURE 3-10 ■ **DWI reversibility.** This patient presented with right hemiparesis at 4 h post onset. Initial DWI at presentation (A) showed a modest area of restricted diffusion consistent with a small core infarct. However, on the subsequent MRI performed at 24 h post iv thrombolysis (B), there has been some resolution of the DWI abnormality, rather than progression to an established infarct.

- To evaluate the size and severity of ischaemia of the penumbra

The following should be considered in this analysis:

- Large core infarcts have a poorer outcome, regardless of penumbra size or severity. Specifically, core volumes greater than 70 mL are associated with adverse outcomes regardless of recanalisation therapy.[43]
- Core infarcts with small penumbra are described as 'matched' defects and carry reduced reperfusion benefit. However, some units proceed with thrombolysis in this situation because of the possibility of partial reversibility of the DWI-positive volume.
- Large areas of salvageable tissue, known as 'mismatch,' are likely to benefit most from recanalisation therapy.[44–46]
- Areas of mildly ischaemic penumbra may reperfuse spontaneously—known as 'benign oligaemia'.
- Appropriate patient selection using penumbral imaging may extend the therapeutic time window beyond 4.5 h.[47–49]

Perfusion Imaging. In the context of stroke, perfusion imaging with CT (CTP) and perfusion weighted MRI (PWI) is most often performed using a first-pass intravenous contrast technique. In PWI, this is achieved using dynamic susceptibility contrast enhancement (DSE-MRI), which relies on the long-range susceptibility effects of gadolinium resulting in a reduction in signal intensity as it transits through brain tissue. By mathematical deconvolution of the time-density (CT) or time-negative signal intensity (MRI) curves which are generated, 3 parameters are usually studied:

- relative cerebral blood volume (rCBV)—essentially the area under the curve
- relative cerebral blood flow (rCBF)—related to the gradient of the curve at contrast arrival
- mean transit time (MTT)—calculated from the Central Volume Principle: MTT = CBV/CBF

These are typically depicted as colour maps. However, there is considerable debate in the literature as to which of the parameters is the most reliable surrogate marker of core and of penumbra. Earlier studies employed first-generation perfusion scanning protocols with shorter acquisition times of 40–50 s which resulted in potential underestimation of both CBV and MTT due to failure to image the whole of the time–density or time signal–intensity curves, Furthermore, standard post-processing algorithms with no correction for the delay in contrast arrival—such as due to a stenosis or haemodynamic instability—exposed the interpretation to underestimation of CBF and overestimation of MTT.[50–54] Whilst new protocols allow for longer acquisition times (60–70 s), and many of the latest-generation post-processing platforms now correct for delay, there is still considerable variability and lack of standardisation in the parameters generated from scanning machines and platforms (or even different versions of the same platform) from different vendors.[55–59] This is particularly true with CT perfusion. Recent reports suggest that newer techniques do allow more accurate and reliable characterisation of the core and penumbra on imaging.[60–62] These are given in Table 3-1.

TABLE 3-1 Thresholds for Determining Infarct Core and Penumbra With CT and MR Perfusion Imaging

	CTP	PWI-MRI
Infarct core	Thresholded CBF (nominally better than CBV)	DWI
Ischaemic penumbra	Thresholded MTT (probably better than CBF)	Thresholded MTT and CBF

As alluded to earlier, the size of the infarct core is the single most important imaging parameter in determining whether recanalisation therapy would be appropriate. Whilst fluorodeoxyglucose (FDG) positron emission tomography (PET) is considered the most accurate, it is clearly not the most practical for clinical use. In descending order, DWI, thresholded CT-CBF, CT-CBV (both from CT perfusion) and CTA-source data are more sensitive and precise than NECT.[63] Unfortunately, for CT perfusion, the threshold at which the CBF should be set to establish the core varies between platforms but is generally 70–85% reduction compared with the normal contralateral side.[61] It remains unclear as to why perfusion imaging derived CBV approximates to the DWI-defined core, when experimentally, CBV rarely falls in an infarct. Additionally, a volume of tissue which has infarcted but then becomes rapidly reperfused may become masked and appear normal on CBV.[64]

Delay-corrected MTT is considered the most reliable biomarker of the penumbra in CT perfusion when appropriately thresholded, at 150% relative to the contralateral normal side.[62] This threshold discriminates between the genuinely 'at-risk' tissue and the region of benign oligaemia. Simultaneous evaluation of CBF should corroborate this as CBF will generally be preserved or only mildly reduced in benign oligaemia, but more significantly diminished in at-risk tissue (Fig. 3-11).

T_{max} is an additional parameter generated by perfusion imaging—at the time of the CBF calculation—and has been used as a penumbra biomarker.[48]

Mismatch is usually accepted as the volume of penumbra, being at least 20% larger than the core.

Angiographic Imaging. Improvements in endovascular device design and the availability of fast, non-invasive angiographic techniques to rapidly identify the site of the occluded vessel are driving a revolution towards intra-arterial thrombolysis and probably, more effectively, endovascular mechanical embolectomy in acute stroke treatment. In comparison with iv tPA therapy, these strategies are not only more successful in recanalising occluded cerebral vessels[65–67] but also are likely to deliver more favourable outcomes in the treatment of strokes from occluded major vessels such as the distal ICA and proximal MCA, and may well prolong the therapeutic window significantly beyond 4.5 h in selected patients. Furthermore, endovascular procedures to recanalise an occluded basilar artery are considered appropriate even up to 18 h. In addition, mechanical embolectomy can be employed when there is a contraindication to tPA, most notably anticoagulant therapy and recent surgery.

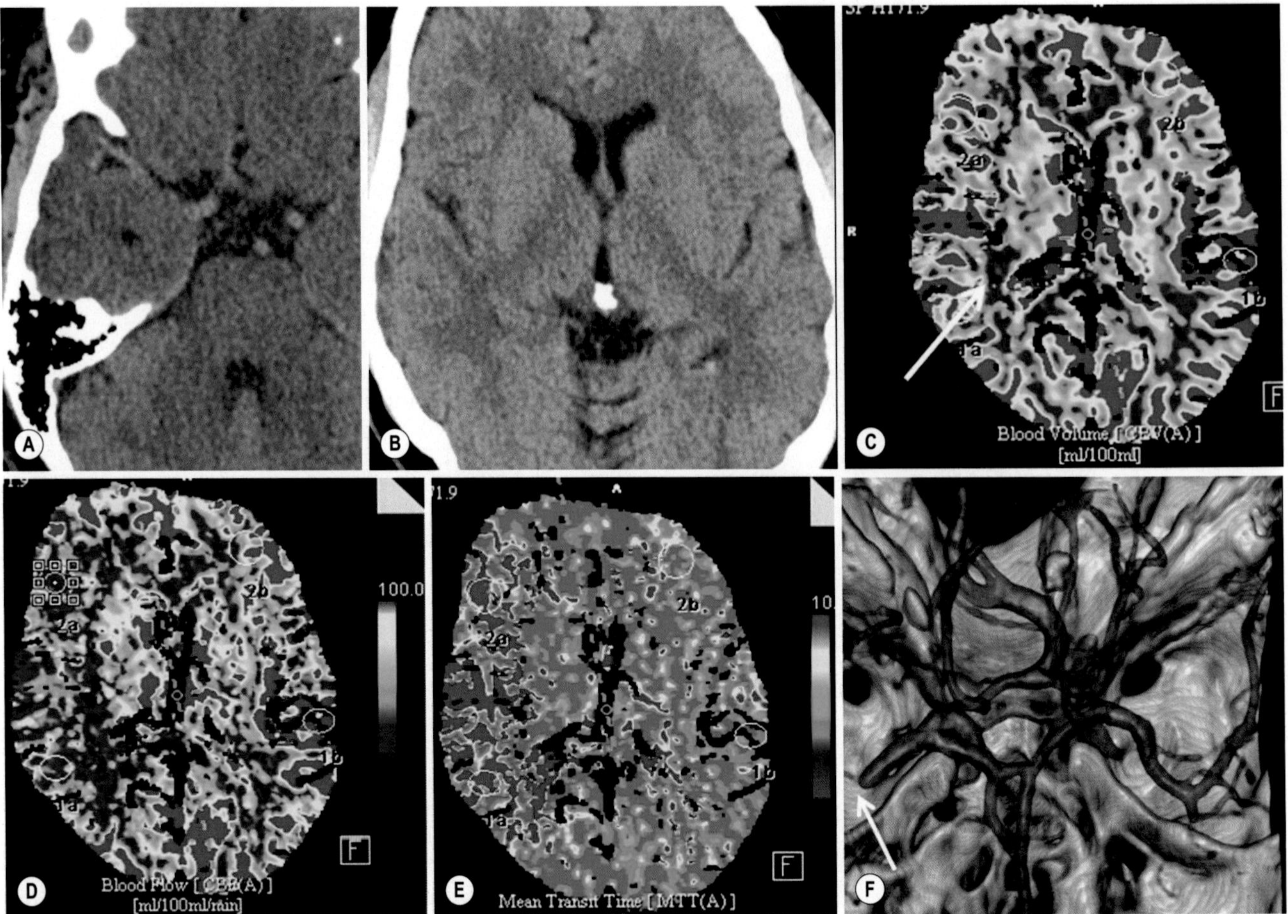

FIGURE 3-11 ■ **Ischaemic penumbra on CT perfusion.** (A, B) Within 2 h of left-sided hemiparesis, the non-contrast enhanced CT was normal. Note that there is no vessel hyperdensity. (C) However, there is a small area of reduced CBV in the right temporo-occipital white matter (white arrow), indicating only a very small 'core' of irreversibly infarcted tissue. (D, E) The CBF and MTT perfusion maps demonstrate a large volume of ischaemic but potentially salvageable tissue, with prolonged transit times (warm colours, E) and reduced cerebral blood flow (cold colours, D). (F) Volume-rendered image from a CT angiogram shows occlusion of the M1 segment of the right middle cerebral artery (white arrow).

In the US, the MERCI™ device has been approved for use up to 8 h post onset.[66] Current technology primarily involves a stent-clot retriever device.

However, procedure-related complication rates are high and there is a paucity of Level 1 data demonstrating a clear overall benefit. Indeed, only one randomised controlled trial has been conducted, evaluating intra-arterial therapy—in this case intra-arterial thrombolysis. This did demonstrate a significant improvement in outcomes compared with intravenous heparin.[68] In several non-randomised control trial open label trials, functional outcomes were poorer than with iv tPA. Longer times to recanalisation (relating to anaesthesia, endovascular access and device deployment) and the selection bias of more severe strokes likely account for much of this.[69]

Nevertheless these techniques are set to become a more common therapeutic option for strokes where the thrombus is in the distal ICA or proximal MCA, or in the basilar artery.[70] Therefore, initial angiographic imaging to identify an appropriate endovascular target is a necessity. As shown above, this can be most effectively achieved using CT, as part of a multimodal examination also delivering penumbral information with CT perfusion. However, data sets are large (typically >200 slices from the aortic arch to the circle of Willis) and reviewing these can take time. By contrast, interpretation of the maximum intensity projection (MIP) images of an MRA is rapid (Figs. 3-12–3-14).

Useful information regarding the extracranial neck arteries is also provided with CT angiography (CTA) or magnetic resonance angiography (MRA). In particular, possible embolic sources in the aortic arch and carotid bifurcation are well demonstrated, as are alternative aetiologies such as vessel dissection.

When acquired correctly (i.e. with saline chase following the iv contrast injection), the thin-slice CT angiographic images of the head (known as the CTA-source data) approximate to relative cerebral blood volume maps. When reviewed on a 35 window width/35 window level setting ('stroke window'), low density on the CTA-source data depicts the infarct core and correlates well with CBV maps from perfusion CT.[63]

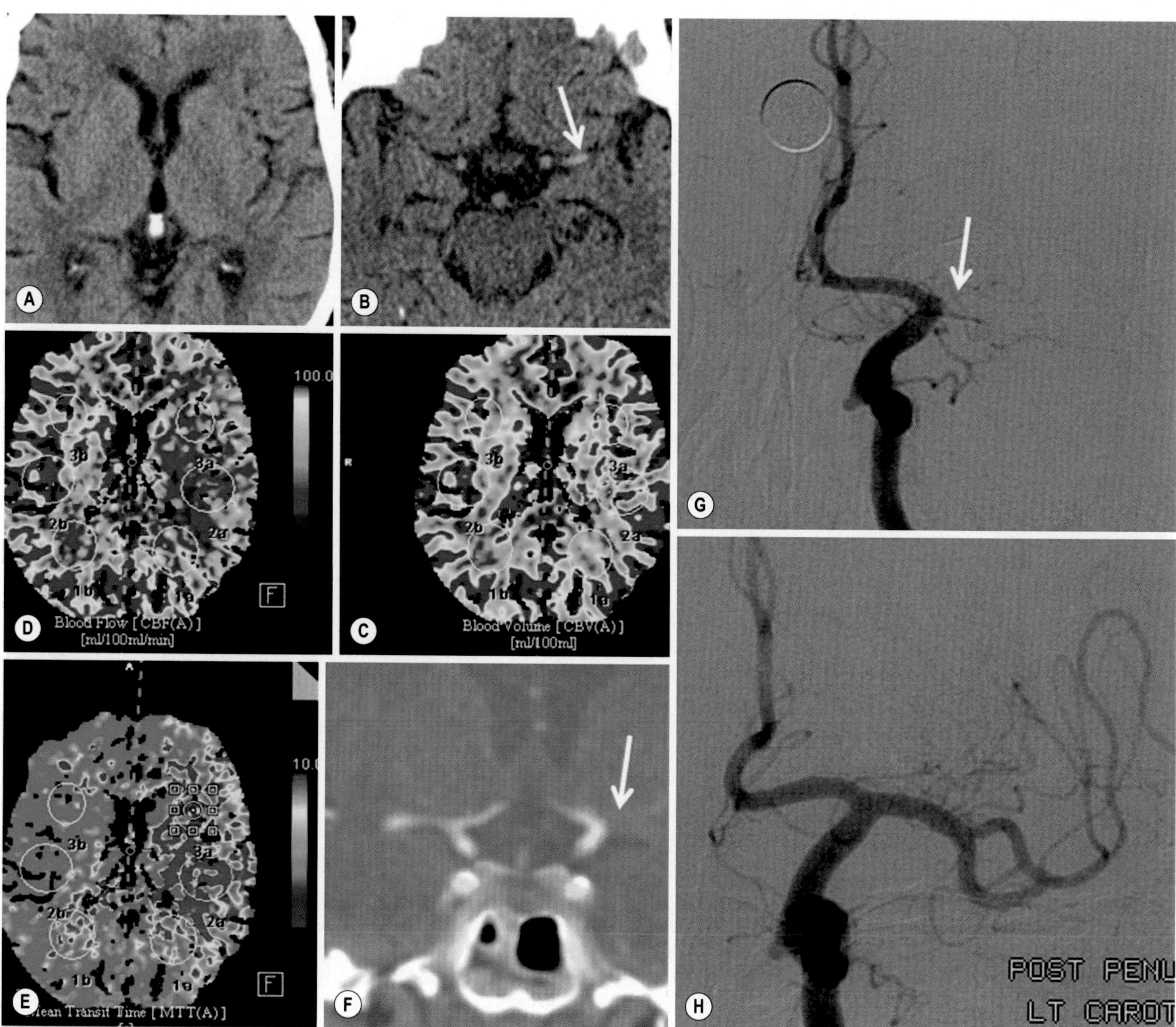

FIGURE 3-12 ■ Mechanical thrombectomy to recanalise an occluded left MCA following identification of a large penumbra using CTP. Within 90 min of the onset of severe right hemiparesis and receptive aphasia, the plain CT showed a hyperdense left M1 segment (B, white arrow) but no parenchymal changes (A). There is also no evidence of a core infarct on the CBV maps (C) but there is significant mismatch with a large penumbra on both CBF (D) and MTT (E) maps. CT angiography confirms occlusion of the left MCA from its origin (F, white arrow), as does the digital subtraction catheter angiogram performed prior to endovascular intervention (G). Following a single pass with a stent clot-retriever device, there has been complete recanalisation of the left MCA (H).

Assessment of Collateral Flow. The importance of perfusion to ischaemic brain tissue via an alternate route is becoming increasingly recognised. This 'collateral' flow—chiefly via leptomeningeal vessels—if adequate is likely to sustain ischaemic tissue for hours or even days after a vessel occlusion. In these areas, CBF and CBV are likely to be preserved whilst the MTT is prolonged. Improved collateral supply is associated with milder deficits, smaller final infarcts and improved outcomes after major vessel occlusions.[71] Imaging the collateral supply is challenging and a number of studies have employed a variety of techniques, from catheter angiography[72] to CTA,[73] MRA[74] and transcranial Doppler ultrasound.[75] CTA is likely to be the most accessible method, as part of the multimodal approach to acute stroke imaging.

Additional Advanced Imaging Techniques. Perfusion imaging, including PET, is also used for elective assessment of haemodynamic reserve and stroke risk. For example, perfusion may be normal at rest despite a significant carotid stenosis but show reduced blood flow following acetazolamide challenge, which is the reverse of normal.[76,77] Single-photon emission computed tomography (SPECT) with ^{99m}Tc-HMPAO will show a perfusion defect as soon as vascular occlusion occurs, although care must be taken in interpretation of HMPAO SPECT studies 10 days or more after the onset of stroke due to hyperfixation of the radiopharmaceutical in infarcted tissue.[78] Quantification of the degree of ischaemia using HMPAO SPECT will predict risk of intracranial haemorrhage following intra-arterial thrombolysis[79]

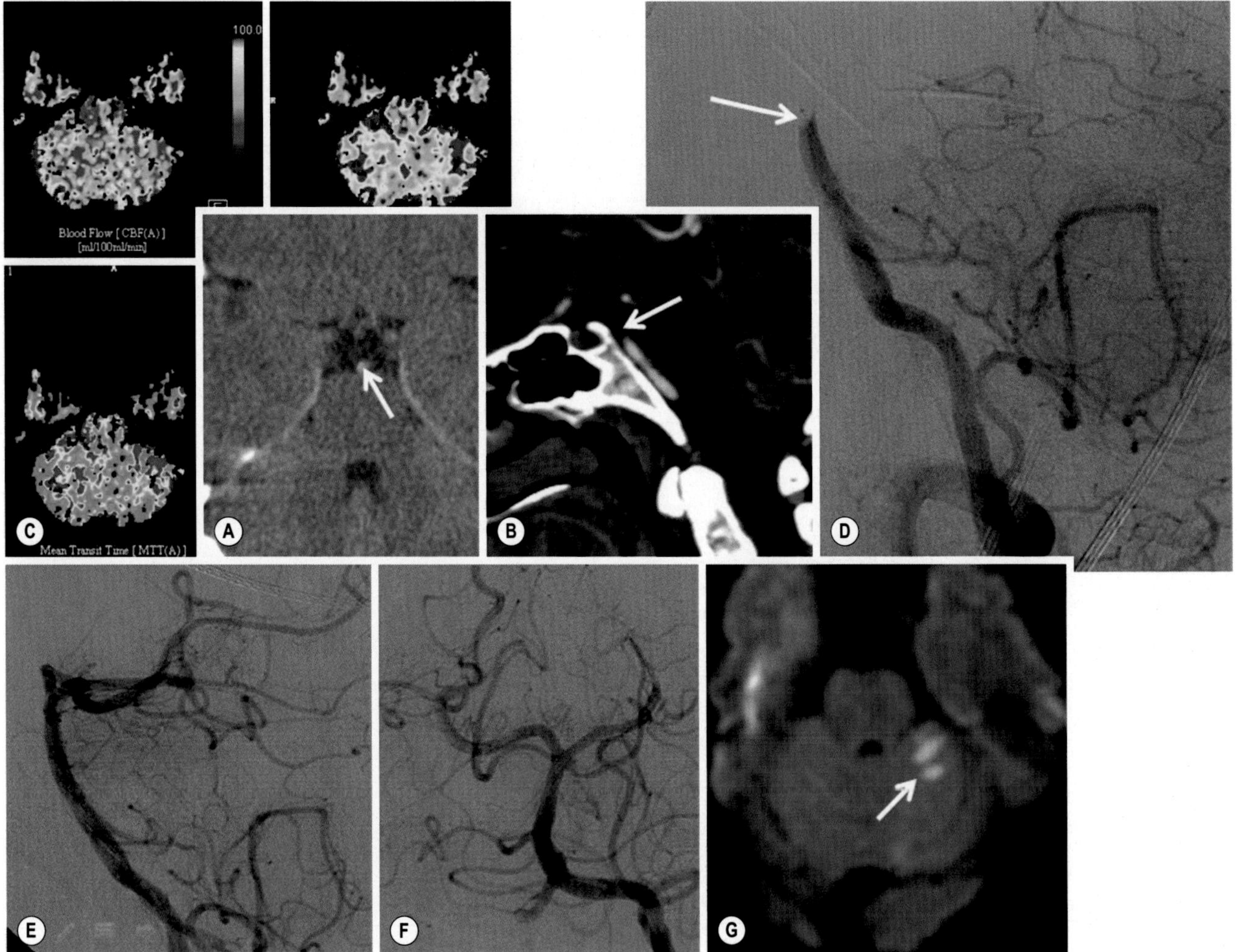

FIGURE 3-13 ■ **Basilar artery thrombectomy.** A young woman presenting with a stuttering progressive reduction in consciousness, a complex ophthalmoplegia and nystagmus was shown to have a hyperdense distal basilar artery on plain CT (A, white arrow). CT angiography confirmed occlusion of the distal basilar artery (B, white arrow) and hypoperfusion was present in the superior aspects of both cerebellar hemispheres on CTP (C, warm colours on MTT). Mechanical thrombectomy, deploying a thrombo-aspirator device, was performed, resulting in complete recanalisation of the basilar artery, shown on digital subtraction angiography following left vertebral artery injection (E and F, compared with D), with total clinical recovery. An MRI performed at 24 h shows only a small infarct in the left superior cerebellar hemisphere (G, white arrow).

but there is currently no practical use for isotope studies in the acute setting.

In addition to the increased sensitivity for acute haemorrhage, SWI also depicts the acutely thrombosed segment of a major intracranial vessel as a prominent, markedly hypointense, expanded, serpiginous structure due to the exaggerated 'blooming' effect.[42] Furthermore, early studies suggest that the ischaemic but potentially salvageable brain tissue may be shown on SWI as tissue with prominent hypointense parenchymal and pial vessels due to engorgement of veins with deoxygenated blood (Figs. 3-15C and 3-15E).[80]

Permeability imaging, which provides imaging biomarkers of the integrity of the blood–brain barrier, can be performed using longer-acquisition CT perfusion or dynamic contrast-enhanced perfusion MRI (DCE-MRI), which is also a first-pass contrast-enhanced perfusion study but evaluates the T1 effects of contrast passage, as opposed to the T2* (susceptibility) effects of DSE described earlier. There is some evidence that increased permeability in infarcted/ischaemic brain tissue is predictive of subsequent haemorrhage following recanalisation therapy in both animal and human experiments.[81–87]

CT or MRI? Penumbral imaging can be achieved effectively on both CT and MR platforms, using perfusion techniques. Despite the superior characterisation of the acute infarct with DWI, whole brain coverage with PWI, rapid visual assessment of vessel occlusion on MRA and at least comparable ability (to NECT) of GRE T2* or SWI to identify acute haemorrhage (Fig. 3-15), multimodal CT appears to have maintained its foothold in most UK neuroscience units. This is largely due to the near-whole head coverage of perfusion CT in machines with 128 slices or more, the rapid acquisition times, much greater access, the reliability of CT angiography (to be discussed later) and rapid more often automated post-processing. Logistical issues regarding immediate access

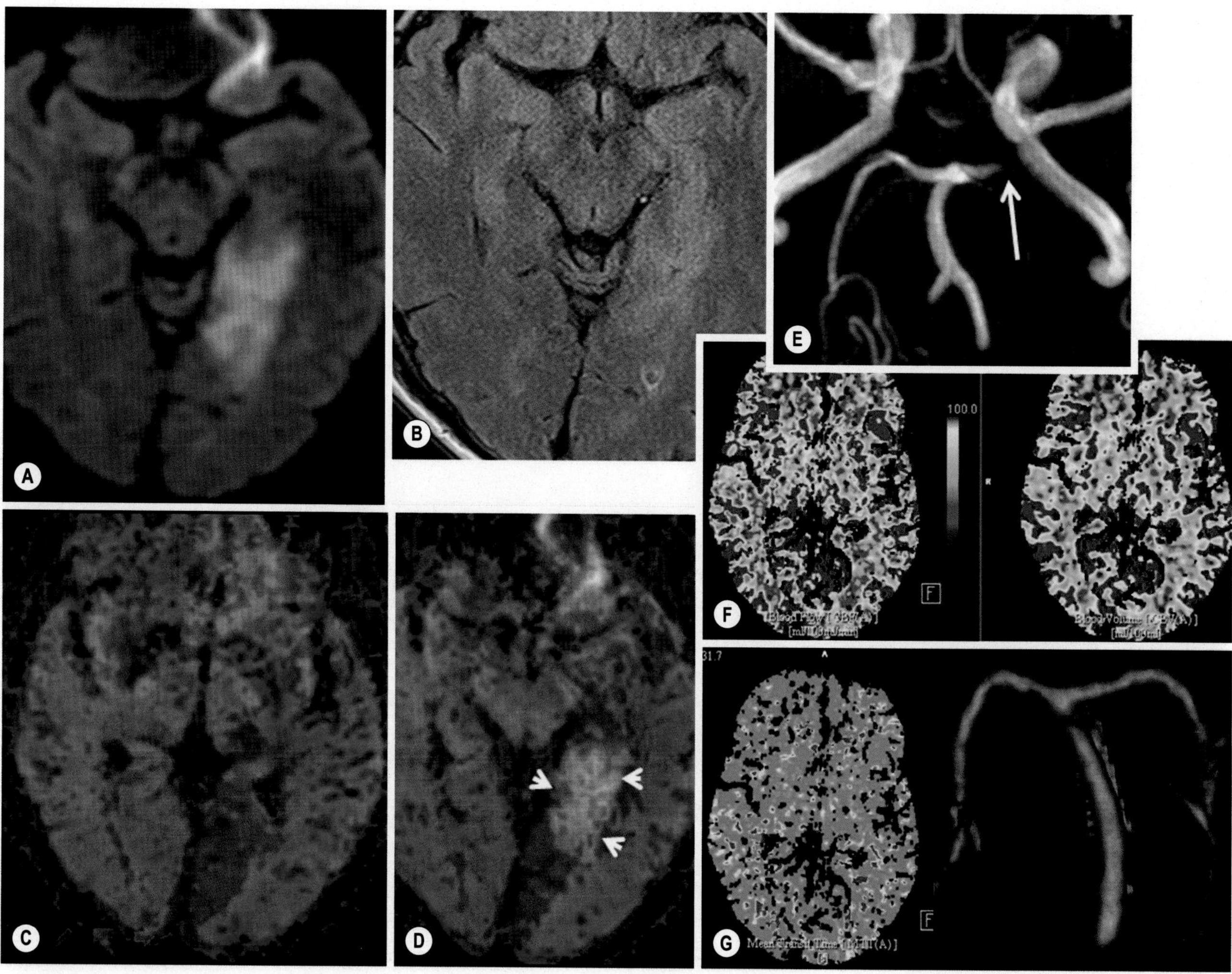

FIGURE 3-14 ■ Recanalisation of the left PCA with intravenous thrombolysis in a patient who woke up with a right hemiparesis and visual disturbance. (A) DWI MRI demonstrates hyperintensity consistent with an acute infarct in the left PCA territory but which is only minimally hyperintense on the FLAIR sequence (B), indicating onset within the last 4.5 h. MRI perfusion fused with DWI shows a significant penumbra with elevated MTT depicted in red against the acute infarct in white (C and D, white arrowheads). The time-of-flight MRA shows severe impairment of flow in the left PCA (E, white arrow), which recanalises completely following iv thrombolysis on CT angiography (G) with restoration of the normal perfusion parameters on CT perfusion (F).

to MRI, prolonged imaging times (not just acquisition, but safety and patient transfers) and post-processing has hampered the role of MRI—particularly evident in the poor recruitment to MRI-based multicentre stroke trials.

CT perfusion techniques also appear to afford more quantitative capability than standard dynamic susceptibility MR perfusion imaging. This permits the utilisation of thresholds for cerebral blood flow and mean transit time to attempt to identify at-risk tissue as discussed earlier. However, there is variability between CT machines, processing platforms and software versions, which precludes the application of this uniformly.

Arterial spin labelling MR perfusion (ASL) provides an assessment of cerebral blood flow without the need for a contrast injection.[88] It is less sensitive to susceptibility and motion effects but is affected by delay phenomena (as with contrast). It is currently a specialised technique, beginning its translation from research environments into clinical practice (Table 3-2).

TABLE 3-2 **Multimodal Stroke Imaging Platforms**

	CT	MRI
Multimodal technique	NECT + CTA + CTP	DWI + PWI + SWI + FLAIR + T1W + CEMRA
Times		
Acquisition	3–5 min	11–13 min
Total imaging time	8–12 min	20–40 min
Post-processing	5 min	5–10 min
Total	13–17 min	25–50 min

NECT = non-contrast-enhanced CT; CTA = CT angiography; CTP = CT perfusion; DWI = diffusion-weighted imaging; PWI = perfusion-weighted MRI; SWI = susceptibility-weighted imaging (for acute haemorrhage); CEMRA = contrast-enhanced MRA.

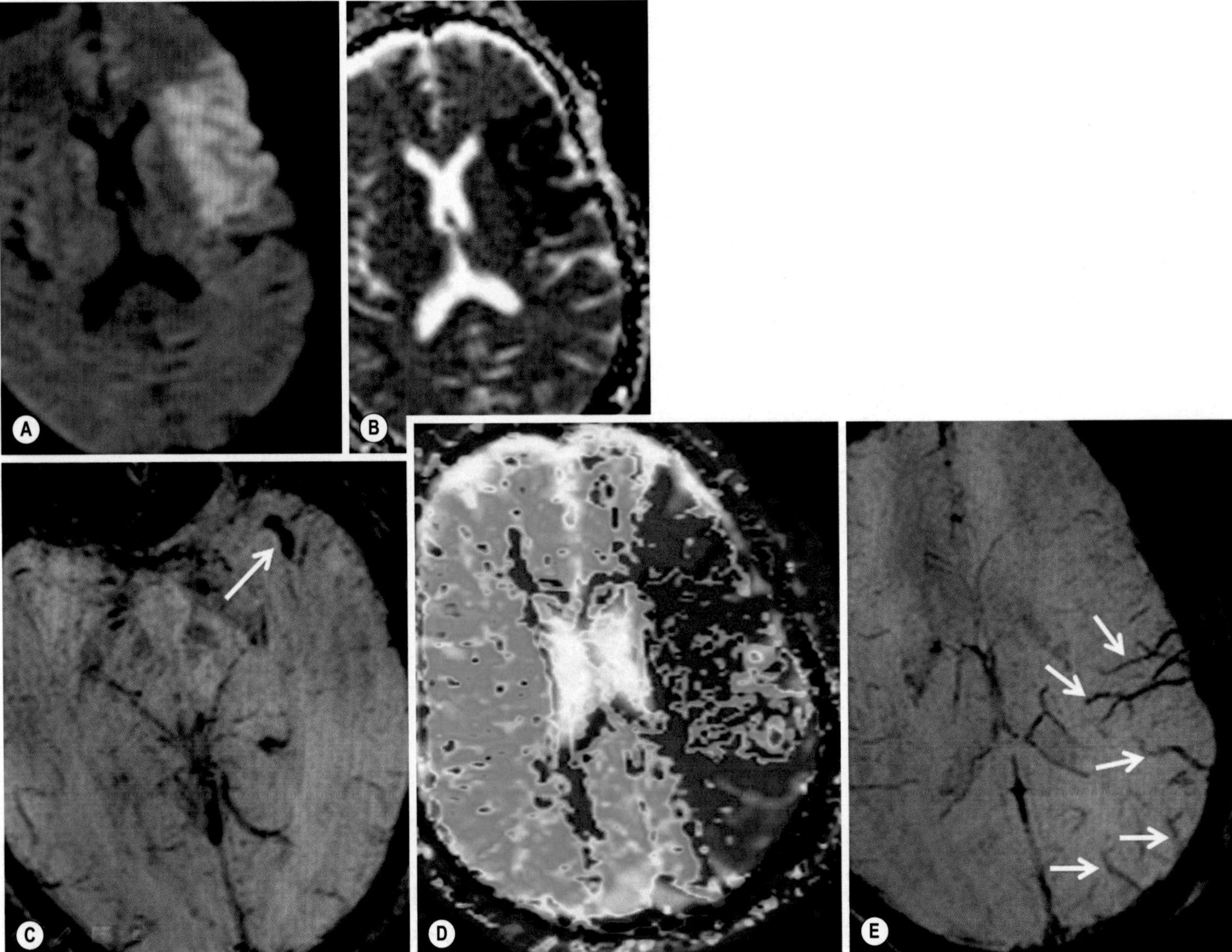

FIGURE 3-15 ■ **Acute stroke MRI imaging.** This patient presented at 5 h following the onset of right hemiparesis and dysphasia. There is an acute left MCA territory infarct represented by parenchymal hyperintensity on DWI (A) and hypointensity on ADC (B). There is a short segment of profound linear hypointensity ('blooming') in the proximal left M2 on SWI (C, white arrow) consistent with intraluminal thrombus. MRI perfusion fused with DWI (D) reveals a significant mismatch with a large area of ischaemic penumbra (red area) in relation to the core infarct (blue area). Prominent hypointense vessels on SWI are also shown in the ischaemic territory beyond the core infarct and may represent the penumbra (E, white arrows). Despite this, this patient was not thrombolysed due to the size of the core infarct and time of presentation.

Multimodal CT can therefore be more easily incorporated into the management of acute stroke patients without substantial detriment to the therapeutic opportunity.

The main clinical application of penumbral imaging in hyperacute stroke is for the assessment of suitability for thrombolytic therapy in:

- Cases presenting 3–6 hours after onset.
- Cases with an unclear time of onset, for example 'wake-up' strokes. That is, where the onset was whilst the patient was asleep and no precise time of onset is known. FLAIR imaging can also be helpful here. The degree of mismatch between the DWI and FLAIR hyperintensity may allow assessment of the volume of infarcted tissue within 6 hours of onset. Tissue infarcted for less than 3 hours is likely to be negative or only very subtly abnormal on FLAIR, whilst tissue infarcted for more than 4.5 h is most likely to be hyperintense on FLAIR (Fig. 3-16).[31,32]
- Clinically severe strokes to determine whether the deficits can be accounted for by a large area of reversible ischaemia (potential benefit with therapy) or a substantial core infarct, where the risk of post-thrombolysis haemorrhage is significantly higher.
- And when considering mechanical thrombectomy as a rescue therapy when iv treatment has failed.

Subacute and Chronic Infarct Imaging Signs

In the **subacute phase** there is structural breakdown and blood–brain barrier disruption. Fluid leaks into the extracellular space, causing well-demarcated low attenuation on CT and T2 hyperintensity on MRI that involves both grey and white matter in large infarcts. The severity and duration of brain swelling depends on infarct size. It usually increases during the first week, persists during the second week and then regresses. Other diagnoses such as tumour or infection should be considered if there is

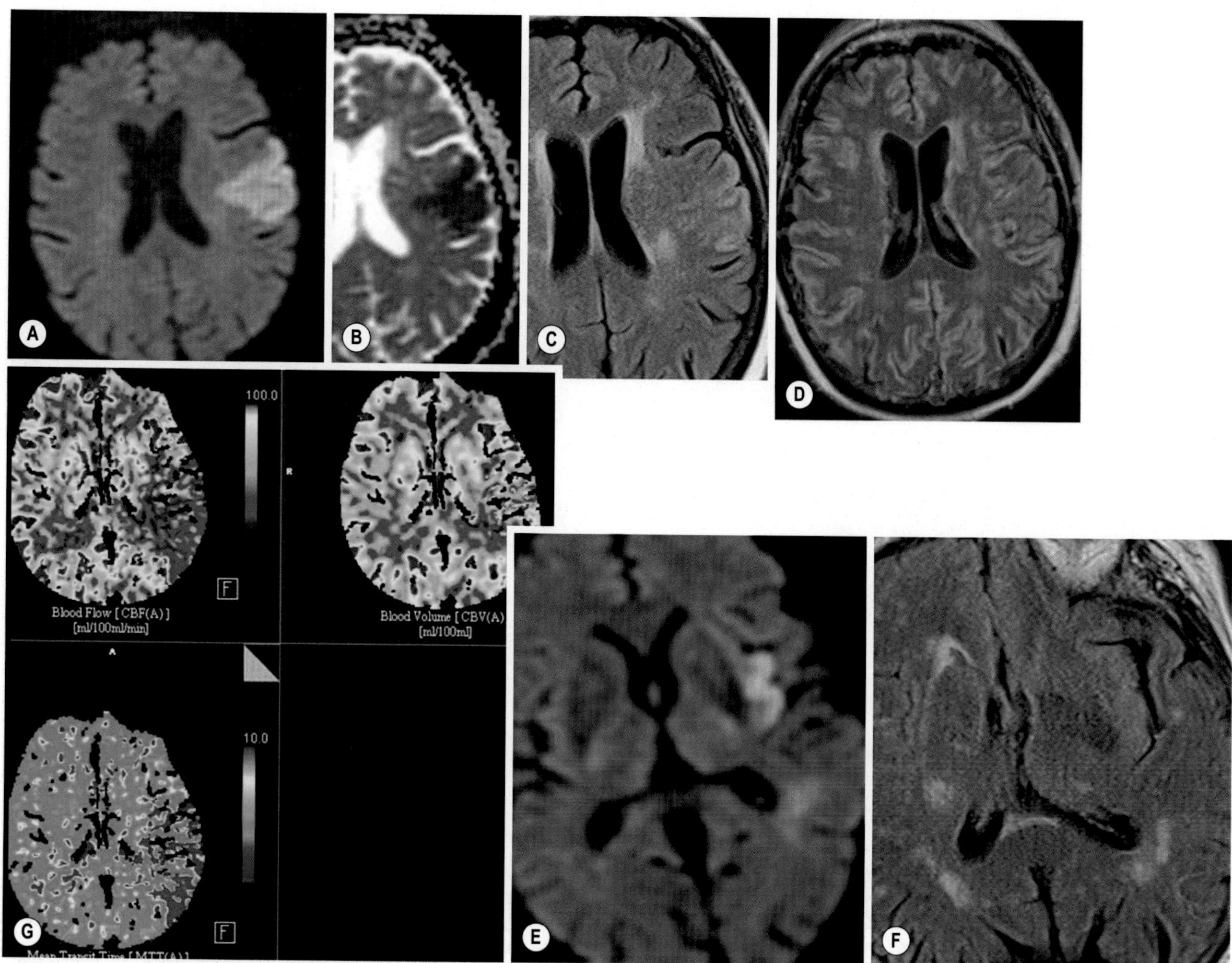

FIGURE 3-16 ■ **Wake-up strokes.** (A–D) This patient presented with a right hemiparesis having woken from sleep. Whilst there is an acute infarct depicted by hyperintensity on the DWI (A) and hypointensity on the ADC map (B), there is also clear cortical hyperintensity in this area on the FLAIR sequence (C). This suggests that the onset was very likely to be longer than 3 h previously and closer to 6 h. MRI perfusion did not demonstrate a significant penumbra, with no CBF deficit (D). This patient was not treated with recanalisation therapy. (E–G) By contrast, this patient who also awoke with symptoms of a left MCA territory infarct, was treated with iv thrombolysis. DWI MRI showed a small core infarct in the left insula (E), which was only minimally hyperintense on FLAIR (F), and therefore considered to be within 4.5 h of inctus. CT perfusion demonstrated mismatch with a moderately large area of potentially reversible ischaemia in the left temporoparietal region (G).

extensive white matter oedema without cortical involvement or prolonged brain swelling.

Contrast enhancement on CT and MR due to blood–brain barrier disruption is common in the subacute stage; indeed on MRI it occurs in almost all cases by the end of the first week[89] and persists for several months. The pattern is variable and therefore not always specific; however, gyriform enhancement, if present, is most characteristic of a cortical infarct (Fig. 3-17F). Lack of enhancement of large cortical lesions on MRI suggests alternative diagnoses such as low-grade glioma.

Haemorrhagic transformation due to secondary bleeding into reperfused ischaemic tissue occurs during the first 2 weeks. It is shown in up to 80% of infarcts on MRI,[90] appearing hyperintense on T1 and hypointense on T2 images, and particularly GRE and SWI images (Fig. 3-18). It is often seen in the basal ganglia and cortex, where it can assume a gyriform pattern. The occurrence and severity of haemorrhagic transformation correlates with the size of the infarct and degree of contrast enhancement in the early stage[91] and its risk is also increased with cardioembolic infarcts, and in the setting of diabetes and thrombolysis treatment. It is worth noting that gyriform cortical T1 shortening (hyperintensity) in the subacute and indeed chronic phases more often represents cortical laminar necrosis—due to the migration and congregation of lipid-laden macrophages—than haemorrhagic transformation. Furthermore, this effect is also observed following other cortical insults such as encephalitis.

Chronically, encephalomalacia and volume loss develop, causing enlargement of adjacent sulci and ventricles. The density on CT and signal intensity on MRI, including FLAIR, approaches that of CSF (Fig. 3-17). Occasionally, and mostly in children, this enecephalomalacia may be cystic in nature, acquiring paradoxical mass effect. Wallerian degeneration is sometimes visible as faint T2 hyperintensity in the ipsilateral corticospinal

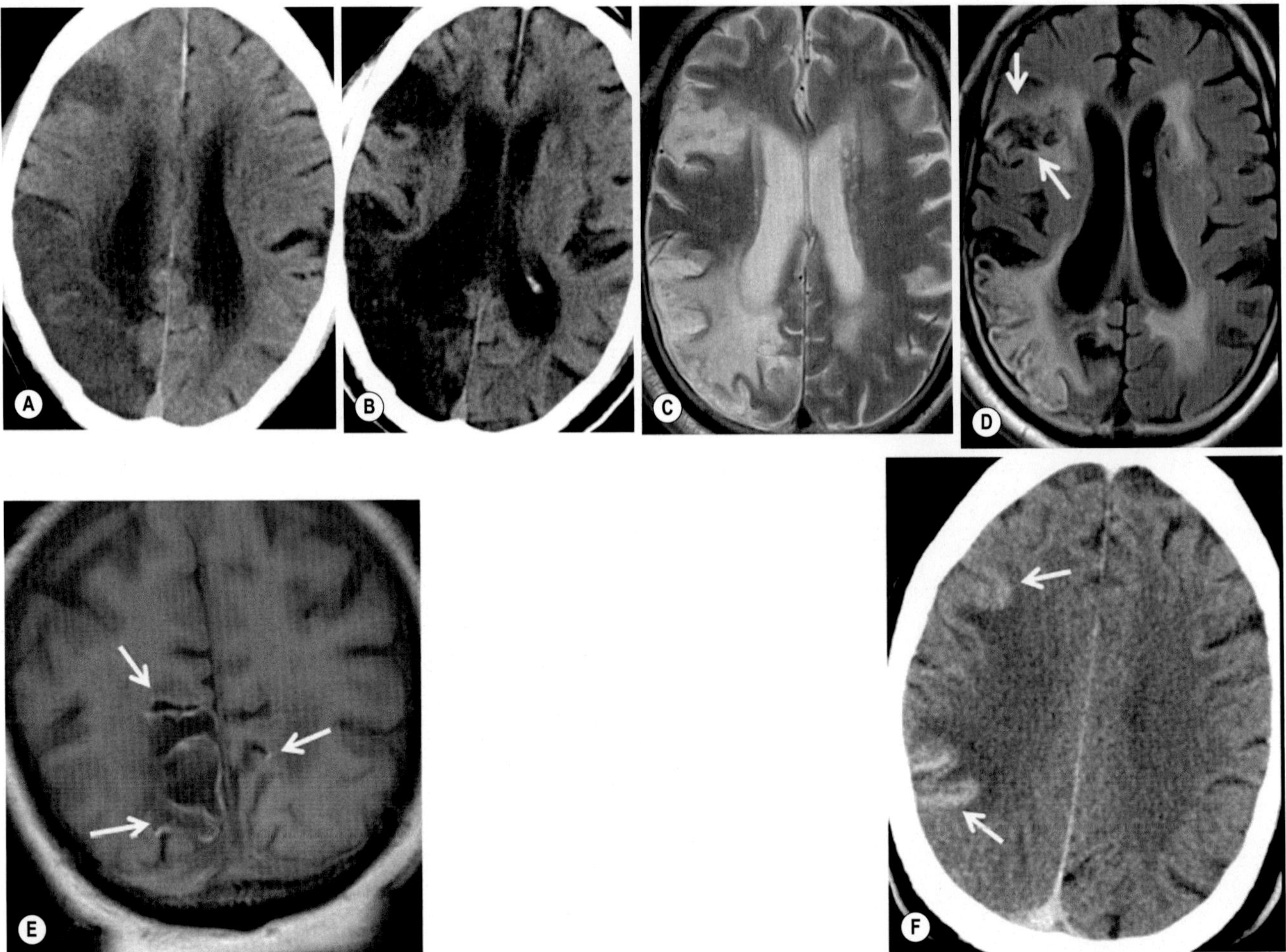

FIGURE 3-17 ■ **Subacute and mature infarcts.** On CT, there is a progressive reduction in attenuation (lower density) with infarct maturation accompanied by increased lesion delineation and volume loss as evidenced by sulcal prominence and ex-vacuo dilatation of the ventricles (A, B). A similar process is depicted on MRI with increased T2 (and FLAIR) hyperintensity (C, D) until the tissue reaches the signal intensity of fluid. At this stage, the infarcted tissue is hypointense on FLAIR with a hyperintense margin of gliosis (D, white arrows). Gyriform cortical T1 hyperintensity in the infarcted tissue develops in the subacute phase, and is known as cortical laminar necrosis (E, white arrows). Gyriform enhancement occurs early in cortical ischaemia due to breakdown of the blood–brain barrier, and may persist for several months (F, white arrows).

tract with related asymmetrical brainstem atrophy. With large middle cerebellar artery infarcts, contralateral cerebellar volume loss is also occasionally observed. Rarely, dystrophic calcification occurs in the very late phase.

On DWI, normalisation of the DWI and ADC signal occurs within 5–10 days ('pseudonormalisation') during which small infarcts can be masked. Larger lesions will still be obvious on structural images. Prolonged restriction of diffusion in small white matter infarcts lasting several weeks has been reported, the explanation for which is not entirely clear.[92] Beyond this period, loss of structural integrity results in increased water mobility and the imaging appearance reverses to low signal on DWI and bright on the ADC map.[93,94] This state is described as 'free diffusion' (Fig. 3-19). In mature infarcts, tissue with very long T2 relaxation times (markedly T2 hyperintense) may appear as high signal on DWI due to T2 effects dominating the signal—the so-called 'T2 shine through' effect. Such areas are easily distinguished from genuinely acutely infarcted tissue as they will also be hyperintense on the ADC map. Another potential pitfall of DWI is acute haemorrhage, which can return a high signal resembling an infarct. However, there is often also a low signal margin produced by susceptibility effects.[95] Analysis of other sequences should indicate the correct diagnosis.

On perfusion imaging, CBV in the infarcted region increases in the early subacute stage[96] due primarily to collateral supply.

Atheromatous Extracranial Vascular Disease

Atheroma can occur at vessel origins (including vertebral arteries), at the carotid bifurcation, and in the distal course of internal carotid or vertebral arteries. The carotid bifurcation is the commonest site and represents a significant source of emboli. Thirty per cent of transient ischaemic attacks progress to cerebral infarction, of which 20% are within the first month, and the majority within the initial few days. Such stenoses are also a cause of hypoperfusion strokes if haemodynamically significant.

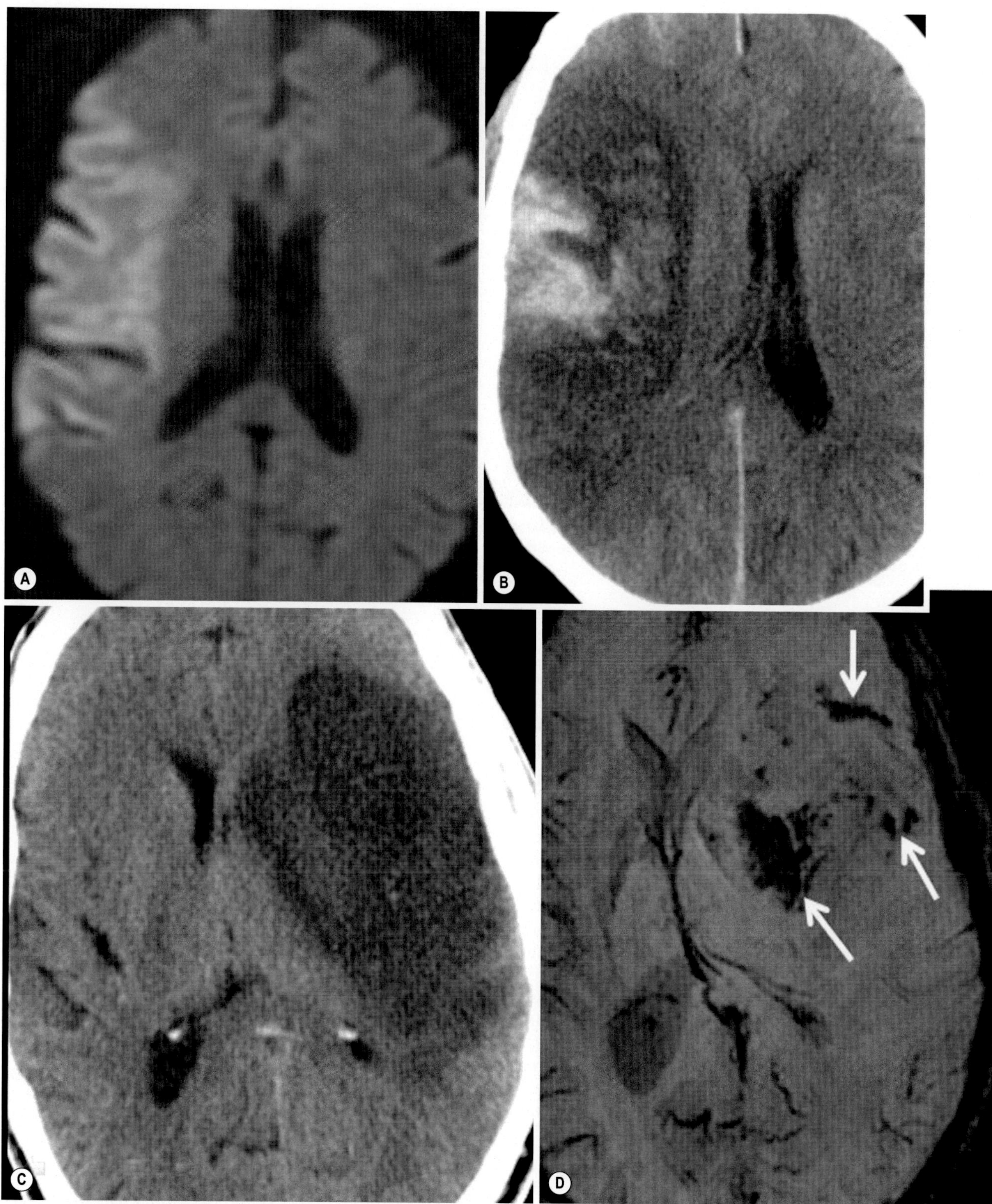

FIGURE 3-18 ■ **Haemorrhagic transformation.** Haemorrhage within an infarct is more common in large infarcts and in those involving the basal ganglia, and following efforts to recanalise occluded major vessels. (A) The DWI of this patient demonstrated a large right MCA territory infarct. Sixty hours after symptom onset, the patient clinically deteriorated. A CT examination revealed a moderate area of acute haemorrhage (hyperdensity) within the infarct, with ipsilateral mass effect and midline shift (B). In (C), a large left MCA territory infarct is complicated by haemorrhagic transformation. Although only subtly hyperdense in the basal ganglia on CT (C), the exquisite sensitivity of SWI to markedly hypointense blood products detects their presence easily (D, white arrows).

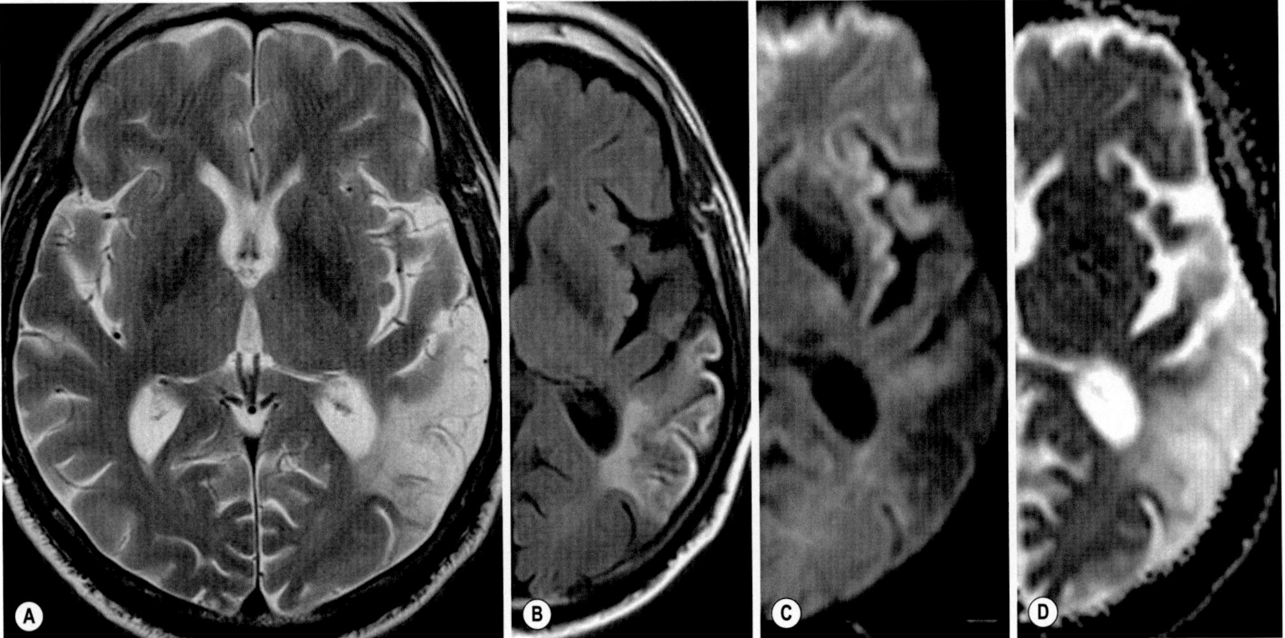

FIGURE 3-19 ■ MR imaging of a patient 6 months after a left MCA territory infarct reveals marked T2 hyperintensity on T2-weighted imaging (A)—which nulls centrally on FLAIR (B)—and free diffusion on DWI (hypointensity on DWI (C) and hyperintensity on ADC (D)). This is associated with local volume loss.

The North American Symptomatic Carotid Endarterectomy Trial (NASCET)[97] and the European Carotid Surgery Trial (ESCT)[98] found that patients with symptomatic 70–99% stenosis of the internal carotid artery benefited from endarterectomy surgery. Stenosis measurements in these trials were performed on conventional catheter angiograms, using slightly different methods, which are illustrated in Fig. 3-20. Surgery also reduces the risk of stroke in asymptomatic carotid stenosis of 70% or more as measured by ultrasound.[99] Symptomatic 50–69% stenoses may be a suitable target for intervention but in both cases the benefits are smaller and the advantages of surgery could more easily be outweighed by poor patient selection or excess morbidity from surgery (or angiography).[100] Carotid intervention should not be considered for a stenosis of less than 50% regardless of symptoms. More recently, the Asymptomatic Carotid Stenosis Trial (ACST) demonstrated that endarterectomy confers a reduction in stroke risk amongst patients younger than 75 years old, with greater than 70% stenosis of the internal carotid artery provided that the operative risk was not higher than in the trial itself.[101,102]

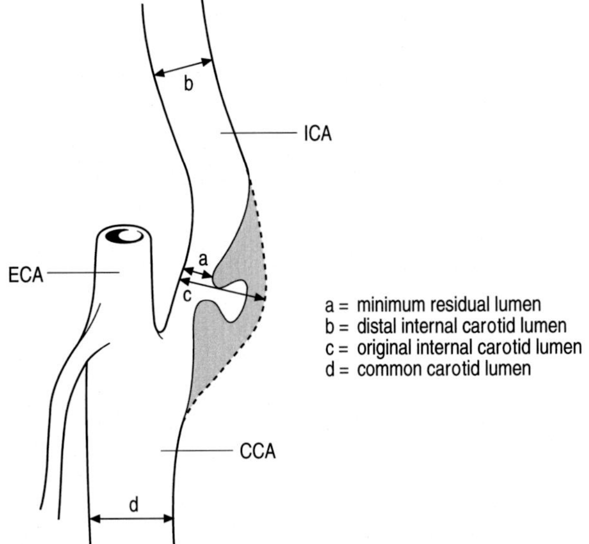

FIGURE 3-20 ■ Different ways of measuring percentage of carotid artery stenosis (adapted from 86): (A) NASCET method = [1 − (*a*/*b*)] × 100; (B) ESCT method = [1 − (*a*/*c*)] × 100; common carotid method = [1 − (*a*/*d*)] × 100.

Imaging Options for Carotid Stenosis

Conventional digital subtraction catheter angiography (DSA) is invasive, potentially hazardous,[103] expensive, and not widely available. Most carotid imaging is now performed with Doppler ultrasound, CTA, MRA performed without exogenous contrast injection such as 2- or 3-dimensional time-of-flight (TOF) methods, or contrast-enhanced MRA (CEMRA) performed dynamically after an intravenous bolus of gadolinium-based contrast.[104] These non-invasive techniques are now very widely available, although access for patients with TIA varies among hospitals,[105] and DSA is no longer in routine use. In both a systematic review of the world literature and individual patient data meta-analysis performed recently in 2009,[106,107] sensitivities and specificities of these techniques were as follows: 70 to 99% stenosis, sensitivity: ultrasound (US), 0.89; CTA, 0.76; MRA, 0.88; CEMRA, 0.94; specificity: US, 0.84; CTA, 0.94; MRA, 0.84; CEMRA, 0.93. Fewer data were available for milder stenoses but accuracy was poorer. Hence, it is widely accepted

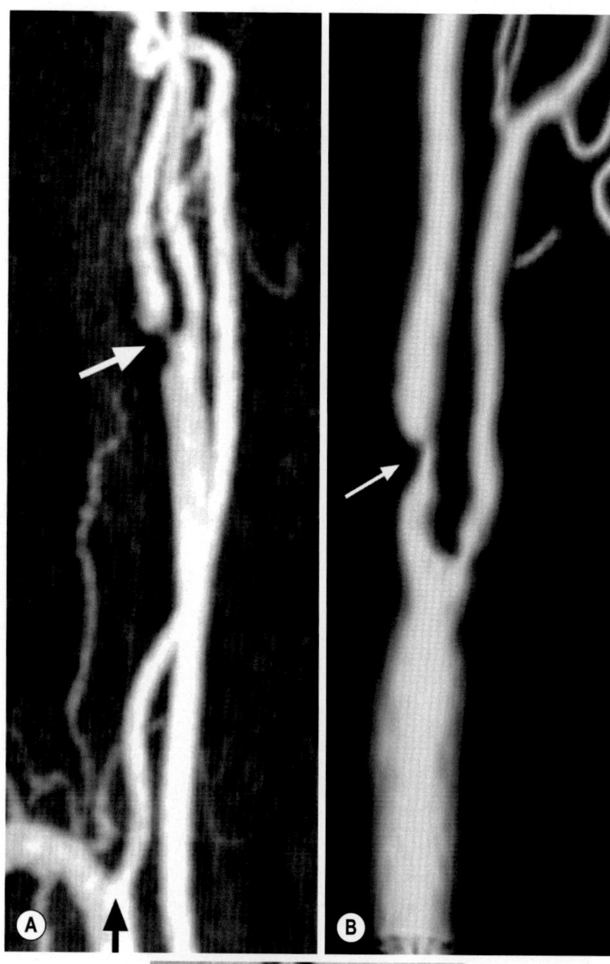

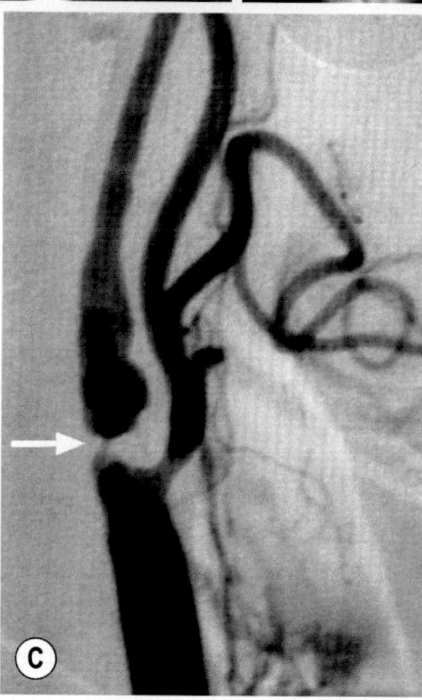

FIGURE 3-21 ■ **Carotid bifurcation atheroma.** Examples of internal carotid artery stenoses (white arrows) from different patients on (A) CEMRA MIP, (B) CTA volume rendering and (C) DSA. Note the right vertebral artery origin is clearly demonstrated (A, black arrow).

that CEMRA is the most accurate method of carotid stenosis evaluation (Fig. 3-21). However, it should be pointed out that in the experience of the authors, CTA performed on 128-multidetector CT is at least as accurate as CEMRA. Indeed, this is supported by the data from very recent case series.

Vessel Plaque Imaging. Ultrasound and MRI techniques are able to identify high-risk plaques with a high risk of rupture and distal embolism.[108,109] Isotope imaging with FDG-PET and ^{11}C-PK11195 detect intraplaque inflammation which is thought to be involved in emboli formation.[110,111]

Imaging Signs

Doppler ultrasound (USS) demonstrates plaque location, extent and morphology. Hyperechoic lesions, typically with acoustic shadowing, represent plaque calcification whilst hypoechoic plaque indicates an increased risk of stroke. Doppler flow velocity and characteristics correlate well with the degree of vascular stenosis but cannot reliably distinguish between complete occlusion and 'trickle' flow. USS may also underestimate the degree of narrowing due to fresh or free-floating thrombus.

A narrowed vessel flow void on MRI indicates stenosis whilst an absent flow void usually indicates occlusion, especially if there is intraluminal high signal. However, this appearance can also represent severely impaired flow distal to a tight stenosis.

There is good correlation between a normal time-of-flight MRA and absence of disease (high specificity). It is, however, rather prone to overestimation of the degree of stenosis. Also, as the technique is heavily flow dependent, turbulence, a reduction in flow and a genuine stenosis can all generate an apparent vessel narrowing. A 'flow-gap' does not differentiate occlusion from very slow flow. Whilst many of the flow-dependent artefacts are significantly reduced by the luminal CEMRA, they are not eliminated. As stated earlier, this technique gives better plaque morphological and extent assessment. However, the ICA distal to a severe stenosis can appear spuriously narrow.

CT angiography (CTA) is a luminal contrast technique and does not suffer from flow-dependent artefacts. It has a very high specificity and, with newer-generation MDCT, affords an excellent assessment of a stenosis. Juxtaluminal hypodensity indicates large fatty plaque and free-floating thrombus—at particular risk of embolism—are well characterised. Furthermore, arterial and slightly delayed phases can usually discriminate between occlusion and trickle-flow defines tandem lesions. Accurate stenosis assessment can be difficult in segments of heavy calcification—not an uncommon problem.

CEMRA and CTA both allow a full assessment of the arterial tree from the aortic arch to the circle of Willis and beyond.

Non-Atheromatous Extracranial Vascular Narrowing

Causes of non-atheromatous extracranial vascular narrowing include arterial dissection, fibromuscular dysplasia (FMD), extrinsic compression (for example, from nasopharyngeal tumours and soft-tissue infection), radiation vasculopathy (with intimal fibrosis and accelerated atherosclerosis) and catheter spasm.

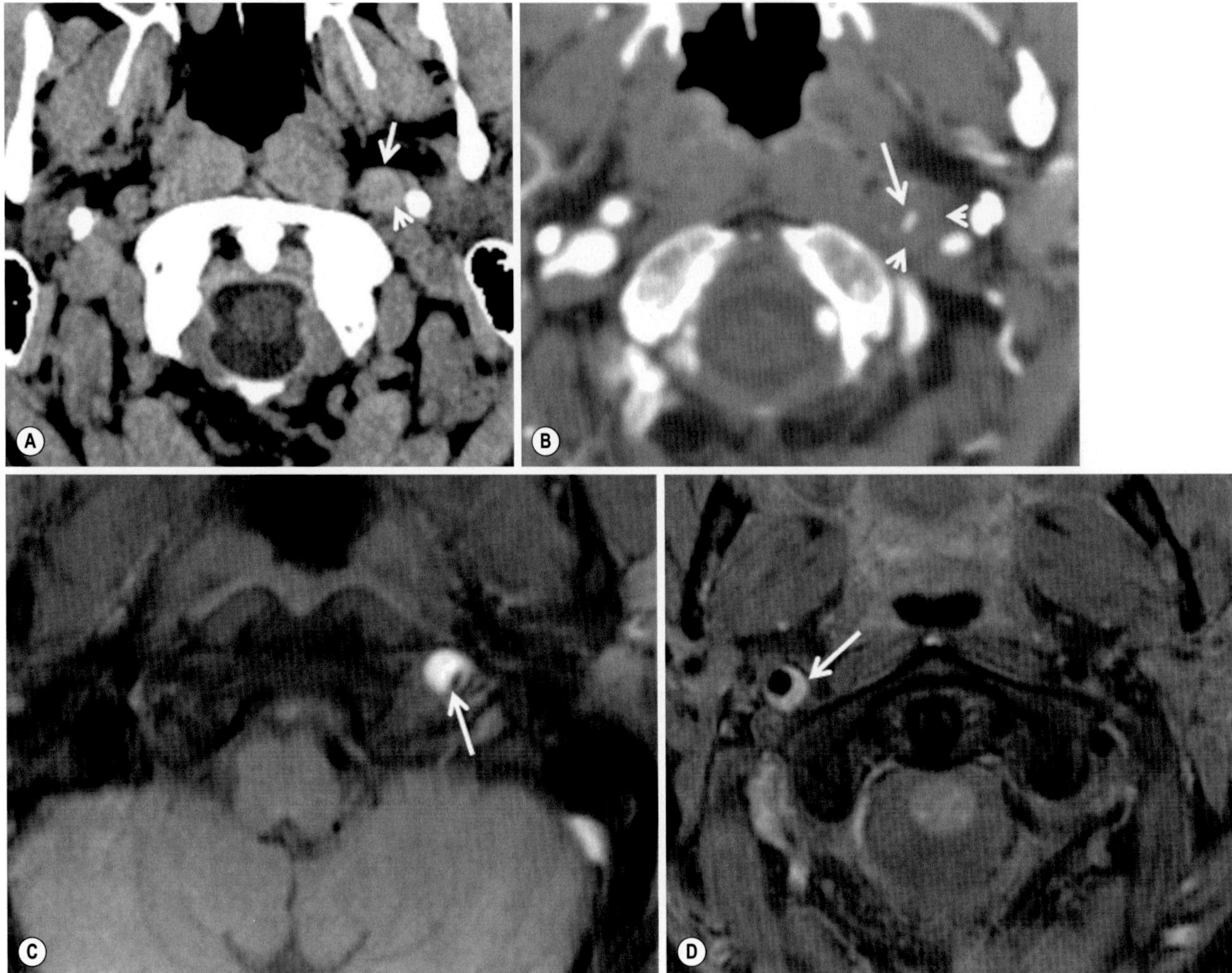

FIGURE 3-22 ■ Carotid artery dissection. A patient presented with neck pain and left-sided Horner's syndrome. Plain non-contrast-enhanced CT at the skull base demonstrated an expanded and heterogenous ICA (A, white arrow) with impression of crescentic hyperdensity (white arrowhead). CT angiography revealed a very narrow-calibre lumen (B, white arrow) within an expanded non-enhancing vessel (white arrowheads). Subsequent fat-saturated T1-weighted MRI shows the hyperintense intramural haemorrhage expanding the left ICA and surrounding the narrowed lumen (C, white arrow), and in another patient with a right ICA dissection (D, white arrow).

Arterial Dissection

Dissection of the cervical arteries is an important cause of stroke, particularly in younger patients, in whom it accounts for 20% of acute ischaemic strokes. Dissection of the internal carotid artery is most common, occurring proximally after the bulb and at the skull base. The vertebral artery is susceptible because of its bony canal and in children due to the arcuate foramen posterior to the lateral mass of C1. Whilst arterial dissection can occur spontaneously, cervical trauma, underlying vasculopathy such as fibromuscular dysplasia and connective tissue disorders such as Ehlers–Danlos syndrome, can precipitate the injury. The risk is also increased amongst patients with migraine, hypertension and in the setting of ilicit drug use.

Carotid artery dissection can occasionally be diagnosed on the routine NECT and axial MRI of the skull base, where an expanded vessel with crescentic hyperdensity on CT, or 'fried egg' appearance on MRI, can be observed. The latter arises from a true lumen with variable patency (ranging from normal flow void to abnormal signal due to occlusion or slow flow) with a surrounding cresecent of intramural haemorrhage in the false lumen. The conspicuity of the T1 hyperintense intramural clot is enhanced on T1 fat-saturated images (Fig. 3-22). Angiographic images typically demonstrate a smooth, tapered reduction of the luminal calibre often with luminal irregularity. The intraluminal flap may also be visible, as may pseudoaneurysmal dilatation. Although DSA classically shows differential opacification and contrast washout in the true and false lumens if they are both patent, most of these features can be shown on MRA or CTA and the diagnosis can usually be made without recourse to DSA. The diagnosis of a vertebral artery dissection is usually more difficult. T1 fat-saturated images are less rewarding in their demonstration of the intramural haematoma due to the signal emanating from the plexus of veins that typically surround the vertebral arteries in their cervical course. Careful scrutiny of the CTA axial images for vessel irregularity, the intimal flap, overall vessel expansion and the possibility of coexisting dissecting aneurysms is warranted.

Fibromuscular Dysplasia (FMD)

FMD occurs predominantly in middle-aged women and most often affects the cervical ICA (75%). The vertebral (12%) and external carotid arteries may also be involved. Disease is bilateral in 60% of cases. Angiographic images, almost always with non-invasive techniques, demonstrate alternating luminal narrowing and dilatation, the resulting appearance often described as a 'string of beads' (Fig. 3-23). This 'corrugation' typically affects the mid ICA, usually 2 cm distal to bulb. Uni- or multifocal tubular stenoses are less common, and where observed, the degree of stenosis is usually modest (less than 40%). FMD can occasionally be observed intracranially and is associated with aneurysms.

Intracranial Vascular Disease

Ischaemic Microangiopathy

There are a number of causes of small vessel disease in the brain (see Table 3-3). By far the most common is ischaemic microangiopathy, the risk factors for which are age, hypertension, diabetes mellitus, hyperlipidaemia and smoking.[112] More than 95% of those over 65 years of age have white matter lesions on MRI, but these are usually limited in extent.[113] Arterioles of the long penetrating arteries become occluded, the outcome probably depending on vessel size. Occlusion of a larger perforating vessel causes a lacunar infarct; blockage of smaller arterioles results in ischaemic demyelination and gliosis. Although highly variable in distribution, it predominantly affects the periventricular and deep cerebral white matter, basal ganglia, thalami and the ventral pons. CT shows white

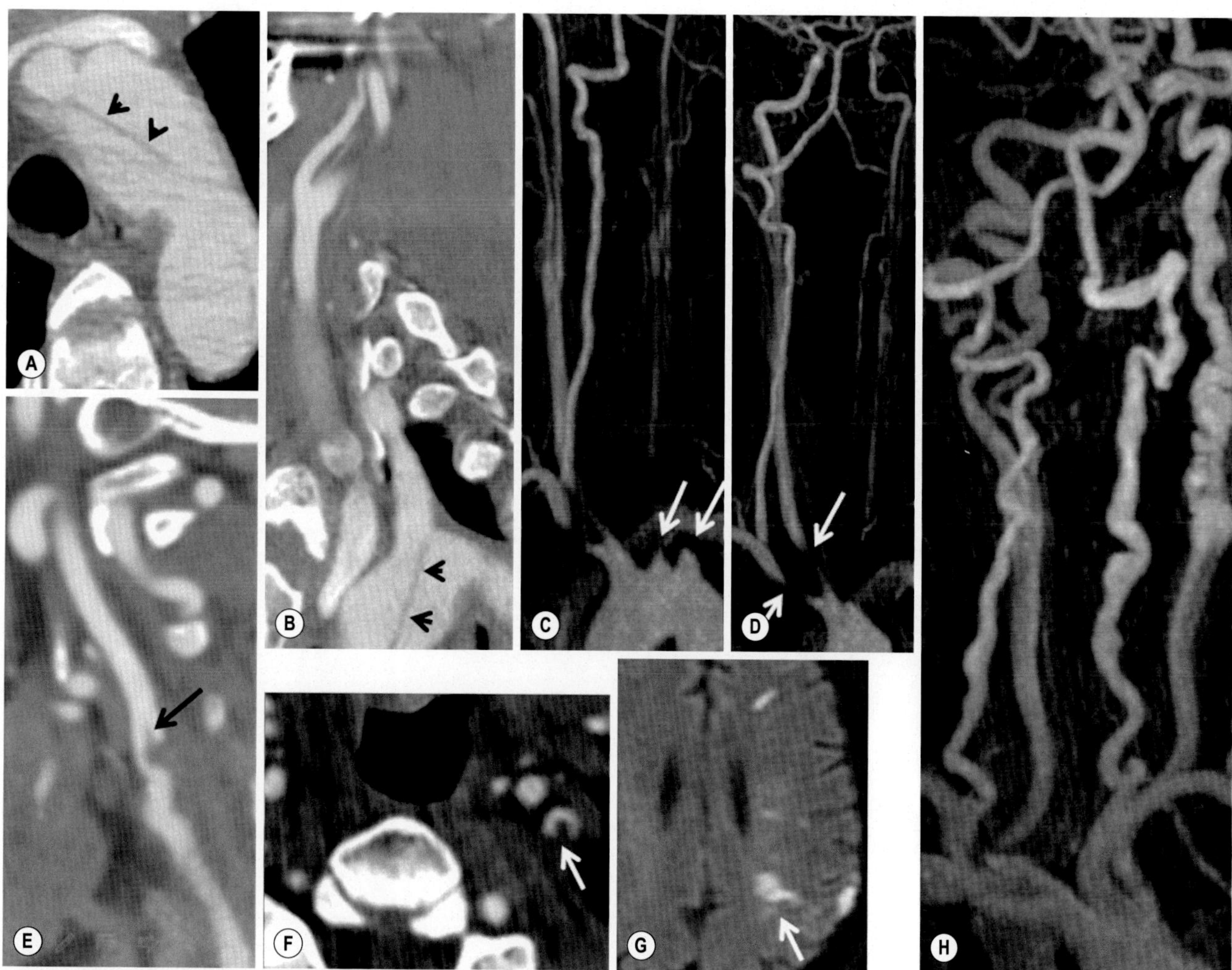

FIGURE 3-23 ■ **Extracranial arterial abnormalities.** An aortic arch dissection extends to involve the origin of the left CCA (A, B). The initimal flap is clearly visible (black arrowheads). Takayasu's arteritis (C, D). This large vessel vasculitis typically affects the great vessel origins, most commonly beginning with the left subclavian artery. In this case, there is occlusion of the left subclavian and common carotid arteries (C, white arrows) with severe stenosis of the right subclavian and common carotid arteries (D, white arrows). Free-floating thrombus (E–G). Low-density atherosclerotic plaque arising from the intima of the vessel wall projects into the lumen of the left internal carotid artery origin (E, black arrow; F, white arrow) and d is associated with small acute embolic infarcts in the left middle cerebral artery territory (G; white arrow) on DWI. Fibromuscular dysplasia. A contrast-enhanced MRA (H) of a 47-year-old female patient reveals extensive 'beading' of the left CCA, left ICA and left vertebral artery, and to a lesser extent right ICA in the neck. This pattern of alternating luminal dilatation and mild narrowings is typical.

matter hypodensities ('leukoariosis') but MRI, particularly FLAIR, is much more sensitive.

Whilst distinguishing an acute infarct from a background of established disease on CT is extremely challenging, DWI will easily identify its site. New infarcts develop every few months in small vessel disease and are clinically silent unless they arise in eloquent areas, although they will be shown on fortuitously timed DWI.[114] It is important to realise that these white matter changes are non-specific and similar appearances may be encountered in other microangiopathic diseases such as vasculitis,[115] and occasionally inflammatory processes affecting the CNS.

TABLE 3-3 **Causes**

Common	Uncommon	Rare
Ischaemic micro-angiopathy	Drug-related hypertension/ vasculopathy	Moya moya
Vasospasm (SAH)	Sickle cell disease	Intravascular lymphoma
	Radiation vasculopathy	Intracranial dissection
	Intracranial atheroma	Intracranial FMD
	Vasculitis	CADASIL
	Amyloid angiopathy	Susac's syndrome
		Neurocutaneous syndromes

Acutely, lacunar infarcts are often rounded with a hazy outline and may fluctuate in size in the subacute phase—most often enlarging. When mature, however, they become sharply delineated, shrink in size—typically less than 1.5 cm diameter—and cavity-like. The gliotic hyperintense rim of a mature lacune on FLAIR differentiates it from a perivascular space.

Ischaemic microangiopathic disease is often associated with microhaemorrhages in the deep nuclei and scattered more peripherally.[116] These are depicted as small foci of susceptibility artefact on T2* GRE and SWI (microbleeds are not visible on CT) (Figs. 3-24 and 3-25). They are also present in around 6% of asymptomatic

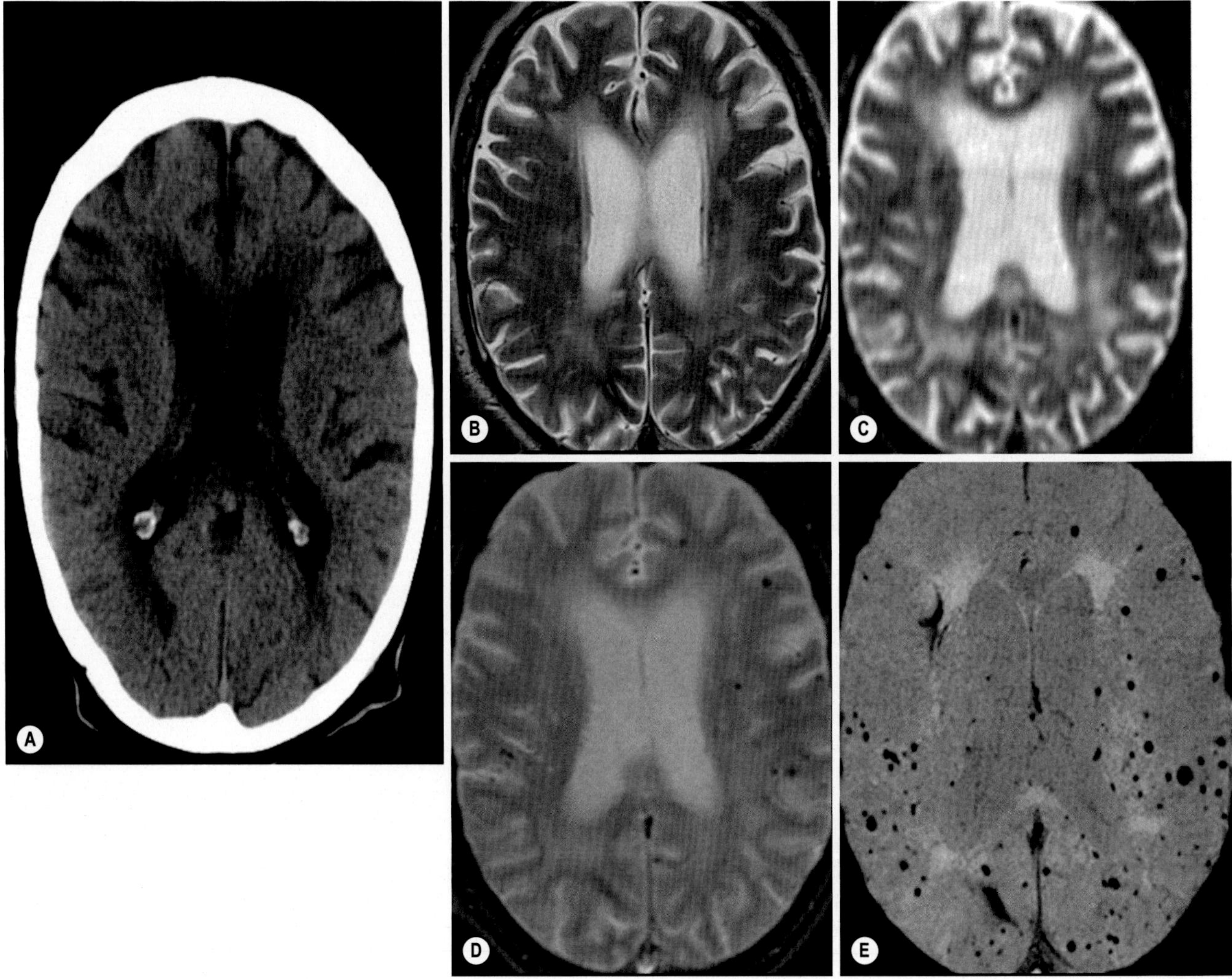

FIGURE 3-24 ■ **Sensitivity to haemosiderin deposition.** No microhaemorrhages are apparent in the brain parenchyma on plain CT in this patient with amyloid angiopathy (A). There is progressively increasing sensitivity to their presence from a standard T2-weighted spin-echo sequence (B), through the b = zero diffusion-weighted acquisition (C), gradient-echo T2* sequence (D) and, finally, susceptibility-weighted imaging (E), which affords exquisite detection of microhaemorrhages by demonstrating multiple foci of susceptibility artefact depicted as marked hypointensity.

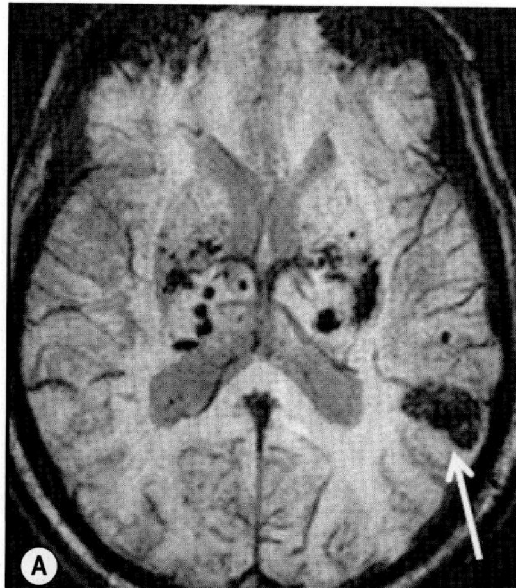

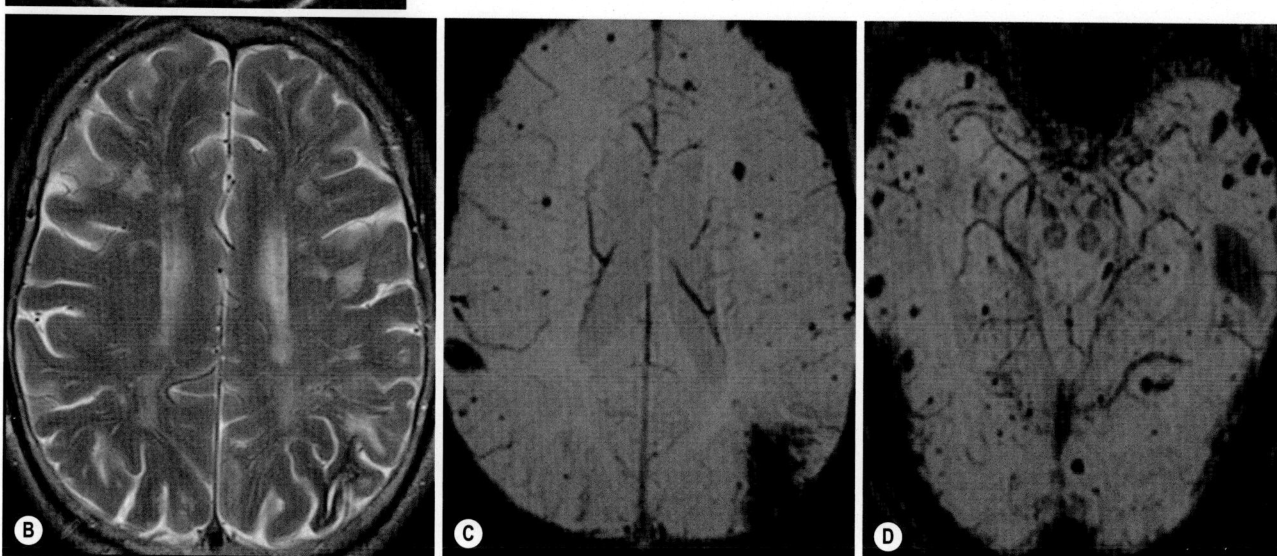

FIGURE 3-25 ■ **Distribution of microhaemorrhages.** Multiple hypertensive microhaemorrhages are shown in the deep grey nuclei in this patient with severe microangiopathic ischaemic disease (A), whilst the distribution of microhaemorrhages is typically more peripheral and lobar in a patient with amyloid angiopathy (B–D). Again, the SWI acquisition (C, D) far exceeds the routine T2-weighted sequence (B) in the sensitivity to such lesions. Note, however, the presence of a previous lobar haemorrhage (A, white arrow).

older people, associated with age, hypertension and radiological extent of small vessel disease.[117] They are a marker of vascular fragility in hypertensive small vessel disease, their distribution mirroring symptomatic haemorrhages. There is some evidence that they present an increased risk for parenchymal haemorrhage in antiplatelet therapy.[118] However, this and the impact of anticoagulation are still under investigation. Similarly, it is not clear whether they increase the risk of post-thrombolysis haemorrhage.[119,120]

Moya Moya

Moya moya is the literal Japanese term for 'puff of smoke', describing the angiographic appearance of abnormal, dilated and irregular collateral vessels that develop secondary to progressive occlusion of the supraclinoid internal carotid arteries. Moya moya represents an idiopathic arteriopathy, which, although primarily involving the supraclinoid ICAs, often progresses to the proximal anterior and middle cerebral arteries, and occasionally the posterior circulation (typically the basilar tip). It is mainly seen in patients from Japan and the Pacific Rim. In advanced cases there may be extensive dural, leptomeningeal and pial collateral circulation. The characteristic vascular changes can also be shown on MRA or CTA and MRI may show associated infarcts. The latter are usually in the borderzones (Fig. 3-26). A moya moya-like pattern may be found in other conditions such as sickle cell disease, Down's syndrome, previous radiotherapy or tuberculous meningitis and Type 1 neurofibromatosis.[80]

Vasculitis

This heterogeneous group of inflammatory diseases mainly affects smaller parenchymal and leptomeningeal vessels. Conditions that cause cerebral vasculitis, other than primary (isolated) angiitis of the central nervous system, include infection, cocaine ingestion and autoimmune diseases such as systemic lupus erythematosus, polyarteritis nodosa, giant cell arteritis and Sjögren's syndrome, sarcoidosis and Wegener's disease.

Appearances on MRI are typically non-specific. White matter hyperintensities with a subcortical distribution are more common and there may be foci of haemorrhage, leptomeningeal enhancement and occasionally infarcts. Medium vessel disease is rare, arising secondarily due to disease of the vasa vasorum. Involved areas may resemble territorial strokes but do not evolve appropriately.

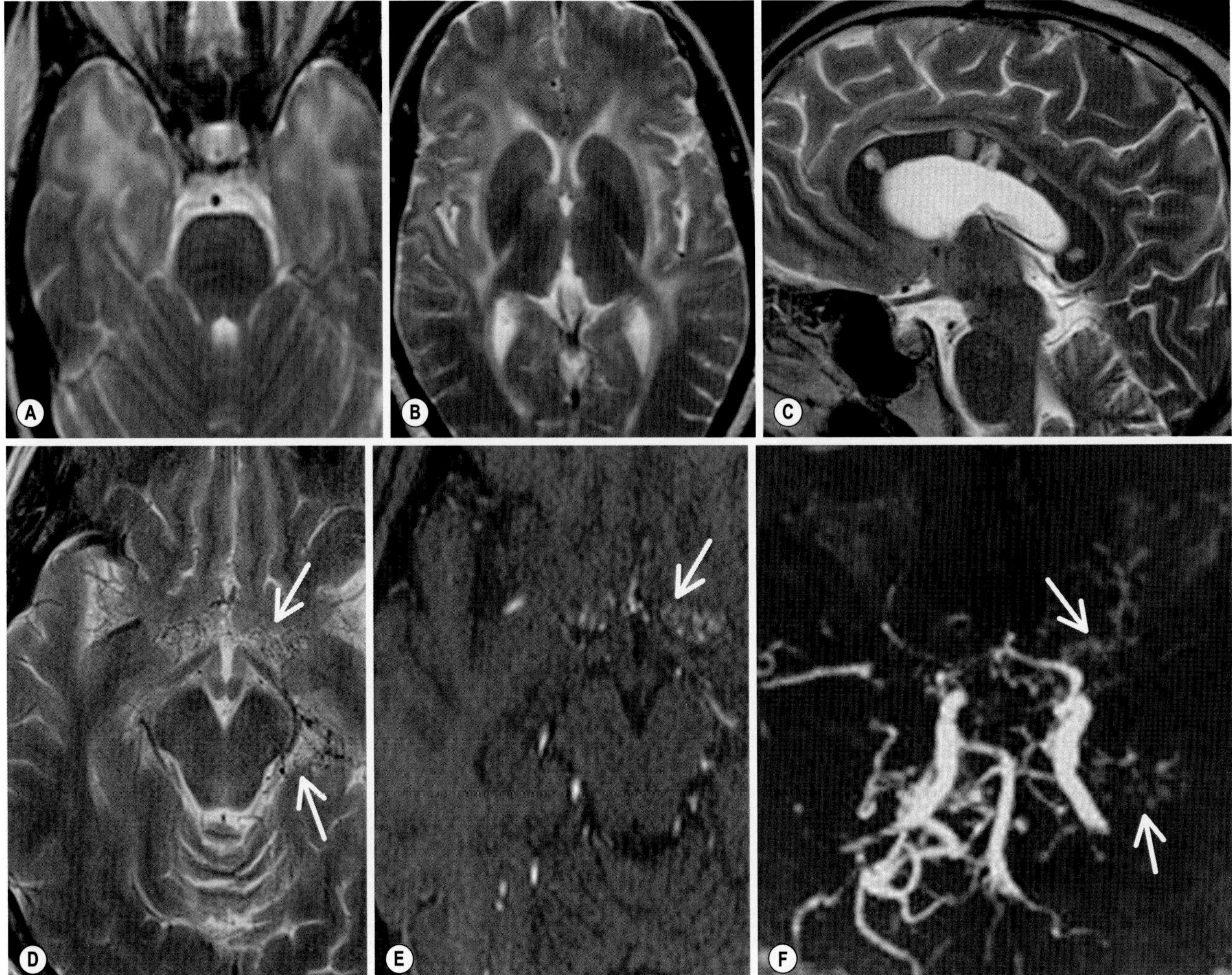

FIGURE 3-26 ■ CADASIL (A, B). Extensive confluent white matter signal abnormality typically involving the anterior temporal lobes and subinsular regions. Basal ganglia involvement and microhaemorrhage are also often noted. Susac's syndrome (C). Small multifocal, often rounded lesions in the corpus callosum in a patient presenting with headache, encephalopathy, retinal branch occlusions and hearing loss. Moya moya syndrome (D–F). There is absence of the normal flow void on the T2-weighted spine-echo image (D) and flow signal on the time-of-flight MRA (axial raw data E, maximum intensity projection F) within both terminal ICAs, middle cerebral arteries, right ACA and left PCA due to the terminal occlusive vasculopathy. In an attempt to compensate, a myriad of fine abnormal collateral vessels have developed in the anterior perforated substance and left choroidal fissure (white arrows).

DSA catheter angiography is superior to MRA and CTA, particularly for smaller, more peripheral vessels. Angiographic signs suggesting a vasculitis include stenoses, occlusion, thromboses or arterial beading, although they are not specific. Aneurysms are also observed. However, angiography is frequently negative and it should not be regarded as the gold standard investigation; a brain or meningeal biopsy is often necessary to make a firm diagnosis.

Cerebral Venous Thrombosis (CVT)

Cerebral venous thrombosis is an easily overlooked diagnosis that should always be considered in the presence of headache, seizures or encephalopathy. Thrombus forms in dural sinuses and/or superficial cortical veins/or extending to internal cerebral veins from straight sinus leading to venous hypertension and haemorrhage. Venousinfarction ensues if anticoagulation is not implemented early.

Cerebral, osseous or air cell infection, local trauma, dehydration, pregnancy, the oral contraceptive pill, smoking and vasculitis (especially Behçet's disease) are not uncommon precipitants but in their absence a thrombophilia screen will be necessary.

Imaging signs pertain both to the thrombosed cortical vein or dural sinus and the 'upstream' parenchyma. An acutely thrombosed sinus, or less commonly superficial cortical vein, typically appears hyperdense and expanded on NECT, and as a hypodense centre within an enhancing periphery in post-contrast CT examinations, especially on CT venography. This is the so-called 'delta' sign. On most MRI sequences, there will loss of the normal flow void, and the thrombosed vessel may be hyperintense on both T1- and T2-weighted imaging. Rarely, very acute thrombus can appear hypointense on T2 and be mistaken for a flow void, and slow flow can result in loss of the flow void, mimicking thrombosis. Loss of flow signal and/or irregularity and severe narrowing indicate thrombus on MR venography. This is a phase contrast angiographic technique where a low-velocity encoding optimises depiction of venous flow. In practice, however, recanalisation versus a hypoplastic sinus versus slow flow can often be difficult to differentiate with MRI and MRV alone. In the authors' opinion, detailed assessment of the NECT and structural MRI images is usually most helpful. SWI can be particularly useful in CVT. In addition to the exaggerated hypointensity and expansion of the thrombosed vein or sinus (described as 'blooming'), multiple prominent serpiginous veins may be observed in the venous territory indicating venous congestion.[121] As mentioned earlier, this sequence is also very sensitive to acute haemorrhage. Phase images generated as part of the SWI sequence may also enable identification of an occluded cortical vein,[122] being hypointense compared with normally patent veins.

The imaging appearance of the parenchymal lesions depends on whether there is venous hypertension or infarction or secondary haemorrhage. Disproportionate parenchymal swelling and oedema (MRI, high T2/FLAIR signal; CT, low density) with early fragmented haemorrhage is typical. The distribution of parenchymal lesions is important: bilateral (although sometimes asymmetric) involvement of the thalami and to a lesser extent basal ganglia is typical in internal cerebral vein and/or straight sinus thrombosis; the posterolateral aspects of the temporal lobe and/or inferior parietal lobule are commonly involved in thrombosis of the vein of Labbé and/or lateral venous sinus; cortical and subcortical lesions, often bilateral but asymmetric, are frequent in superior sagittal sinus occlusion (Figs. 3-27 and 3-28).

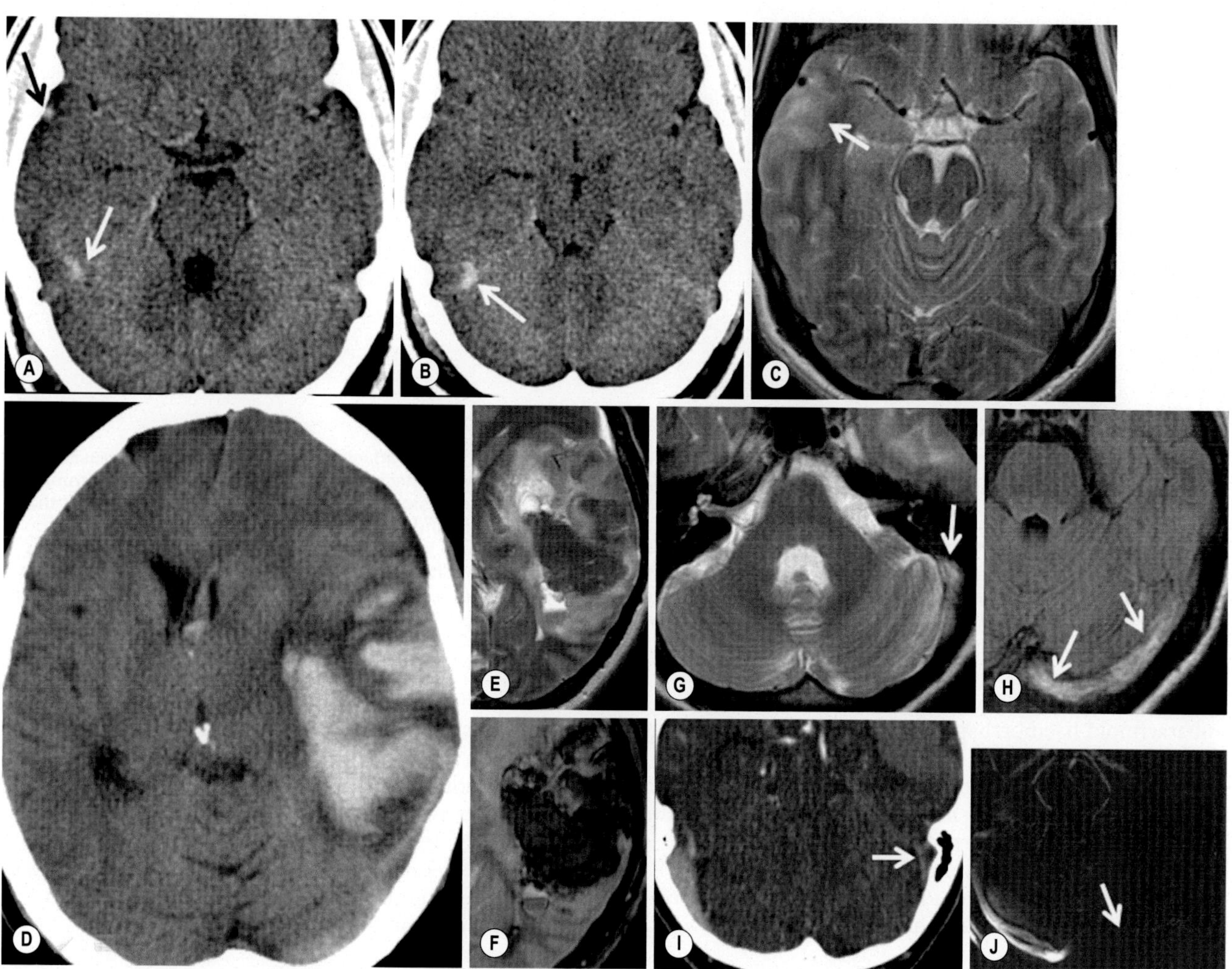

FIGURE 3-27 ■ **Cerebral venous thrombosis.** (A–C) This young male patient presented with headache and seizures. Serpiginous hyperdensity on CT within a vessel on the surface of the right temporal lobe (A, black arrow) and approaching the right lateral venous sinus (A, B, white arrows) is consistent with the 'string sign' of cortical venous thrombosis—in this case, involving the right vein of Labbé. There is a small area of early venous ischaemia in the anterolateral aspect of the right temporal lobe on T2-weighted MRI (C, white arrow). Lateral venous thrombosis. (D–J) A large acute parenchymal haemorrhage in the left frontal and temporal lobes was discovered on plain CT (D) in this patient who presented with seizures and encephalopathy. Hypointensity on the T2-weighted MRI (E) and SWI (F) are consistent with acute blood products. There is a considerable degree of surrounding parenchymal oedema shown as high signal intensity on T2W. A causative left lateral sinus thrombosis is identified on T2W (G, white arrow) and FLAIR (H, white arrows) with loss of the normal related signal void and confirmed by a filling defect within the left lateral sinus on the CT venogram (I, white arrow; compare with right lateral sinus) and absence of flow-related signal in this sinus on MR venography (J, white arrow).

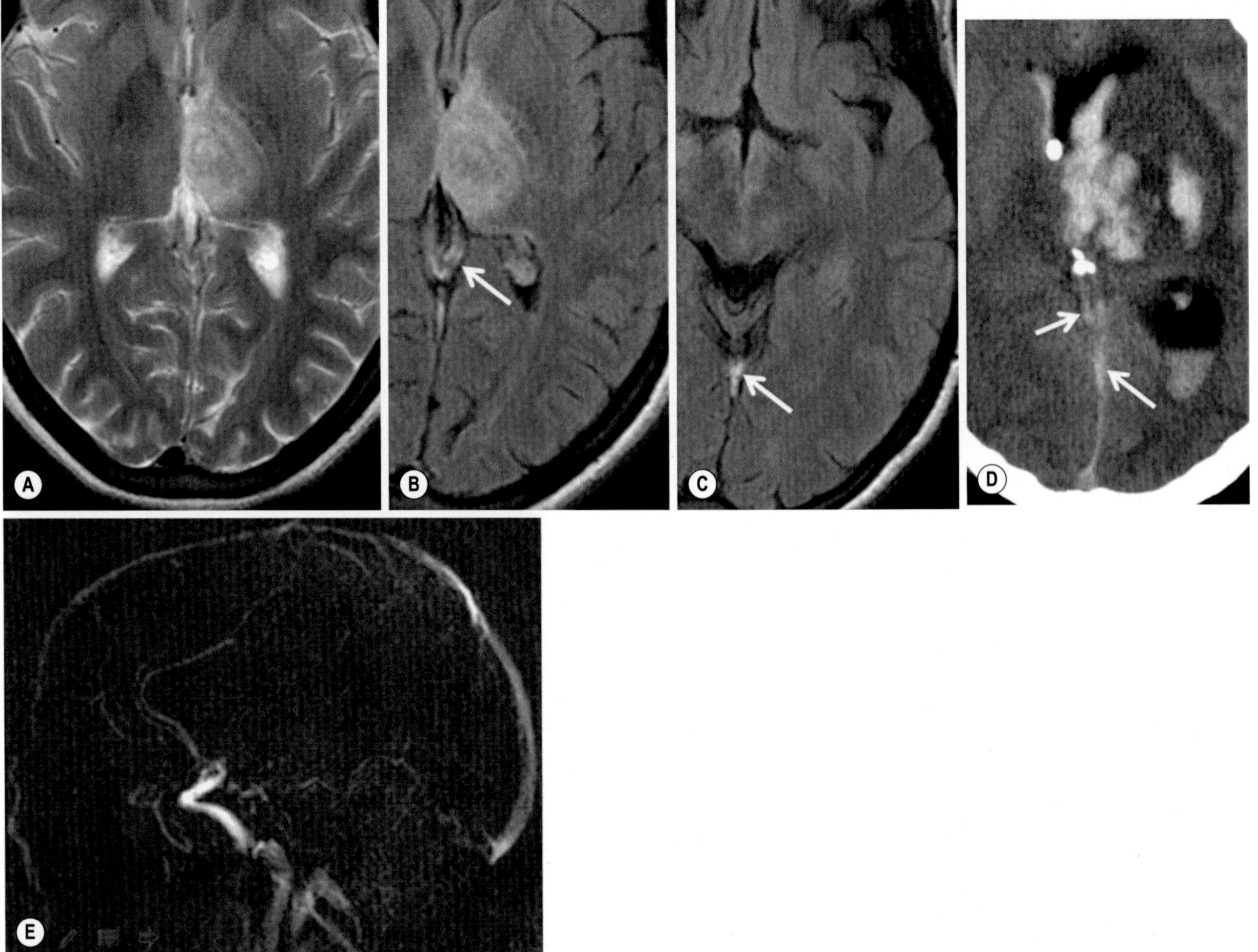

FIGURE 3-28 ■ **Deep venous thrombosis.** (A–E) This young female patient presented with headache and right-sided hemiparesis whilst playing in a prolonged hockey competition in summer, followed by reduced consciousness. The initial MRI examination (A, C) demonstrates signal abnormality and swelling consistent with venous hypertension, oedema and ischaemia in the left thalamus. There is abnormal signal within and expansion of the left internal cerebral vein and straight sinus on FLAIR (B, C, white arrows) in keeping with thrombus. The MR venogram does not show any flow in the deep venous system (E). A clinical deterioration is accompanied by haemorrhage and venous infarction in the left thalamus (D), with additional involvement of the left lentiform nucleus and right thalamus. Intraventricular haemorrhage and hydrocephalus has developed. There is persistent hyperdensity within both internal cerebral veins and the proximal straight sinus (D, white arrows).

Subarachnoid haemorrhage is also often observed in this setting.

Overall, CVT is a difficult diagnosis to make and often requires more than one investigation. Scrutiny of the initial NECT is usually rewarding. CT venography is optimal for major dural venous sinus thrombosis, whilst MRI/V is more likely to identify subtle parenchymal lesions and thrombosis of the internal cerebral veins, straight sinus and cortical veins. On MRI, assessment of all of the major venous structures on all sequences is important as individual sequences can be misleading. Although, DSA catheter angiography is now rarely required, it most accurately defines the extent of disease and most reliably demonstrates recanalisation. Most commonly, it is utilised as a prelude to endovascular therapy if there is clinical deterioration despite medical management.

NON-TRAUMATIC INTRACRANIAL HAEMORRHAGE

Intracranial haemorrhage can be traumatic or spontaneous (non-traumatic) and is usually described in relation to the anatomical compartment in which it occurs.

SUBARACHNOID HAEMORRHAGE (SAH)

The incidence of SAH has remained stable over the last 30-40 years and is quoted at 9 per 100,000 person-years.[123]

Classically, SAH presents with a sudden-onset severe headache. In almost half of patients a period of unresponsiveness occurs, with 30% patients developing a focal neurological deficit. Severe acute-onset headaches are not uncommon. The majority will be innocuous and it should be noted that with this isolated symptom only 10% of patients will have had a subarachnoid haemorrhage.[124] However, with mortality rates approaching 50% and a post ictus dependency rate of 30%,[125] SAH and subsequently acute severe-onset headaches cannot be taken lightly.

Spontaneous SAH is most commonly due to a vascular abnormality, with a ruptured aneurysm accounting for approximately 80% (Table 3-4).

TABLE 3-4 Causes of Subarachnoid Haemorrhage

- Aneurysm (80%)
- Non-aneurysmal perimesencephalic (10%)
- Traumatic

Rare Causes

- Arteriovenous malformations
- Dural venous sinus or cortical vein thrombosis
- Intracranial dissection
- Drug abuse—cocaine
- Pseudoaneurysms—vaso-occlusive disorders with flow aneurysm on collateral vessels. Mycotic aneurysms
- Reversible cerebrovascular vasoconstrictive syndrome

In 10% no structural or vascular abnormality is demonstrated. This most frequently occurs when the subarachnoid blood is confined to the perimesencephalic area of the basal cisterns and is termed 'non-aneurysmal perimesenchephalic SAH'. These patients (who by definition have a negative catheter angiogram) have a very good long-term prognosis.[126] The risk of further bleeding is thought to be no higher than that in the general population. Variations in venous anatomy found with this pattern of SAH suggest a venous origin.[127] Rarer causes of SAH such as vascular malformations, venous thrombosis and drug abuse account for a much smaller proportion of cases.

Initial Investigation of Acute SAH

NECT is positive for SAH in 98% within 12 h of ictus onset[128] but this falls to less than 75% by the third day.[129] Acute SAH causes increased density of the cerebrospinal fluid (CSF) spaces on CT (assuming sufficient elevation of the CSF haematocrit). Most aneurysms are located on or close to the circle of Willis and blood is therefore seen in the basal cisterns, although the entire intracranial subarachnoid space may be opacified and intraventricular blood is common. In some cases the distribution of the surrounding blood may indicate the aneurysm location (Fig. 3-29).

A lumbar puncture should be performed when there is a strong clinical suspicion of SAH but a negative CT. Ideally this should take place at least 6 h, and ideally 12 h, following the ictus. This enables red blood cell lysis to

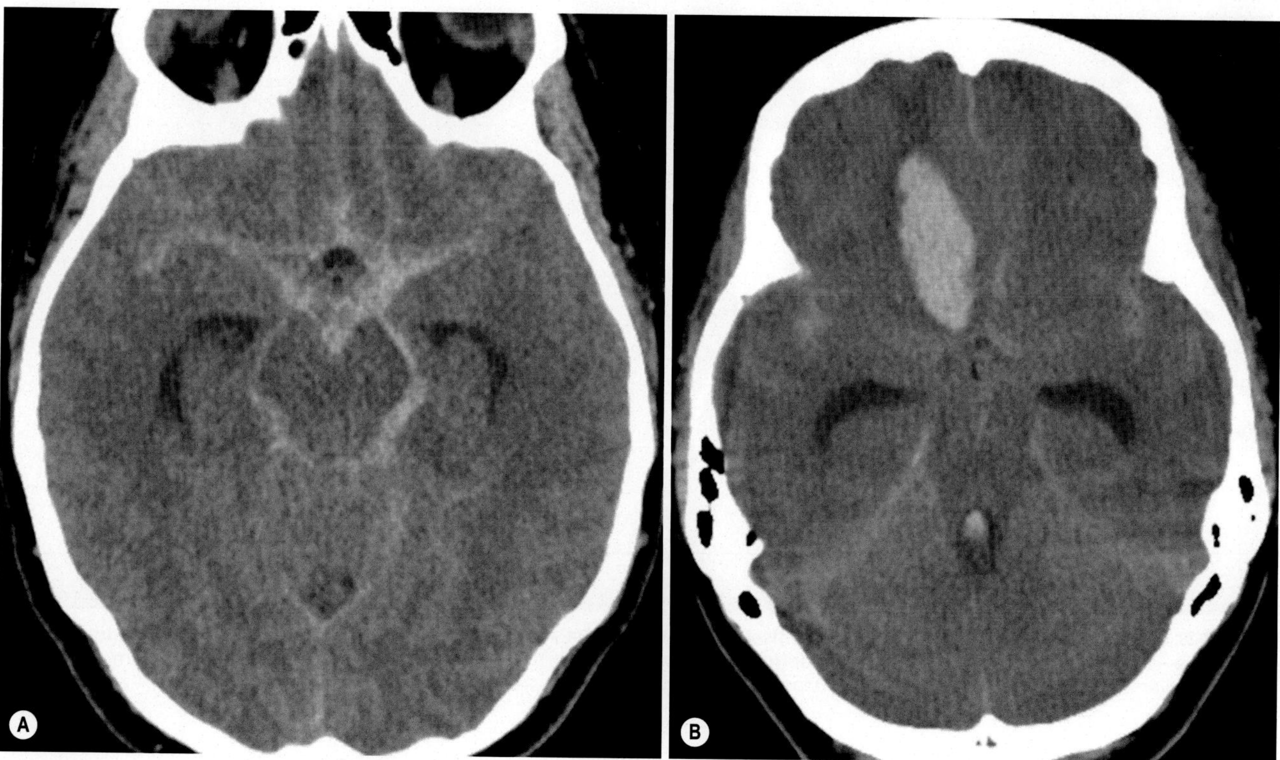

FIGURE 3-29 ■ Distributions of acute SAH. (A) Diffuse SAH within basal cisterns. (B) SAH with a focal parenchymal haematoma in the right inferior temporal lobe. This is very suggestive of an anterior communicating complex aneurysm—note the temporal horn dilatation in keeping with hydrocephalus.

Continued on following page

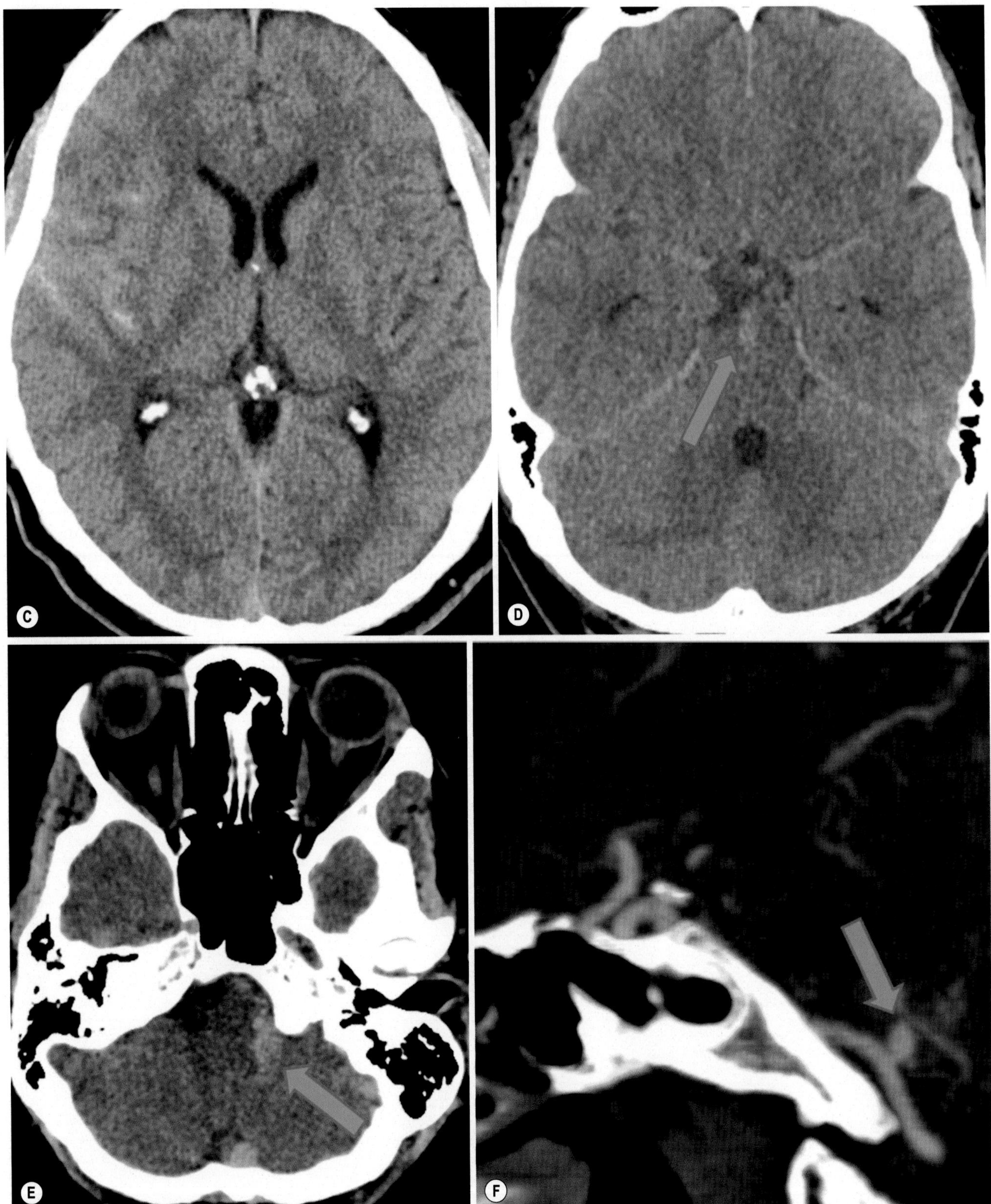

FIGURE 3-29, Continued ■ (C) SAH in the right sylvian fissure suggests an MCA anuerysm. (D) Small amount of SAH in the interpeduncular fossa—in keeping with a non-aneurysmal perimesencephalic SAH. (E) SAH adjacent to left side of the brainstem suggests a PICA aneurysm. (F) CTA confirms a PICA aneurysm.

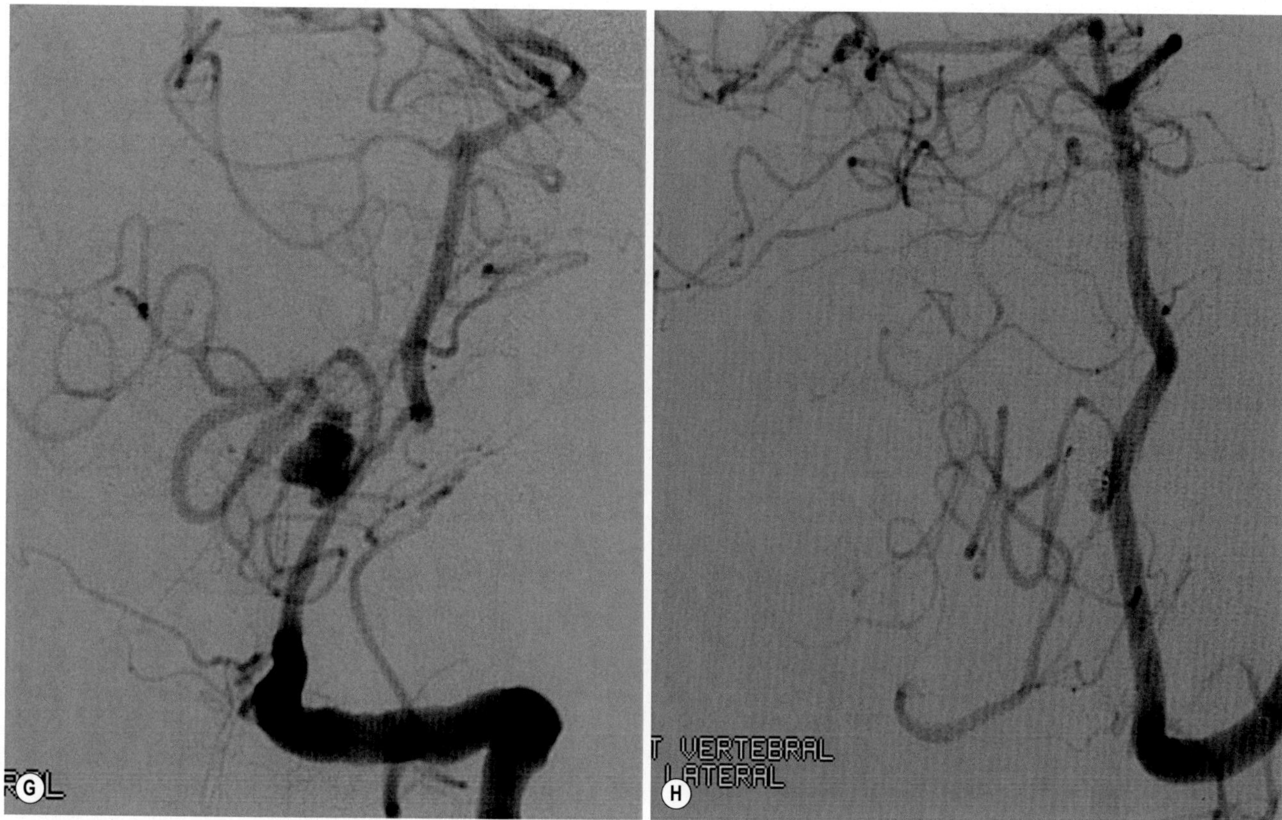

FIGURE 3-29, Continued ■ (G) DSA demonstrates the same PICA aneurysm. (H) Aneurysm is excluded from the circulation by endovascular insertion of platinum coils.

occur and thus blood degredation products such as bilirubin can be detected.[130,131]

Spin-echo MRI sequences are unreliable in SAH but by using a T2* gradient-echo or FLAIR sequence, sensitivities of 94–100% and 81–87% can be achieved in the acute (less than 4 days) and subacute (more than 4 days) periods, respectively.[132] The susceptibility effects of paramagnetic iron cause low signal on gradient-echo sequences; on FLAIR the CSF appears high signal due to the presence of increased protein. FLAIR may remain positive for up to 45 days after a haemorrhage,[133] at a time when the blood has long since become invisible on CT. However, FLAIR imaging is less sensitive at low CSF red blood cell concentrations following normal CT.[134]

Abnormal signal within the sulcal spaces on FLAIR sequences is not specific for SAH. Supplemental inspired oxygen,[135] leptomeningeal vascular engorgement and contrast medium leakage into the subarachnoid space after an acute infarct[136] can all cause the CSF to return high signal on FLAIR. CSF flow and pulsation artefact within the basal cisterns and at the foramen magnum is a common cause of artefactual abnormal signal which is commonly encountered in daily practice.

In the subacute period, CT and MRI will demonstrate a number of the complications associated with acute SAH. Of these, communicating hydrocephalus and ischaemia secondary to vasospasm are the most important. It is very common to see mild dilatation of the ventricles, particularly the temporal horns, at diagnosis. Indeed it may be a useful clue to the diagnosis if the presence of blood is not obvious. It usually resolves over several days, but may progress and necessitate CSF diversion. Vasospasm usually occurs between 4 and 11 days after the haemorrhage and is a significant cause of morbidity during this period.[137] It is more likely if the initial CT shows a large amount of subarachnoid blood.

MRI in chronic repeated SAH may show evidence of superficial siderosis with haemosiderin staining of the leptomeninges, particularly around the midbrain and in the posterior fossa. Such patients often present with symptoms related to the lower cranial nerves, ataxia or gradual cognitive decline. Location of an occult bleeding site is often not possible in these cases. The haemosiderin staining is often best appreciated on T2* GRE or SWI imaging (Fig. 3-30C).

Aneurysmal SAH

Aetiologically, cerebral aneurysms account for the majority of acute SAH cases. Aneurysms may be saccular, fusiform, or dissecting.[138] Fusiform aneurysms can be regarded as an extreme form of focal ectasia in hypertensive arteriosclerotic disease. Intracranial aneurysms can also develop following an arterial dissection or following direct vessel wall infection.

The majority are saccular aneurysms, which are usually round or lobulated and arise from arterial bifurcations, predominantly in the circle of Willis. Giant aneurysms, by definition, measure over 25 mm in diameter and account for approximately 5% of all cerebral aneurysms. They

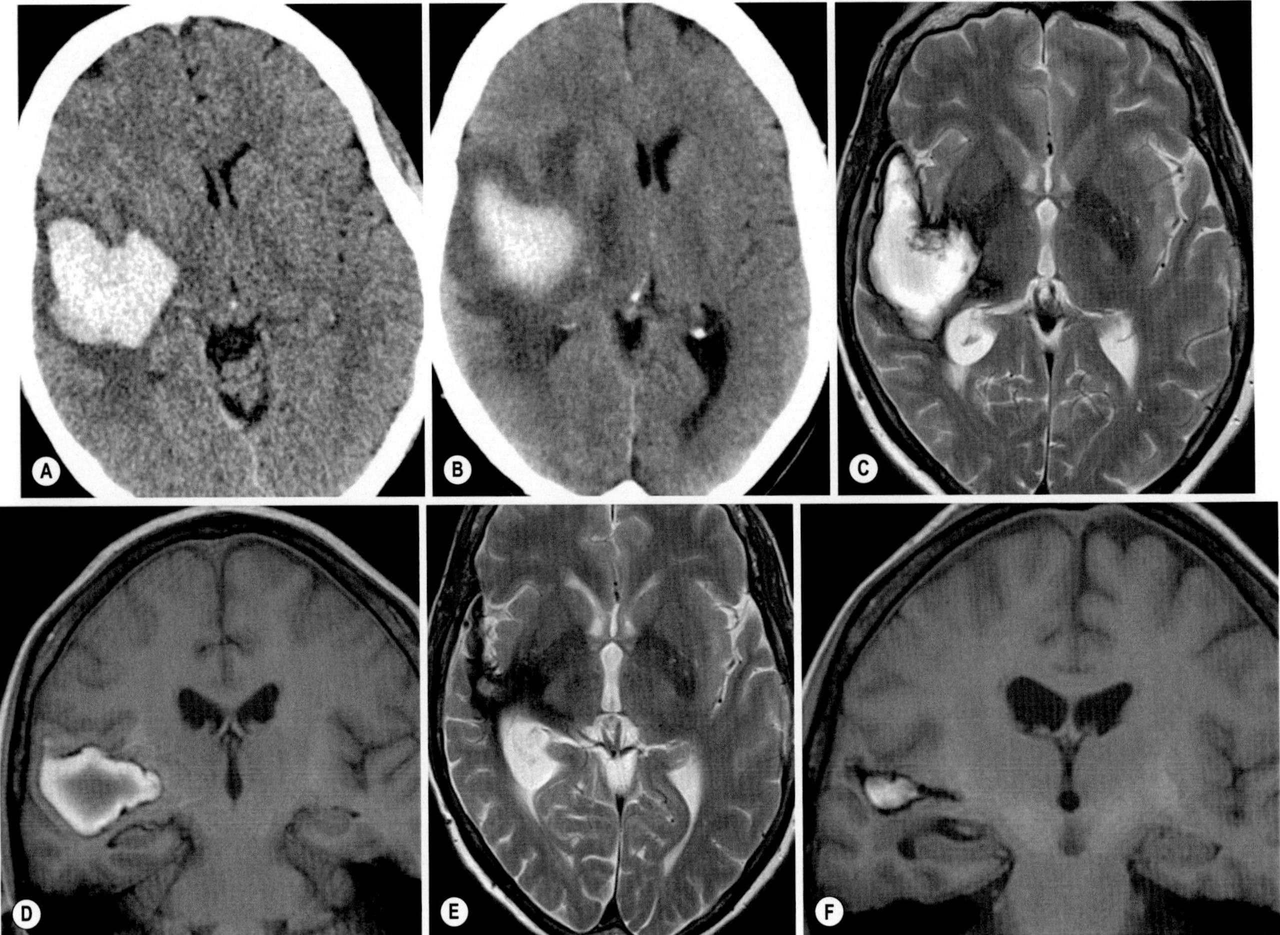

FIGURE 3-30 ■ **Evolution of intraparenchymal haemorrhage.** (A) Acute primary haematoma on CT. Note the homogeneous appearance with only a small peripheral rim of hypodensity. (B) Two weeks later the haematoma is less hyperdense but there is more surrounding oedema. (C, D) MRI at 1 month. The haematoma remains prominant but the surrounding oedema has resolved. There is a peripheral haemosiderin rim. There is T1 shortening (D) predominantly in the periphery. (E, F) At 5 months there has been shrinkage of the haematoma cavity which still shows residual T1 shortening (F). There is adjacent parenchymal haemosiderin staining with local loss of volume evidenced by the enlarged trigone of the right lateral ventricle.

often contain layers of organised thrombus. Aneurysms tend to present with SAH or mass effect on adjacent structures, most commonly a posterior communicating artery aneurysm resulting in extrinsic compression upon the cisternal segment of the third cranial nerve. Around 90% of intracranial aneurysms arise from the carotid circulation, the remaining 10% from vertebral or basilar arteries.[138] The anterior and posterior communicating arteries give rise to approximately one-third each of all intracranial aneurysms, with another 20% from middle cerebral arteries and 5% from the basilar termination. The remainder arises from other vessel origins and bifurcations. It should be remembered that 20% of aneurysms are multiple.

Aneurysmal SAH will often diffuse quickly throughout the CSF spaces giving little clue to its site of origin. More focal cisternal or parenchymal haematomas can be helpful in localising the source of the haemorrhage. A clot in the septum pellucidum, possibly extending into one or other frontal lobe, is virtually diagnostic of an aneurysm of the anterior communicating artery. Aneurysms of the distal anterior cerebral artery related to pericallosal branches are less common. Aneurysms of the MCA bleed into the sylvian fissure, sometimes with a clot in the temporal lobe. Aneurysms of the posterior communicating artery (which arise from the internal carotid artery at the origin of this vessel) are a frequent cause of SAH but can also present with an isolated third nerve palsy due to pulsatile pressure on the nerve.

Aneurysms of the posterior circulation are commonly located at the basilar artery termination and if they rupture blood may be seen in the interpeduncular fossa, brainstem or thalami; prognosis is frequently poor. The second commonest site in the posterior circulation is at the origin of one of the posterior inferior cerebellar arteries. They often haemorrhage into the ventricular system via the fourth ventricle and the haematoma localises around the craniocervical junction and the spinal subarachnoid space.

Larger aneurysms are shown on standard structural CT and MRI. On CT they appear as rounded enhancing lesions. Giant aneurysms have an enhancing lumen and a wall of variable thickness that often contains laminated thrombus and may be calcified. On spin-echo MRI sequences a patent aneurysm appears as an area of flow void. Areas of increased signal intensity within the aneurysm may represent mural thrombus or turbulent, slow flow.

Surrounding white matter oedema suggests a mycotic aneurysm, particularly if very extensive. Mycotic aneurysms are caused by septic emboli and tend to occur peripherally, typically on the branches of the MCA. They commonly present with haemorrhage, usually with a peripheral intraparenchymal clot, which, while not specific, is highly suggestive of such a lesion in a patient with known septicaemia or bacterial endocarditis.

Angiography in Acute SAH

The investigation of acute SAH requires expedient evaluation of the intracranial arterial circulation.

Digital subtraction catheter angiography (DSA) remains the gold standard for the imaging of intracranial aneurysms and vascular malformations. Its high spatial and temporal resolution allows accurate characterisation of the smallest aneurysms and enables endovascular treatment or surgical planning. Three-dimensional angiography rotational angiography (3D DSA) has further improved accuracy as it helps to resolve aneurysms which may be obscured by overlying vessels.[139–141] It reduces the need for multiple angiographic runs and provides high-resolution 3D images of the cerebral vessels that show the relationship of an aneurysm to adjacent vessels. Manipulation at the workstation permits the image to be rotated and viewed from any angle. This technique, however, is invasive, with an approximately 0.5–2% complication rate.[142,143] It is costly, requires specialist operator skills and equipment and is largely confined to neurosciences centres.

The last decade has seen dramatic advances in non-invasive imaging of aneurysms. Modern multidetector CT scanners with sophisticated post-processing computer software now provide fast, non-invasive intracranial angiographic data which approaches the sensitivity of catheter angiography. Results of several systematic reviews and meta-analysis show that CT angiography has a very high diagnostic value for the detection of intracranial aneurysms, particularly those of 3 mm[144–146] and over in size. Smaller aneurysms, particularly at the skull base, can be difficult to resolve. However, recent publications on multidetector scanners (320 detector rows) often using bone subtraction algorithms showed equivalent sensitivity and specificities with 3D DSA.[147–150]

Given its availability, speed and accuracy, CTA is the standard initial investigation of choice for investigating SAH in the acute setting. It takes only a few minutes to prepare the patient and plan the examination and on a multidetector CT system the whole head is imaged in less than 10 s. This is ideal in patients with SAH, who are often restless and unwell. It provides rapid diagnosis and enables endovascular and surgical treatment planning. This may negate the need for diagnostic catheter angiography prior to treatment, although catheter angiography is still required when the treatment strategy is not clear.

It is essential to methodically review source images on a workstation, in addition to multiplanar reformats and 3D surface renderings. Particular care should be taken close to the skull base, where adjacent bone may reduce the conspicuity of small aneurysms. CTA images can be degraded by vasospasm or inadequate opacification if the images are not acquired during the arterial phase of contrast enhancement. It is apparent on visual inspection when this is the case. The images can be rotated in multiple planes (like in 3D DSA), allowing for accurate evaluation of the anatomy of an aneurysm and its neck. However, the greatest benefit of CTA is its ease of use. It seems superficially attractive to consider devolving CTA to the general hospital environment. However, accurate interpretation requires experience in neurovascular radiology and CTA is part of the overall care of SAH patients, which is currently delivered in a neuroscience environment.

Practice varies in patients with a negative CTA following acute SAH. There is a body of opinion that a single technically adequate CTA is sufficient following a classical perimesencephalic SAH.[151] Some institutions now rely solely on CTA for all diagnostic imaging in SAH. However, in most centres it remains routine practice to confirm a negative CTA result with DSA. It is also used if for any reason aneurysm anatomy is not adequately displayed on CTA. Other vascular causes of SAH such as small vascular malformations are also more accurately assessed with this method.

CT angiography should be performed as soon as possible following SAH since the aneurysm re-bleed rate is greatest during the first 48 h and vasospasm can adversely affect the quality of angiograms performed several days after the haemorrhage. If a negative angiogram is marred by vasospasm, a repeat study is indicated.

Aneurysms can be treated by surgical clipping or endovascular coiling. The latter is performed via a microcatheter placed in the aneurysm sac through which a number of electrically detachable platinum coils with or without a gel coating are deployed (Figs. 3-31 and 3-32). The coiling may be assisted by the use of a catheter-mounted balloon or insertion of a stent across the aneurysm neck to prevent the coil ball prolapsing into the parent vessel. A multicentre randomised comparison of surgical clipping and endovascular coiling showed superior outcomes at 1 year for coiling over clipping (death or dependency 23.5 vs 30.9%; absolute risk reduction 7.4%). This difference was maintained at 7 years with a lower risk of epilepsy but more episodes of re-bleeding in the coiled group.[152] There is still a role for surgical clipping if the anatomy of the aneurysm is unfavourable for endovascular treatment.

Imaging of Incidental Intracranial Aneurysms

Increasingly, saccular aneurysms are discovered incidentally on scans for other indications and this represents a management problem. A large-scale study, International Study of Unruptured Intracranial Aneurysms (ISUIA) suggests that the annual risk of haemorrhage from

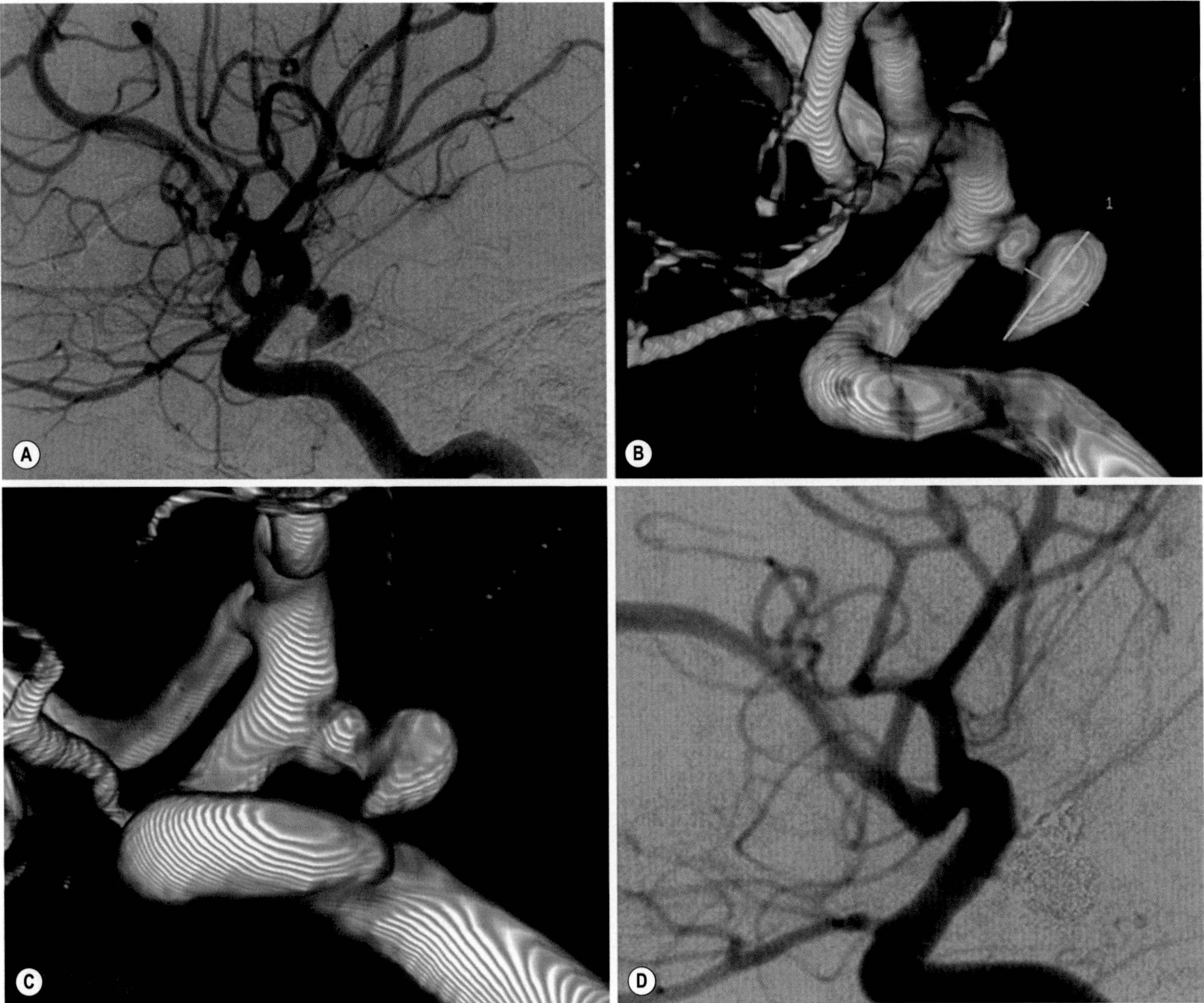

FIGURE 3-31 ■ A 37-year-old female patient presents with an acute-onset painful right third nerve palsy with pupil involvement. CT angiography demonstrated the presence of a lobulated posterior communicating artery (Pcomm) aneurysm. (A) The Pcomm aneurysm is demonstrated at DSA. (B, C) The size and position of the aneurysm neck is further appreciated with the volume-rendered images from the 3D rotational DSA. (D) After endovascular coiling, the aneurysm is completely excluded from the circulation.

small incidental aneurysms is substantially lower than previously thought and the risks of elective intervention higher.[153,154] Current data indicate that there is no benefit from treating aneurysms of the anterior circulation that are 7 mm or less in diameter, regardless of the patient's age, if there is no prior history of SAH. The difference between the risks of haemorrhage and treatment may favour intervention for larger or posterior circulation aneurysms (including posterior communicating aneurysms) depending on aneurysm size and remaining life expectancy.[154]

With no ionising radiation, MRA is considered to be the preferred method of imaging for intracranial aneurysms in the non-acute setting. These include screening of patients with two first-degree relatives who have suffered subarachnoid haemorrhage or those with connective tissue disorders who are at higher risk of aneurysm formation. It is also the preferred method of investigation for follow-up of incidental aneurysms and increasingly in follow-up assessment of endovascularly treated aneurysms.[155–157] Three-dimensional TOF MRA is the most widely accepted technique because it provides good spatial resolution and is relatively insensitive to signal dropout from turbulent flow. Resolution is further improved at higher field strengths and a number of studies have shown accurate detection of aneurysms down to the size of 1 mm,[158–160] although aneurysms less than 3 mm and those at the carotid siphon are those most easily missed. Like CTA, MRA images can be easily manipulated on the work station. Recent SAH may cause image degradation on TOF MRA due to T1 shortening from haemorrhage. Giant aneurysms are rarely visualised in their full extent on 3D TOF MRA because of slow and turbulent flow in their fundus. The lumen is properly opacified on CTA, which also shows mural thrombus and the aneurysm wall.

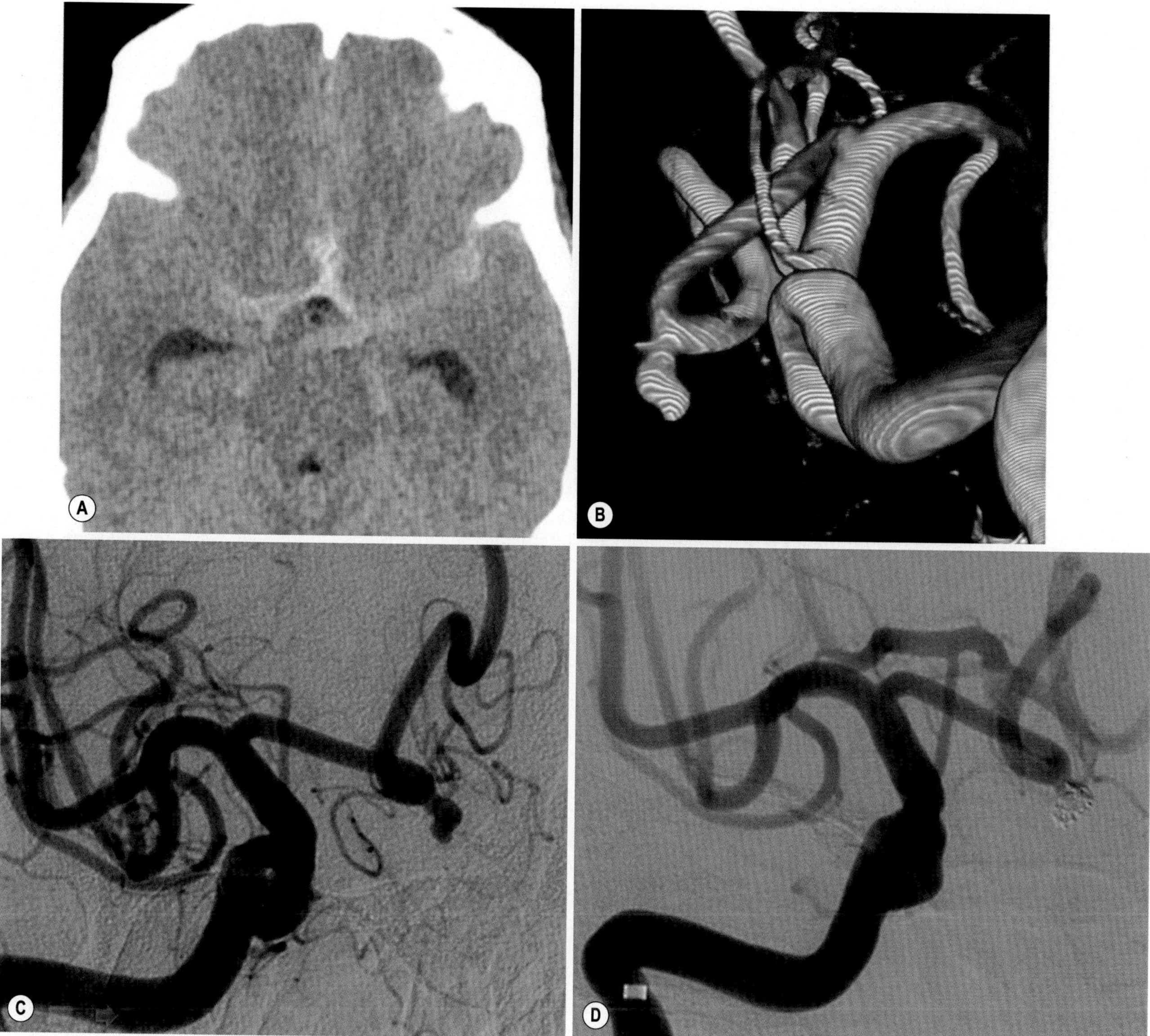

FIGURE 3-32 ■ A 50-year-old presents with an acute-onset headache. (A) NCECT demonstrates acute subarachnoid blood. (B, C) 3D DSA characterises the lobulated anterior communicating artery aneurysm prior to endovascular coiling where it is completely excluded from the circulation (D).

INTRACEREBRAL HAEMORRHAGE

Non-traumatic intracerebral haemorrhage accounts for 10–15% of all strokes. It has a higher mortality rate than other types of stroke, with less than 40% of patients surviving the first year. Primary haemorrhage occurs most commonly in the elderly from the rupture of small perforating vessels damaged by atherosclerotic hypertensive change or amyloid angiopathy. This accounts for up to 80% of spontaneous parenchymal haemorrhage. The preferential sites of hypertensive haemorrhage are the striato-capsular/thalamo-capsular regions, pons and cerebellum.[161–164] Larger hypertensive bleeds in the basal ganglia can extend into the ventricles or subarachnoid spaces. Peripheral or lobar haemorrhages in the elderly are suggestive of amyloid angiopathy, particularly if they are multifocal.[165] Both pathologies are often accompanied by a background of microbleeds.[166] These are best identified on T2* gradient-echo or susceptibility-weighted imaging. Hypertensive microbleeds tend to have a central predominance, whereas those associated with amyloid angiopathy are most often peripheral (Fig. 3-30).

Secondary haemorrhage can be due to a coagulopathy (usually on a background of hypertensive or amyloid angiopathy), underlying vascular malformation, haemorrhagic transformation of arterial and venous infarction (Fig. 3-33) and tumour. 'Recreational' drugs such as cocaine and ecstasy[167] and vasculitis are other rare but important causes.

Intracranial haemorrhage caused by aneurysms is usually associated with SAH, but very occasionally a ruptured aneurysm can cause an apparently isolated intracerebral clot (particularly if the surrounding subarachnoid space has been 'sealed off' by preceding SAH). This should be considered whenever a parenchymal haematoma extends to involve the sylvian fissure or basal cistern.

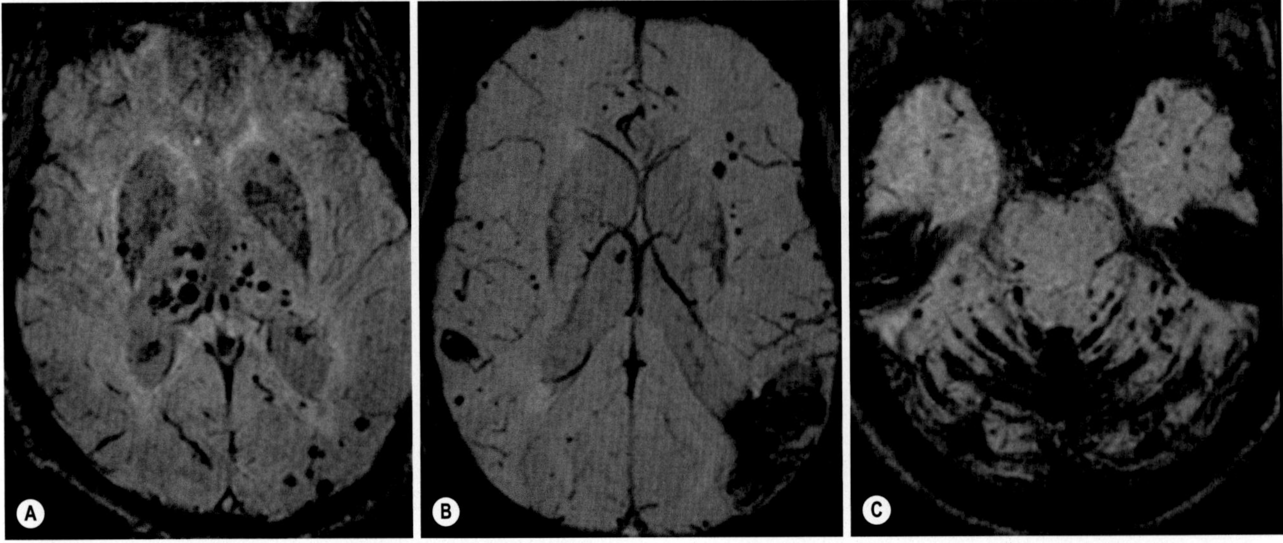

FIGURE 3-33 ■ SWI images demonstrate (A) cerebral microhaemorrhages related to hypertension. Note the predominantly ganglionic distribution. (B) Small lobar haemorrhages and predominantly peripheral microhaemorrhages in a patient with amyloid angiopathy. (C) Extensive haemosiderin staining over the cerebellar folia in a patient with siderosis of unknown aetiology.

TABLE 3-5 **Temporal MR Characteristics of Parenchymal Haematomas**[169]

Time	Stage	Biochemical form	SI on T1-weighted image	SI on T2-weighted image
Immediately to several hours	Hyperacute	Oxyhaemoglobin in RBC	↔	↑
1 to 3 days	Acute	Deoxyhaemoglobin in RBC	↔ ↓	↓↓
3 to 7 days	Early subacute	Methaemoglobin in RBC	↑↑	↓↓
1 to several weeks	Subacute to chronic	Extracellular methaemoglobin	↑↑	↑↑
Weeks to indefinitely	Remote	Ferritin and haemosiderin	↓	↓↓

SI = Signal intensity relative to grey matter.

Appearance on CT and MRI

Acute parenchymal haemorrhage is reliably detected on CT, appearing as increased density. Calcified or highly proteinaceous material and contrast enhancement of tumours can reach a similar density to fresh blood clot, but the clinical context or correlation with unenhanced images should prevent confusion. Hyperacute, unclotted blood will appear less dense, which may cause a blood–fluid level to be visible. This appearance is most commonly due to haemorrhage from coagulopathies (usually anticoagulant medication). Very rarely in severely anaemic patients with a haematocrit level below 20% haematomas can be isodense to the surrounding brain.[168] Deep or extensive haemorrhage may extend into the ventricles, forming a haematoma, or a blood–fluid level in the occipital horns, which are dependent with the patient supine.

Typically an acute primary parenchymal haematoma is homogeneous with only a fine rim of surrounding low density. Extensive oedema at presentation suggests an underlying abnormality. Features favouring a neoplastic haemorrhage are a more complex structure, extensive surrounding vasogenic oedema and enhancing areas not immediately adjacent to the blood clot. In some cases the diagnosis can only be made after follow-up studies.

Over the course of several days, an untreated haematoma becomes less dense, from the periphery towards the centre, and therefore appears smaller, although the surrounding oedema usually increases. The time of ictus is important, as small haemorrhages can look identical to infarcts on CT by 8–9 days, which clearly has important treatment ramifications. MRI will help to distinguish between the two. Vasogenic oedema may develop in the surrounding white matter and should contrast medium be given at this stage, it usually produces a halo of enhancement. After several weeks, the blood products become hypodense and are eventually absorbed to leave a focal, often slit-like, cavity or area of atrophy.

The MRI appearance of intracerebral haemorrhage changes over time as red cells break down and degrade, ultimately taken up by macrophages as haemosiderin.[169] These physiological phenomena result in a relatively characteristic temporal pattern of MRI appearances on T1 and T2 spin-echo sequences (Table 3-5).[169] Factors such as protein and water content, fibrin formation and clot retraction can alter the sequence and timing of changes in appearance on MRI (Fig. 3-34).

Gradient-echo and more recently susceptibility-weighted imaging[170,171] is much more sensitive to the magnetic field inhomogeneities induced by blood degredation products than spin-echo sequences. This applies to both acute and old haemorrhage (deoxyhaemoglobin and haemosiderin, respectively).

Angiography in Intracerebral Haemorrhage

The indications for angiography in intraparenchymal haemorrhage are determined by clinical factors as much as imaging appearance. It is unlikely a treatable vascular abnormality will be found in a basal ganglia bleed in an elderly hypertensive patient, whereas a haemorrhage in the same location in a young, normotensive patient warrants further investigation with angiography to exclude an arteriovenous malformation (AVM). It is also noteworthy that some 'recreational' drugs are associated with aneurysm formation and rupture, so angiography is often appropriate in such patients.[167]

The timing of angiography depends on the size and mass effect of the haematoma. CTA is used in the emergency setting for the detection of ruptured AVMs and aneurysms as it is much easier and quicker to perform in very sick patients. It allows the neurosurgeons to assess the location and extent of the vascular abnormality and to plan their surgical approach prior to evacuation of the haematoma. In a stable patient not requiring urgent haematoma evacuation it is usually preferable to defer angiography until the haematoma has resolved because smaller vascular lesions can be compressed by an acute haematoma and not be apparent angiographically. It is not yet established that a small arteriovenous fistula or malformation can be reliably excluded using CTA/MRA, so DSA is still preferred for elective investigation of such patients. Dynamic contrast-enhanced CTA and MRA studies which are time resolved are demonstrating good results in comparative studies with catheter angiography in patients with vascular malformations.[172–174]

ARTERIOVENOUS MALFORMATIONS

Intracranial vascular malformations can be classified according to the presence or otherwise of arteriovenous shunting.[175] The former comprises cerebral (or subpial) AVMs and dural fistulae; the latter includes developmental venous anomalies (DVAs), cavernous angiomas ('cavernomas') and capillary telangiectasias. DSA is still the method of choice for the investigation of cerebral AVMs and dural fistulae. Cavernous angiomas and telangiectasias are angiographically occult or 'cryptic' vascular malformations which tend to have characteristic appearances on MRI.

Cerebral (subpial) AVMs are probably congenital anomalies consisting of direct arteriovenous shunts without a normal intervening capillary bed. Some are essentially fistulous—direct shunting from an artery to a vein; others have a plexiform nidus or a combination of the two. They lie within the brain substance or cerebral sulci and are supplied by branches of the internal carotid artery or vertebrobasilar system, sometimes recruiting additional supply from meningeal arteries. Cerebral haemorrhage is the commonest clinical presentation, others being epilepsy, headache or focal neurological deficit.

They are usually detectable on CT or MRI as serpiginous areas of high density (with marked contrast enhancement) or mixed signal, respectively. CT may show calcification and the MR signal comprises areas of flow void and high signal, which may represent thrombosis or flow-related enhancement. There may be haemorrhage at different stages of evolution. AVMs may be surrounded by areas of ischaemic damage that are low attenuation on CT and hyperintense on T2-weighted MRI. Dilated feeding arteries and early opacification of draining veins indicating shunting are the angiographic hallmarks of these lesions (Fig. 3-35).

Dural arteriovenous fistulae are direct shunts between branches of the external carotid artery or meningeal branches of the cerebral vessels and dural sinuses. They are thought to be acquired and may be due to prior venous thrombosis. The clinical presentation depends on their location and venous drainage pattern.[176,177] Lesions shunting into the cavernous sinus commonly present with proptosis. Shunting into the transverse or sigmoid sinus may cause pulsatile tinnitus. Intracranial haemorrhage, which may be intracerebral, subarachnoid or subdural, usually occurs in lesions that reflux into cortical veins. They may go undetected on MRI or CT unless there are enlarged dural sinuses or cortical veins. MRA or CTA may show abnormal vessels more clearly but intra-arterial angiography is still required to make a definitive diagnosis (Fig. 3-36).

Angiography for an AVM or dural fistula should include injections of all possible feeding vessels using a high frame rate to improve delineation of the nidus, which otherwise can be obscured by overlying veins in rapidly shunting lesions. There may be associated aneurysms, either on the feeding arteries or within the nidus and venous drainage may be via deep and/or superficial systems. There may be venous varices or stenoses. There is an increased risk of haemorrhage in AVMs with the presence of intranidal aneurysms, a single draining vein, deep venous drainage and venous stenoses.[177–179] CTA and MRA show the components of an AVM[177] and increasingly dynamic contrast-enhanced MR and CT angiography can provide the temporal information only previously available from DSA.[173,174,180,181]

The treatment options for cerebral AVMs include surgery, radiosurgery and endovascular embolisation. More than one technique may be used in combination.

Cavernous angiomas are mulberry-like lesions consisting of vascular spaces with little intervening tissue and haemorrhage of different ages. The incidence of clinically symptomatic haemorrhage remains uncertain, but is less frequent than with cerebral AVMs or dural fistulae. A previous bleed and infratentorial location are the main prognostic factors for recurrent haemorrhage. Lesions in

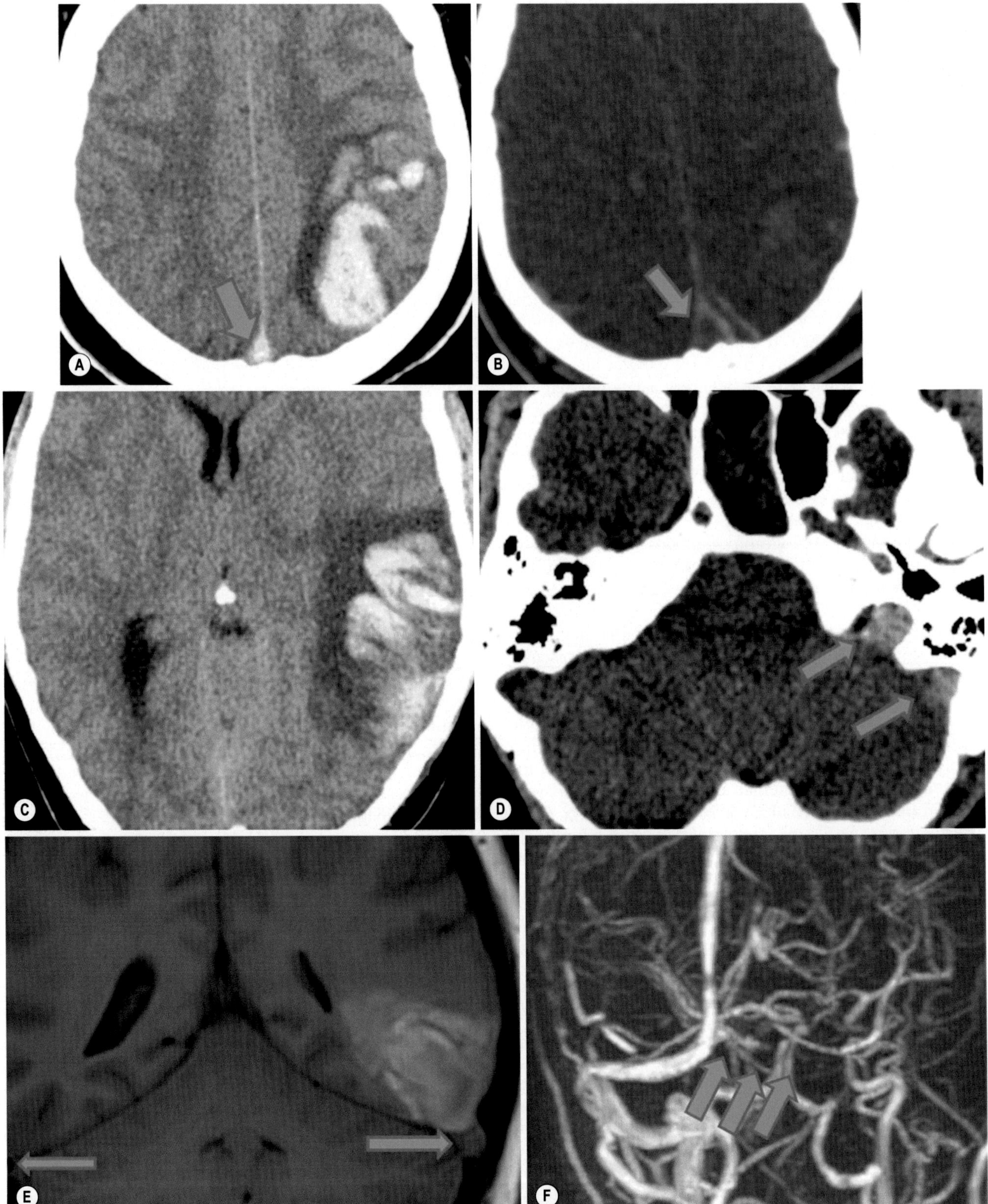

FIGURE 3-34 ■ (A) Fragmented parenchymal haemorrhage in dural venous sinus thrombosis (DVST). Note the hyperdense superior sagittal sinus on the NCET. (B) The venographic study shows absence of contrast enhancement within the sinus 'empty delta sign'. (C) The parieto-temporal location suggests lateral venous sinous/vein of Labbé thrombosis. (D) The hyperdense left lateral transverse sinus and sigmoid sinus is seen on the NCET. (E) Same patient as (C, D): coronal T1 FSE with parenchymal T1 shortening in keeping with haemorrhage. Note the attenuated left-sided venous sinus flow void (arrows). (F) The 3D MRV does not demonstrate any flow with the left transverse or sigmoid sinus. This can be a normal variant which should be confirmed with structural MRI imaging. In DVST there will be attenuation of the normal dural sinus flow void and it is usually hyperintense on the T2-dependent sequences although this is dependent on the age of the blood products. CT will also demonstrate the presence of a sinus grooving the occipital bone rather than showing true hypoplasia.

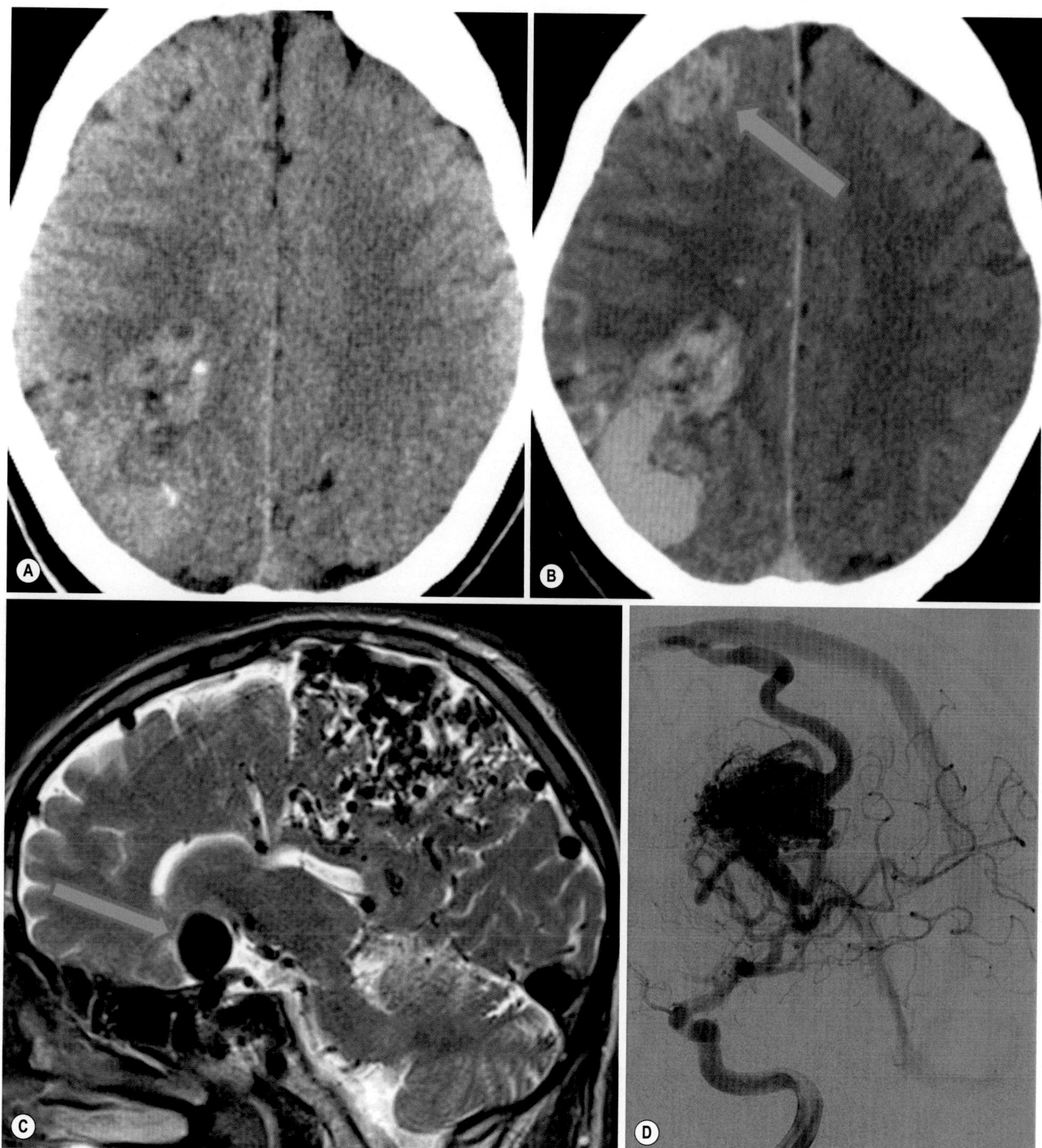

FIGURE 3-35 ■ CT in a young female patient who presented with a seizure. (A) Unenhanced study shows lobulated hyperdensity with focal areas of calcification. (B) Following contrast administration there is avid enhancement in two distinct areas of the right frontal and parietal lobes. The appearances are typical of an AVM. Multiple AVMs suggest hereditary haemorrhagic telangiectasia (HHT). In this case there was no parenchymal haemorrhage. (C) MRI in a different patient shows a diffuse parietal AVM with large superficial draining veins. Note the large flow aneurysm related to the terminal ICA (arrow). (D) DSA shows an AVM with a compact nidus. It is supplied by branches of the middle cerebral artery and drains via both the superficial and deep venous systems.

or close to the cerebral cortex may cause epilepsy. They are occasionally intraventricular or arise on a cranial nerve. They appear as relatively well-defined, dense or calcified lesions on CT, which may show patchy contrast enhancement. On MRI they appear multilobular with mixed but predomiantly elevated T2 signal intensity centrally surrounded by a dark haemosiderin rim.[182] Not surprisingly, susceptibility-based sequences are the most sensitive.[171,172] They may be multiple, particularly in familial cases.[183] In many clinical situations the discovery of a cavernoma represents an incidental finding (Fig. 3-37).

Developmental venous anomalies are not malformations but represent a benign variation in venous

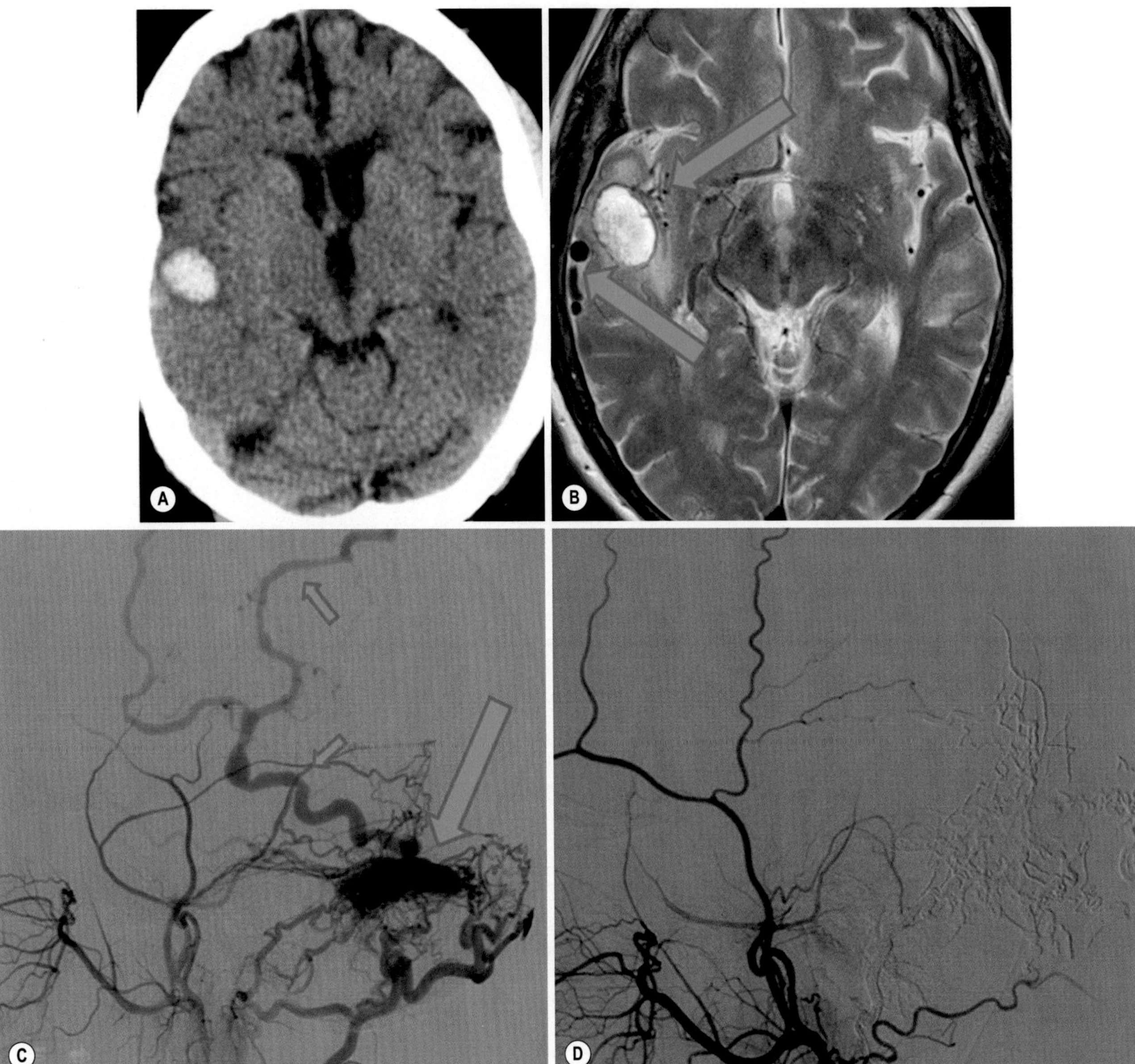

FIGURE 3-36 ■ (A) CT demonstrates small right temporal haemorrhage. (B) T2W MRI shows the haemorrhage but also demonstrates the presence of prominent local vessels (arrows). (C) DSA injection of the external carotid circulation shows a fistulous connection between ECA branches (occipital and meningeal) with an isolated transverse sinus (long arrow). There is retrograde venous drainage via a hyprotrophied vein of Labbé and the vein of Trolard (short arrows) into the superior sagittal sinus. (D) The fistula has been embolised using a liquid embolic agent.

drainage. They may be found with cavernomas. They consist of radially arranged, dilated transmedullary veins that have a typical 'caput medusa' appearance on the venous phase of conventional angiograms. They may drain into the superficial or deep venous system. They are readily diagnosed by contrast-enhanced CT or MRI.[182]

Capillary telangiectasias are benign nests of dilated capillaries with normal brain tissue in between. They are usually found on postmortem examinations and are occasionally visible on MRI as areas of very subtle T2 hyperintensity or ill-defined enhancement. They do not cause haemorrhage.

SUBDURAL AND EXTRADURAL HAEMORRHAGE

Acute subdural and extradural haematomas are almost always post-traumatic.

Occasionally, rupture of a cerebral aneurysm may cause an acute subdural haematoma, most frequently a posterior communicating artery aneurysm lying next to the free edge of the tentorium cerebelli. A dural arteriovenous fistula may also bleed into the subdural space. Angiography is therefore indicated following a spontaneous acute subdural haematoma, particularly in a young patient.

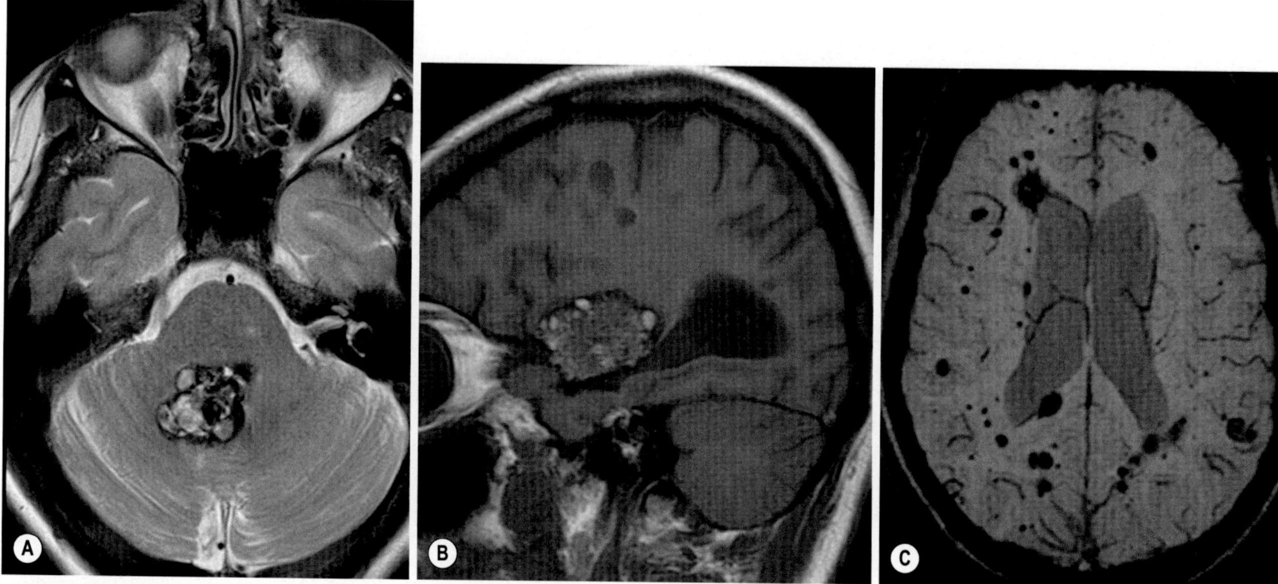

FIGURE 3-37 ■ (A) Posterior fossa cavernoma has a 'popcorn' appearance with a peripheral haemosiderin ring. (B) Sagittal T1W image again shows peripheral haemosiderin ring. There are locules of T1 shortening in keeping with blood degradation products. (C) SWI image demonstrates numerous areas of susceptibility 'blooming' related to blood products from multifocal cavernomas.

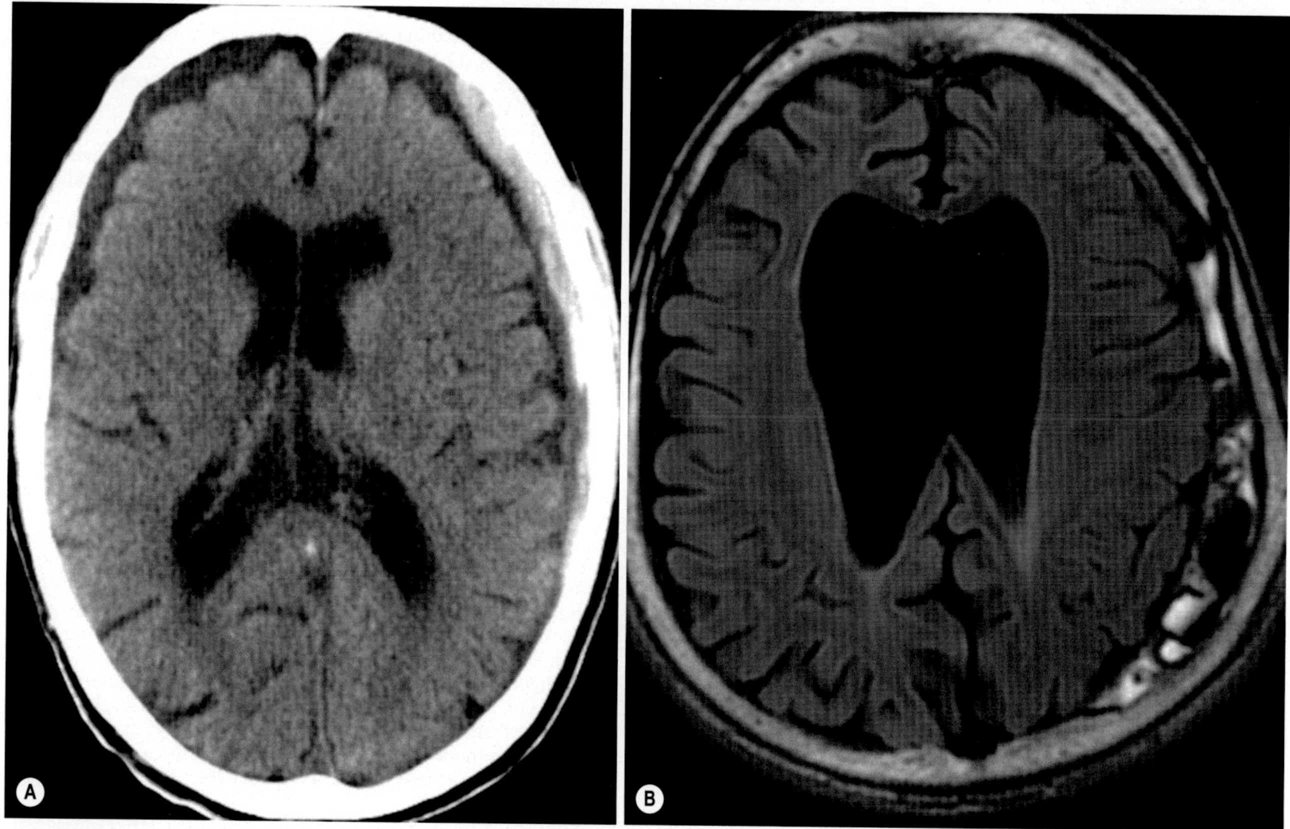

FIGURE 3-38 ■ (A) Shallow bilateral convexity chronic subdural haematomas. The increased density over the left convexity suggests a more acute component. (B) A larger left convexity chronic subdural haematoma on FLAIR. Note the local left hemispheric sulcal effacement.

Chronic subdural haematomas represent a different entity. These are frequently bilateral and occur in elderly patients or alcoholics with underlying brain atrophy, patients on anticoagulants or following shunting for hydrocephalus. The underlying mechanism is thought to be leakage from bridging cortical veins following minor trauma. They may present with increasing confusion and a reduction in conscious level. Burr holes for drainage of a chronic subdural collection, sometimes under a local anaesthetic, are one of the few neurosurgical operations performed on the very elderly (Fig. 3-38).

On CT they appear to be of lower density than the brain but may contain areas of high density, or even fluid levels, due to more recent haemorrhage. The MRI appearance evolves in a similar pattern to intraparenchymal haemorrhage. Chronic subdural haematomas continue to give high signal on T2-weighted images, while returning low signal on T1-weighted images, without becoming isointense to CSF, because of their higher protein content. Repeated episodes of bleeding can produce variable changes of signal intensity analogous to the variable density changes on CT. A pseudomembrane, which forms around chronic subdural haematomas, may show marked contrast enhancement or haemosiderin staining.

Shallow subdural fluid collections and occasionally overt haemorrhage may also develop around the cerebral hemispheres and cerebellum secondary to mild brain descent in the low CSF volume syndrome.[184] In this condition patients usually present with postural headache that is worse on standing and relieved by lying down. There is sometimes a history of vigorous Valsalva, lumbar puncture or other spinal intervention. The MRI features, other than subdural collections, are diffuse dural thickening shown best on FLAIR or contrast-enhanced T_1-weighted images and mild cerebellar ectopia. These changes resolve after successful treatment.

REFERENCES

1. Mant J, Wade DT, Winner S. Health care needs assessment: stroke. In: Stevens A, Raftery J, Mant J, et al, editors. Health Care Needs Assessment: The Epidemiologically Based Needs Assessment Reviews, First series. 2nd ed. Oxford: Radcliffe Medical Press; 2004. pp. 141–244.
2. Lloyd-Jones D, Adams R, Carnethon M, et al. Heart disease and stroke statistics—2009 update: a report from the American Heart Association Statistics Committee and Stroke Statistics Subcommittee. Circulation 2009;119(3):e21–181.
3. Lovett JK, Dennis MS, Sandercock PAG, et al. Very early risk of stroke after a first transient ischemic attack. Stroke 2003;34: e138–40.
4. Fairhead JF, Mehta Z, Rothwell PM. Population-based study of delays in carotid imaging and surgery and the risk of recurrent stroke. Neurology 2005;65:371–5.
5. Ovbiagele B, Kidwell CS, Saver JL. Epidemiological impact in the United States of a tissue-based definition of transient ischemic attack. Stroke 2003;34:919–24.
6. Calvet D, Touze E, Oppenheim C, et al. DWI lesions and TIA aetiology improve the prediction of stroke after TIA. Stroke 2009;40(1):187–92.
7. Ueda T, Yuh W, Taoka T. Clinical application of perfusion and diffusion MR imaging in acute ischemic stroke. J Magn Reson Imaging 1999;10:305–9.
8. Markus HS. Cerebral perfusion and stroke. J Neurol Neurosurg Psychiatry 2004;75:353–61.
9. Halpin SFS. Brain imaging using multislice CT: a personal perspective. Br J Radiol 2004;77:20–6.
10. Powers WJ. Cerebral hemodynamics in ischemic cerebrovascular disease. Ann Neurol 1991;29:231–40.
11. Hakim AM, Pokrupa RP, Villanueva J, et al. The effect of spontaneous reperfusion on metabolic function in early human cerebral infarcts. Ann Neurol 1987;21:279–89.
12. Marchal G, Furlan M, Beaudouin V, et al. Early spontaneous hyperperfusion after stroke. A marker of favourable tissue outcome? Brain 1996;119:409–19.
13. Marchal G, Young AR, Baron JC. Early postischemic hyperperfusion: Pathophysiologic insights from positron emission tomography. J Cereb Blood Flow Metab 1999;19:467–82.
14. Adams HP, Benixden BH, Kapelle LJ, et al. Classification of subtype of acute ischaemic stroke. Definitions for use in a multicentre clinical trial. TOAST. Trial of Org 10172 in Acute Stroke Treatment. Stroke 1993;24(1):35–41.
15. Caplan LR. 'Top of the basilar' syndrome. Neurology 1980;30: 72–9.
16. NINDS Study Group. Tissue plasminogen activator for acute ischemic stroke. N Engl J Med 1995;333:1581–7.
17. Hacke W, Kaste M, Bluhmki E, et al. ECASS Investigators. Thrombolysis with alteplase 3 to 4.5 hours after acute ischemic stroke. N Engl J Med 2008;359:1317–29.
18. Wahlgren N, Ahmed N, Davalos A, et al. Thrombolysis with alteplase for acute ischaemic stroke in the Safe Implementation of Thrombolysis in Stroke-Monitoring Study (SITS-MOST): an observational study. Lancet 2007;369(9558):275–82.
19. London Cardiac and Stroke Networks. National audit shows London hospitals top in stroke care 210. Available at <http://www.slcsn.nhs.uk/files/stroke/events/general/pmlss.updates.pdf>.
20. Chen ZM, Sandercock PAG, Pan HC, et al, on behalf of the CAST and IST collaborative groups. Indications for early aspirin use in acute ischaemic stroke. A combined analysis of 40,000 randomised patients from the Chinese Acute Stroke Trial and the International Stroke Trial. Stroke 2000;31:1240–9.
21. Blight A, Pereira AC, Brown MM. A single consultation cerebrovascular disease clinic is cost effective in the management of transient ischaemic attack and minor stroke. J R Coll Physicians Lond 2000;34:452–5.
22. Smith WS, Tsao JW, Billings ME, et al. Prognostic significance of angiographically confirmed large vessel intracranial occlusion in patients presenting with acute brain ischemia. Neurocrit Care 2006;4(1):14–17.
23. Barber PA, Demchuk AM, Hudon ME, et al. Hyperdense Sylvian fissure MCA 'dot' sign: a CT marker of acute ischemia. Stroke 2001;32:84–8.
24. Kummer R, Meyding-Lamade U, Forsting M, et al. Sensitivity and prognostic value of early CT in occlusion of the middle cerebral artery trunk. Am J Neuroradiol 1994;15:9–15.
25. Bryan RN, Levy LM, Whitlow WD, et al. Diagnosis of acute cerebral infarction: comparison of CT and MR imaging. Am J Neuroradiol 1991;12:611–20.
26. Barber PA, Demchuk AM, Zhang J, et al, for the ASPECTS study group. Hyperacute stroke: the validity and reliability of a novel quantitative CT score in predicting outcome prior to thrombolytic therapy. Lancet 2000;355:1670–4.
27. Barber PA, Hill MD, Eliasziw M, et al. Imaging of the brain in acute ischaemic stroke: comparison of computed tomography and magnetic resonance diffusion-weighted imaging. J Neurol Neurosurg Psychiatry 2005;76:1528–33.
28. Coutts SB, Demchuk AM, Barber PA, et al. Interobserver variation of ASPECTS in real time. Stroke 2004;35:e103–5.
29. Toyoda K, Masahiro I, Fukuda K. Fluid-attenuated inversion recovery intra-arterial signal: an early sign of hyperacute cerebral ischemia. Am J Neuroradiol 2001;22:1021–9.
30. Karonen JO, Partanen PLK, Vanninen RL, et al. Evolution of MR contrast enhancement patterns during the first week after acute ischemic stroke. Am J Neuroradiol 2001;22:103–11.
31. Ebinger M, Galinovic I, Rozanski M, et al. Fluid-attenuated inversion recovery evolution within 12 hours from stroke onset: a reliable tissue clock? Stroke 2010;41(2):250–5.
32. Aoki J, Kimura K, Iguchi Y, et al. FLAIR can estimate the onset time in acute ischemic stroke patients. J Neurol Sci 2010; 293(1–2):39–44.
33. Zimmerman RD. Stroke wars: Episode IV. CT strikes back. Am J Neuroradiol 2004;25:1304–9.
34. Na DG, Kim EY, Ryoo JW, et al. CT sign of brain swelling without concomitant parenchymal hypoattenuation: comparison with diffusion- and perfusion-weighted MR imaging. Radiology 2005;235:992–8.
35. Mullins ME, Schaefer PW, Sorensen AG, et al. CT and conventional and diffusion-weighted MR imaging in acute stroke: Study in 691 patients at presentation to the emergency department. Radiology 2002;224:353–60.
36. Chemmanam T, Campbell BC, Christensen S, et al. EPITHET Investigators: Ischaemic diffusion lesion reversal is uncommon

and rarely alters perfusion-diffusion mismatch. Neurology 2010; 75:1040–7.

37. Olivot JM, Mylnash M, Thijs VN, et al. Relationships between cerebral perfusion and reversibility of acute diffusion lesions in DEFUSE: insights from RADAR. Stroke 2009;40:1692–7.
38. Yoo AJ, Hakimelahi R, Rost NS, et al. Diffusion weighted imaging reversibility in the brainstem following recanalisation of acute basilar artery occlusion. J Neurointerv Surg 2010;2(3): 195–7.
39. Liang L, Korogi Y, Sugahara T, et al. Detection of intracranial hemorrhage with susceptibility-weighted MR sequences. AJNR Am J Neuroradiol 1999;20:1527–34.
40. Fiebach JB, Schellinger PD, Gass A, et al. Stroke magnetic resonance imaging is accurate in hyperacute intracerebral haemorrhage: a multicenter study on the validity of stroke imaging. Stroke 2004;35:502–6.
41. Kidwell CS, Chalela JA, Sayer JL, et al. Comparison of MRI and CT for detection of acute intracerebral haemorrhage. JAMA 2004;292:1823–30.
42. Mittal S, Wu Z, Neelavalli J, Haacke EM. Susceptibility weighted imaging: Technical aspects and clinical applications, part 2. Am J Neuroradiol 2009;30:232–52.
43. Yoo AJ, Verduzco LA, Schaefer PW, et al. MRI based selection for intra-arterial stroke therapy: value of pretreatment diffusion weighted imaging lesion volume in selecting patients with acute stroke who will benefit from early recanalisation. Stroke 2009; 40:2046–54.
44. Karonen JO, Vanninen RL, Liu Y, et al. Combined diffusion and perfusion MRI with correlation to single-photon emission CT in acute ischemic stroke. Ischemic penumbra predicts infarct growth. Stroke 1999;30:1583–90.
45. Barber PA, Darby DG, Desmond PM, et al. Prediction of stroke outcome with echoplanar perfusion- and diffusion-weighted MRI. Neurology 1998;51:418–26.
46. Schlaug G, Benfield A, Baird AE, et al. The ischemic penumbra: Operationally defined by diffusion and perfusion MRI. Neurology 1999;53:1528–37.
47. Hacke W, Albers G, Al-Rawi Y, et al. The Desmoteplase in Acute Ischemic Stroke Trial (DIAS): a phase II MRI-based 9-hour window acute stroke thrombolysis trial with intravenous desmoteplase. Stroke 2005;36:66–73.
48. Albers GW, Thijs VN, Wechsler L, et al. Magnetic resonance imaging profiles predict clinical response to early reperfusion: the diffusion and perfusion imaging evaluation for understanding stroke evolution (DEFUSE) study. Ann Neurol 2006;60: 508–17.
49. Davis SM, Donnan GA, Parsons MW, et al. Effects of alteplase beyond 3 h after stroke in the Echoplanar Imaging Thrombolytic Evaluation Trial (EPITHET): a placebo-controlled randomised trial. Lancet Neurol 2008;7:209–309.
50. Schaefer PW, Roccatagliata L, Ledezma C, et al. First-pass quantitative CT perfusion identifies thresholds for salvageable penumbra in acute stroke patients treated with intra-arterial therapy. Am J Neuroradiol 2006;27:20–5.
51. Murphy BD, Fox AJ, Lee DH, et al. Identification of penumbra and infarct in acute ischemic stroke using computed tomography perfusion-derived blood flow and blood volume measurements. Stroke 2006;37:1771–7.
52. Schaefer PW, Mui K, Kamalian S, et al. Avoiding 'pseudoreversibility' of CT-CBV infarct core lesions in acute stroke patients after thrombolytic therapy: the need for algorithmically 'delay-corrected' CT perfusion map postprocessing software. Stroke 2009;40:2875–8.
53. Calamante F, Gadian DG, Connelly A. Delay and dispersion effects in dynamic susceptibility contrast MRI: Simulations using singular value decomposition. Magn Reson Med 2000;44: 466–73.
54. Wu O, Østergaard L, Koroshetz WJ, et al. Effects of tracer arrival time on flow estimates in MR perfusion-weighted imaging. Magn Reson Med 2003;50:856–64.
55. Kudo K, Sasaki M, Yamada K, et al. Differences in CT perfusion maps generated by different commercial software: quantitative analysis by using identical source data of acute stroke patients. Radiology 2009;254:200–9.
56. Wintermark M, Albers GW, Alexandrov AV, et al. Acute stroke imaging research roadmap. Stroke 2008;39:1621–8.
57. Konstas AA, Lev MH. CT perfusion imaging of acute stroke: the need for arrival time, delay insensitive, and standardized postprocessing algorithms? Radiology 2010;254:22–5.
58. Rose SE, Janke AL, Griffin M, et al. Improving the prediction of final infarct size in acute stroke with bolus delay-corrected perfusion MRI measures. J Magn Reson Imaging 2004;20:941–7.
59. Rose SE, Janke AL, Griffin M, et al. Improved prediction of final infarct volume using bolus delay-corrected perfusion-weighted MRI: Implications for the ischemic penumbra. Stroke 2004;35: 2466–71.
60. Copen WA, Schaefer PW, Wu O. MR perfusion imaging in acute ischemic stroke. Neuroimaging Clin N Am 2011;21(2): 259–83.
61. Kamalian S, Kamalian S, Maas MB, et al. CT cerebral blood flow maps optimally correlate with admission diffusion-weighted imaging in acute stroke but thresholds vary by postprocessing platform. Stroke 2011;42(7):1923–8.
62. Kamalian S, Kamalian S, Konstas AA, et al. CT perfusion mean transit time maps optimally distinguish benign oligemia from true 'at-risk' ischemic penumbra, but thresholds vary by postprocessing technique. Am J Neuroradiol 2012;33(3):545–9.
63. Schramm P, Schellinger PD, Klotz E, et al. Comparison of perfusion computed tomography and computed tomography angiography source images with perfusion-weighted imaging and diffusion-weighted imaging in patients with acute stroke of less than 6 hours' duration. Stroke 2004;35:1652–7.
64. Nagar VA, McKinney AM, Karagulle AT, Truwit CL. Reperfusion phenomenon masking acute and subacute infarcts at dynamic perfusion CT: Confirmation by fusion of CT and diffusion-weighted MR images. Am J Roentgenol 2009;193:1629–38.
65. Miteff F, Faulder KC, Goh AC, et al. Mechanical thrombectomy with a self-expanding retrievable intracranial stent (Solitaire AB): experience in 26 patients with acute cerebral artery occlusion. Am J Neuroradiol 2011;32(6):1078–81.
66. Smith WS, Sung G, Starkman S, et al. Safety and efficacy of mechanical embolectomy in acute ischemic stroke: results of the MERCI trial. Stroke 2005;36(7):1432–8.
67. Smith WS. Safety of mechanical thrombectomy and intravenous tissue plasminogen activator in acute ischemic stroke. Results of the multi Mechanical Embolus Removal in Cerebral Ischemia (MERCI) trial part I. Am J Neuroradiol 2006;27(6): 1177–82.
68. Furlan A, Higashida R, Wechsler L, et al. Intra-arterial prourokinase for acute ischemic stroke. The PROACT II study: a randomized controlled trial. Prolyse in Acute Cerebral Thromboembolism. JAMA 1999;282(21):2003–11.
69. Josephson SA, Saver JL, Smith WS; Merci and Multi Merci Investigators. Comparison of mechanical embolectomy and intraarterial thrombolysis in acute ischemic stroke within the MCA: MERCI and Multi MERCI compared to PROACT II. Neurocrit Care 2009;10(1):43–9.
70. Almekhlafi MA, Menon BK, Freiheit EA, et al. A meta-analysis of observational intra-arterial stroke therapy studies using the Merci device, Penumbra system, and retrievable stents. Am J Neuroradiol 2013;34(1):140–5.
71. Miteff F, Levi CR, Bateman GA, et al. The independent predictive utility of computed tomography angiography collateral status in acute ischemic stroke. Brain 2009;132:2231–8.
72. Higashida RT, Furlan AT, Roberts H, et al. Trial design and reporting standards for intra-arterial thrombolysis for acute ischemic stroke. Stroke 2003;34:e109–37.
73. Tan LIY, Demchuk AM, Hopyan M. CT angiography clot burden score and collateral score: correlation with clinical and radiological outcomes in acute middle cerebral artery infarct. Am J Neuroradiol 2009;30:525–31.
74. Lee KY, Latour LL, Luby M, et al. Distal hyperintense vessels on FLAIR: an MRI marker for collateral circulation in acute stroke. Neurology 2009;72:1134–9.
75. Silvestrini M, Balucani A, Luzzi S, et al. Early activation of intracranial collateral vessels influences the outcome of spontaneous internal carotid artery dissection. Stroke 2011;42:139–43.
76. Guckel FJ, Brix G, Schmiedek P, et al. Cerebrovascular reserve capacity in patients with occlusive cerebrovascular disease: assessment with dynamic susceptibility contrast-enhanced MR imaging and the acetazolamide stimulation test. Radiology 1996;201: 405–12.

77. Kuwabara Y, Ichiya Y, Sasaki M. PET evaluation of cerebral hemodynamics in occlusive cerebrovascular disease pre- and post-surgery. J Nucl Med 1998;39:760–5.
78. Sperling B, Lassen N. Cerebral blood flow by SPECT in ischaemic stroke. In: Deyn PD, Diercks R, Alave A, Pickut B, editors. A Textbook of SPECT in Neurology and Psychiatry. London: John Libbey; 1999.
79. Alexandrov A, Masdeu J, Devous S. Brain single-photon emission CT with HMPAO and safety of thrombolytic therapy in acute ischemic stroke. Stroke 1997;28:1830–4.
80. Kao HW, Tsai FY, Hasso AN. Predicting stroke evolution: comparison of susceptibility weighted MR imaging with MR perfusion. Eur Radiol 2012;22(7):1397–403.
81. Hom J, Dankbaar JW, Soares BP, et al. Blood-brain barrier permeability assessed by perfusion CT predicts symptomatic hemorrhagic transformation and malignant edema in acute ischemic stroke. Am J Neuroradiol 2011;32(1):41–8.
82. Lin K, Kazmi KS, Law M, et al. Measuring elevated microvascular permeability and predicting hemorrhagic transformation in acute ischemic stroke using first-pass dynamic perfusion CT imaging. Am J Neuroradiol 2007;28:1292–8.
83. Aviv RI, d'Esterre CD, Murphy BD, et al. Hemorrhagic transformation of ischemic stroke: prediction with CT perfusion. Radiology 2009;250:867–77.
84. Kassner A, Roberts T, Taylor K, et al. Prediction of hemorrhage in acute ischemic stroke using permeability MR imaging. Am J Neuroradiol 2005;26:2213–17.
85. Bang OY, Buck BH, Saver JL, et al. Prediction of hemorrhagic transformation after recanalization therapy using T2*-permeability magnetic resonance imaging. Ann Neurol 2007;62: 170–6.
86. Ding G, Jiang Q, Li L, et al. Detection of BBB disruption and haemorrhage by Gd-DTPA enhanced MRI after embolic stroke in rat. Brain Res 2006;1114(1):195–203.
87. Jiang Q, Ewing JR, Ding GL, et al. Quantitative evaluation of BBB permeability after embolic stroke in rat using MRI. J Cereb Blood Flow Metab 2005;25(5):583–92.
88. Zaharchuk G. Arterial spin label imaging of acute ischaemic stroke and transient ischaemic attack. Neuroimaging Clin N Am 2011;21(2):285–301.
89. Karonen JO, Partanen PLK, Vanninen RL, et al. Evolution of MR contrast enhancement patterns during the first week after acute ischemic stroke. Am J Neuroradiol 2001;22:103–11.
90. Mayer TE, Schuffe-Altedorneburg G, Droste DW, et al. Serial CT and MRI of ischaemic cerebral infarcts: frequency and clinical impact of haemorrhagic transformation. Neuroradiology 2000;42:233–9.
91. Mayer TE, Schuffe-Altedorneburg G, Droste DW, et al. Serial CT and MRI of ischaemic cerebral infarcts: frequency and clinical impact of haemorrhagic transformation. Neuroradiology 2000;42: 233–9.
92. Geijer B, Lindgren A, Brockstedt S, et al. Persistent high signal on diffusion weighted MRI in the late stages of small cortical and lacunar ischaemic lesions. Neuroradiology 2001;43: 115–22.
93. Provenzale J, Sorensen G. Diffusion-weighted MR imaging in acute stroke: theoretic considerations and clinical applications. AJR Am J Roentgenol 1999;173:1459–67.
94. Burdette J. Cerebral infarction: time course of signal intensity changes on diffusion-weighted images. AJR Am J Roentgenol 1998;171:791–5.
95. Morita N, Harada M, Yoneda K, et al. A characteristic feature of acute haematomas in the brain on echo-planar diffusion-weighted imaging. Neuroradiology 2002;44:907–11.
96. Kim JH, Shin T, Chung JD, et al. Temporal pattern of blood volume change in cerebral infarction: evaluation with dynamic contrast-enhanced T2-weighted MR imaging. AJR Am J Roentgenol 1998;170:765–70.
97. North American Symptomatic Carotid Endarectomy trial collaborators. Beneficial effect of carotid endarterectomy in symptomatic patients with high grade carotid stenosis. N Engl J Med 1991;325:445–53.
98. European Carotid Surgery Trialists' collaborative group. MRC European carotid surgery trial: interim results for symptomatic patients with severe (70–99%) or with mild (0–29%) carotid stenosis. Lancet 1991;337:1235–43.
99. Halliday A, Mansfield A, Marro J, et al. Prevention of disabling and fatal strokes by successful carotid endarterectomy in patients without recent neurological symptoms: randomised controlled trial. Lancet 2004;363:1491–502.
100. Chaturvedi S, Bruno A, Feasby T, et al. Carotid endarterectomy—An evidence based review. Neurology 2005;65:794–801.
101. Halliday A, Mansfield A, Marro J, et al. Prevention of disabling and fatal strokes by successful carotid endarterectomy in patients without recent neurological symptoms: randomised controlled trial. Lancet 2004;363:1491–502.
102. Halliday A, Harrison M, Hayler E, et al. ACST Collaborative Group. 10 year stroke prevention after successful endarterectomy for ACST-1: a multicentre randomized trial. Lancet 2010; 376(9746):1074–84.
103. Davies KN, Humphrey PRD. Complications of cerebral angiography in patients with symptomatic carotid territory ischaemia screened by carotid ultrasound. J Neurol Neurosurg Psychiatry 1993;56:967–72.
104. Osarumwense D, Pararajasingam R, Wilson P, et al. Carotid artery imaging in the United Kingdom: a postal questionnaire of current practice. Vascular 2005;13:173–7.
105. Leys D, Ringelstein EB, Kaste M, Hacke W. Facilities available in European hospitals treating stroke patients. Stroke 2007;38: 2985–91.
106. Wardlaw JM, Chappell FM, Best JJK, et al; on behalf of the NHS Research & Development Health Technology Assessment Carotid Stenosis Imaging Group. Non-invasive imaging compared with intra-arterial angiography in the diagnosis of symptomatic carotid stenosis: a meta-analysis. Lancet 2006;367:1503–12.
107. Chappell FM, Wardlaw JM, Young GR, et al. Accuracy of noninvasive tests for carotid stenosis—an individual patient data meta-analysis. Radiology 2009;251:493–502.
108. Madani A, Beletsky V, Tamayo A, et al. High-risk asymptomatic carotid stenosis: ulceration on 3D ultrasound vs TCD microemboli. Neurology 2011,77.744–50.
109. Parmar JP, Rogers WJ, Mugler JP III, et al. Magnetic resonance imaging of carotid atherosclerotic plaque in clinically suspected acute transient ischemic attack and acute ischemic stroke. Circulation 2010;122:2031–8.
110. Kwee RM, Truijman MT, Mess WH, et al. Potential of integrated [18F] fluorodeoxyglucose positron-emission tomography/CT in identifying vulnerable carotid plaques. Am J Neuroradiol 2011; 32:950–4.
111. Gaemperli O, Shalhoub J, Owen DR, et al. Imaging intraplaque inflammation in carotid atherosclerosis with 11C-PK11195 positron emission tomography/computed tomography. Eur Heart J 2012;33(15):1902–10.
112. Murray AD, Staff RT, Shenkin SD, et al. Brain white matter hyperintensities: Relative importance of vascular risk factors in nondemented elderly people. Radiology 2005;237:251–7.
113. Longstreth WT, Manolio TA, Arnold A, et al; for the Cardiovascular Health Study Collaborative Research Group. Clinical correlates of white matter findings on cranial magnetic resonance imaging of 3301 elderly people. Stroke 1996;27:1274–82.
114. O'Sullivan M, Rich PM, Barrick TR, et al. Frequency of subclinical lacunar infarcts in ischemic leukoaraiosis and CADASIL. AJNR Am J Neuroradiol 2003;24:1348–54.
115. Pomper M, Miller T, Stone H, et al. CNS vasculitis in autoimmune disease: MR imaging findings and correlation with angiography. AJNR Am J Neuroradiol 1999;20:75–85.
116. Kwa VI, Franke CL, Verbeeten B Jr. Silent intracerebral microhemorrhages in patients with ischemic stroke. Amsterdam Vascular Medicine Group. Ann Neurol 1998;44:372–7.
117. Roob G, Schmidt R, Kapeller P, et al. MRI evidence of past cerebral microbleeds in a healthy elderly population. Neurology 1999;52:991–4.
118. Gregoire SM, Jager HR, Yousry TA, et al. Brain microbleeds as a potential risk factor for antiplatelet-related intracerebral haemorrhage: hospital based, case-control study. J Neurol Neurosurg Psychiatry 2010;81(6):679–84.
119. Kakuda W, Thijs VN, Lansberg MG, et al. Clinical importance of microbleeds in patients receiving IV thrombolysis. Neurology 2005;65:1175–8.
120. Kidwell CS, Saver JL, Villablana JP, et al. Magnetic resonance imaging detection of microbleeds before thrombolysis. Stroke 2002;33:95–8.

121. Tang PH, Chai J, Chan YH, et al. Superior sagittal sinus thrombosis: subtle signs on neuroimaging. Ann Acad Med Singapore 2008;37:397–401.
122. Chatterjee S, Thomas B, Kesavadas C, Kapilamoorthy TR. Susceptibility-weighted imaging in differentiating bilateral medial thalamic venous and arterial infarcts. Neurol India 2010;58: 615–17.
123. de Rooij NK, Linn FH, van der Plas JA, et al. Incidence of subarachnoid haemorrhage: a systematic review with emphasis on region, age, gender and time trends. J Neurol Neurosurg Psychiatry 2007;78(12):1365–72.
124. Linn FH, Rinkel GJ, Algra A, van Gijn J. Headache characteristics in subarachnoid haemorrhage and benign thunderclap headache. J Neurol Neurosurg Psychiatry 1998;65(5):791–3.
125. Hop JW, Rinkel GJ, Algra A, van Gijn J. Case fatality rates and functional outcome after early subarachnoid haemorrhage. A systematic review. Stroke 1997;28:660–4.
126. Rinkel GJ, Wijdicks EF, Hasan D, et al. Outcome in patients with subarachnoid haemorrhage and negative angiography according to pattern of haemorrhage on computed tomography. Lancet 1991;338:964–8.
127. van der Schaaf IC, Velthius BK, Gouw A, et al. Venous drainage in perimesencephalic haemorrhage. Stroke 2004;35:1614–18.
128. van der Wee N, Rinkel GJ, Hasan D, et al. Detection of subarachnoid haemorrhage on early CT: is lumbar puncture still needed after a negative scan? J Neurol Neurosurg Psychiatry 1995;58: 357–9.
129. Adams HP Jr, Kassell NF, Torner JC, et al. CT and clinical correlations in recent aneurysmal subarachnoid hemorrhage: a preliminary report of the Cooperative Aneurysm Study. Neurology 1983;33:981–8.
130. Van Gijn J, Rinkel GJE. How to do it: investigate the CSF in a patient with sudden headache and a normal CT brain scan. Pract Neurol 2005;5:362–5.
131. Van Gijn J, Rinkel GJ. Subarachnoid haemorrhage: diagnosis, causes and management. Brain 2001;124:249–78.
132. Mitchell P, Wilkinson ID, Hoggard N, et al. Detection of subarachnoid haemorrhage with magnetic resonance imaging. J Neurol Neurosurg Psychiatry 2001;70:205–11.
133. Mohamed M, Heasely DC, Yagmurlu B, et al. Fluid-attenuated inversion recovery MR imaging and subarachnoid hemorrhage: Not a panacea. Am J Neuroradiol 2004;25:545–50.
134. Noguchi K, Ogawa T, Seto H, et al. Subacute and chronic subarachnoid hemorrhage: diagnosis with fluid-attenuated inversion-recovery MR imaging. Radiology 1997;203:257–62.
135. Deliganis AV, Fisher DJ, Lam AM, et al. Cerebrospinal fluid signal intensity increase on FLAIR MR images in patients under general anesthesia: the role of supplemental O_2. Radiology 2001;218: 152–6.
136. Dechambre SD, Duprez T, Grandin CB, et al. High signal in cerebrospinal fluid mimicking subarachnoid haemorrhage on FLAIR following acute stroke and intravenous contrast medium. Neuroradiology 2000;42:608–11.
137. Kassell NF, Sasaki T, Colohan ART, et al. Cerebral vasospasm following aneurysmal subarachnoid hemorrhage. Stroke 1985;16: 562–72.
138. Osborn AG. Diagnostic Cerebral Angiography. 2nd ed. Washington, DC: Lippincott Williams & Wilkins; 1999. p. 462.
139. Anxionnat R, Bracard S, Ducrocq X, et al. Intracranial aneurysms: clinical value of 3D digital subtraction angiography in the therapeutic decision and endovascular treatment. Radiology 2001;218: 799–808.
140. Sugahara T, Korogi Y, Nakashima K, et al. Comparison of 2D and 3D digital subtraction angiography in evaluation of intracranial aneurysms. Am J Neuroradiol 2002;23(9):1545–52.
141. Van Rooij WJ, Sprengers ME, de Gast AN, et al. 3D rotational angiography; the new gold standard in the detection of additional intracranial aneurysms. Am J Neuroradiol 2008;29:976–9.
142. Cloft HJ, Joseph GJ, Dion JE. Risk of cerebral angiography in patients with subarachnoid haemorrhage, cerebral aneurysm and arteriovenous malformation: a meta-analysis. Stroke 1999;30: 317–20.
143. Willinsky RA, Taylor SM, TerBrugge K, et al. Neurologic complications of cerebral angiography: prospective analysis of 2,899 procedures and review of the literature. Radiology 2003;227: 522–8.
144. White PM, Wardlaw JM, Easton V. Can noninvasive imaging accurately depict intracranial aneurysms? A systemic review. Radiology 2000;217(2):361–70.
145. Chappell ET, Moure FC, Good MC. Comparison of computed tomographic angiography with digital subtraction angiography in the diagnosis of cerebral aneurysms: a meta-analysis. Neurosurgery 2003;52(3):624–31.
146. Westerlaan HE, van Dijk JM, Jansen-van der Weide MC, et al. Intracranial aneurysms in patients with subarachnoid haemorrhage: CT angiography as a primary examination tool for diagnosis—systemic review and meta-analysis. Radiology 2011; 258(1):134–45.
147. Villablanca JP, Jahan R, Hooshi P, et al. Detection and characterisation of very small cerebral aneurysms by using 2D and 3D helical CT angiography. AJNR Am J Neuroradiol 2002;23: 1187–98.
148. Lu L, Zhang LJ, Poon CS, et al. Digital subtraction CT angiography for detection of intracranial aneurysms: comparison with three-dimensional digital subtraction angiography. Radiology 2012;262(2):605–12.
149. Luo Z, Wang D, Sun X, et al. Comparison of the accuracy of subtraction CT angiography performed on 320-detector row volume CT with conventional CT angiography for diagnosis of intracranial aneurysms. Eur J Radiol 2012;81(1): 118–22.
150. Wang H, Li W, He H, et al. 320-Detector row CT angiography for detection and evaluation of intracranial aneurysms: Comparison with conventional digital subtraction angiography. Clin Radiol 2013;68(1):e15–20.
151. Ruigrok YM, Rinkel GJ, Buskens E, et al. Perimesencephalic hemorrhage and CT angiography: A decision analysis. Stroke 2000;31:2976–83.
152. Molyneux AJ, Kerr RSC, Yu L-M, et al. International subarachnoid aneurysm trial (ISAT) of neurosurgical clipping versus endovascular coiling in 2143 patients with ruptured intracranial aneurysms: a randomised comparison of effects on survival, dependency, seizures, rebleeding, subgroups, and aneurysm occlusion. Lancet 2005;366:809–17.
153. Wiebers DO, Whisnant JP, Huston J 3rd, et al. International Study of Unruptured Intracranial Aneurysms Investigators. Unruptured intracranial aneurysms: natural history, clinical outcome and risks of surgical and endovascular treatment. Lancet 2003;362:103–10.
154. Vindlacheruvu RR, Mendelow AD, Mitchell P. Risk-benefit analysis of the treatment of unruptured intracranial aneurysms. J Neurol Neurosurg Psychiatry 2005;76:234–9.
155. Deutschmann HA, Augustin M, Simbrunner J, et al. Diagnostic accuracy of 3D time-of-flight MR angiography compared with digital subtraction angiography for follow-up of coiled intracranial aneurysms: influence of aneurysm size. Am J Neuroradiol 2007;28(4):628–34.
156. Kwee TC, Kwee RM. MR angiography in the follow-up of intracranial aneurysms treated with Guglielmi detachable coils: systematic review and meta-analysis. Neuroradiology 2007;49(9): 703–13.
157. Pierot L, Portefaix C, Gauvrit JY, Boulin A. Follow-up of coiled intracranial aneurysms: comparison of 3D time-of-flight MR angiography at 3T and 1.5T in a large prospective series. Am J Neuroradiol 2012;33(11):2162–6.
158. Okahara M, Kiyosue H, Yamashita M, et al. Diagnostic accuracy of magnetic resonance angiography for cerebral aneurysms in correlation with 3D-digital subtraction angiographic images: a study of 133 aneurysms. Stroke 2002;33:1803–8.
159. Li M-H, Li YD, Tan HQ, et al. Contrast-free MRA at 3.0T for the detection of intracranial aneurysms. Neurology 2011;77: 667–76.
160. Dennis MS, Burn JP, Sandercock PA, et al. Long-term survival after first-ever stroke: the Oxfordshire Community Stroke Project. Stroke 1993;24:796–800.
161. Qureshi AI, Tuhrim S, Broderick JP, et al. Spontaneous intracerebral hemorrhage. N Engl J Med 2001;344:1450–60.
162. Sacco S, Marini C, Toni D, et al. Incidence and 10-year survival of intracerebral hemorrhage in a population-based registry. Stroke 2009;40:394–9.
163. Qureshi AI, Medelow AD, Hanley DF. Intracerebral haemorrhage. Lancet 2009;373(9675):1632–44.

164. Keep RF, Hua Y, Xi G. Intracerebral haemorrhage: mechanisms of injury and therapeutic targets. Lancet Neurol 2012;11(8): 720–31.
165. Greenberg SM. Cerebral amyloid angiopathy: prospects for clinical diagnosis and treatment. Neurology 1998;51:690–4.
166. Greenberg SM, Vernooij MW, Cordonnier C, et al. Microbleed Study Group. Cerebral microbleeds: a guide to detection and interpretation. Lancet Neurol 2009;8(2):165–74.
167. McEvoy A, Kitchen N, Thomas D. Intracerebral haemorrhage in young adults: the emerging importance of drug abuse. Br Med J 2000;320:1322–4.
168. Gaskill-Shipley M. Routine CT evaluation of acute stroke. Neuroimaging Clin North Am 1999;9:411–22.
169. Bradley WG Jr. Hemorrhage and hemorrhagic infections in the brain. Neuroimaging Clin North Am 1994;4:707–32.
170. Haacke EM, Mittal S, Wu Z, et al. Susceptibility-weighted imaging: technical aspects and clinical applications, part 1. Am J Neuroradiol 2009;30(1):19–30.
171. Mittal S, Wu Z, Neelavalli J, Haacke EM. Susceptibility-weighted imaging: technical aspects and clinical applications, part 2. Am J Neuroradiol 2009;30(2):232–52.
172. Coley SC, Romanowski CAJ, Hodgson TJ, et al. Dural arteriovenous fistulae: non-invasive diagnosis with dynamic MR digital subtraction angiography. Am J Neuroradiol 2002;23:404–7.
173. Brouwer PA, Bosman T, van Walderveen MA, et al. Dynamic 320-section CT angiography in cranial arteriovenous shunting lesions. Am J Neuroradiol 2010;31(4):767–70.
174. Nishimura S, Hirai T, Sasao A, et al. Evaluation of dural arteriovenous fistulas with 4D contrast-enhanced MR angiography at 3T MRI. Am J Neuroradiol 2010;31(1):80–5.
175. Valavanis A. The role of angiography in the evaluation of cerebral vascular malformations. Neuroimaging Clin North Am 1996;6: 679–704.
176. Rodesch G, Lasjaunias P. Physiopathology and semeiology of dural arteriovenous shunts. Rivista di Neuroradiologia 1992;5: 11–21.
177. Gandhi D, Chen J, Pearl M, et al. Intracranial dural arteriovenous fistulas: classification, imaging findings, and treatment. Am J Neuroradiol 2012;33(6):1007–13.
178. Meisel HJ, Mansmann U, Alvarez H, et al. Cerebral arteriovenous malformations and associated aneurysms: analysis of 305 cases from a series of 662 patients. Neurosurgery 2000;46:793–800.
179. Mast H, Young WL, Koennecke HC, et al. Risk of spontaneous hemorrhage after diagnosis of cerebral arteriovenous malformation. Lancet 1997;350:1065–8.
180. Jager HR, Grieve JP. Advances in non-invasive imaging of intracranial vascular disease. Ann R Coll Surg Engl 2000; 82:1–5.
181. Hadizadeh DR, von Falkenhausen M, Gieseke J, et al. Cerebral arteriovenous malformation: Spetzler-Martin classification at subsecond-temporal-resolution four-dimensional MR angiography compared with that at DSA. Radiology 2008;246(1):205–13.
182. Wilms G, Demaerel P, Bosmans H, et al. MRI of non-ischemic vascular disease: aneurysms and vascular malformations. Eur Radiol 1999;9:1055–60.
183. Brunereau L, Labauge P, Tournier-Lasserve E, et al. Familial form of intracranial cavernous angioma: MR imaging findings in 51 families. Radiology 2000;214:209–16.
184. Goadsby PJ, Boes C. New daily persistent headache. J Neurol Neurosurg Psychiatry 2002;72(suppl 2):ii6–9.

CHAPTER 4

INTRACRANIAL INFECTIONS

Daniel J. Scoffings • Julia Frühwald-Pallamar • Majda M. Thurnher • H. Rolf Jäger

CHAPTER OUTLINE

BACTERIAL INFECTIONS

Bacterial Meningitis

The causes of bacterial meningitis are age-dependent; in adults the most common causes are *Streptococcus pneumoniae* and *Neisseria meningitidis*. Bacteria can reach the meninges by haematogenous dissemination, spread from an adjacent focus of infection (such as sinusitis or otomastoiditis) or through congenital or acquired structural defects in the skull. Clinical manifestations include fever, headache, photophobia, lethargy and confusion. Imaging is frequently normal in patients with uncomplicated bacterial meningitis and is not necessary for its diagnosis, which requires analysis of a sample of cerebrospinal fluid (CSF) obtained by lumbar puncture (LP). The issue of whether neuroimaging is necessary before LP can be a matter of dispute between referring clinicians and radiologists. Although computed tomography (CT) can show findings that contraindicate LP, such as effacement of the basal cisterns and cerebellar tonsillar herniation, a normal CT does not imply that LP can be performed without the risk of causing tonsillar herniation.[1] The guidelines of the National Institute for Health and Clinical Excellence (NICE) in the United Kingdom are that CT is indicated when there are focal neurological signs or with a reduced or fluctuating level of consciousness, but that treatment should not be delayed in order to obtain imaging.[2]

Imaging is often normal in patients with uncomplicated bacterial meningitis but some abnormalities may be observed. Subtle distension of the subarachnoid spaces by inflammatory exudate has been reported, but can be difficult to appreciate in the very young and in older subjects, both of whom have relatively prominent basal cisterns. Leptomeningeal contrast enhancement, which follows the surface of the brain and extends into the sulci and basal cisterns, may be seen and is better detected by contrast-enhanced magnetic resonance imaging (MRI) than by contrast-enhanced CT. Leptomeningeal enhancement can be difficult to distinguish from contrast enhancement in normal blood vessels and the detection of abnormal enhancement of the leptomeninges may be improved by the use of a post-contrast fluid-attenuated inversion recovery (FLAIR) sequence, which is less sensitive to vascular enhancement.[3] An unenhanced FLAIR sequence may also show increased signal intensity in the subarachnoid spaces, most often over the frontal convexities and in the sylvian fissures, as a result of increased protein concentration in the CSF, causing failure of signal suppression by the inversion pulse (Fig. 4-1).[4] This FLAIR hyperintensity is non-specific, however, and can also be seen with subarachnoid haemorrhage, with malignant meningitis and in patients receiving large doses of supplemental oxygen. In a minority of cases (probably less than 10%) diffusion-weighted imaging (DWI) can show multiple foci of high signal intensity in the subarachnoid spaces; these are typically nodular and are associated with increased signal intensity on the FLAIR sequences in most cases. The finding of subarachnoid high signal on DWI has been reported to be associated with a poor prognosis.[5]

Complications of bacterial meningitis include hydrocephalus, most often of the communicating type, brain abscess, subdural empyema and ventriculitis (see below). Focal parenchymal lesions may also be observed on DWI, principally secondary to vasculopathy of arteries surrounded by inflammatory exudate, and have been classified into four patterns: large vessel territory infarcts, perforator territory infarcts, multiple bilateral lesions in the cortex and subcortical white matter and multiple bilateral lesions restricted to the cerebral cortex.[6]

Cerebritis and Brain Abscess

In immunocompetent patients most brain abscesses are bacterial, streptococci accounting for the majority. In 20–40% no causative organism is identified. Brain abscesses arise by haematogenous dissemination, penetrating trauma or direct spread from contiguous infection. The site of an abscess depends on its cause: frontal sinusitis will result in an abscess in or beneath the adjacent frontal lobe, whereas mastoiditis will give rise to a temporal lobe or cerebellar lesion. Blood-borne infection can occur

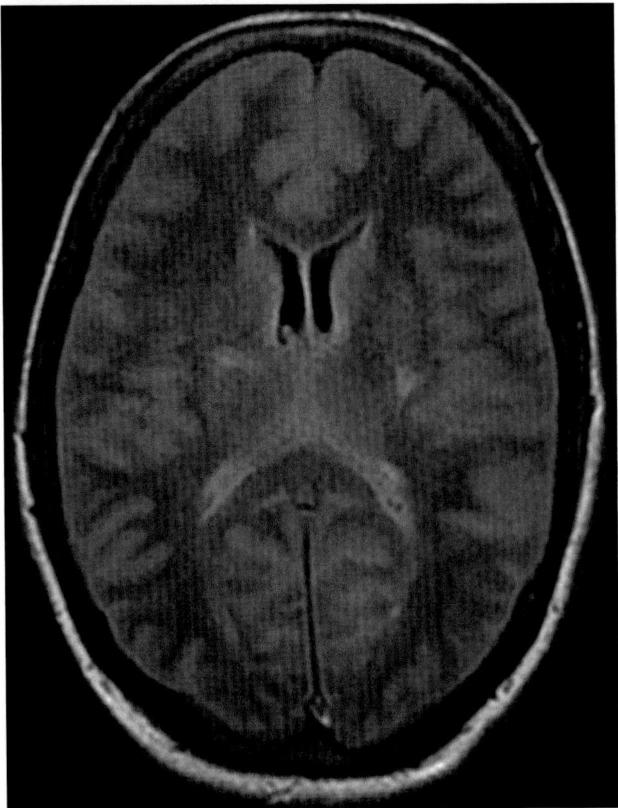

FIGURE 4-1 ■ ***Listeria* meningitis in a renal transplant recipient.** Axial fluid-attenuated inversion recovery (FLAIR) image shows failure of CSF suppression in the sulci as a result of pus in the subarachnoid space, manifesting as abnormal high signal intensity.

anywhere in the brain, but has a predilection for the territory of the middle cerebral arteries, particularly the frontoparietal region. A thorough search for a predisposing factor should be made; a cardiac cause is frequently overlooked (occult endocarditis and septal defects). Abscesses are frequently subcortical or periventricular. Four stages of development are described: early and late cerebritis and early and late capsule formation. Patients present with fever (in 50%), headache and focal neurological deficits. Brain abscesses are multiple in 10–50%.[7]

On CT, cerebritis appears as ill-defined low attenuation; enhancement is usually absent at the early stage but can appear irregular and peripheral in late cerebritis and may progress centrally on delayed images. With capsule formation the abscess shows central low attenuation, because of pus or necrotic debris and a rim of slightly higher attenuation surrounded by low-attenuation vasogenic oedema. After contrast medium, a ring of enhancement corresponds to the capsule. The enhancing rim typically has a smooth inner margin and shows thinning of its medial aspect.[8] In contrast to cerebritis, the centre of the abscess never enhances on delayed images. The degree of enhancement is diminished in patients who are immunocompromised or are on corticosteroid therapy.[9] Abscesses rarely contain gas; when present this is most often caused by surgical intervention or communication with a cranial air space such as the paranasal sinuses or mastoid air cells. It is only rarely because of a gas-forming organism.

On MRI, the signal of the abscess centre is intermediate between that of CSF and white matter on T1-weighted images and iso- or slightly hyperintense to CSF on T2-weighted images. On T2 sequences the abscess rim is relatively hypointense (Fig. 4-2); it may be slightly hyperintense to white matter on T1 images.[10] The abscess rim often appears markedly hypointense on susceptibility-weighted imaging (SWI); this is thought to be the result of free radicals produced by phagocytosis.[11] A 'dual rim' sign of concentric outer hypointensity and inner hyperintensity relative to the abscess core can also be seen on SWI.[12] The pattern of rim enhancement is similar to that shown by CT, the outer margin rim more often being smooth than lobulated.[13] Surrounding vasogenic oedema is of low signal on T1 and high signal on T2 images. The abscess centre is of high signal on DWI and low signal on maps of apparent diffusion coefficient (ADC), because of restricted diffusion in the viscous pus (Fig. 4-2). The degree of restriction of diffusion is inversely correlated with the viable cell count within the abscess centre.[14]

Though typical, the appearance of a brain abscess as a rim-enhancing mass is non-specific and may be mimicked by metastasis, glioblastoma and resolving haematoma. A thick, irregular rind of enhancement is more suggestive of tumour. Abscesses are more likely to show small satellite lesions. Despite initial hopes that restricted diffusion would reliably distinguish abscess from tumour, reduced ADC has been subsequently reported in metastases and glioblastomas. Dynamic contrast-enhanced perfusion MRI may help distinguish between brain abscess and tumour; abscesses have a lower relative cerebral blood volume in their enhancing rim than gliomas.[15]

The management of brain abscesses can require both medical and neurosurgical therapy. CT diagnosis has been responsible for a marked reduction in the mortality of brain abscesses. Follow-up imaging is recommended at biweekly intervals or when new symptoms arise. Sufficient treatment is indicated by resolution of rim enhancement or disappearance of the low signal rim on T2 images. Treatment response may be better assessed with DWI than conventional MRI; low signal on DWI correlates with a good clinical response, whereas increasing signal implies reaccumulation of pus.[16]

Epidural Abscess and Subdural Empyema

An intracranial epidural abscess is a collection of pus between the inner table of the skull and the endosteum of the skull, which forms the outer layer of the dura mater. Abscesses mainly arise by direct spread from a contiguous focus of infection, most often sinusitis or otomastoiditis, less often as a complication of dental sepsis or after craniotomy. *Streptococcus milleri* is the most frequent causative organism. As intracranial epidural abscesses are typically slow-growing, the clinical presentation is often insidious, usually with fever and headache. CT and MRI show a lentiform collection of fluid constrained by the dura at the sites of cranial sutures. Accordingly, when anteriorly located as a complication of frontal

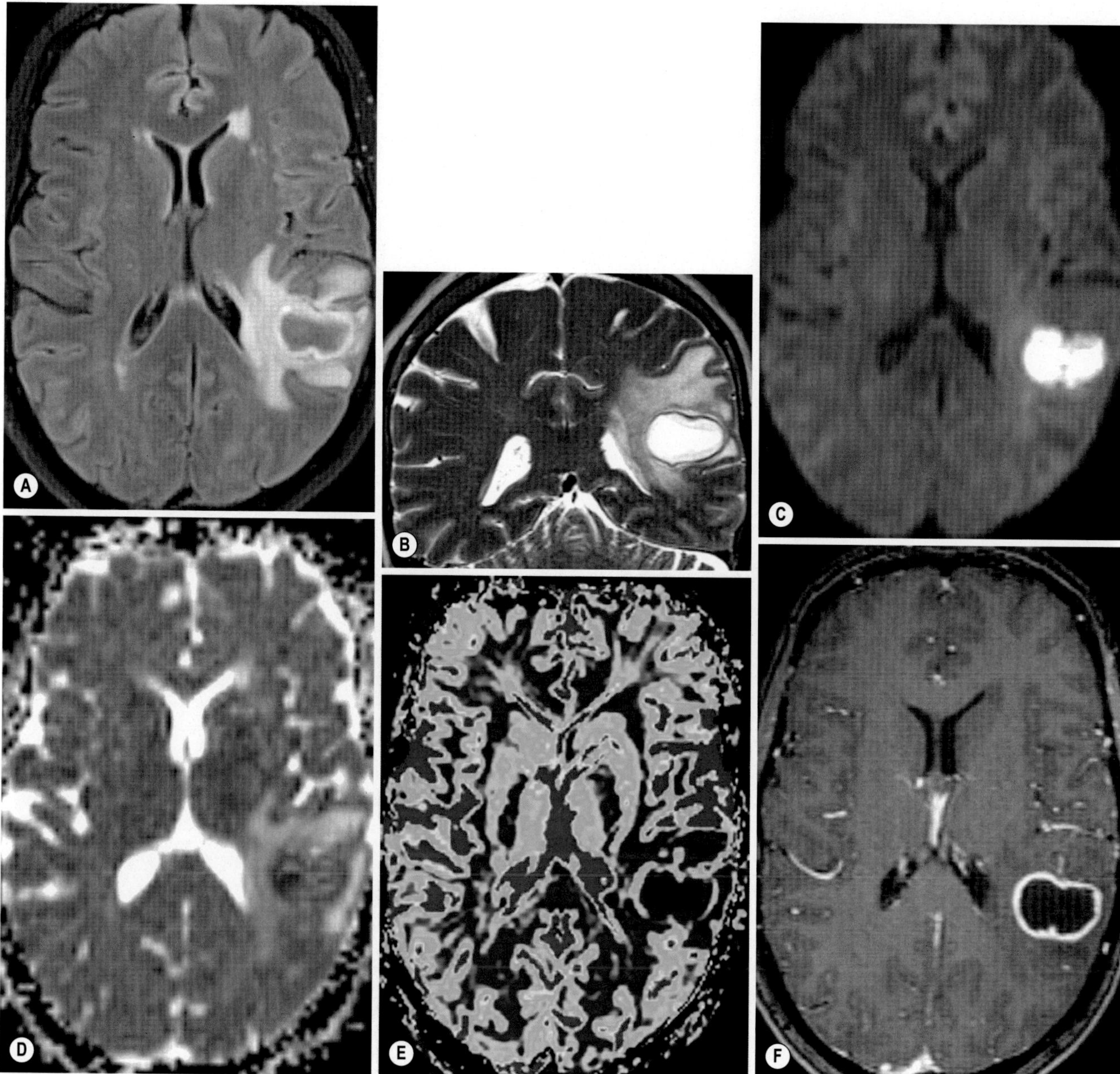

FIGURE 4-2 ■ **Pyogenic brain abscess in a 40-year-old female patient.** (A) Axial FLAIR image shows a ring-like low-signal-intensity lesion with marked perifocal oedema in the left hemisphere. (B) Coronal T2 image shows the lesion has a high-signal-intensity centre with a low-signal-intensity capsule. (C, D) On trace DWI (C), high signal was detected in the abscess cavity, with relatively low ADC values (D). (E) On the perfusion MRI, low relative cerebral blood volume (rCBV) was seen in the cavity, with a thin rim of increased perfusion in the capsule. (F) On post-contrast T1, a peripheral ring-like enhancement was observed.

sinusitis they can cross the midline, in contrast to subdural empyemas which do not cross the midline. The fluid within the epidural abscess is of slightly higher attenuation than CSF on CT and is hyperintense on T2 and FLAIR images and is slightly hyperintense compared to CSF on T1.[17] The dura at the deep margin of an epidural abscess typically shows thick and slightly irregular contrast enhancement (Fig. 4-3). Similar to cerebral abscesses, the pus within an epidural abscess can show restricted diffusion, appearing hyperintense on DWI and hypointense on ADC maps.[18] In patients with fever after a neurosurgical operation, normal and expected sterile fluid collections in the epidural space can be hard to distinguish from an epidural abscess, but a serial increase in the attenuation of the fluid suggests infection. DWI has been found to be less sensitive and specific in the postoperative setting.[19]

A subdural empyema is a collection of pus in the potential space between the inner layer of the dura mater and the arachnoid mater. Empyemas occur more commonly than epidural abscesses. As with epidural abscesses, the most frequent predisposing causes are sinusitis and otogenic infection; head trauma, surgery and haematogenous spread are less common. Headache, fever, focal neurological deficit and meningism are the most frequent clinical features at presentation. The CT and MRI

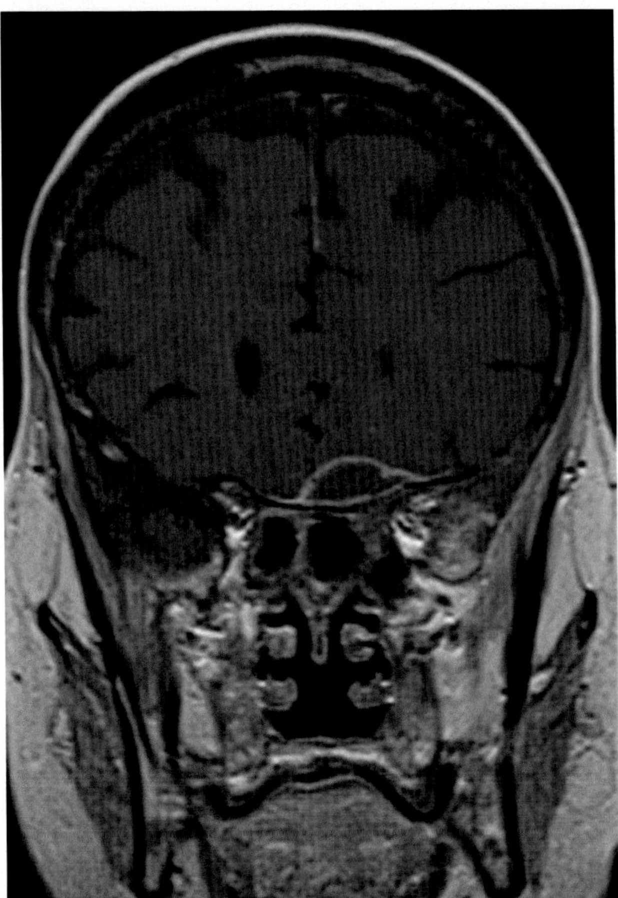

FIGURE 4-3 ■ **Epidural abscess.** Coronal T1 spin-echo image shows a left subfrontal epidural fluid collection surrounded by an enhancing rim of dura.

appearances of subdural empyema are of a crescentic fluid collection overlying the cerebral convexity or in the interhemispheric fissure alongside the falx cerebri. The margins of the collection may be irregular and scalloped, as a result of loculation. Although contrast enhancement at the deep margin of a subdural empyema is a characteristic finding, it can be subtle or absent in the early stages of infection. The adjacent brain may show oedema or cortical contrast enhancement. The CT attenuation and MRI signal characteristics of a subdural empyema are the same as for an epidural abscess (Fig. 4-4).

Ventriculitis

Ventriculitis is uncommon. Causes include trauma, intraventricular rupture of an abscess, shunt infection and haematogenous spread of infection to the ependyma or choroid plexus. The most frequent imaging finding is intraventricular debris, which is slightly hyperattenuating compared to CSF on CT and is of increased signal on FLAIR and DWI sequences with low signal intensity on ADC maps (Fig. 4-5). Periventricular and subependymal high signal and enhancement of the ventricular margins are less common although are still present in most cases.[20,21] The affected ventricles are usually dilated.

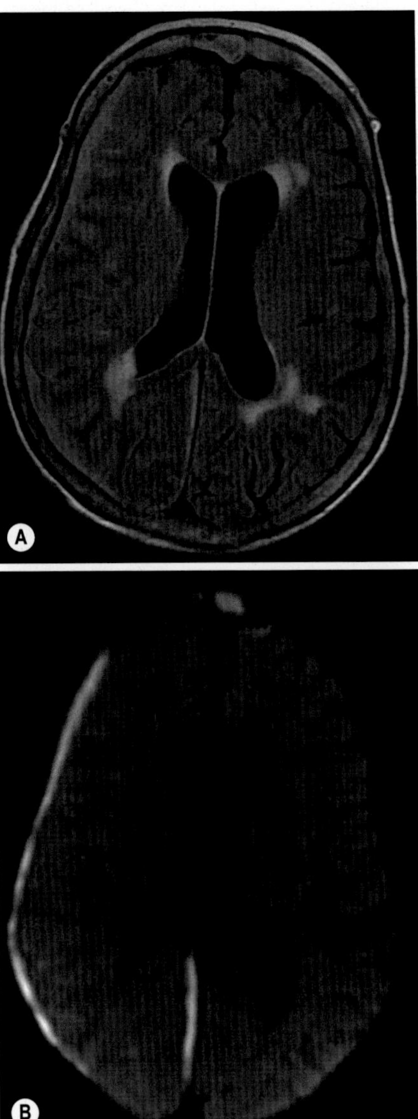

FIGURE 4-4 ■ **Subdural empyema.** (A) Axial FLAIR image shows a right cerebral convexity and posterior parafalcine fluid collection of higher signal intensity than ventricular CSF. (B) DWI shows restricted diffusion within the subdural collection.

Tuberculosis

Involvement of the central nervous system (CNS) occurs in 5% of cases of tuberculosis; most patients are younger than 20 years. Of patients with CNS tuberculosis, the chest radiograph is abnormal in 45–60%.[7] Tuberculous meningitis is the most frequent manifestation of tuberculous CNS infection. In the early stages of the disease a diffuse pattern of leptomeningeal enhancement is common, with a later predilection for the basal leptomeninges, most frequently in the interpeduncular cistern of the midbrain.[22] CT shows obliteration of the basal cisterns by isoattenuating or slightly hyperattenuating exudate, which enhances diffusely after IV contrast medium. The most sensitive and specific CT criteria for tuberculous meningitis are linear enhancement of the middle cerebral artery cisterns, obliteration by contrast of the CSF spaces around normal vascular enhancement,

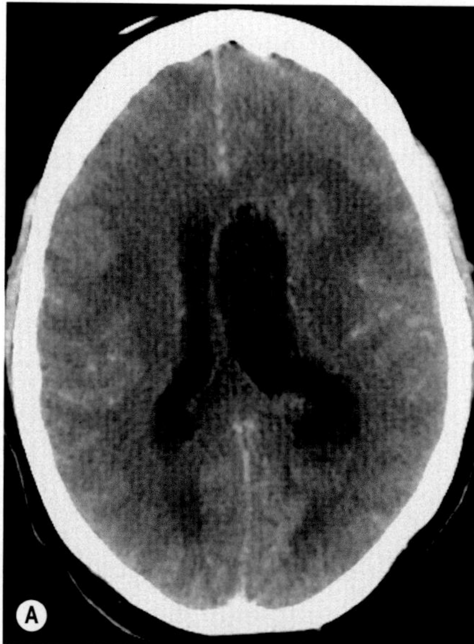

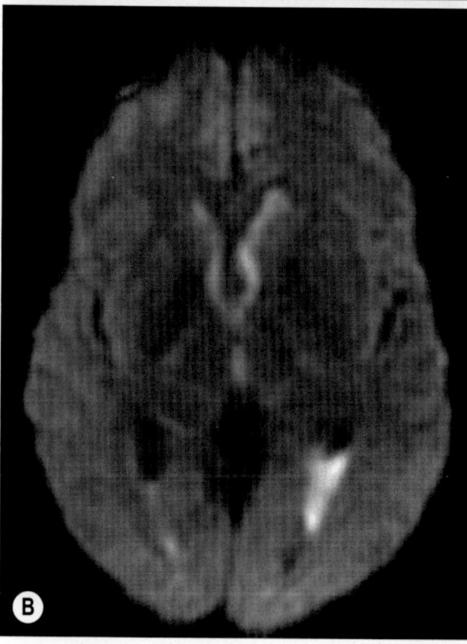

FIGURE 4-5 ■ **Pyogenic ventriculitis.** (A) Axial CT shows dilated lateral ventricles that contain intermediate attenuation debris. There is a rim of low-attenuation interstitial oedema surrounding the ventricles. (B) DWI at a more caudal level shows restricted diffusion in the debris.

Y-shaped enhancement at the junction of the suprasellar and middle cerebral artery cisterns and asymmetry of enhancement.[23] The meningeal exudate obstructs the resorption of CSF and so causes communicating hydrocephalus, resulting in dilatation of the lateral, third and fourth ventricles. This is seen in 50% of adults and 85% of children.[7] Less often, non-communicating hydrocephalus can occur because of obstruction of the outlet foramina of the fourth ventricle. Arteritis of the penetrating arteries within the subarachnoid space affected by areas of tuberculous meningitis can result in infarctions of the basal ganglia, internal capsules and brainstem. With healing, calcification of the affected meninges may be seen rarely.

MRI depicts the basal meningeal enhancement, hydrocephalus and perforator territory infarcts with greater sensitivity than CT (Fig. 4-6). The differential diagnosis for tuberculous meningitis includes fungal meningitis, neurosarcoid and carcinomatous meningitis.

Tuberculomas (parenchymal granulomas) occur most often at the junction of white and grey matter (Fig. 4-7). On CT they appear as small rounded lesions isoattenuating or hypoattenuating to normal brain, with variable amounts of surrounding vasogenic oedema. Contrast enhancement is homogeneous when lesions are solid and shows rim enhancement when central caseation or liquefaction occurs. The 'target sign' of central high attenuation with rim enhancement is not pathognomonic for tuberculoma. On MRI small, non-caseated, tuberculomas show low signal intensity on T1 sequences and high signal on T2 sequences. Caseation of tuberculomas results in low signal intensity on T2 (Fig. 4-7). On DWI tuberculomas may show elevated or restricted diffusion. Tuberculomas may calcify when healed, but, as with meningeal disease, this is uncommon.[24]

Tuberculous abscesses are uncommon; they may resemble tuberculomas but are usually larger and have a thinner enhancing rim. The enhancing rim of a tuberculous abscess is more often lobulated than smooth, whereas, similar to pyogenic abscesses, the non-enhancing core of a tuberculous abscess typically shows restricted diffusion.[13]

Neurosyphilis

CNS involvement can occur at any stage of syphilis; in human immunodeficiency virus (HIV) infection its course may be more aggressive. Meningovascular syphilis causes a small-vessel endarteritis that appears as arterial segmental 'beading' on angiography, with associated infarcts in the basal ganglia. Cerebral gummas are rare, typically arise from the meninges and appear as mass lesions with variable MR signal characteristics and enhancement.[25]

FUNGAL INFECTIONS

Fungal infections of the CNS are uncommon in immunocompetent patients, occurring most frequently in patients with acquired immunodeficiency syndrome (AIDS) or in transplant recipients. As with bacterial infections, fungi can cause meningitis (Fig. 4-8), epidural abscess or subdural empyema, cerebritis (Fig. 4-8), brain abscesses (Fig. 4-9) and granulomas. The imaging appearances of these manifestations are for the most part non-specific and do not suggest fungal infection as the cause. Fungal abscesses are a possible exception; one study found fungal abscesses to show intracavitary projections from their walls which were not present in bacterial or tuberculous abscesses. Unlike the bacterial and tuberculous abscesses, none of the fungal abscesses showed restricted diffusion in their non-ehancing core.[13] The type of CNS involvement has been reported to vary with the fungal species; meningitis is more common with small unicellular organisms such as *Candida* and *Cryptococcus* (Fig. 4-8), whereas cerebritis, granulomas and abscesses are more frequently caused by hyphal organisms such as *Aspergillus*.[26]

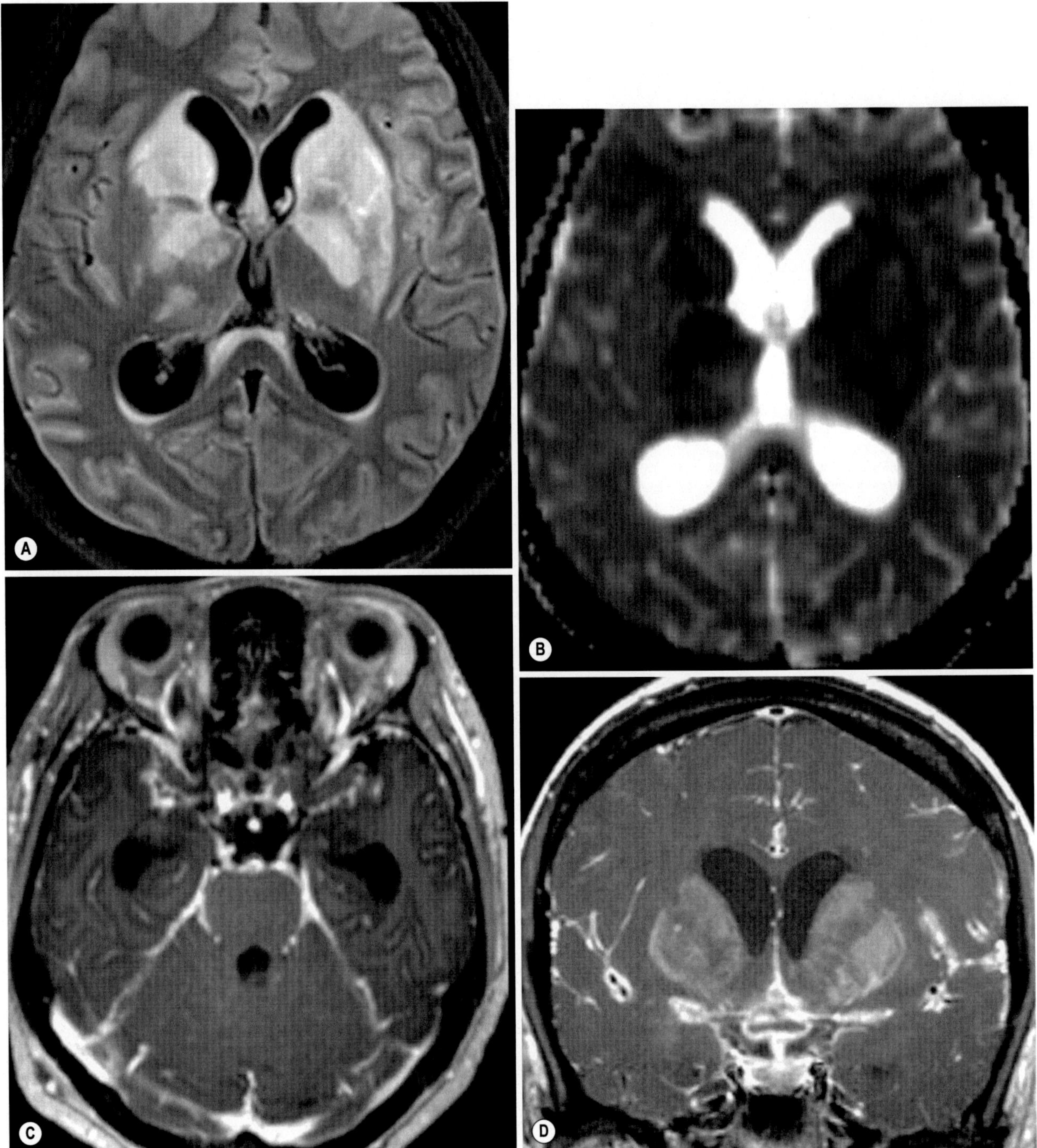

FIGURE 4-6 ■ Cerebral tuberculosis in a 27-year-old female patient. (A) Axial FLAIR image shows bilateral high-signal-intensity abnormalities in the basal ganglia regions. The ventricular system is mildly enlarged. (B) On the ADC map, low ADC values were measured, indicating restricted diffusion in the subacute infarctions. (C, D) On axial (C) and coronal (D) post-contrast T1 images, marked meningeal enhancement was detected, consistent with tuberculous meningitis.

VIRAL INFECTIONS

Herpes Simplex Encephalitis

Herpes simplex type 1 is the most frequent cause of viral encephalitis in adults and is often fatal without treatment. It results from reactivation of latent infection in the trigeminal ganglion or from reinfection by the olfactory route. Although early reports observed that CT appears normal in the first 3 to 5 days after onset, a more recent study with modern CT equipment showed that abnormalities were visible in the majority of patients within 3 days.[27] CT shows low attenuation and swelling in the anteromedial temporal lobe and inferior frontal lobe, with less frequent involvement of the insula and cingulate gyrus. The abnormalities are initially unilateral but often progress to become bilateral. Haemorrhage is seen as a late feature and not usually a prominent finding. Contrast

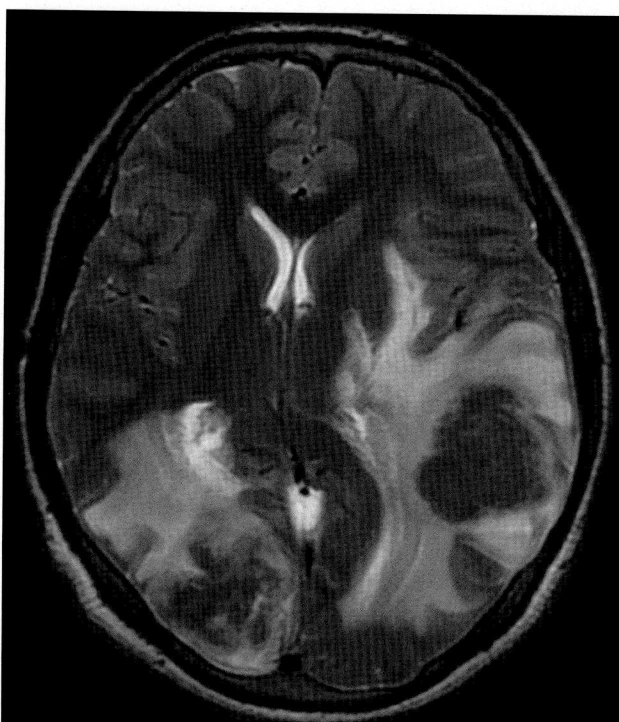

FIGURE 4-7 ■ **Tuberculomas.** Axial T2 fast spin-echo image shows large, hypointense, bilateral caseating granulomas. The extensive surrounding high signal in the cerebral white matter is caused by vasogenic oedema.

enhancement within the affected areas may be patchy or gyriform. MRI is more sensitive; T2 and FLAIR sequences show high signal and swelling within 2 days of onset (Fig. 4-10). The abnormal signal is mainly cortical, with secondary involvement of the subjacent white matter. MRI is also more sensitive than CT to foci of haemorrhage, particularly with the use of T2* gradient echo or SWI. Diffusion-weighted imaging shows cortical hyperintensity with greater sensitivity than conventional MRI.

Other Viral Encephalitides

Imaging appearances in most other viral encephalitides are less characteristic than in the case of herpes simplex encephalitis. Japanese encephalitis, caused by a flavivirus, is an exception and most often manifests as areas of hyperintensity on T2 and FLAIR sequences in the thalami, basal ganglia and brainstem—particularly in the substantia nigra. Other viral infections of the CNS, such as West Nile virus and tick-borne encephalitis, have a predilection for the basal ganglia, thalami and brainstem but, like the clinical presentation, the imaging is often non-specific and does not suggest a particular virus.[28]

Human Immunodeficiency Virus (HIV) and Acquired Immunodeficiency Syndrome (AIDS)

Infection by HIV merits a more detailed coverage in view of its high prevalence and global importance. Here we discuss the direct impact of the HIV on the brain and the associated complications of progressive multifocal leukoencephalopathy (PML) and immune reconstitution inflammatory syndrome (IRIS). Opportunistic infections, which can occur in AIDS, such as cryptococcal infection and toxoplasmosis, are discussed under the headings of 'Fungal Infections' and 'Parasitic Infections', respectively.

The HIV/AIDS pandemic is now in its fourth decade and UNAIDS estimates that, in 2011, a total of 34.2 million people were living with HIV infection. Prognosis has dramatically improved since the introduction of combination antiretroviral therapy (cART) and HIV/AIDS has been transformed from a death sentence into a manageable illness. However, in 2011, still less than 25% of all HIV-infected people had access to antiretroviral therapy or had virologic suppression from receipt of such therapy.[29]

Opportunistic infections (OIs) are still of concern in undiagnosed and untreated patients with HIV/AIDS. For those with access to cART, there has been a dramatic decline in the incidence of OIs and neurocognitive and vascular CNS complications of HIV have become the major causes of morbidity.

HIV Encephalopathy

The HIV virus invades peripheral macrophages, endogenous microglial cells and astrocytes. Direct neuronal invasion is very rare and neuronal injury, which may be partially reversible, occurs as a consequence of the release of toxic viral gene products as well as pro-inflammatory cytokines, including tumour necrosis factor, quinolinic acid and platelet activating factor.[30]

The neuroradiological correlates of HIV encephalopathy (HIVE) are areas of hyperintense signal on T2 and FLAIR images which can be either ill-defined, diffuse and symmetrical (Fig. 4-11), or patchy and scattered; involvement of the deep grey matter is also seen (Fig. 4-11).[30] The MRI appearances are thought to reflect an increase of water content and serum proteins in the brain parenchyma as a result of increased vascular permeability in the presence of circulating cytokines and/or a loss of myelin.

Advanced MRI techniques such as diffusion tensor imaging, MR perfusion imaging and MR spectroscopy can be used to investigate more subtle effects of HIV on the brain parenchyma and provide quantitative measures.[31]

Brain volume loss is a feature of more advanced HIVE and was one of the most prominent imaging features in the pre-cART era. Cerebral atrophy caused by HIV is not diffuse but has a predilection for specific regions such as the basal ganglia, thalamus, corpus callosum and frontal lobes.[32]

HIVE is typically associated with various degrees of cognitive impairment and a new classification of HIV-associated neurocognitive disorders (HAND) was proposed in 2007,[33] distinguishing the following:

1. Asymptomatic neurocognitive impairment (ANI) where patients have abnormal neuropsychological tests but are not impaired in their everyday life.
2. Mild cognitive impairment (MND) with mildly impaired functioning.

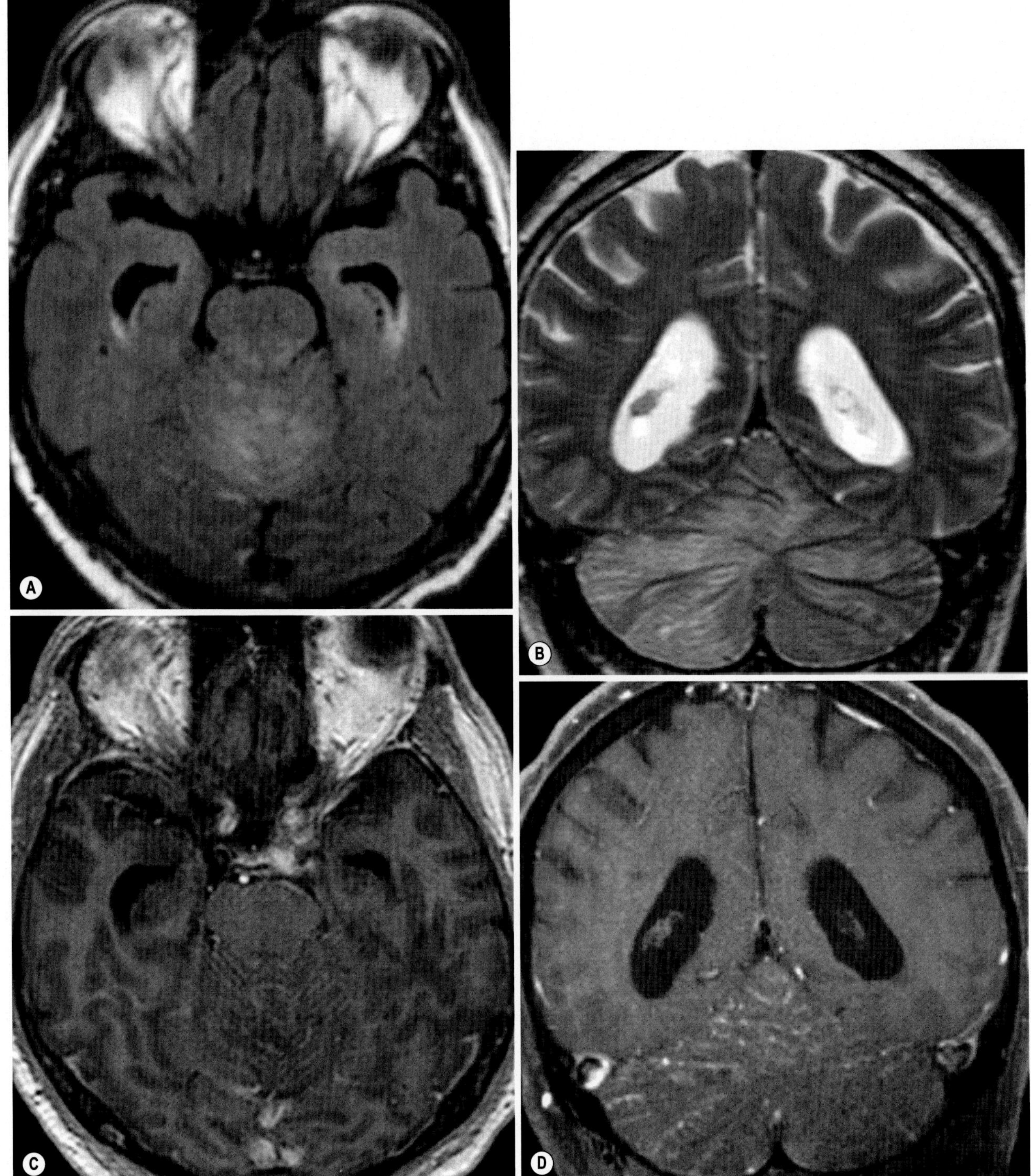

FIGURE 4-8 ■ ***Crypotcoccus neoformans* meningitis and cerebellitis in a renal transplant recipient.** (A) Axial FLAIR images show high signal intensity of the subarachnoid spaces in the region of the cerebellar vermis. (B) High signal in the cerebellum on both sides was demonstrated on the coronal T2 MR image. (C, D) Strong leptomeningeal enhancement is nicely shown on axial and coronal post-contrast T1 images.

3. HIV-associated dementia (HAD), which corresponds to the former AIDS dementia complex.

Before the introduction of cART, the prevalence of HAD was around 16%, with an annual incidence of 7% among patients with advanced HIV infection. In the era of cART, this is now rare but milder forms of cognitive impairment present a major cause of morbidity.

HIV and Vascular Disease

HIV patients have an increased risk of stroke and ischaemic stroke is far more frequent than haemorrhagic stroke.[34] There is a cumulative increase in risk according to the duration of cART.[35] Several mechanisms contribute to the increase of non-haemorrhagic stroke in HIV

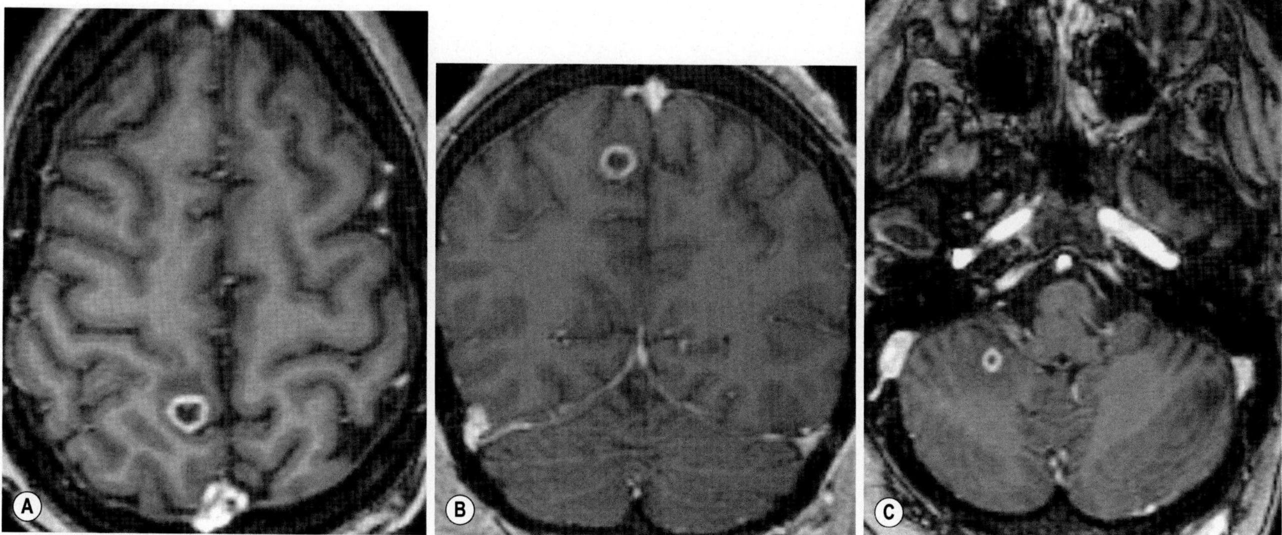

FIGURE 4-9 ■ Multiple fungal abscesses in an 8-year-old bone marrow transplant recipient. On axial (A, C) and coronal (B) post-contrast T1 MR images, FLAIR ring-like enhancing focal lesions were detected in the right cerebellum and right parietal region.

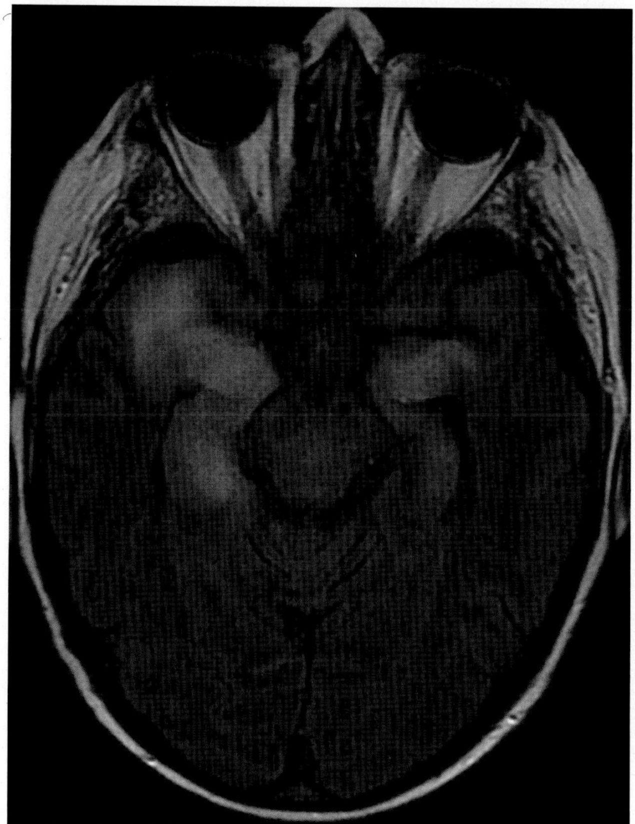

FIGURE 4-10 ■ Herpes simplex encephalitis. Axial FLAIR image shows asymmetrical swelling and increased signal intensity in the anteromedial temporal lobes, more severe on the right.

including endothelial dysfunction in the presence of chronic inflammation, coagulopathies, such as HIV-associated thrombocytopaenia and the atherogenic effect of certain antiretroviral drugs. HIV infection can cause accelerated atherosclerosis and/or vasculitis of the extracranial and intracranial vessels. Immune-mediated vascular damage can also lead to the formation of aneurysms, which are more common in young male patients (Fig. 4-12).

Progressive Multifocal Leukoencephalopathy

PML is a form of progressive demyelination caused by reactivation of a latent *John Cunningham virus* (*JC papovavirus*) infection in immunocompromised patients, typically seen in HIV patients with a CD4 count less than 100/mm^3. PML can also occur in other forms of immunocompromise and in patients receiving immunosuppressive drugs.[36] Clinical presentation can be with gradual cognitive impairment and personality disturbances, or acutely with focal neuropathy and seizures.

The lesions are typically hyperintense on T2 and FLAIR images and hypointense on T1-weighted images, have ill-defined borders and involve predominantly the subcortical or cerebellar white matter. DWI shows a characteristic peripheral hyperintense rim corresponding to the front line of active demyelination around a central area of necrosis (Fig. 4-13). Grey matter involvement and lesion enhancement have been demonstrated, particularly in patients in immune recovery.

Immune Reconstitution Inflammatory Syndrome (IRIS)

Immune reconstitution inflammatory syndrome (IRIS) is defined as a paradoxical deterioration in clinical status attributable to the recovery of the immune system during cART.[37] HIV/AIDS treatment with cART leads to an increase in CD4 cell count/function, and a recovery of the immune system, which can instigate an intense inflammatory response to dead or latent organisms, days to months after commencement of treatment. CD8 cell infiltration in the leptomeninges, perivascular spaces,

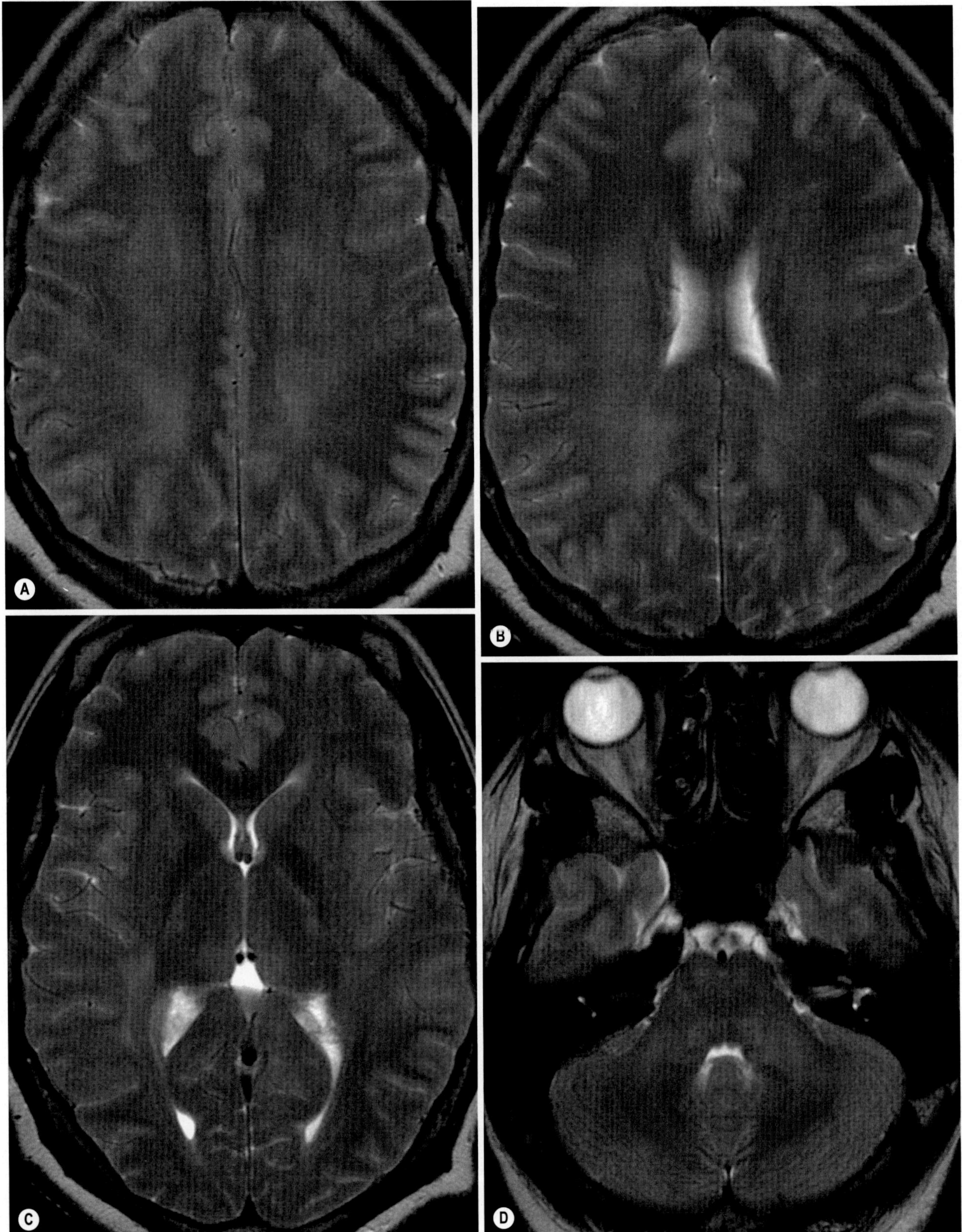

FIGURE 4-11 ■ **HIV encephalopathy.** T2 images showing a diffuse, ill-defined, symmetrical signal intensity increase of the white matter in the centrum semiovale (A), in periventricular white matter (B), in the thalami, caudate nuclei, right optic radiation and internal capsules (C) and in the middle cerebellar peduncles (D). These appearances are typical for HIVE and are potentially reversible with cART.

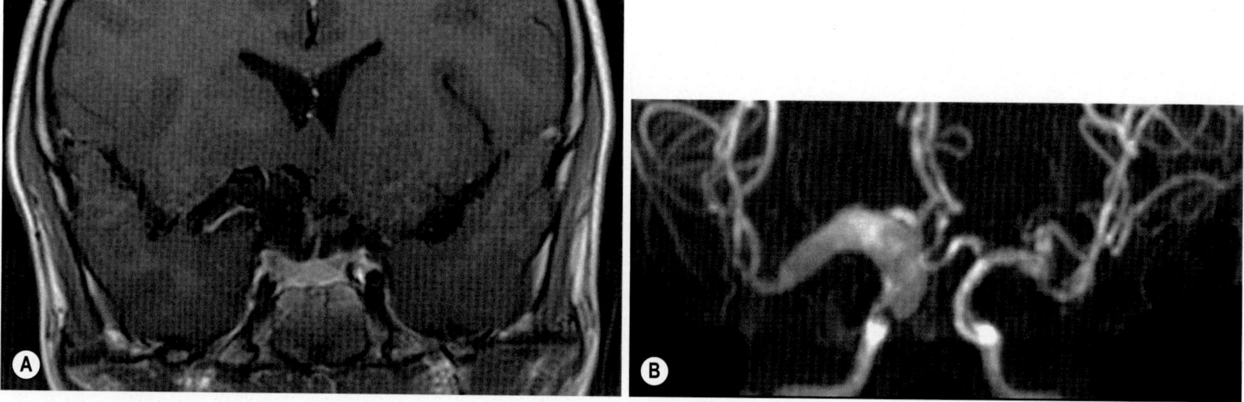

FIGURE 4-12 ■ HIV vasculitis in a 15-year-old man with vertically transmitted HIV infection. The coronal contrast-enhanced T1 (A) shows fusiform dilatation of the right distal internal carotid artery and of both middle cerebral arteries with some enhancement of the wall of the right middle cerebral artery. The extent of fusiform aneurysmal dilatation of the intracranial vessels is well demonstrated on the time-of-flight MRA (B).

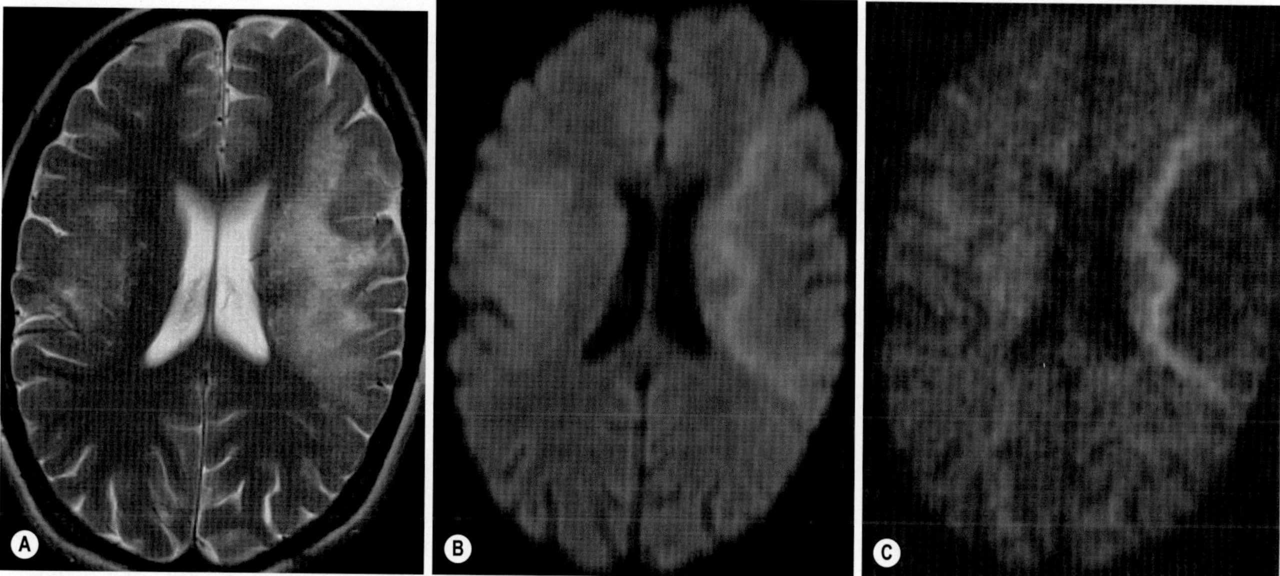

FIGURE 4-13 ■ Progressive multifocal leukoencephalopathy (PML). The T2 image (A) demonstrates widespread hyperintense signal change in the left, and to a lesser extent, right corona radiata. The involvement of the subcortical U fibres is typical for PML. DWI with $b = 1000$ (B) demonstrates a hyperintense edge of the lesion medially, particularly on the left, which is more clearly seen on the DWI with $b = 3000$ (C) and corresponds to the zones of active demyelination.

blood vessels and parenchyma is the pathological hallmark of CNS-IRIS. Risk factors include a rapid drop in viral load or increase in CD4 count and young age. The most commonly associated organisms are the JC virus (PML-IRIS) and *Cryptococcus* but an inflammatory response to other viruses (varicella-zoster virus, cytomegalovirus, HIV), *Candida*, *Mycobacterium tuberculosis* or *Toxoplasma gondii* can also occur.

Clinical presentation is diverse and depends upon the associated OI and extent of disease. Any patient who has commenced cART within the preceding 8 weeks presenting with new CNS symptoms or progressive cognitive dysfunction despite good viral control should be investigated for HIV-related IRIS. Recognition of IRIS in cART-treated patients allows adaptation of medical management, which can improve outcome and prevent death from IRIS-related illness, overall improving prognosis.[37]

Imaging features of CNS-IRIS are a transient increase in parenchymal high signal on FLAIR and T2 sequences, or hypoattenuation on CT, and contrast enhancement (Fig. 4-14). Mass effect and restricted diffusion can also occur. CNS-IRIS is associated with an improved long-term outcome if the acute inflammatory response can be contained.

PARASITIC INFECTIONS

There are many parasitic infections which can involve the brain. Some of these are very rare and only the most important parasitic infections will be discussed here.

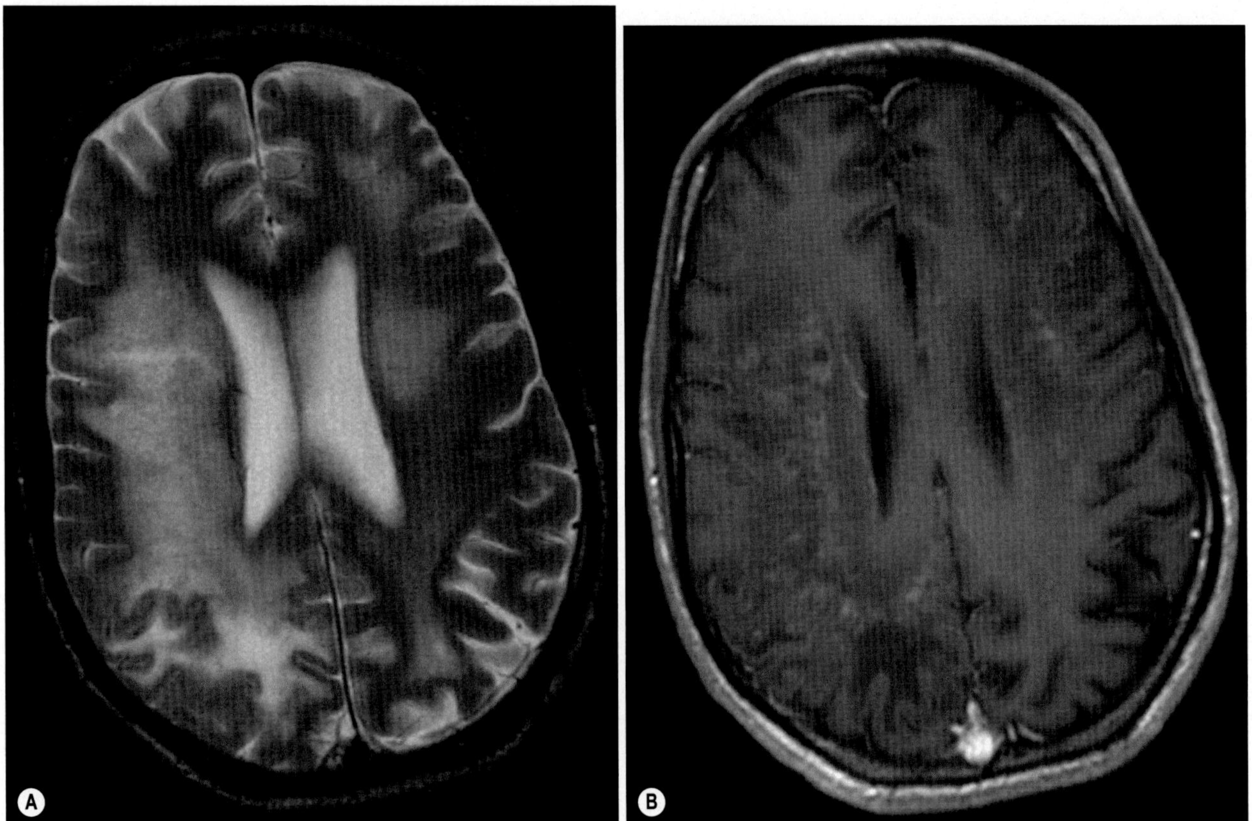

FIGURE 4-14 ■ Immune reconstitution inflammatory syndrome (PML-IRIS) in a 40-year-old HIV-infected patient with PML and low CD4 count at presentation. MRI was performed 8 weeks after treatment with cART. The T2 image (A) demonstrates widespread, confluent hyperintense signal change in the white matter of both cerebral hemispheres, extending into the subcortical U fibres, which is typical for PML. The contrast-enhanced T1 (B) demonstrates hypointense lesions with ill-defined enhancement that is more marked around the periphery and consistent with inflammatory response of a partially recovered immune system.

Toxoplasmosis

Toxoplasma gondii is an intracellular protozoan that infects humans via direct contact with feline excrement or ingestion of raw or undercooked vegetables, pork or lamb. In healthy patients, the acute infection is asymptomatic and becomes latent within the neuroparenchyma. The latent infection is reactivated in patients with a compromised immune system, most commonly in HIV patients with a low CD4 count (below 100 cells/mm^3).

Typical CT and MRI findings are ring-enhancing abscesses centred in the basal ganglia, thalamus and at the corticomedullary junction, with variable degrees of perilesional oedema and mass effect (Fig. 4-15). Enhancement can also be nodular or can be absent if the patient is severely immunocompromised. On non-enhanced MRI, the abscesses appear hyperintense on T2/FLAIR sequences and hypointense on T1 images, unless there has been haemorrhage which causes peripheral T1 shortening. The characteristic 'target sign' of toxoplasmosis on T2 images is caused by central hyperintensity (fluid), peripheral hypointensity (mural blood) and an outer ring of hyperintense perilesional oedema.

The main radiological differential diagnosis is primary CNS lymphoma of the immunocompromised. Lymphoma shows typically restricted diffusion on DWI, whereas toxoplasmosis has a wide range of diffusion characteristics, which can overlap with lymphoma. The latter shows also a much higher tracer uptake on thallium-201 SPECT and ^{18}F-FDG. In clinical practice, the diagnosis of toxoplasmosis is often made by the response to empirical treatment with pyrimethamine–sulfadiazine and folic acid, which should lead to a decrease of lesion size within 10 days.

Cysticercosis

Neurocysticercosis is the most important parasitic disease of the CNS worldwide and is common in Central and South America, India, Africa and Eastern Europe. It is caused by the encysted larvae of the tapeworm *Taenia solium*, which develop after ingestion of eggs in undercooked pork or faeco-oral transmission between humans. Larvae are disseminated by haematogenous spread to neural, muscular and ocular tissues. Symptoms occur approximately 5 years after initial infection and are non-specific, 50–70% presenting with epilepsy.

Neurocysticercosis larvae can spread to the brain parenchyma, subarachnoid space and ventricles. The parenchymal form is the most common, followed by the intraventricular form; mixed types can occur.[38]

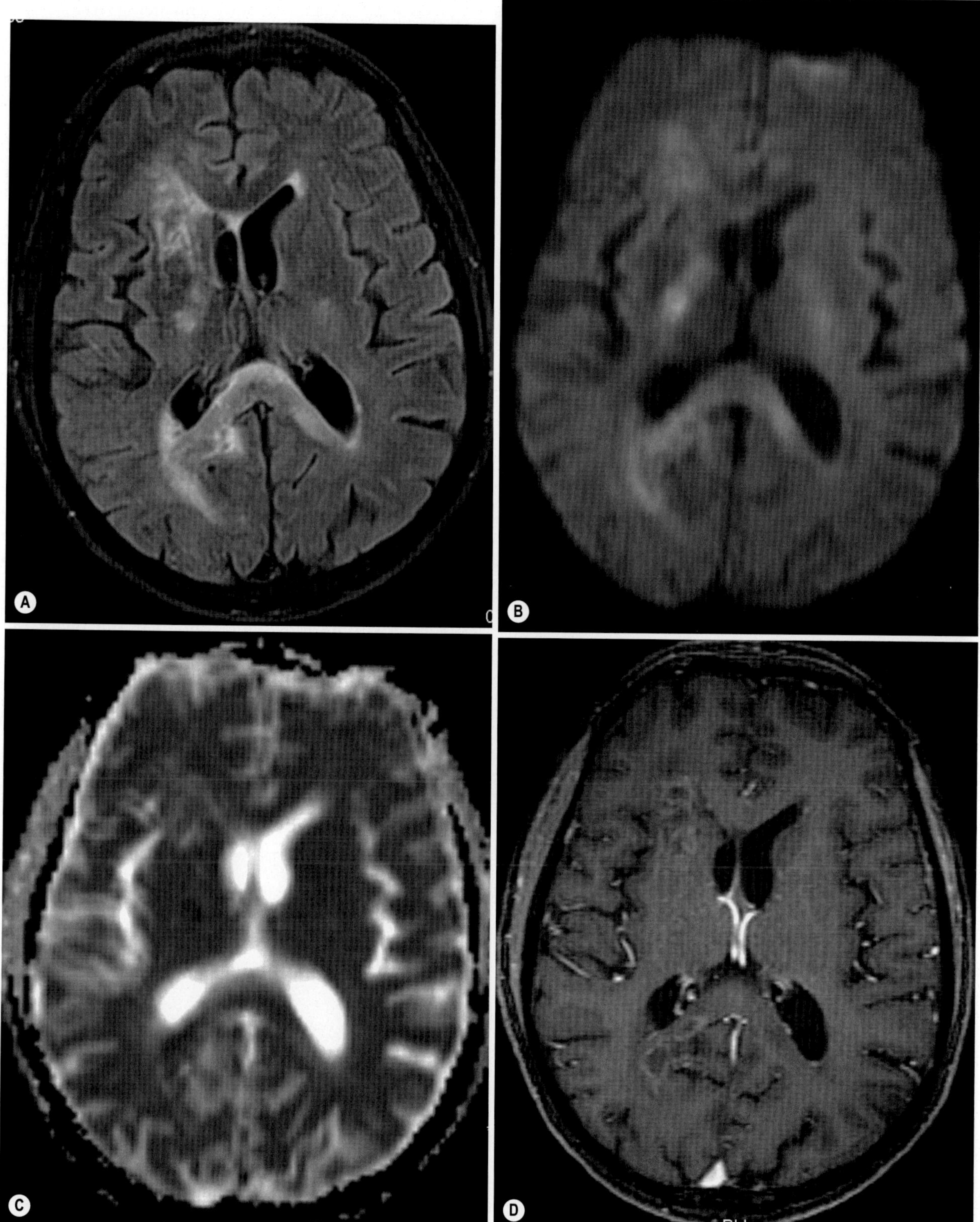

FIGURE 4-15 ■ Cerebral toxoplasmosis in a 50-year-old, HIV-infected male patient. (A) Axial FLAIR image shows signal intensity abnormalities in the right frontal periventricular region, as well as in the right part of the splenium of the corpus callosum. (B, C) High signal was noted on the trace DWI (B), with relatively low ADC values (C). (D, E) Peripheral, irregular enhancement of the lesions was demonstrated on axial (D) and coronal (E) post-contrast MR images.

Continued on following page

On imaging, one can distinguish four stages of *parenchymal neurocysticercosis*:[39]

1. *Vesicular stage*. This stage consists of a viable larva with a scolex (worm head). The cysts are thin-walled and show no or little enhancement and there is no perilesional oedema. The cyst fluid has similar signal characteristics to CSF and water diffusion is unrestricted. The scolex can appear hyperintense on T1, FLAIR and DWI images (Fig. 4-16).
2. *Colloidal vesicular stage*. This is the stage where larva breaks down and an immune response from the host is instigated. Ring-enhancing lesions with perilesional oedema and mass effect are typical imaging findings (Figs. 4-17A, B). Compared to the vesicular stage, the cyst content is more proteinaceous and appears consequently more hyperintense on T1 and FLAIR images.
3. *Granular nodular stage*. As the larva dies, the cyst collapses and the host response is marked with thick enhancing cyst walls and progression of surrounding oedema (Figs. 4-17C, D).
4. *Calcified nodular stage*. This is the non-active form of neurocysticercosis. The oedema resolves and small calcified lesions of 2–10 mm diameter are seen. Contrast enhancement and oedema are unusual for this stage but may occur in the context of seizure activity.

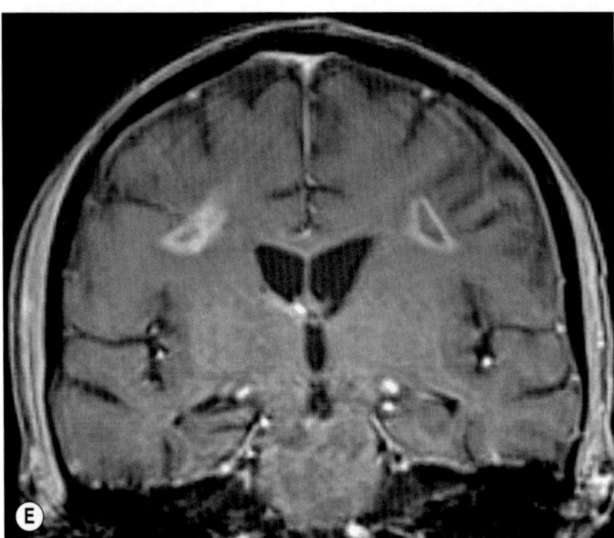

FIGURE 4-15, Continued

Intraventricular cysticercosis is the second most common form of neurocysticercosis and larvae are more frequently found in the fourth and third ventricles than in the lateral ventricles. Intraventricular cysts can cause obstruction to the CSF flow and hydrocephalus, which may present acutely. *Subarachnoid cysticercosis* can involve the basal cisterns, sylvian fissures and cerebellopontine angle regions. *Racemose cysticercosis* is a rare form of subarachnoid cysticercosis where multiple clustered cysts are separated by septae, causing a 'bunch of grapes' appearance. The racemose form can lead to large cystic lesions, which may be associated with local meningeal nodular enhancement.[39]

Echinococcus (Hydatid Disease)

There are two main types of hydatid disease: cystic echinococcosis and aveolar echinococcosis, the latter being much less common. Carnivores such as dogs are

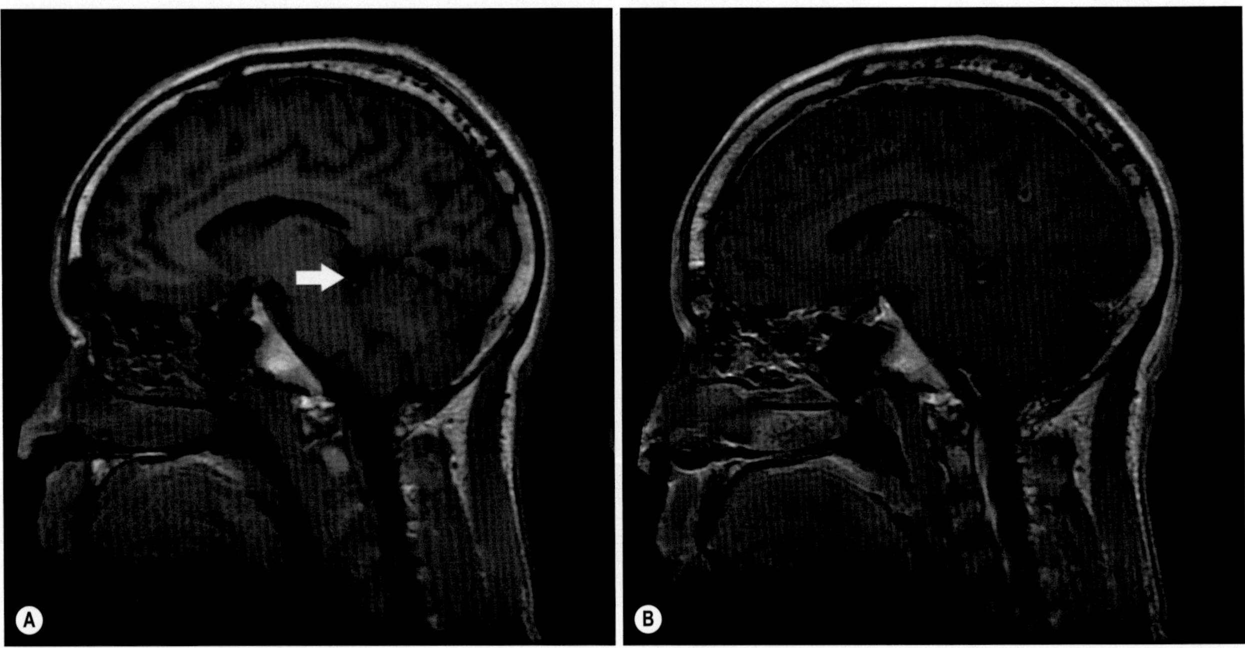

FIGURE 4-16 ■ **Neurocysticercosis.** Sagittal T1 (A), contrast-enhanced T1 (B), axial T2 (C) and coronal FLAIR image (D) in a patient with extensive parenchymal and subarachnoid (arrows) cysticercosis. Most of the lesions are in the vesicular stage showing thin-walled cysts with little or no enhancement and a scolex (worm head) in the centre of the cyst. There is no oedema.

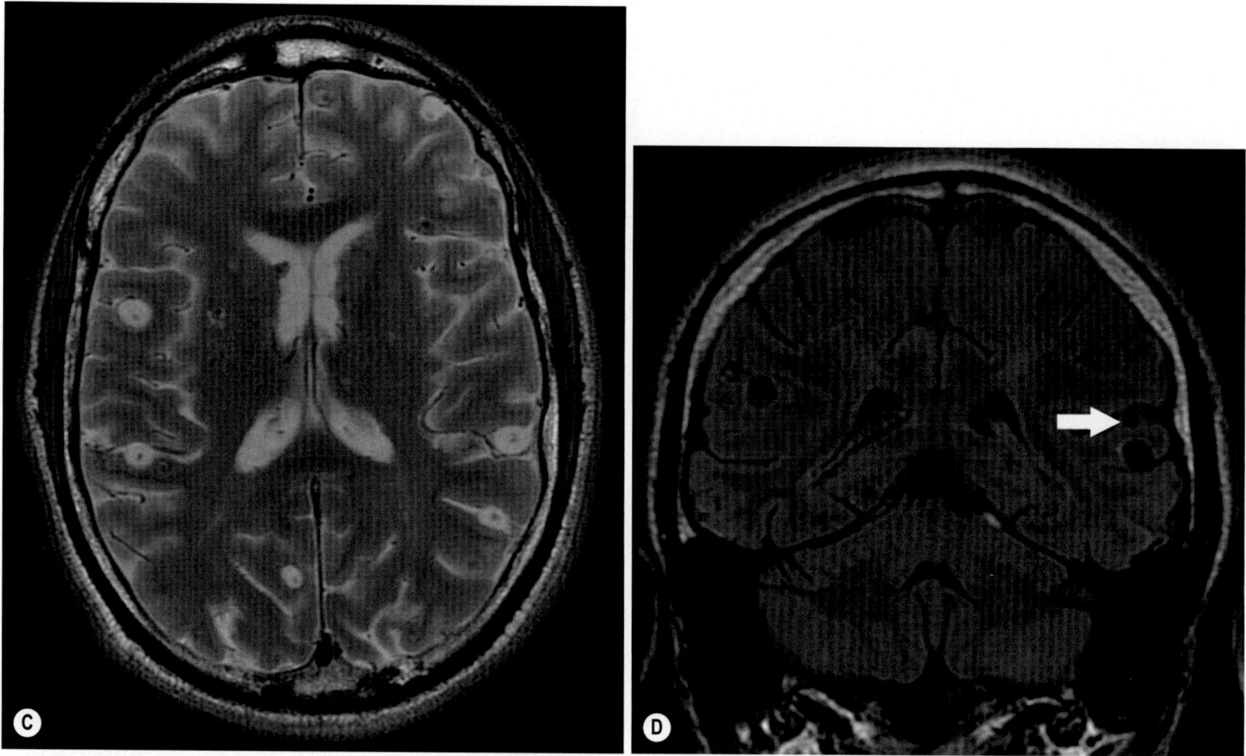

FIGURE 4-16, Continued

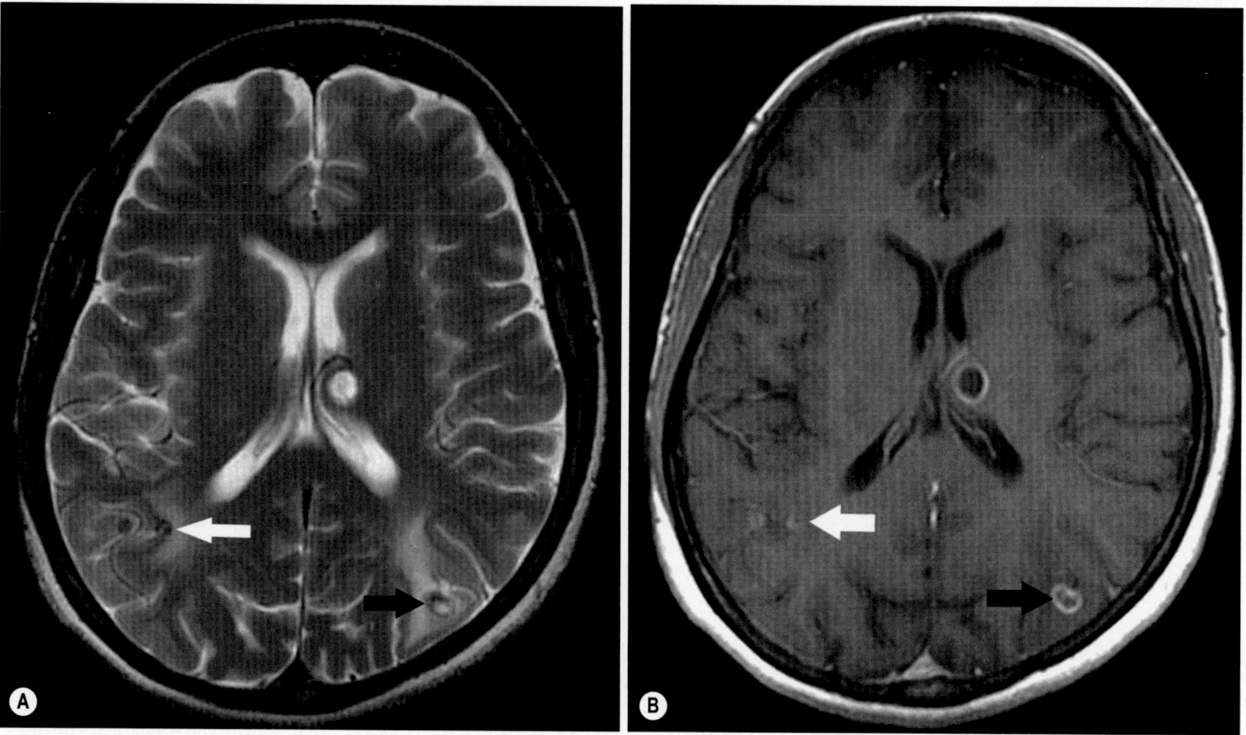

FIGURE 4-17 ■ **Neurocysticercosis.** T2 image (A) and contrast-enhanced T1 image (B) showing the vesicular stage (lesion in the left lateral ventricle), colloidal vesicular stage (black arrows) and calcified nodular stage (white arrows) of cysticercosis.

Continued on following page

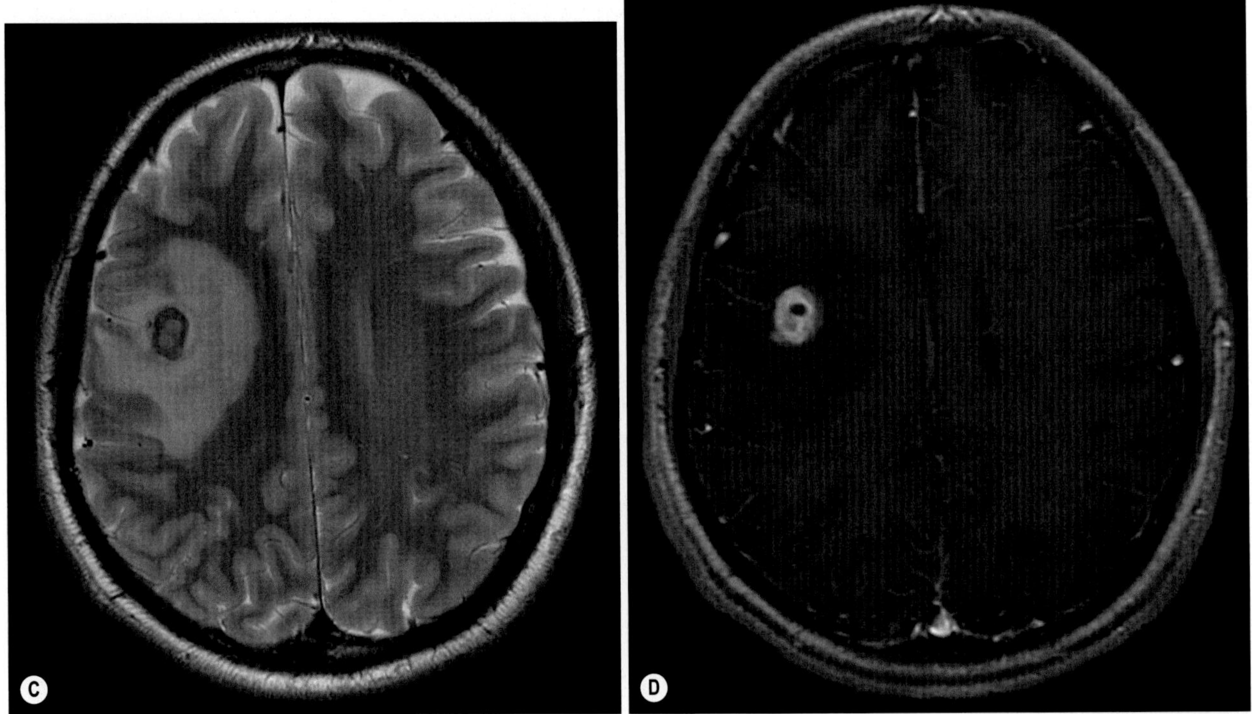

FIGURE 4-17, Continued ■ T2 image (C) and enhanced T1 image (D) demonstrating the granular nodular stage with a partially collapsed cyst associated with marked immune reaction from the host evidenced by a thick enhancing wall and marked surrounding oedema.

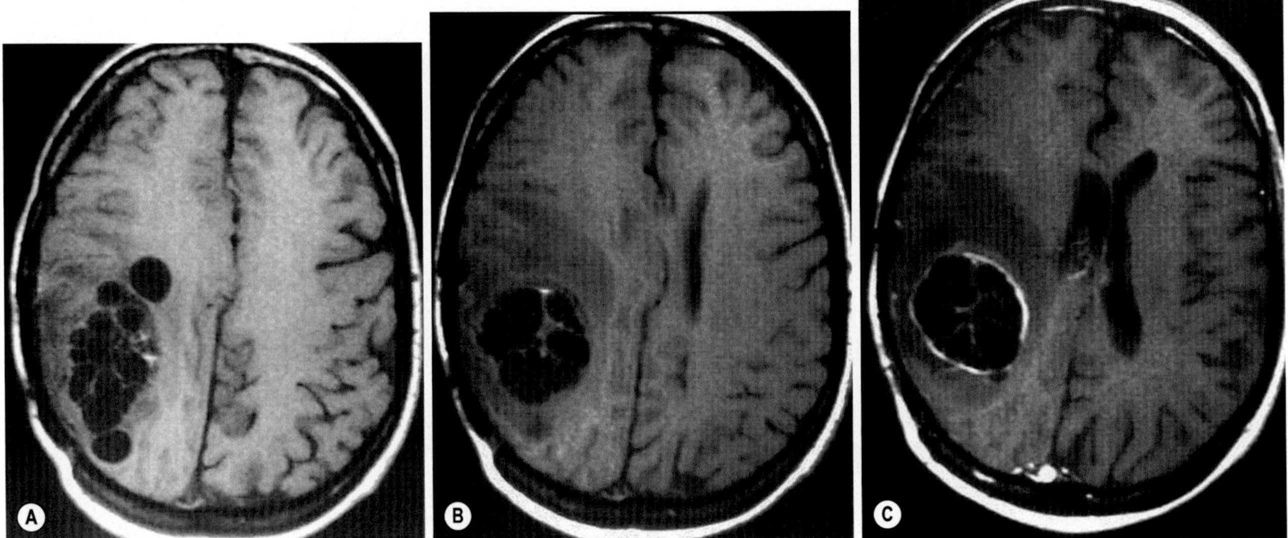

FIGURE 4-18 ■ ***Echinococcus* (hydatid).** Non-enhanced T1 (A, B) show multiple well-defined cysts corresponding to a hydatid cyst with multiple daughter cysts. There is also some associated oedema which appears hypointense. The contrast-enhanced T1 (C) demonstrates a thin outer rim of enhancement, which together with the oedema indicates that this is an active hydatid cyst.

definitive hosts to the *Echinococcus* (or hydatid) tapeworm. Herbivores such as sheep and cattle are intermediate hosts and humans are accidental hosts, infected by faeco-oral transmission. CNS involvement is seen in approximately 4% of patients with primary hepatic or pulmonary infestation.

Cystic echinococcosis in the brain is usually the result of haematogenous spread of embryos from the gastrointestinal tract and usually manifests itself as large, isolated, unilocular, well-defined and relatively thin-walled cysts. Small daughter cysts may be arranged peripherally within a large maternal cyst and this is considered to represent a pathognomonic sign of a hydatid cyst.[38] The cyst fluid appears similar to CSF on CT and MRI. In active cysts, a thin rim of enhancement and surrounding oedema may be detectable on MRI (Fig. 4-18). At a late stage CT may show calcification, which is an indicator that the cyst is dead.

Alveolar echinococcosis has a high mortality rate and the imaging features are of numerous irregular

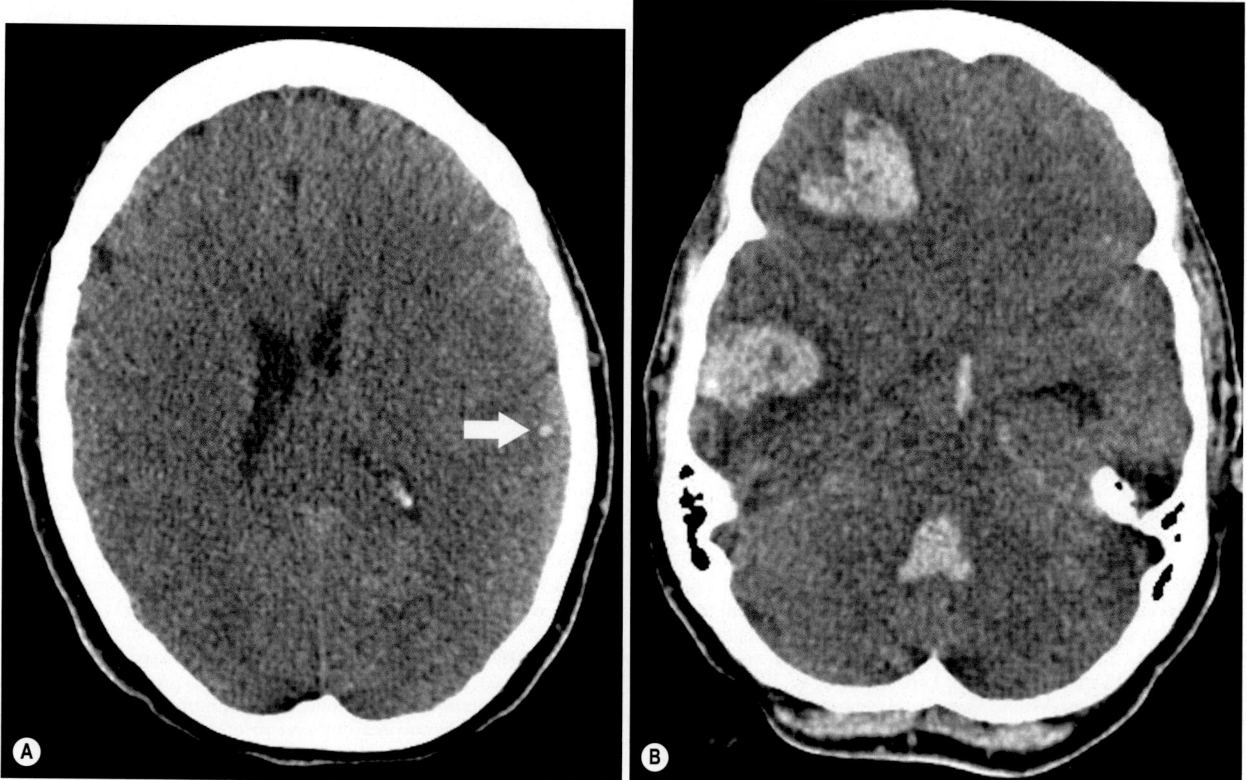

FIGURE 4-19 ■ Cerebral *Plasmodium falciparum* malaria in a 40-year-old woman with a state of confusion with reduced conscious level. The initial CT (A) performed on admission shows a small bleed peripherally in the left frontal lobe (arrow). An emergency CT performed 24 h later (B) shows multiple intraparenchymal and intraventricular haemorrhages and brain swelling with obliteration of the basal cisterns.

small cysts. Heterogeneous, nodular and cauliflower-like enhancement has been reported.

Malaria

With increasing travel to endemic regions, one must be aware of cerebral involvement in malaria, which occurs in about 2% of patients with *Plasmodium falciparum* infection. Cerebral malaria is a serious and life-threatening condition with a mortality rate of 20–50%. Early diagnosis and treatment are essential. Symptoms are often non-specific and include raised intracranial pressure, seizures, altered consciousness and stroke.

The infected erythrocytes cause occlusion of the cerebral capillaries and imaging findings include cortical and subcortical ischaemic lesions, cerebral oedema, microhaemorrhages, which are best seen on susceptibility-weighted imaging,[40] and macrohaemorrhages (Fig. 4-19).

REFERENCES

1. Hughes DC, Raghavan A, Mordekar SR, et al. Role of imaging in the diagnosis of acute bacterial meningitis and its complications. Postgrad Med J 2010;86:478–85.
2. National Institute for Health and Clinical Excellence. Bacterial meningitis and meningococcal septicaemia: management of bacterial meningitis and meningocococcal septicaemia in children and young people younger than 16 years in primary and secondary care. CG102. London: National Institute for Health and Clinical Excellence; 2010.
3. Parmar H, Sitoh Y-Y, Anand P, et al. Contrast-enhanced FLAIR imaging in the evaluation of infectious leptomeningeal diseases. Eur J Radiol 2006;58:89–95.
4. Kamran S, Bari Bener A, Alper D, et al. Role of fluid-attenuated inversion recovery in the diagnosis of meningitis: comparison with contrast-enhanced magnetic resonance imaging. J Comp Assist Tomogr 2004;28:68–72.
5. Kawaguchi T, Sakurai K, Hara M, et al. Clinico-radiological features of subarachnoid hyperintensity on diffusion-weighted images in patients with meningitis. Clin Radiol 2012;67:306–12.
6. Katchanov J, Siebert E, Endres M, Klingebiel R. Focal parenchymal lesions in community-acquired bacterial meningitis: a clinico-radiological study. Neuroradiology 2009;51:723–9.
7. Roos KL. Principles of Neurologic Infectious Disease. New York: McGraw-Hill; 2005.
8. Stevens EA, Norman D, Kramer RA, et al. Computed tomographic brain scanning in intraparenchymal pyogenic abscesses. Am J Roentgenol 1978;130:111–14.
9. Enzmann DR, Britt RH, Placone R. Staging of human brain abscesses by computed tomography. Radiology 1983;146:703–8.
10. Haimes A, Zimmerman RD, Morgello S, et al. MR imaging of brain abscesses. Am J Roentgenol 1989;152:1073–85.
11. Lai PH, Chang HC, Chuang TC, et al. Susceptibility-weighted imaging in patients with pyogenic brain abscesses at 1.5T: characteristics of the abscess capsule. Am J Neuroradiol 2012;33:910–14.
12. Toh CH, Wei K-C, Chang C-N, et al. Differentiation of pyogenic brain abscesses from necrotic glioblastoma with use of susceptibility-weighted imaging. Am J Neuroradiol 2012;33:1534–8.
13. Luthra G, Parihar A, Nath K, et al. Comparative evaluation of fungal, tubercular and pyogenic brain abscesses with conventional and diffusion MR imaging and proton MR spectroscopy. Am J Neuroradiol 2007;28:1332–8.
14. Tomar V, Yadav A, Rathore RKS, et al. Apparent diffusion coefficient with higher b-value correlates better with viable cell count

quantified from the cavity of brain abscess. Am J Neuroradiol 2011;32:2120–5.
15. Holmes TM, Petrella JR, Provenzale JM. Distinction between cerebral abscesses and high-grade neoplasms by dynamic susceptibility contrast perfusion MRI. Am J Roentgenol 2004;183:1247–52.
16. Cartes-Zumelzu FW, Stavrou I, Castillo M, et al. Diffusion-weighted imaging in the assessment of brain abscess therapy. Am J Neuroradiol 2004;25:1310–17.
17. Rich PM, Deasy NP, Jarosz JM. Intracranial dural empyema. Br J Radiol 2000;73:1329–36.
18. Tsuchiya K, Osawa A, Katase S, et al. Diffusion-weighted MRI of subdural and epidural empyemas. Neuroradiology 2003;45:220–3.
19. Farrell CJ, Hoh BL, Pisculli ML, et al. Limitations of diffusion-weighted imaging in the diagnosis of postoperative infections. Neurosurgery 2008;62:577–83.
20. Fujikawa A, Tsuchiya K, Honya K, et al. Comparison of MRI sequences to detect ventriculitis. Am J Roentgenol 2006;187: 1048–53.
21. Fukui MB, Williams RL, Mudigonda S. CT and MR imaging features of pyogenic ventriculitis. Am J Neuroradiol 2001;22: 1510–16.
22. Öztoprak Î, Gümüs C, Öztoprak B, Engin A. Contrast medium-enhanced MRI findings and changes over time in stage I tuberculous meningitis. Clin Radiol 2007;62:1206–15.
23. Pryzbojewksi S, Andronikou S, Wilmhurst J. Objective CT criteria to determine the presence of abnormal basal enhancement in children with suspected tuberculous meningitis. Paediar Radiol 2006; 36:687–96.
24. Bernaerts A, Vanhoenacker FM, Parizel PM, et al. Tuberculosis of the central nervous system: overview of neuroradiological findings. Eur Radiol 2003;12:1876–90.
25. Brightbill TC, Ihmedian IH, Post MJD, et al. Neurosyphilis in HIV-positive and HIV-negative patients: neuroimaging findings. Am J Neuroradiol 1995;16:703–11.
26. Mathur M, Johnson CE, Sze G. Fungal infections of the central nervous system. Neuroimaging Clin N Am 2012;22: 609–32.
27. Noguchi T, Yoshiura T, Hiwatashi A, et al. CT and MRI findings of human herpesvirus 6-associated encephalopathy: comparison with findings of herpes simplex virus encephalitis. Am J Roentgenol 2011;194:754–60.
28. Rath TJ, Hughes M, Arabi M, Shah GV. Imaging of cerebritis, encephalitis and brain abscess. Neuroimaging Clin N Am 2012; 22:585–607.
29. Piot P, Quinn TC. Responses to the AIDS pandemic—a global health model. N Engl J Med 2013;368:2210–18.
30. Manji H, Jäger HR, Winston A. HIV, dementia and antiretroviral drugs: 30 years of an epidemic. J Neurol Neurosurg Psychiatry 2013;84(10):1126–37.
31. Thurnher MM, Donovan Post MJ. Neuroimaging in the brain in HIV-1-infected patients. Neuroimaging Clin N Am 2008;18: 93–117.
32. Chiang MC, Dutton RA, Hayashi KM, et al. 3D pattern of brain atrophy in HIV/AIDS visualised using tensor based morphometry. Neuroimage 2007;34:44–60.
33. Antori A, Arendt G, Brew JT, et al. Updated research nosology for HIV-associated neurocognitive disorders. Neurology 2007;69: 1789–99.
34. Benjamin LA, Bryer A, Emsley HC, et al. HIV infection and stroke: current perspectives and future directions. Lancet Neurol 2012; 11:878–90.
35. Islam FM, Wu J, Jansson J, et al. Relative risk of cardiovascular disease among people living with HIV: a systematic review and meta-analysis. HIV Med 2012;13:453–68.
36. Yousry TA, Major EO, Ryschkewitsch C, et al. Evaluation of patients treated with natalizumab for progressive multifocal leukoencephalopathy. N Engl J Med 2006;354:924–33.
37. Post MJD, Thurnher MM, Clifford DB, et al. CNS-immune reconstitution inflammatory syndrome in the setting of HIV infection, part 1: overview and discussion of progressive multifocal leukoencephalopathy-immune reconstitution inflammatory syndrome and cryptococcal-immune reconstitution inflammatory syndrome. Am J Neuroradiol 2013;34:1297–307.
38. Abdel Razek AA, Watcharakorn A, Castillo M. Parasitic diseases of the central nervous system. Neuroimaging Clin N Am 2011;21: 815–41.
39. Kimura-Hayama ET, Higuera JA, Corona-Cedillo R, et al. Neurocysticercosis: radiologic-pathologic correlation. Radiographics 2010;30:1705–19.
40. Nickerson JP, Tong KA, Raghavan R. Imaging cerebral malaria with a susceptibility-weighted MR sequence. Am J Neuroradiol 2009;30:e85–6.

CHAPTER 5

Inflammatory and Metabolic Disease

Alex Rovira • Pia C. Sundgren • Massimo Gallucci

CHAPTER OUTLINE

IDIOPATHIC INFLAMMATORY-DEMYELINATING DISORDERS OF THE CENTRAL NERVOUS SYSTEM

Idiopathic inflammatory-demyelinating diseases (IIDDs) represent a broad spectrum of central nervous system disorders that can be differentiated on the basis of severity, clinical course and lesion distribution, as well as imaging, laboratory and pathological findings. The spectrum includes monophasic, multiphasic and progressive disorders, ranging from highly localised forms to multifocal or diffuse variants.

Relapsing-remitting and secondary progressive multiple sclerosis (MS) are the two most common forms of IIDDs.[1] MS can also have a progressive course from onset (primary progressive and progressive relapsing MS). Fulminant forms of IIDDs include a variety of disorders that have in common the severity of the clinical symptoms, an acute clinical course and atypical findings on MR imaging. The classic fulminant IIDD is Marburg's disease. Baló's concentric sclerosis, Schilder's disease and acute disseminated encephalomyelitis can also present with acute and severe attacks.

Some IIDDs have a restricted topographical distribution, such as Devic's neuromyelitis optica, which can have a monophasic or, more frequently, a relapsing course. Other types of IIDDs occasionally present as a focal lesion that may be clinically and radiographically indistinguishable from a brain tumour. It is difficult to classify these tumefactive or pseudotumoural lesions within the spectrum of IIDDs. Some cases have a monophasic, self-limited course, while in others the tumefactive plaque is the first manifestation or appears during a typical relapsing form of MS. MR imaging of the brain and spine is the imaging technique of choice for diagnosing these disorders, and, together with the clinical and laboratory findings, can accurately classify them.[2]

Multiple Sclerosis

MS is a chronic, persistent inflammatory-demyelinating disease of the central nervous system (CNS), characterised pathologically by areas of inflammation, demyelination, axonal loss and gliosis scattered throughout the CNS. MS has a predilection for the optic nerves, brainstem, spinal cord and cerebellar and periventricular white matter.

MS is one of the most common neurological disorders and the second cause of disability in Western countries in young adults of Caucasian origin. It is relatively common in Europe, the United States, Canada, New Zealand and parts of Australia, but rare in Asia, and in the tropics and subtropics of all continents. Multiple sclerosis is twice as common in women as in men; men have a tendency for later disease onset, with a poorer prognosis. The incidence of MS is low in childhood, increases rapidly after the age of 18, reaches a peak between 25 and 35, and then slowly declines, becoming rare at 50 and older.[3]

The aetiology of MS is still unknown, but it most likely results from an interplay between as-yet unidentified environmental factors and susceptibility genes.

The clinical course of MS can follow different patterns over time, but is usually characterised by acute episodes of worsening (relapses, bouts), gradual progressive deterioration of neurological function, or a combination of both these features (relapsing MS). In a relatively small percentage of patients, the disease has a progressive course from onset, without acute relapses (primary progressive MS).

Relapsing MS accounts for 85% of all MS. This clinical form typically presents as an acute clinically isolated syndrome attributable to a monofocal or multifocal CNS demyelinating lesion. The presenting lesion usually affects the optic nerve (optic neuritis), spinal cord (acute transverse myelitis), brainstem (typically an internuclear ophthalmoparesis) and cerebellum (clumsiness and gait ataxia). Over the following years, patients usually experience episodes of acute worsening of neurological function, followed by variably complete recovery (relapsing-remitting (RR) course). Clinical and subclinical activity is frequent in this form. After several years of the RR course, more than 50% of untreated patients will develop progressive disability with or without occasional relapses, minor remissions and plateaus (secondary progressive (SP) course).[1]

As long as the aetiology of MS remains unknown, causal therapy and effective prevention are not possible. Immunomodulatory drugs such as beta-interferon, glatiramer acetate, natalizumab and fingolimod can alter the course of the disease, particularly in the RR form, by reducing the number of relapses and the accumulation of lesions as seen on MR imaging, and by influencing the impact of the disease on disability. Patients with the SP form of MS, continuing relapses of activity and pronounced progression of disability may also benefit from immunomodulatory or immunosuppressive therapy.

Primary progressive forms (PPMS) comprise approximately 10% of MS cases. This form of MS begins as a progressive disease with occasional plateaus and relapses, and temporary minor improvements. Progressive-relapsing MS follows a progressive course like PPMS, but shows clear acute relapses that may or may not be followed by full recovery.[1] Compared to patients with the more frequent relapsing forms of MS, patients with PPMS have smaller T_2 lesion loads, smaller T_2 lesions, slower rates of new lesion formation and minimal gadolinium enhancement on brain MRI, despite their accumulating disability. The presence of extensive cortical damage, diffuse white matter tissue damage and prevalent involvement of the spinal cord may partially explain this discrepancy between the MR abnormalities and the severity of the clinical disease. Because patients with PPMS may have less inflammation than those with relapsing MS, they may be less likely to respond to immunomodulatory therapies.

MR Imaging

Brain. MR imaging is the most sensitive imaging technique for detecting MS plaques throughout the brain and spinal cord. Proton density (PD) or T_2-weighted MR images show areas of high signal intensity in the periventricular white matter in 98% of MS patients. MS plaques are generally round to ovoid in shape and range from a few millimetres to more than 1 cm in diameter. They are typically discrete and focal at the early stages of the disease, but become confluent as the disease progresses, particularly in the posterior hemispheric periventricular white matter (Fig. 5-1). MS plaques tend to affect the deep white matter rather than the subcortical

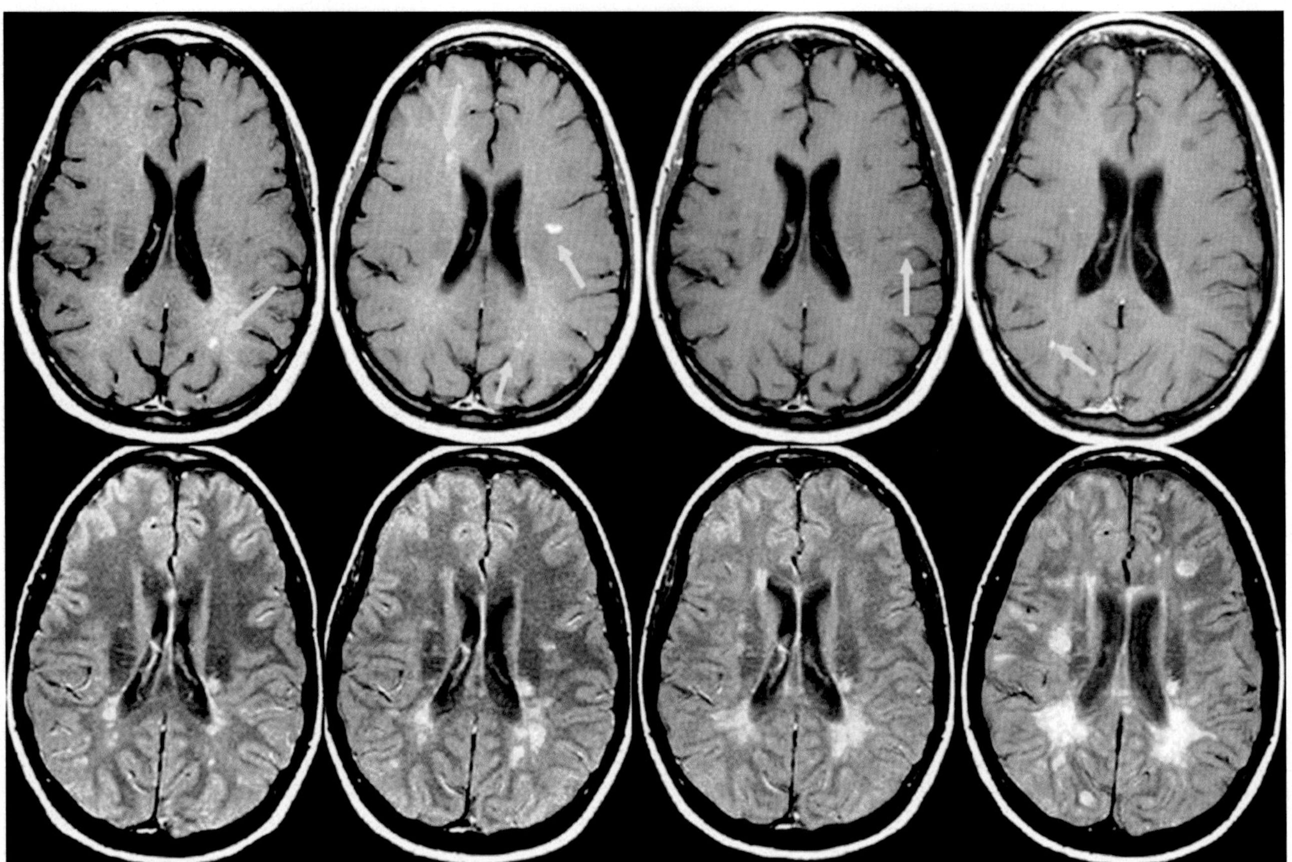

FIGURE 5-1 ■ Relapsing form of multiple sclerosis. Serial, contrast-enhanced T_1-weighted (top row) and FLAIR (bottom row) MR images of the brain obtained yearly in a patient with a typical relapsing form of MS and progressive disability. Note the new lesions that appeared during this three-year follow-up, some of them showing gadolinium enhancement (arrows).

white matter, whereas small vessel ischaemic lesions tend to involve the subcortical white matter more than the periventricular white matter.[4,5] The total T_2 lesion volume of the brain increases by approximately 5 to 10% each year in the relapsing forms of MS.[6]

Both acute and chronic MS plaques appear bright on PD- and T_2-weighted sequences, reflecting their increased tissue water content. The signal increase indicates oedema, inflammation, demyelination, reactive gliosis and/or axonal loss in proportions that differ from lesion to lesion. The vast majority of MS patients have at least one ovoid periventricular lesion, whose major axis is oriented perpendicular to the outer surface of the lateral ventricles (Fig. 5-2). The ovoid shape and perpendicular orientation derive from the perivenular location of the demyelinating plaques (Dawsons' fingers).

Multiple sclerosis lesions tend to affect specific regions of the brain, including the periventricular white matter situated superolateral to the lateral angles of the ventricles, the callososeptal interface along the inferior surface of the corpus callosum, the cortico-juxtacortical regions, and the infratentorial regions. Focal involvement of the periventricular white matter in the anterior temporal lobes is typical for MS and rarely seen in other white matter disorders (Fig. 5-3). The lesions commonly found at the callososeptal interface are best depicted by sagittal fast-FLAIR images; so this sequence is highly recommended for diagnostic MR imaging studies (Fig. 5-4).

Histopathological studies have shown that a substantial portion of the total brain lesion load in MS is located within the cerebral cortex. Presently available MR imaging techniques are not optimal for detecting cortical lesions because of poor contrast resolution between normal-appearing grey matter (NAGM) and the plaques in question, and because of the partial volume effects of the subarachnoid spaces and CSF surrounding the cortex. Cortical lesions are better visualised by 2D or 3D fast-FLAIR sequences and newer MR techniques such as 3D double inversion recovery (DIR) MR sequences which selectively suppress the signal from white matter and cerebrospinal fluid (Fig. 5-5).[7]

Juxtacortical lesions that involve the 'U' fibres are seen in two-thirds of patients with MS. They are a rather characteristic finding in early stages of the disease, and are best detected by fast-FLAIR (Fig. 5-6) sequences.

Multiple sclerosis frequently affects the brainstem and cerebellum, leading to acute clinical syndromes, such as trigeminal neuralgia, internuclear ophthalmoplegia, vertigo and ataxia. Later on, chronic damage to the

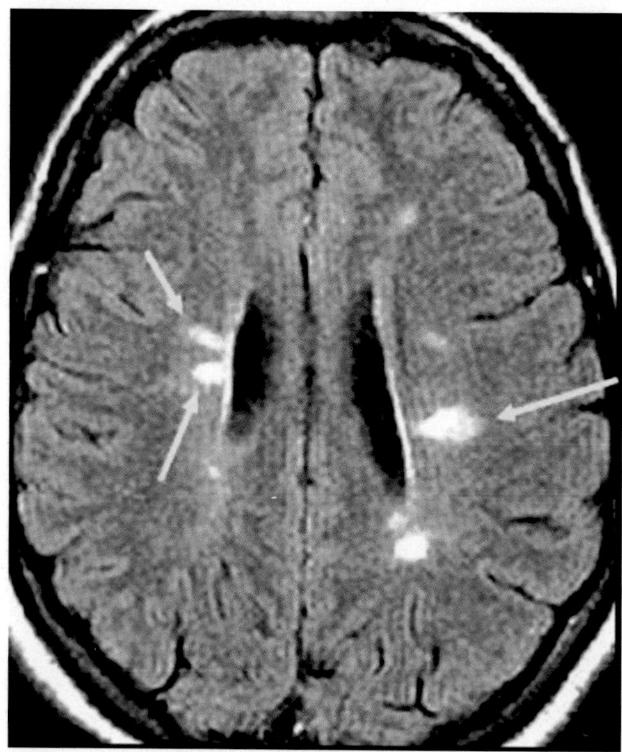

FIGURE 5-2 ■ **Relapsing-remitting MS.** Transverse fast-FLAIR MR image shows typical ovoid demyelinating plaques (arrows), whose major axis is perpendicular to the ventricular wall.

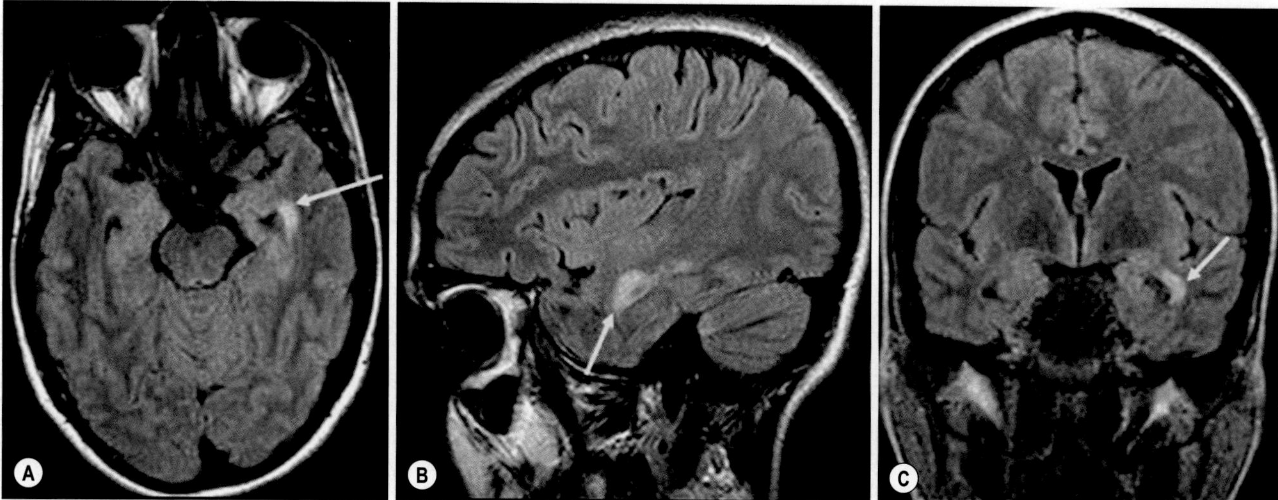

FIGURE 5-3 ■ **(A–C) Relapsing-remitting MS.** Transverse, sagittal and coronal fast-FLAIR MR images depict typical demyelinating plaques affecting the anterior temporal periventricular white matter on the left side (arrows).

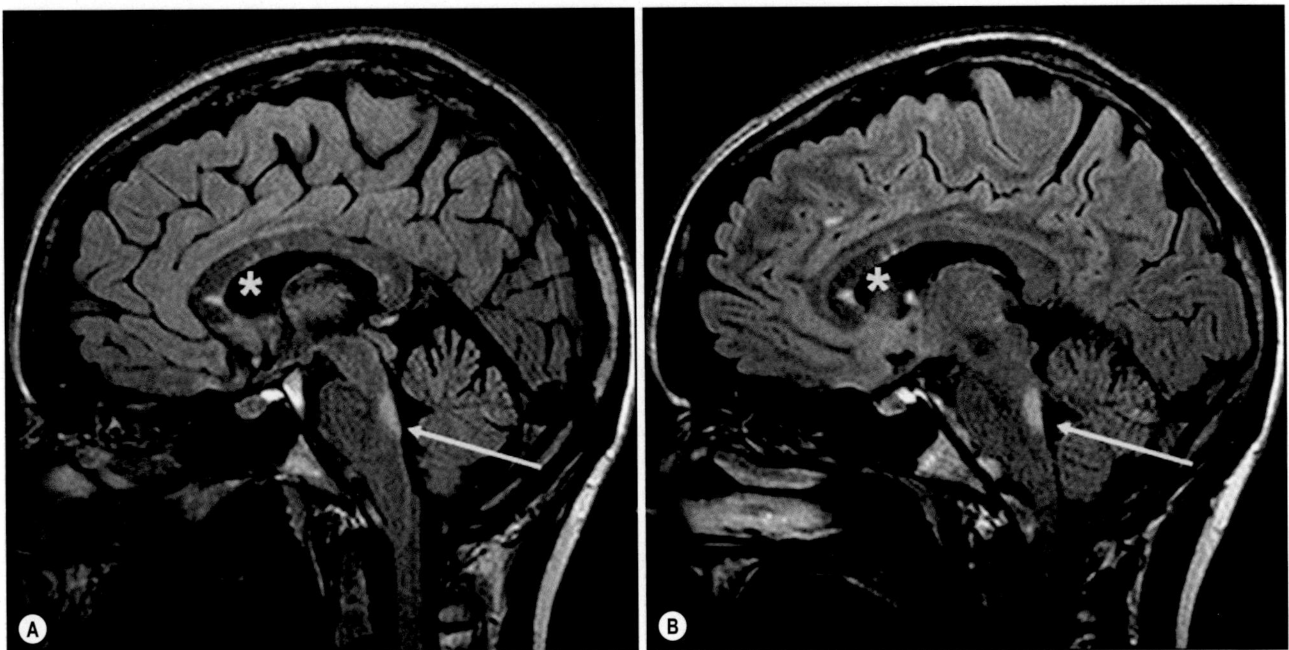

FIGURE 5-4 ■ (A, B) Clinically isolated syndrome of the brainstem (internuclear ophthalmoplegia). Sagittal fast-FLAIR MR images show the symptomatic lesion located in the floor of the IV ventricle (arrows), and subclinical lesions on the callososeptal interface (asterisks).

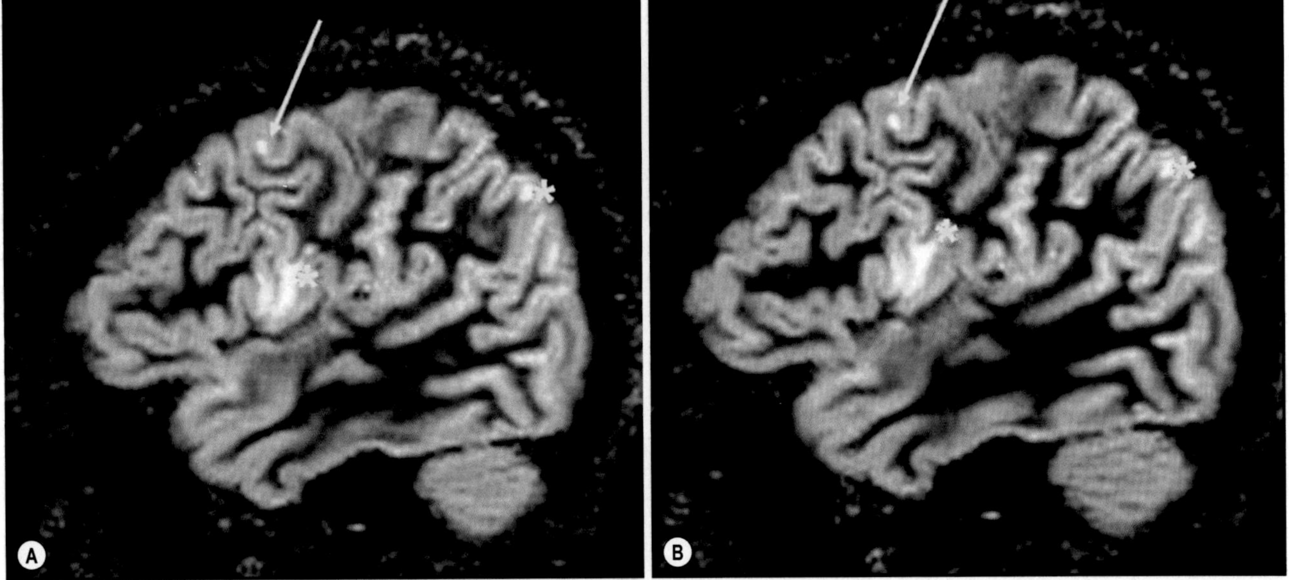

FIGURE 5-5 ■ (A, B) Relapsing-remitting MS. Sagittal double inversion recovery MR images show small hyperintense lesions involving the posterior frontal cortex (arrow) and multiple juxtacortical lesions affecting the inferior frontal and parietal lobes (asterisks).

posterior fossa causes chronic disabling symptoms such as ataxia and oculomotor disturbances. Acute symptomatic lesions appear as well-defined, hyperintense focal lesions that enhance with contrast administration on T_1-weighted images (Fig. 5-7).

Posterior fossa lesions preferentially involve the floor of the fourth ventricle, the middle cerebellar peduncles and the brainstem. Most brainstem lesions are contiguous with the cisternal or ventricular cerebrospinal fluid spaces, and range from large confluent patches to solitary, well-delineated paramedian lesions or discrete 'linings' of the cerebrospinal fluid border zones. Predilection for these areas is a key feature that helps to identify MS plaques and to differentiate them from focal areas of ischaemic demyelination and infarction that preferentially involve the central pontine white matter. Because of their short acquisition time and greater sensitivity, PD- and T_2-weighted fast spin-echo sequences are preferred over conventional spin-echo or fast-FLAIR sequences for detecting posterior fossa lesions.

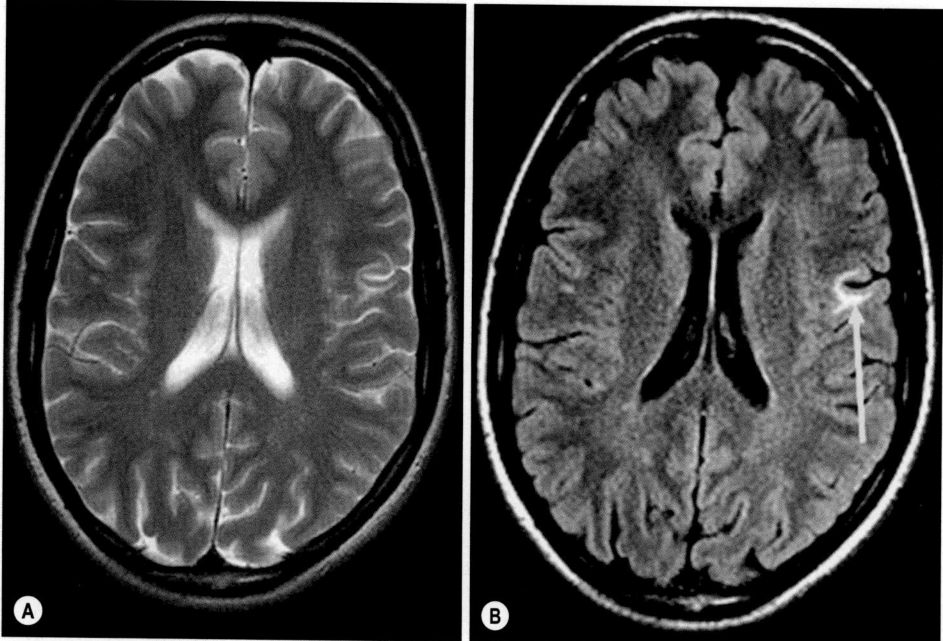

FIGURE 5-6 ■ **Relapsing-remitting MS.** Transverse fast spin-echo T_2-weighted (A) and fast-FLAIR (B) MR images. A juxtacortical lesion involving the inferior frontal lobe is better depicted on the fast-FLAIR image as compared to the fast spin-echo image (arrow).

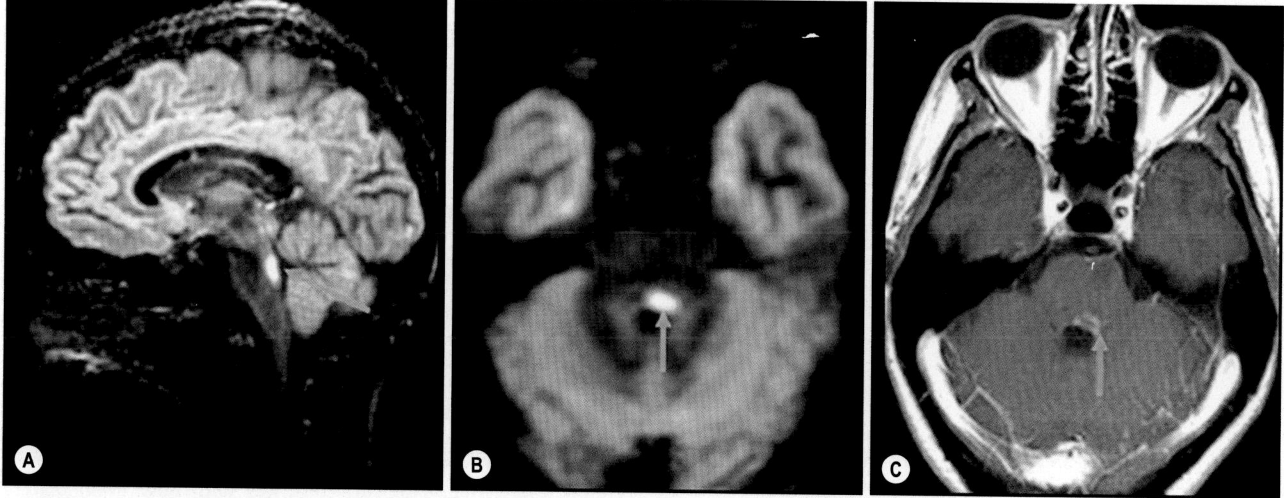

FIGURE 5-7 ■ **Clinically isolated syndrome of the brainstem (internuclear ophthalmoplegia).** Sagittal (A) and transverse (B) double inversion recovery (DIR) and contrast-enhanced T_1-weighted (C) MR images. The symptomatic lesion is clearly seen on the DIR sequence as a well-defined focal hyperintense area affecting the left medial longitudinal fasciculus and showing contrast uptake (arrows).

Approximately 10–20% of T_2 hyperintensities are also visible on T_1-weighted images as areas of low signal intensity compared with normal-appearing white matter. These so-called 'T_1 black holes' have a different pathological substrate that depends, in part, on the lesion age. The hypointensity is present in up to 80% of recently formed lesions and probably represents marked oedema, with or without myelin destruction or axonal loss. In most cases the acute (or wet) 'black holes' become isointense within a few months as inflammatory activity abates, oedema resolves and reparative mechanisms like remyelination become active. Less than 40% evolve into persisting or chronic black holes,[8] which correlate pathologically with the most severe demyelination and axonal loss, indicating areas of irreversible tissue damage. Chronic black holes are more frequent in patients with progressive disease than in those with RR disease (Fig. 5-8), and are more frequent in the supratentorial white matter as compared with the infratentorial white matter. They are rarely found in the spinal cord and optic nerves.

MS lesions of the spinal cord resemble those in the brain. The lesions can be focal (single or multiple) or diffuse, and mainly affect the cervical cord segment. On sagittal images, the lesions characteristically have a cigar shape and rarely exceed two vertebral segments in length. On cross-section they typically occupy the lateral and

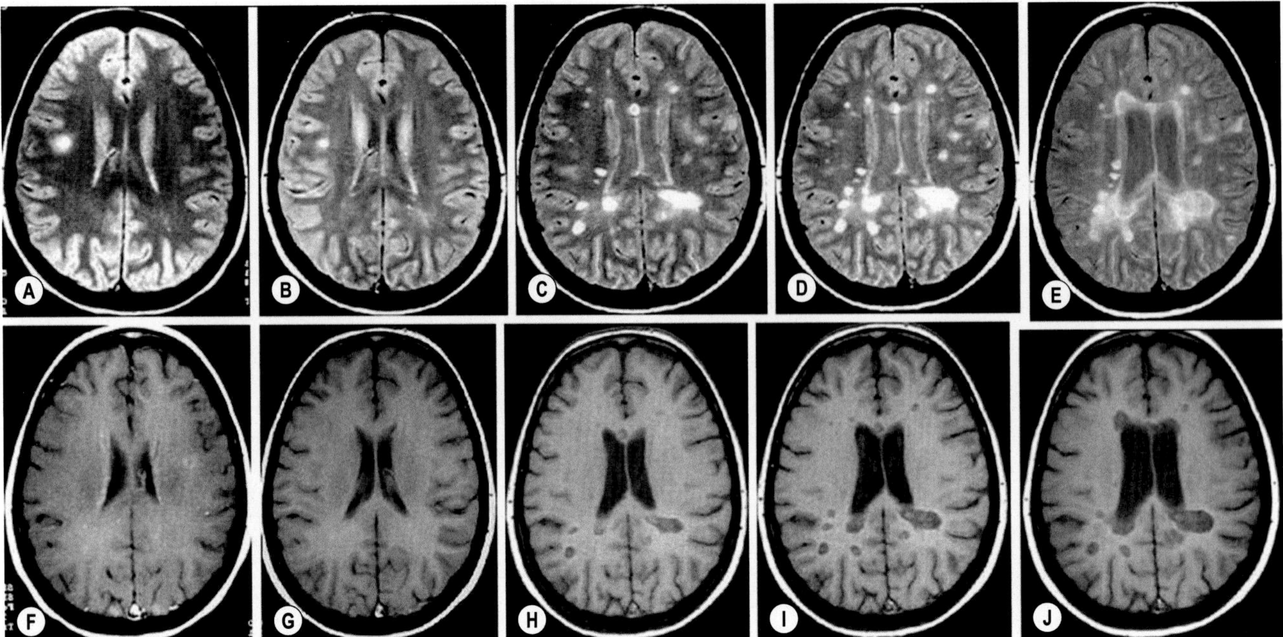

FIGURE 5-8 ■ Serial MR images obtained on a biyearly basis in a patient with a relapsing form of MS. Transverse proton-density-weighted (A–E) and T_1-weighted (F–J) MR images. In addition to the increasing number of plaques within the hemispheric white matter, observe the increase in number and size of irreversible black holes and progressive brain volume loss.

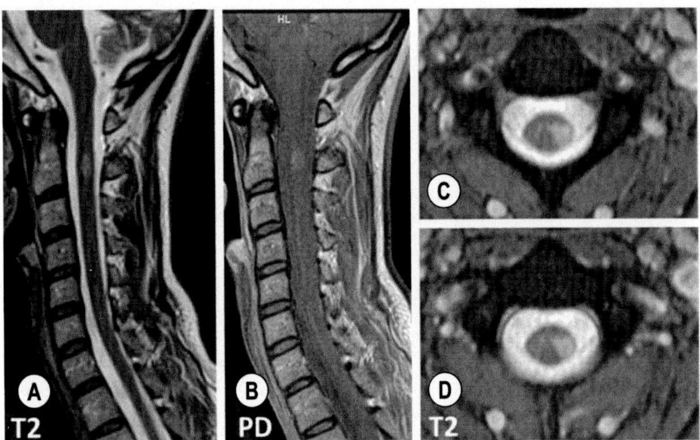

FIGURE 5-9 ■ (A–D) Relapsing-remitting MS with plaques in the cervical spinal cord. Sagittal T_2 and proton-density and transverse T_2 MR images. Observe the small focal lesion that does not exceed two vertebral segments in length and does not affect more than half the cross-sectional area of the cord.

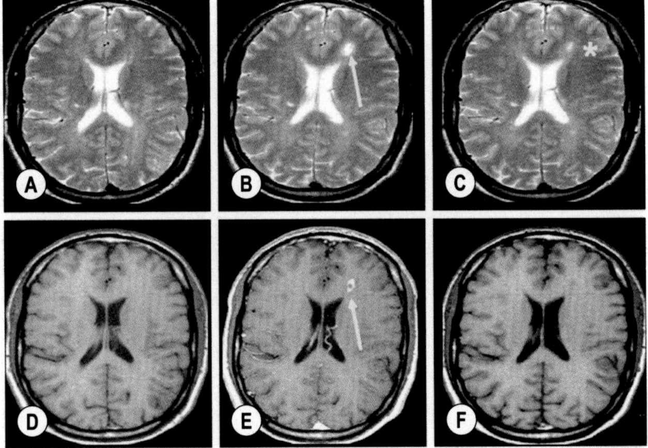

FIGURE 5-10 ■ Relapsing-remitting MS with new brain plaque formation. Transverse T_2-weighted (A–C) and contrast-enhanced T_1-weighted (D–F) brain MR images obtained serially at monthly intervals. Observe formation of a new plaque in the left frontal white matter showing transient contrast uptake (arrows). With cessation of inflammatory activity, the T_2 lesion decreased in size, but left a persistent hyperintense footprint on the T_2-weighted image (asterisk).

posterior white matter columns, extend to involve the central grey matter, and rarely occupy more than one-half the cross-sectional area of the cord[9] (Fig. 5-9).

Acute spinal cord lesions can produce a mild-to-moderate mass effect with cord swelling and may show contrast enhancement. Active lesions are rarer in the spinal cord than the brain, and are almost always associated with new clinical symptoms. The prevalence of cord abnormalities is as high as 74–92% in established MS, and depends on the clinical phenotype of MS. In clinically isolated syndromes, the prevalence of spinal cord lesions is lower, particularly if there are no spinal cord symptoms. Nevertheless, asymptomatic cord lesions are found in 30–40% of patients with a clinically isolated syndrome. In relapsing-remitting MS, the spinal cord lesions are typically multifocal. In secondary progressive MS, the abnormalities are more extensive and diffuse and are commonly associated with spinal cord atrophy. In primary progressive MS, cord abnormalities are quite extensive as compared with brain abnormalities. This discrepancy may help to diagnose primary progressive MS in patients with few or no brain abnormalities.

Longitudinal and cross-sectional MR studies have shown that the formation of new MS plaques is often associated with contrast enhancement, mainly in the acute and relapsing stages of the disease[10] (Fig. 5-10).

The gadolinium enhancement varies in size and shape, but usually lasts from a few days to weeks, although steroid treatment shortens this period. Incomplete ring enhancement on T_1-weighted gadolinium-enhanced images, with the open border facing the grey matter of the cortex or basal ganglia, is a common finding in active MS plaques and is a helpful feature for distinguishing between inflammatory-demyelinating lesions and other focal lesions such as tumours or abscesses[11] (Fig. 5-11).

Focal enhancement can be detected before abnormalities appear on unenhanced T_2-weighted images, and can reappear in chronic lesions with or without a concomitant increase in size. Although enhancing lesions also occur in clinically stable MS patients, their number is much greater when there is concomitant clinical activity. Contrast enhancement is a relatively good predictor of further enhancement and of subsequent accumulation of T_2 lesions, but shows no (or weak) correlation with progression of disability and development of brain atrophy.

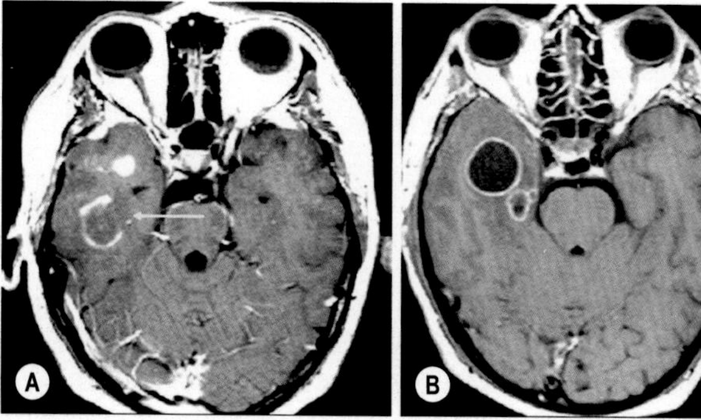

FIGURE 5-11 ■ **Ring-enhancing pattern of contrast uptake.** Contrast-enhanced T_1-weighted MR images obtained in a patient with relapsing-remitting MS (A) and a patient with glioblastoma multiforme (B). Both patients have focal lesions in the right temporal lobe. However, an incomplete ring-enhancing pattern of contrast uptake with the open margin facing the cortical grey matter of the hippocampus (arrow) is only seen in the patient with MS. In glioblastoma, the multiforme lesions show a complete ring of enhancement, despite contact with the cortical grey matter.

In relapsing-remitting and secondary progressive MS, enhancement is more frequent during relapses and correlates well with clinical activity. For patients with primary progressive MS, serial T_2-weighted studies show few new lesions and little or no enhancement with conventional doses of gadolinium, despite steady clinical deterioration.[12] Contrast-enhanced T_1-weighted images are routinely used in the study of MS to provide a measure of inflammatory activity in vivo. The technique detects disease activity 5–10 times more frequently than clinical evaluation of relapses, suggesting that most of the enhancing lesions are clinically silent. Subclinical disease activity with contrast-enhancing lesions is four to ten times less frequent in the spinal cord than the brain, a fact that may be partially explained by the large volume of brain as compared with spinal cord. High doses of gadolinium and a long post-injection delay can increase the detection of active spinal cord lesions.

Optic neuritis (ON) can usually be diagnosed clinically. MR imaging is not necessary to confirm the diagnosis, unless there are atypical clinical features (e.g. no response to steroids, long-standing symptoms). In these situations, brain and optic nerve MR imaging should be performed to rule out an alternative diagnosis, such as a compressive lesion.[13] Coronal fat-saturated T_2-weighted images are the most sensitive MR technique for depicting signal abnormalities. Focal thickening of the affected optic nerve reflects demyelination and inflammation (Fig. 5-12), which may persist for long periods despite improvements in vision and visual-evoked potential findings. Intense optic nerve enhancement seen on fat-suppressed contrast-enhanced T_1-weighted images is a consistent feature of acute ON (Fig. 5-12). The length of the enhancing optic nerve segment on axial images correlates with the severity of visual impairment, but does not predict the degree of visual recovery. In MS, signal abnormalities may also be seen in the absence of acute attacks of ON.

Atrophy of the brain and spinal cord is an important part of MS pathology, and a clinically relevant component of disease progression.[14] Although this process is more severe in the progressive forms of the disease, it

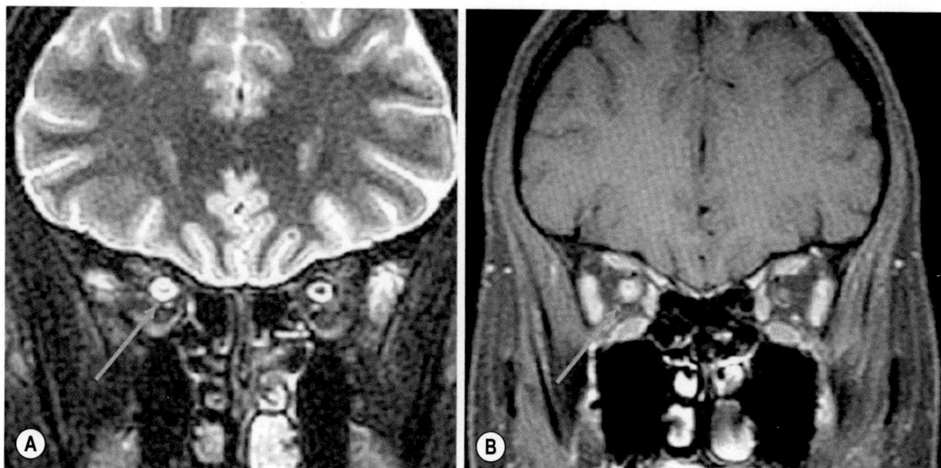

FIGURE 5-12 ■ **Right optic neuritis.** Coronal fat-suppressed T_2-weighted fast spin-echo (A) and fat-suppressed contrast-enhanced T_1-weighted MR images. There is hyperintensity of the right optic nerve, with diffuse enhancement (arrows) (B).

may also occur early in the disease process (Fig. 5-8). In fact, early atrophy seems to predict subsequent development of physical disability better than do measures of lesion load. The aetiology of CNS atrophy is multifactorial and likely reflects demyelination, Wallerian degeneration, axonal loss and glial contraction. CNS atrophy, which involves both grey and white matter, is a progressive phenomenon that worsens with increasing disease duration, and progresses at a rate of 0.6–1.2% of brain loss per year. Quantitative measures of whole-brain atrophy, acquired by automated or semi-automated methods, display this progressive loss of brain tissue bulk in vivo in a sensitive and reproducible manner. Subcortical brain atrophy is particularly well correlated to neuropsychological impairment, which can be explained by a disruption of frontal-subcortical circuits. Spinal cord atrophy is better correlated with motor disability.

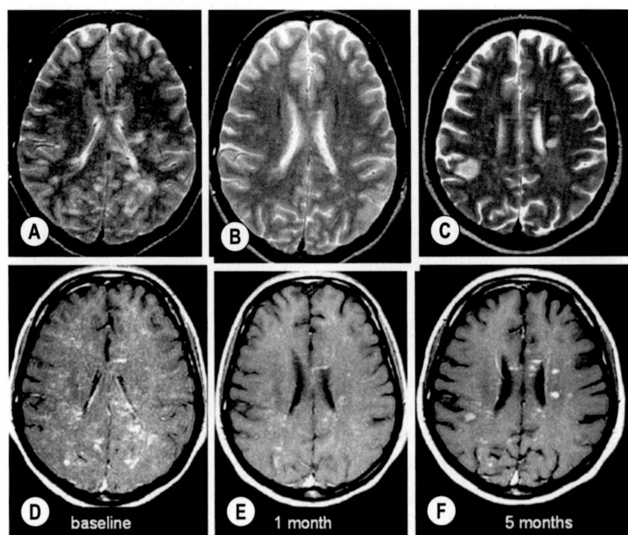

FIGURE 5-13 ■ **Marburg's disease.** Serial T_2-weighted (A–C) and contrast-enhanced T_1-weighted (D–F) MR images of the brain obtained in a patient with a final diagnosis of fulminant IIDD. Note multiple contrast-enhanced focal lesions diffusely involving the cerebral white matter. Some of the lesions are persistent, whereas others are new. The patient died 5 months after symptoms onset.

Multiple Sclerosis Variants

Marburg's Disease

Marburg's disease (MD) (also termed malignant MS) is a rare, acute MS variant that occurs predominantly in young adults. It is characterised by a confusional state, headache, vomiting, gait unsteadiness and hemiparesis. This entity has a rapidly progressive course with frequent, severe relapses leading to death or severe disability within weeks to months, mainly from brainstem involvement, or mass effect with herniation. Most of the patients who survive subsequently develop a relapsing form of MS. Because MD is often preceded by a febrile illness, this disease may also be considered a fulminant form of acute disseminated encephalomyelitis, if has a monophasic course. Pathologically, Marburg's lesions are more destructive than those of typical MS or acute disseminated encephalomyelitis and are characterised by massive macrophage infiltration, acute axonal injury and tissue necrosis. Despite the destructive nature of these lesions, areas of remyelination are often observed. In MD, MRI typically shows multiple focal T_2 lesions of varying size, which may coalesce to form large white matter plaques disseminated throughout the hemispheric white matter and brainstem (Fig. 5-13). Mild-to-moderate perilesional oedema is often present and the lesions may show peripheral enhancement.[2] A similar imaging pattern is also seen in acute disseminated encephalomyelitis.

Schilder's Disease

Schilder's disease (SD) is a rare acute or subacute disorder that can be defined as a specific clinical-radiological presentation of IIDD. It commonly affects children and young adults. The clinical spectrum of SD includes psychiatric predominance, acute intracranial hypertension, intermittent exacerbations and progressive deterioration. Imaging studies show large ring-enhancing lesions involving both hemispheres, sometimes symmetrically, and located preferentially in the parieto-occipital regions. These large, focal demyelinating lesions can resemble a brain tumour, an abscess or even adrenoleucodystrophy. MR features that suggest possible SD include large and relatively symmetrical involvement of brain hemispheres, incomplete ring enhancement, minimal mass effect, restricted diffusivity and sparing of the brainstem (Fig. 5-14).[2] Histopathologically, SD consistently shows well-demarcated demyelination and reactive gliosis with relative sparing of the axons. Microcystic changes and even frank cavitation can occur. The clinical and imaging findings usually show a dramatic response to steroids.

Baló's Concentric Sclerosis

Baló's concentric sclerosis (BCS) is thought to be a rare, aggressive variant of MS that can lead to death in weeks to months. The pathological hallmarks of the disease are large demyelinated lesions showing a peculiar pattern of alternating layers of preserved and destroyed myelin. One possible explanation for the concentric alternating bands in this variant of MS may be that sublethal tissue injury is induced at the edge of the expanding lesion, which would then stimulate the expression of neuroprotective proteins to protect the rim of periplaque tissue from damage, thereby resulting in alternative layers of preserved and non-preserved myelinated tissue.[15]

These alternating bands can be identified with T_2 MR imaging, which typically shows concentric hyperintense bands corresponding to areas of demyelination and gliosis, alternating with isointense bands corresponding to normal myelinated white matter (Figs. 5-15 and 5-16). This pattern can appear as multiple concentric layers (onion skin lesion), as a mosaic, or as a 'floral' configuration. The centre of the lesion usually shows no layering because of massive demyelination. Contrast enhancement and decreased diffusivity are frequent in the outer rings (inflammatory edge) of the lesion (Fig. 5-16). On MR imaging, this Baló pattern can be isolated, multiple or

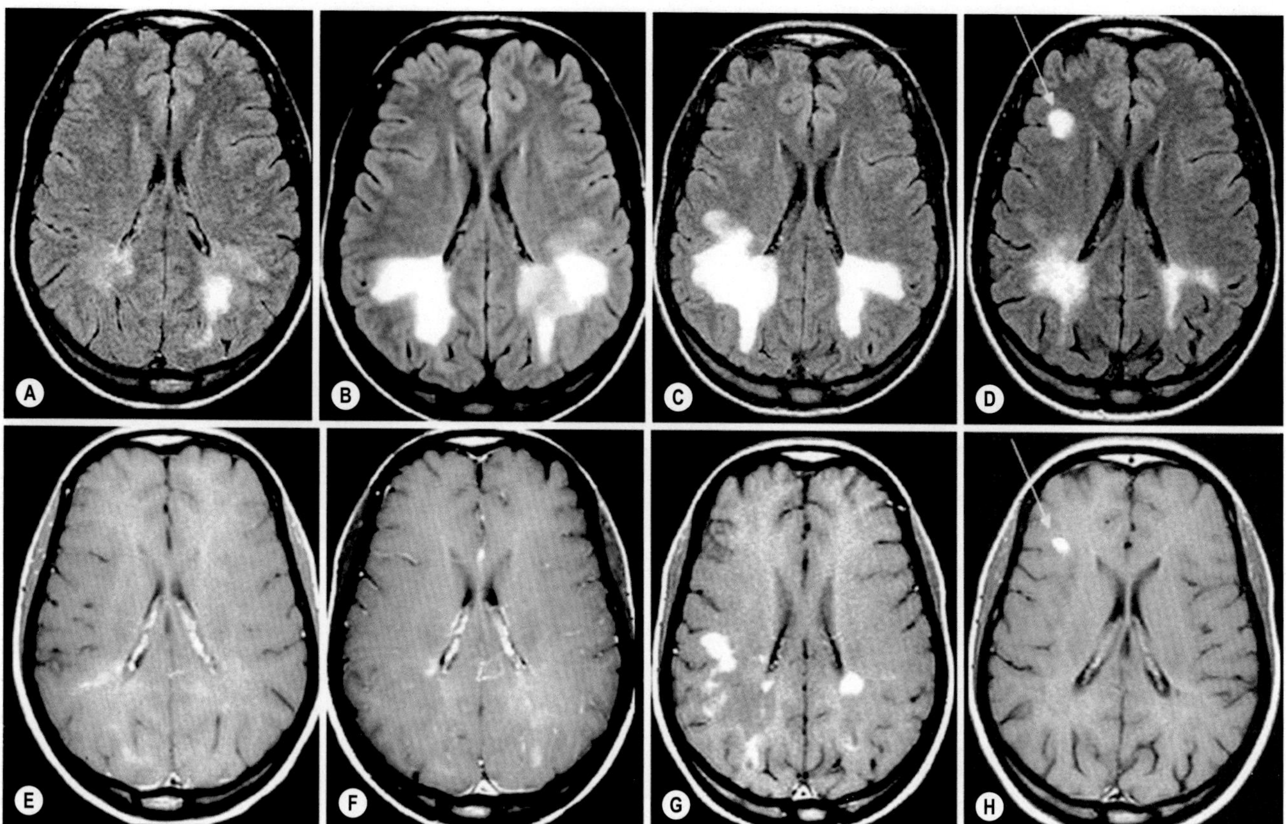

FIGURE 5-14 ■ **Schilder's disease.** Serial brain MR images in a patient with Schilder's disease who later developed clinically definite MS. Transverse fast-FLAIR images (A–D) and contrast-enhanced T_1-weighted (E–H) images obtained serially over 6 months. Note the progressive appearance of large, bilateral, almost symmetrical lesions in the posterior periventricular white matter. Despite considerable extension of the lesions, there is no mass effect. The 6-month image obtained during an episode of optic neuritis shows a new contrast-enhancing lesion in the right frontal white matter (arrows). A final diagnosis of relapsing-remitting MS was established.

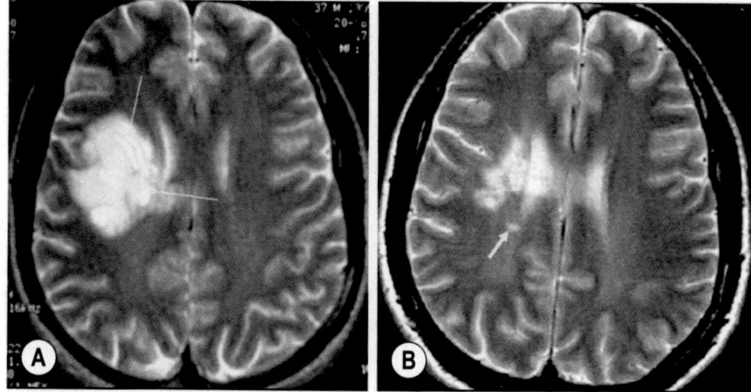

FIGURE 5-15 ■ **Baló-like lesion in a patient who converted to MS.** Transverse T_2-weighted MR image of the brain shows a large focal lesion within the right frontal white matter. The striking lamellated pattern of alternating bands of demyelination and relatively normal white matter, reflecting either spared or remyelinated regions, is clear in this image (arrows) (A). Note partial resolution of the large hemispheric lesion in a follow-up MR image obtained 4 years after symptoms onset, and the presence of a new T_2 lesion (arrow) (B).

mixed with typical MS-like lesions. Although Baló's concentric sclerosis was initially described as an acute, monophasic and rapidly fatal disease that resembled Marburg's disease, large Baló-like lesions are frequently identified on MR imaging in patients with a classical acute or chronic MS disease course, or in acute disseminated encephalomyelitis, with a non-fatal course.

Tumefactive or Pseudotumoural IIDDs

Infrequently, IIDDs present as single or multiple focal lesions that can be clinically and radiographically indistinguishable from a brain tumour. This situation represents a diagnostic challenge, and may require biopsy for definitive diagnosis, despite the clinical suspicion of demyelination. Given the hypercellular nature of these lesions, however, even the biopsy specimen may resemble a brain tumour. Large reactive astrocytes with fragmented chromatin (Creutzfeldt–Peters cells) are often present.

In some cases, pseudotumoural IIDDs are the first clinical and radiological manifestation of MS. More commonly, tumefactive demyelinating plaques affect patients with a known diagnosis of MS (Fig. 5-17). In rare cases, pseudotumoural IIDDs have a relapsing course, with single or multiple pseudotumoural lesions appearing over time in different locations. On CT or MR imaging the pseudotumoural plaques usually present as large, single or multiple focal lesions within the cerebral hemispheres. Clues that can help to differentiate these lesions from a brain tumour are the relatively minor mass effect and the presence of *incomplete* ring enhancement on

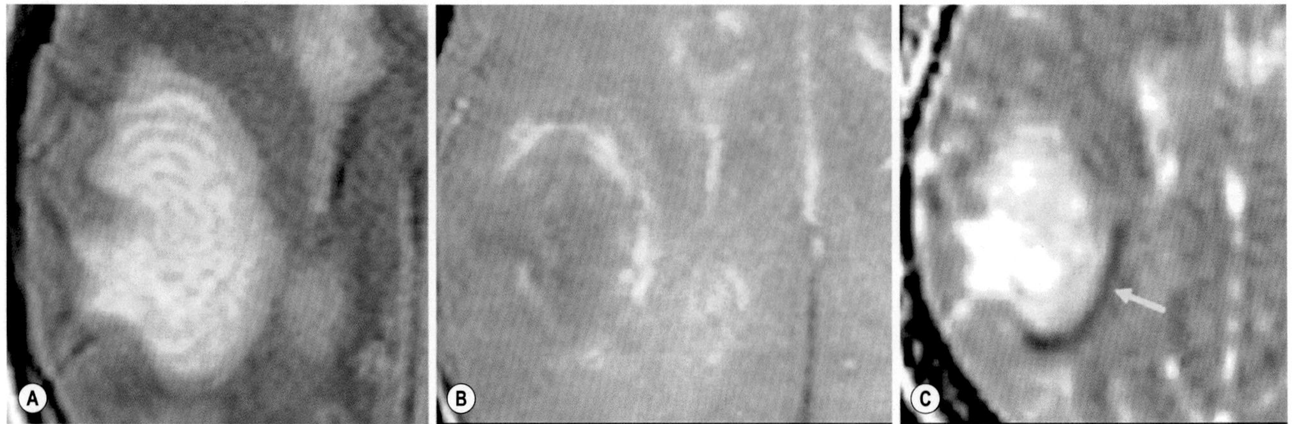

FIGURE 5-16 ■ Baló-like lesion in patients with acute disseminated encephalomyelitis. Transverse T_2-weighted (A) and contrast-enhanced T_1-weighted (B) MR images, and apparent diffusion coefficient (ADC) map. Observe the alternating concentric bands, peripheral contrast uptake and decreased peripheral diffusivity (C).

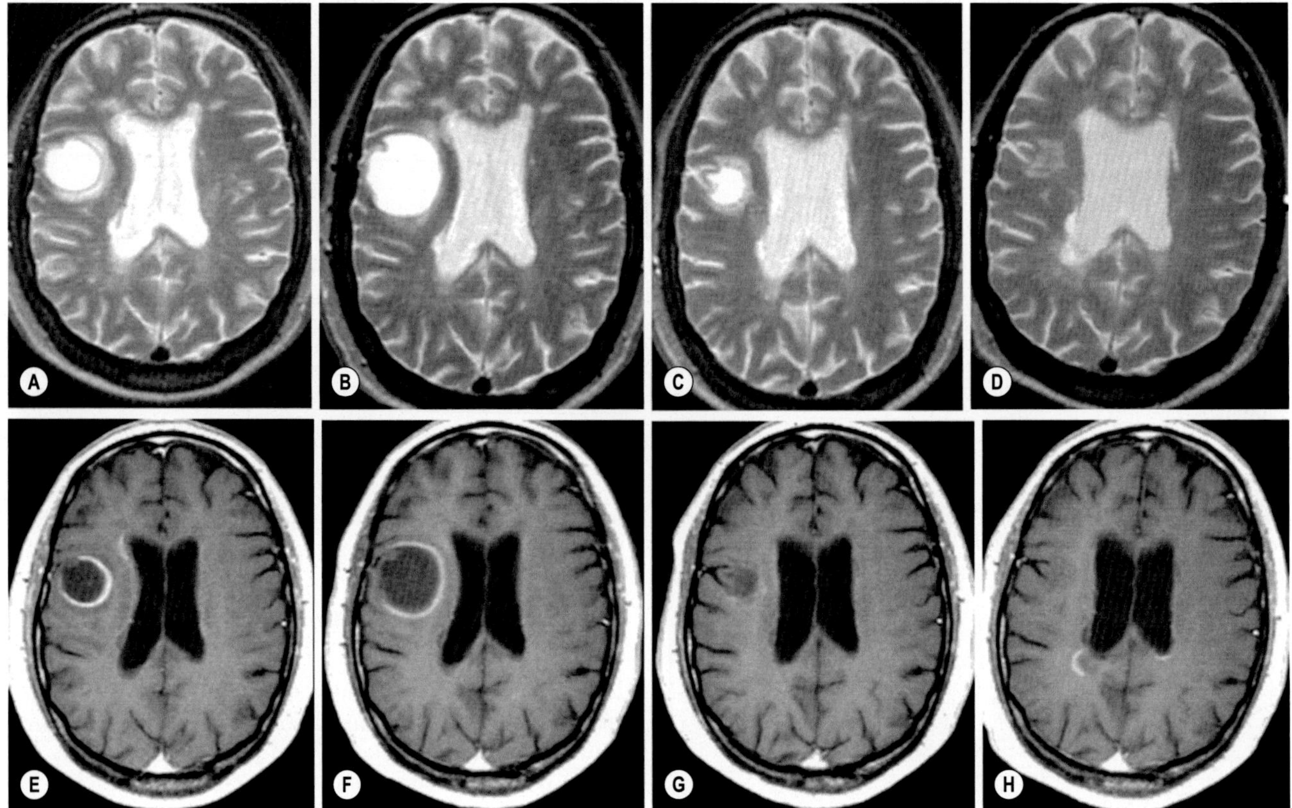

FIGURE 5-17 ■ Tumefactive form of relapsing-remitting MS. T_2-weighted (A–D) and contrast-enhanced T_1-weighted (E–H) serial MR images of the brain acquired over 12 months in a patient with the relapsing-remitting form of MS. Note the initial increase, and later decrease in size of the right frontal lobe pseudotumoural lesion, which is almost imperceptible on the 12-month imaging. The lesion shows an open ring-enhancing pattern of contrast uptake, with the open margin facing the grey matter. This pseudotumoural lesion was asymptomatic.

gadolinium-enhanced T_1-weighted images, with the open border facing the grey matter of the cortex or basal ganglia (Fig. 5-18),[16] sometimes associated with a rim of peripheral hypointensity on T_2-weighted sequences.

Devic's Neuromyelitis Optica

Devic's neuromyelitis optica (NMO) is an uncommon and topographically restricted form of IIDD that is best considered to be a distinct disease rather than a variant of MS. NMO is characterised by severe unilateral or bilateral optic neuritis and complete transverse myelitis, which occur simultaneously or sequentially within a varying period of time (weeks or years), without clinical involvement of other CNS regions. The incidence and prevalence of NMO are unknown, but the condition likely accounts for less than 1% of IIDDs in Caucasians. NMO affects females almost exclusively.

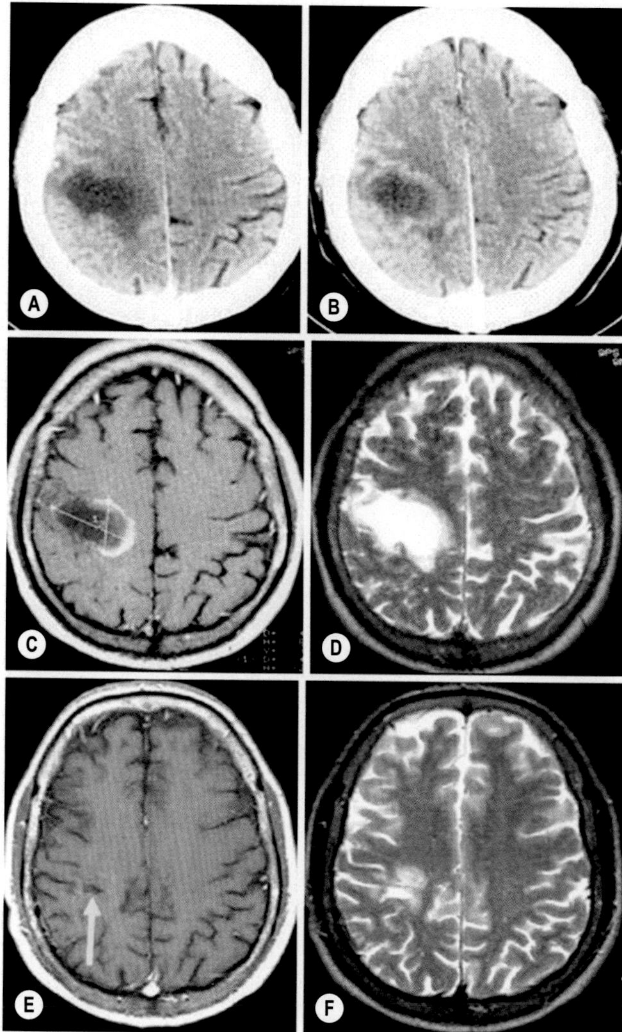

FIGURE 5-18 ■ **Tumefactive inflammatory demyelinating lesion.** Unenhanced and contrast-enhanced brain CT (A, B) and T_2-weighted and contrast-enhanced T_1-weighted MR images (C, D) show a posterior frontal lesion with minimal surrounding vasogenic oedema and no mass effect. Observe the ring-enhancing pattern of contrast uptake, with the open margin facing the cortical grey matter. A follow-up brain MR imaging performed one year later (E, F) shows almost complete resolution of the lesion. The necrotic focus (arrow) in the subcortical white matter corresponds to the site of a brain biopsy, which confirmed the diagnosis of inflammatory demyelinating lesion.

Approximately 85% of patients have a relapsing course with severe acute exacerbations and poor recovery, accumulating increasing neurological impairment and a high risk of respiratory failure and death due to cervical myelitis.[17]

Clinical features alone are insufficient to diagnose NMO; CSF analysis and MR imaging are usually required to confidently exclude other disorders. Cerebrospinal fluid pleocytosis (>50 leucocytes/mm^3) is often present, while CSF oligoclonal bands are seen less frequently (20–40%) than in MS patients (80–90%).

A serum autoantibody marker for NMO (NMO-IgG) has been recently developed. The target antigen of NMO-IgG is aquaporin-4, a water channel located on

TABLE 5-1 Revised Diagnostic Criteria for Devic's Neuromyelitis Optica (NMO)[18]

Definite NMO:

- Optic neuritis
- Acute myelitis
- At least two of three supportive criteria:
  - Contiguous MRI spinal cord lesion extending over ≥3 vertebral segments
  - Brain MRI findings do not meet diagnostic criteria for multiple sclerosis
  - NMO-IgG seropositive status

the foot process of the astrocyte. It is associated with tight endothelial junctions and cerebral microvessels and plays a critical role in maintaining fluid homeostasis in the CNS. This autoantibody is reported to have a sensitivity of 73% and a specificity of 91% for NMO. It may be helpful for distinguishing this form of IIDD from MS and may predict relapse and conversion to NMO in patients presenting with a single attack of longitudinally extensive myelitis. Wingerchuk et al. have proposed a revised set of criteria for diagnosing NMO (Table 5-1).[18] These new criteria remove the absolute restriction on CNS involvement beyond the optic nerves and spinal cord, allow any interval between the first events of optic neuritis and myelitis, and emphasise the specificity of longitudinally extensive spinal cord lesions on MR imaging and NMO-IgG seropositive status.

Devic's neuromyelitis optica is a B-cell-mediated disorder that can coexist with diverse systemic autoimmune diseases, such as systemic lupus erythematosus, Sjögren's syndrome and autoimmune thyroiditis. The presence of prodromal factors such as fever, infections and autoimmune abnormalities suggest that previous infectious-inflammatory events may be involved in the pathogenesis of the disease.[19]

MR imaging of the spinal cord shows extensive cervical or thoracic tumefactive myelitis, involving more than three vertebral segments on sagittal and much of the cross-section on axial T_2-weighted images, which sometimes enhance with gadolinium for several months (Fig. 5-19). In some cases, the spinal cord lesions are small at the onset of symptoms, mimicking those in MS, and then progress in extent over time. These lesions are usually located centrally, can progress to atrophy and necrosis, and may lead to syrinx-like cavities on T_1-weighted images (Fig. 5-20). MR imaging of the brain can demonstrate unilateral or bilateral optic nerve enhancement during acute optic neuritis. In contrast to MS, white matter lesions are absent or few in the early stages, and are non-specific. Over the next years serial studies may reveal an increasing number of cerebral white matter lesions but < 10% ever meet MR imaging criteria for MS. Paediatric cases sometimes show diencephalic (hypothalamic), brainstem, or cerebral hemispheric lesions, which should be considered atypical for MS[20] (Fig. 5-21). Hypothalamic lesions seem to be relatively specific for NMO, and may be associated with clinical and laboratory evidence of hypothalamic endocrinopathy.

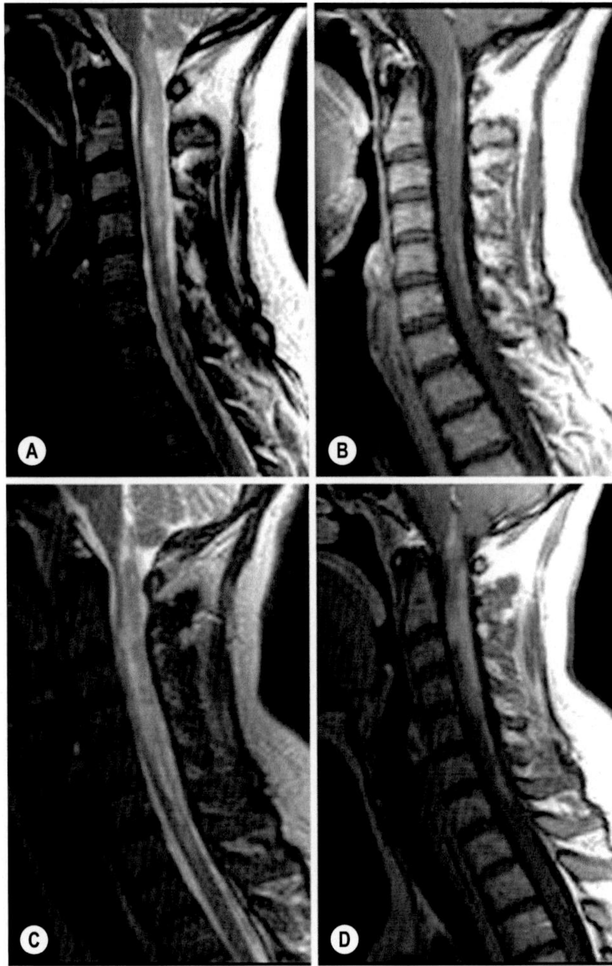

FIGURE 5-19 ■ Devic's neuromyelitis optica (NMO). Sagittal fast spin-echo T_2-weighted and contrast-enhanced T_1-weighted MR images of the cervical spinal cord obtained serially over a period of 4 months. Baseline examination (A, B) shows a large spinal cord lesion extending to the brainstem. Follow-up MR image acquired 4 months later (C, D) shows lesion extension to the thoracic cord and persistent and more extensive contrast uptake.

Acute Disseminated Encephalomyelitis

Acute disseminated encephalomyelitis (ADEM) is a severe, immune-mediated inflammatory disorder of the CNS that is usually triggered by an inflammatory response to viral or bacterial infections and vaccinations.[21] It predominantly affects the white matter of the brain and spinal cord. In the absence of specific biological markers, the diagnosis of ADEM is based on the clinical and radiological features (Table 5-2). Although ADEM usually has a monophasic course, recurrent or multiphasic forms

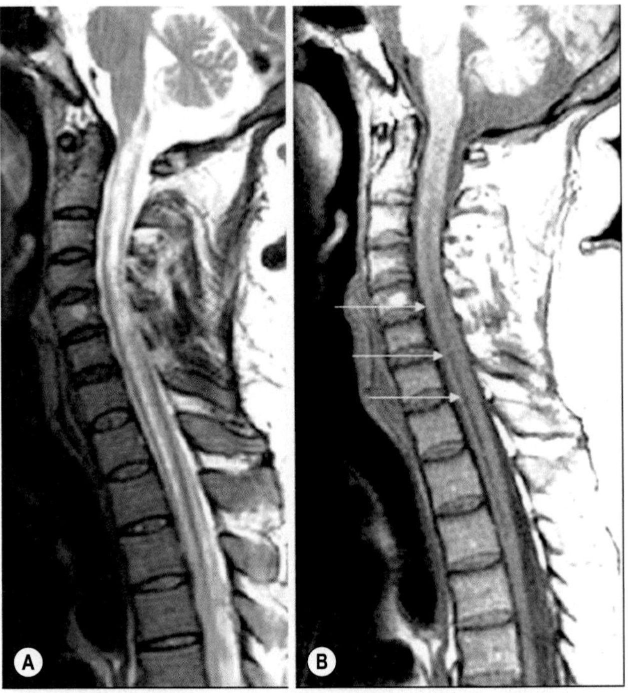

FIGURE 5-20 ■ (A, B) Devic's neuromyelitis optica (NMO). Sagittal T_2-weighted and T_1-weighted MR images of the cervicodorsal spinal cord showing a long syrinx-like spinal cord lesion extending to the lower medulla (arrows).

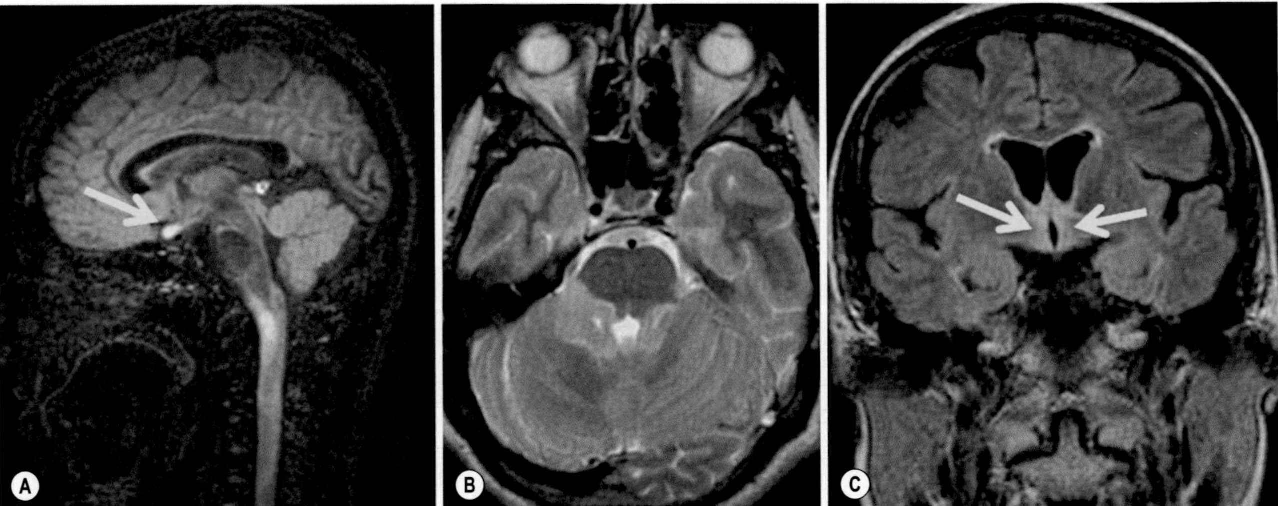

FIGURE 5-21 ■ Devic's neuromyelitis optica (NMO). Brain MRI showing hyperintense T_2 lesions (arrows) involving the optic chiasm and proximal segment of the cervical cord (A), the brainstem (B) and hypothalamic region (C).

TABLE 5-2 **Clinical, Biological and Radiological Differences between Acute Disseminated Encephalomyelitis (ADEM) and Multiple Sclerosis (MS)**

	ADEM	MS
Age	≤10 years	>10 years
Gender	Male = female	Male < female
Prior flu	Very frequent	Variable
Encephalopathy	Required	Rare
Attacks	Fluctuate over 3 months	Separated by >1 month
Large MRI lesions	Frequent	Rare
Lesion margins	Poorly defined	Well defined
Deep grey matter	Frequently involved	Rarely involved
Spinal cord lesions	Extensive	Small
Longitudinal MRI	Resolution	New lesions
CSF white blood cell count >50	Frequent	Very rare
CSF oligoclonal bands	Variable	Frequent

have been reported, raising diagnostic difficulties in distinguishing these cases from MS.

Acute disseminated encephalomyelitis affects children more commonly than adults, and in contrast to MS, shows no sex preponderance. The estimated incidence is 0.8 per 100,000 population per year. In 50–75% of cases, the clinical onset of disease is preceded by viral or bacterial infections, usually non-specific upper respiratory tract infections. ADEM may also develop following a vaccination (postimmunisation encephalomyelitis). Although ADEM is relatively rare, it is becoming increasingly important, since vaccination schedules have expanded over the past years, particularly for children. Typically, there is a latency of 7 to 14 days between a febrile illness and the onset of neurological symptoms. In the case of vaccination-associated ADEM, this latency period may be longer.

Patients commonly present with non-specific polyfocal symptoms, which developed subacutely over a period of days, frequently associated with encephalopathy that is relatively uncommon in MS and defined as an alteration in consciousness (e.g. stupor, lethargy) or behavioral change unexplained by fever, systemic illness or postictal symptoms. In general, the disease is self-limiting and the prognostic outcome favourable. Neurological symptoms usually developed subacutely over a period of days and lead to hospitalisation within a week. Although ataxia, altered level of consciousness and brainstem symptoms are frequently present in both paediatric and adult cases, certain signs and symptoms appear to be age-related. In childhood ADEM, long-lasting fever and headaches occur more frequently, while in adult cases, motor and sensory deficits predominate. According to the International Most of ADEM have a monophasic course, although a small proportion (<4%) of patients have a multiphasic course defined as a new encephalopathic event consistent with ADEM, separated by three months after the initial illness but not followed by any further events. The second ADEM event can involve either new or a re-emergence of prior neurologic symptoms, signs and MRI findings. Relapsing disease following ADEM that occurs beyond a second encephalopathic event is no longer consistent with multiphasic ADEM but rather indicates a chronic disorder, most often leading to the diagnosis of MS or NMO (22). Not infrequently, an ADEM attack is the first manifestation of the classical relapsing form of MS. In fact, 30% of patients who meet the ADEM criteria at initial presentation ultimately receive a diagnosis of MS. Hence, ADEM is likely to be overdiagnosed on the basis of the initial clinical presentation and MR findings. For this reason, presumptive diagnoses of ADEM mandates close clinical and MR imaging follow-up.

Unlike lesions in MS, the lesions of ADEM are often large, patchy and poorly marginated on MR imaging. There is usually asymmetrical involvement of the subcortical and central white matter and cortical grey–white junction of cerebral hemispheres, the cerebellum, brainstem and spinal cord (Fig. 5-22). The grey matter of the thalami and basal ganglia is frequently affected, particularly in children, typically in a symmetrical pattern.[23] Lesions confined to the periventricular white matter and corpus callosum are less common than in MS. Contrast enhancement is not a common feature in ADEM. The spinal cord is involved in less than 30% of ADEM patients,[23] predominantly in the thoracic region (Fig. 5-22). The cord lesion is typically large, causes swelling of the cord and shows variable enhancement. Most ADEM patients show partial or complete of the MR imaging abnormalities within a few months after treatment. This evolution is positively associated with a final diagnosis of ADEM. Because ADEM is usually a monophasic disease, the focal lesions would be expected to appear and mature simultaneously and to resolve or remain unchanged, with no new lesions on follow-up MR images. Not infrequently, however, new lesions are seen on follow-up MRI within the first month after the initial attack. Most MR lesions appear early in the course of the disease, supporting the clinical diagnosis, In some cases there may be a delay of more than 1 month between the onset of symptoms and the appearance of lesions on MR imaging. Therefore, a normal brain MR imaging obtained within the first days after the onset of neurological symptoms suggestive of ADEM does not exclude this diagnosis.

Acute Disseminated Encephalomyelitis Variants

Bickerstaff's Encephalitis. Bickerstaff's encephalitis is a rare acute syndrome considered to be a subgroup of ADEM, in which inflammation appears to be confined to the brainstem.[24] The syndrome consists of localised encephalitis of the brainstem, commonly preceded by a febrile illness, and has a benign prognosis. T_2-weighted MR imaging usually shows an extensive high-signal-intensity lesion involving the midbrain, the pons and sometimes the thalamus. The clinical outcome is good and parallels resolution of the MR imaging lesions (Fig. 5-23). The pathogenesis of Bickerstaff's encephalitis is uncertain; however, the absence of CSF oligoclonal bands

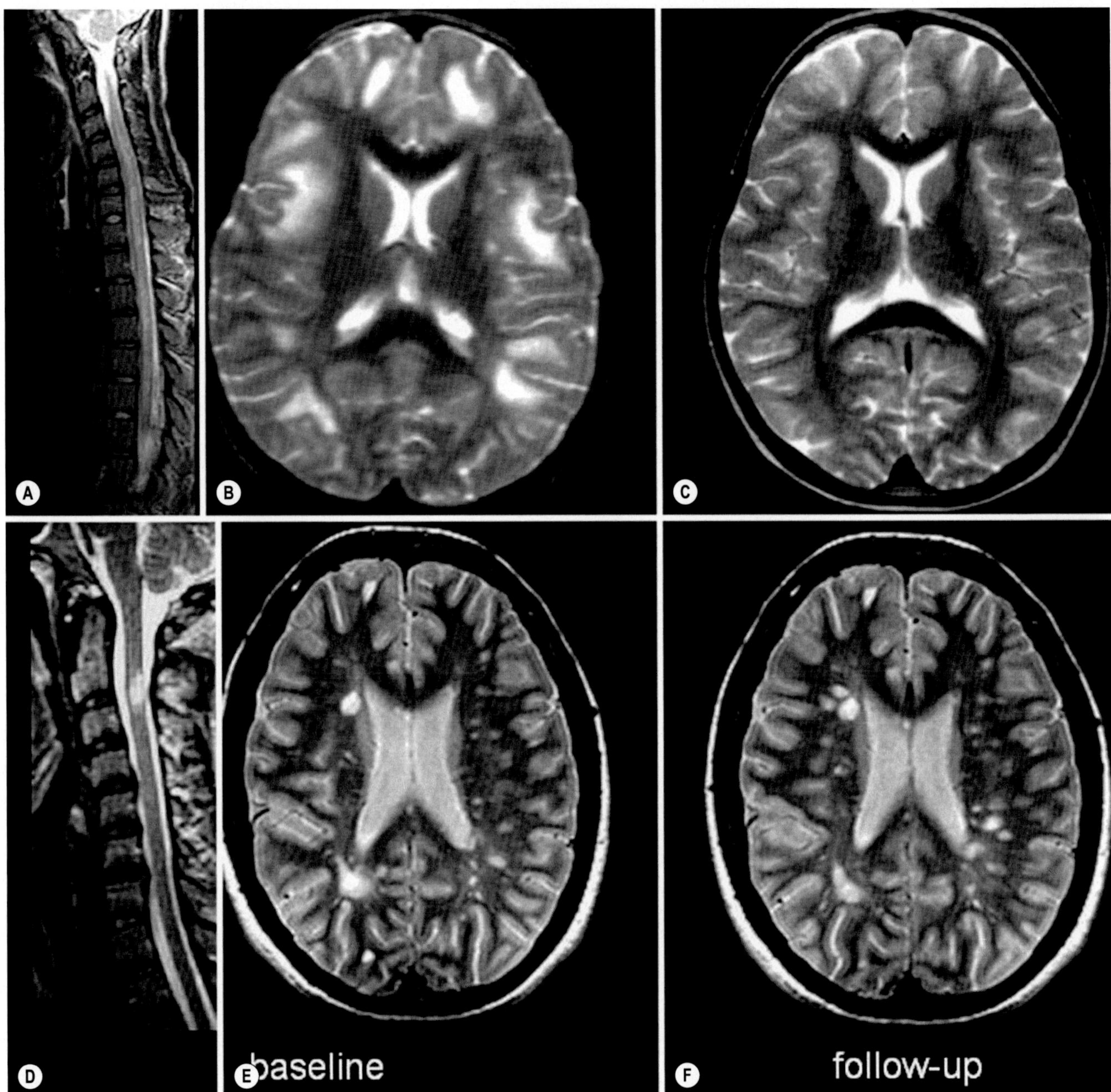

FIGURE 5-22 ■ MR imaging differences between acute disseminated encephalomyelitis (ADEM) (A–C) and multiple sclerosis (MS) (D–F). Spinal cord lesions are extensive in ADEM and are usually associated with large, poorly defined subcortical white matter lesions on brain MR imaging. In MS, symptomatic cord lesions are usually small and commonly associated with subclinical white matter brain lesions of the type seen in MS. In ADEM, longitudinal studies usually show resolution of lesions, while in MS, new lesions appear (arrows).

and resolution of the clinical symptoms and MR imaging lesions suggest an inflammatory origin and make demyelination unlikely.

Acute Disseminated Necrohaemorrhagic Leucoencephalitis. Acute disseminated necrohaemorrhagic leucoencephalitis (acute haemorrhagic encephalomyelitis or Hurst's disease) is an uncommon condition that has been observed in patients of all ages. It is thought to be a hyperacute form or the maximal variant of ADEM. This usually fatal disease manifests clinically with abrupt onset of fever, neck stiffness, hemiplegia or other focal signs, seizures and decreasing level of consciousness.[21] At autopsy, the brain is congested and swollen, sometimes asymmetrically, and herniation is frequent. Multiple petechial haemorrhages are distributed diffusely throughout the brain. The perivascular lesions chiefly consist of ball-like or ring haemorrhages surrounding necrotic venules, sometimes with fibrinous exudates within the vessel wall or extending into adjacent tissue. Perivenous demyelinating lesions, identical to those occurring in ADEM, may also be present. Perivascular cuffs of mononuclear cells, often with neutrophils, are seen. T_2*-weighted MR sequences show large regions

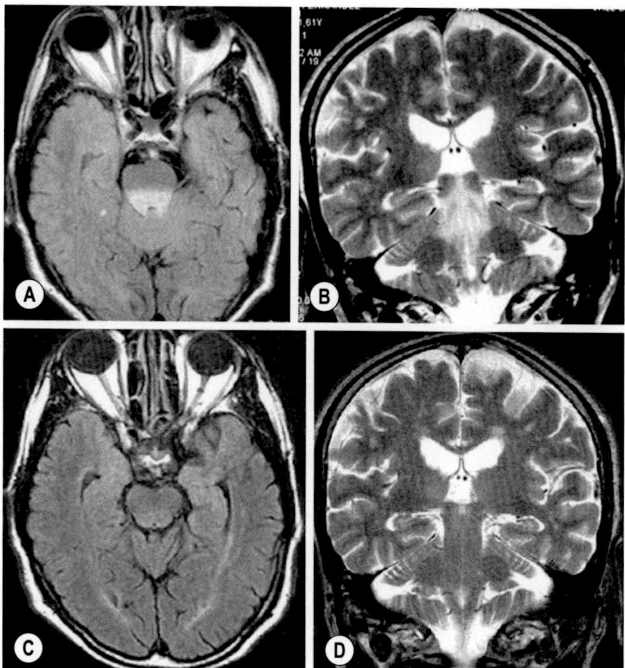

FIGURE 5-23 ■ **Bickerstaff's encephalitis.** Initial brain MR imaging (transverse fast-FLAIR and coronal fast spin-echo T_2-weighted sequences) shows an extensive brainstem lesion (A, B) that fully resolved in a follow-up study obtained 2 months later (C, D).

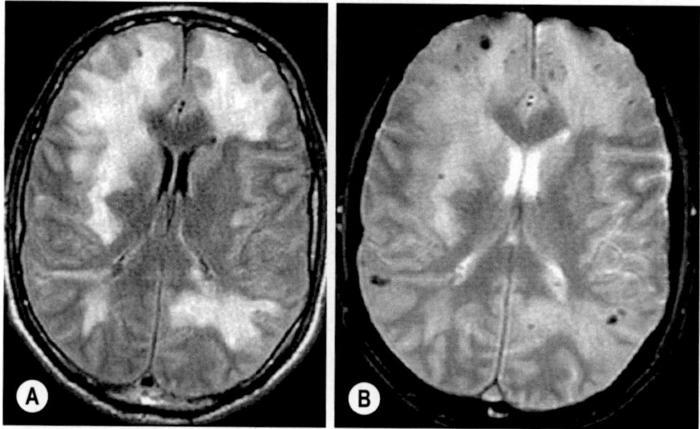

FIGURE 5-24 ■ **Acute haemorrhagic leucoencephalitis (Hurst's encephalitis).** Axial FLAIR MR image shows an extensive abnormal signal affecting the periventricular and subcortical white matter (A), with acute haemorrhagic foci visualised as markedly hypointense areas within the white matter lesions on the T_2*-weighted gradient-echo MR image (B).

of demyelination and petechial haemorrhages in the peripheral white matter of both cerebral hemispheres (Fig. 5-24).

PRIMARY AND SECONDARY VASCULITIS

Central Nervous System Vasculitis

There are many different causes of central nervous system (CNS) vasculitis and the diagnosis should always be suspected in patients who present with severe headache, focal or multifocal neurological dysfunction, altered cognition or consciousness, and non-specific MR or CT imaging findings. More often the angiographic picture is more convincing but the definitive diagnosis can only be made after confirmation by CNS biopsy. Since the distribution of the CNS vasculitis can be segmented and focal, a positive biopsy is enough to confirm the diagnosis, while one single negative biopsy does not exclude it.[25] Vasculitis has been reported to be responsible for 3–5% of strokes occurring in patients younger than 50 years of age. The CNS vasculitis can be divided into primary and secondary. There are no exact numbers of the incidence rate of either the primary or secondary vasculitides of the CNS. However, primary CNS vasculitis is relatively uncommon but has a generally poor prognosis.

Primary Central Nervous System Vasculitis

Primary angiitis of the CNS (PACNS) is a rare and severe idiopathic disorder limited to the central nervous system that results in multifocal inflammation of predominantly small arteries, but can also involve medium-sized leptomeningeal, cortical and subcortical arteries, and veins of the cortex and leptomeninges.

Its hallmark is a striking inflammatory alteration of the affected vessel wall. The mean age of onset is 50 years, and men are affected twice as commonly as women. The most frequent initial symptoms of PACNS are headaches and encephalopathy. Strokes or persistent neurological deficits occur in 40% of patients with PACNS, and transient ischaemic attacks have been reported in 30–50% of patients but occur in less than 20% of patients at the onset of disease.[26] Less commonly, seizures may also occur as the presenting symptom. MRI of the brain is abnormal in more than 90% of patients, but the patterns are not specific and are seen predominantly in the subcortical white matter, followed by the deep grey and white matter, and the cerebral cortex (Fig. 5-25). Other less common findings are infarcts, mass lesions, and confluent white matter lesions, which can be mistaken for multiple sclerosis, or cortical laminar necrosis. However, intracranial haemorrhages are infrequent.[27] Parenchymal and leptomeningeal enhancement can be seen in up to 35% of patients. The cerebrospinal fluid (CSF) analysis is abnormal in 80–90% of the patients with modest, non-specific elevations in total protein level or white blood cell count. Angiography has a low sensitivity and low specificity. Common findings are those seeing in other forms of vasculitis, including single or multiple areas of segmental narrowing and dilatations along the course of a vessel, and vascular occlusions (Fig. 5-26).

The most frequent mimic of PACNS is a group of disorders known collectively as the reversible cerebral vasoconstriction syndromes (RCVS). Features that are more suggestive of RVCS are acute thunderclap headache, with normal CSF analysis. The final diagnosis of PACNS is established by brain biopsy. The typical biopsy specimen reveals segmental inflammation of small arteries and arterioles, intimal proliferation and fibrosis, with sparing of the media, and in some cases multinucleate

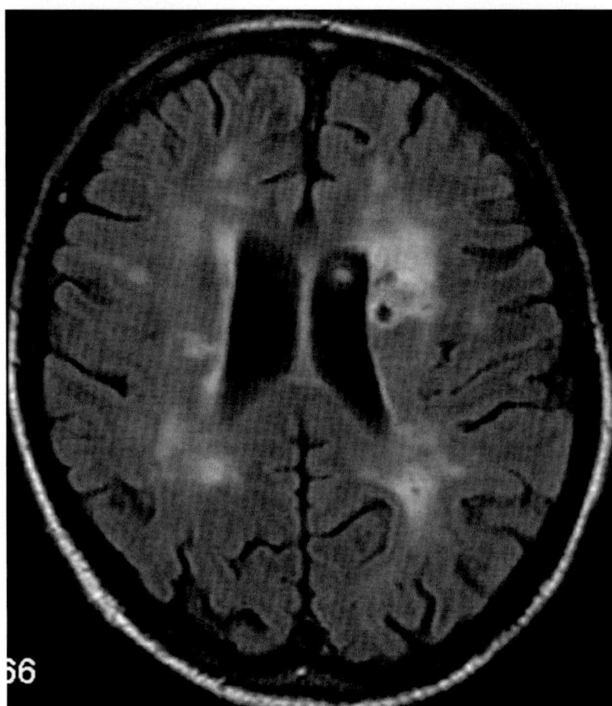

FIGURE 5-25 ■ Axial fluid-attenuated inversion recovery (FLAIR) image demonstrating diffuse increased signal in the periventricular, deep and subcortical white matter in a patient diagnosed with primary angiitis of the CNS (PACNS).

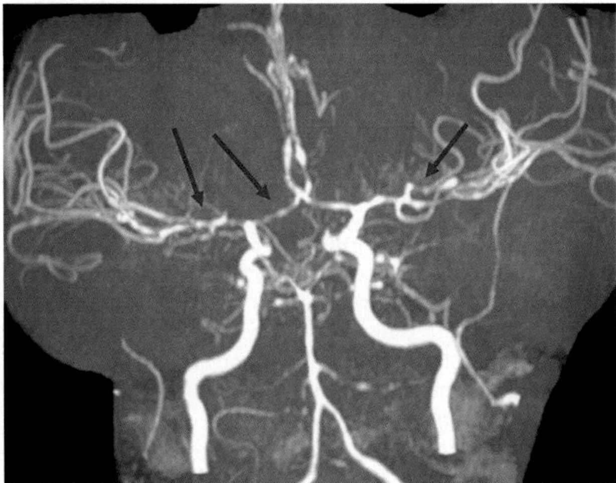

FIGURE 5-26 ■ MR angiography (MRA) of the intracranial vessels demonstrates narrowing and irregularities of the right middle cerebral artery and of other medium-sized intracranial vessels.

giant Langerhans cells.[28] Since PACNS is fatal if untreated, patients with biopsy-proven PACNS are treated with cyclophosphamide and prednisone.

Secondary Central Nervous System Vasculitis

Secondary CNS vasculitis of the nervous system caused by an underlying disease is more commonly seen than the primary vasculitides and may involve either the CNS or the peripheral nervous system (PNS) or both. They can be further classified into a systemic disorder or infection with or without evidence of systemic vasculitis. One of those related to infection is the one caused by the varicella-zoster virus that might present fever, headache, seizures or stroke-like symptoms due to with encephalitis secondary to vasculitis in large or small vessels. MRI might demonstrate multiple areas of ischaemic and haemorrhagic infarcts of varying size, involving both the grey and white matter. Human immunodeficiency virus and herpes virus infections are other less common viral causes of secondary CNS vasculitis. Uncommonly, CNS vasculitis has been reported in association with some malignant conditions and drug abuse, including amphetamines and related sympathomimetic agents, cocaine and opioids.

Primary Systemic Vasculitis with Central Nervous System Involvement

CNS vasculitis can occur as a systemic manifestation of other primary small, medium or large vessel vasculitits such as giant cell arteritis, Takayasu's arteritis, Kawasaki's disease, Wegener's granulomatosis, polyarteritis nodosa, and Churg–Strauss syndrome.

Giant Cell Arteritis. The most common form of primary systemic vasculitis is giant cell arteritis (temporal arteritis) defined as a granulomatous arteritis of the aorta and its major branches often involving the extracranial branches of the carotid artery such as the temporal artery. It usually occurs in patients older than 50 years. Most common neurological complications are retinal ischaemia, ischaemic optic neuropathy and diplopia secondary to ischaemia of the extraocular muscles. Stroke might occur, even if uncommon, secondary to the involvement of the posterior intracranial circulation. There is a known association with polymyalgia rheumatica and the combination of increased CRP value with an elevated ESR has a high diagnostic specificity.[29] A daily dose of corticosteroids is the classic treatment.

Takayasu's Arteritis. Takayasu's arteritis is a granulomatous arteritis of the aorta and its major branches and is considered a form of giant cell arteritis, affecting younger individuals under 50 years of age. CNS involvement is fairly common and is seen in up to one-third of the patients secondary to carotid artery stenosis, and cerebral hypoperfusion.

Kawasaki's Disease. Kawasaki's disease, generally affecting infants and children, is an acute febrile vasculitis that predominantly involves medium-sized arteries. However, large, and small arteries might also be affected. Its aetiology is still unknown even if an infectious cause has been suggested. Neurological symptoms include seizures, facial palsy and, rarely, cerebral infarction.

Wegener's Granulomatosis. Wegener's granulomatosis is an inflammatory multisystem disorder characterised by necrotising granulomas in the upper and lower respiratory tract, with or without focal segmental glomerulonephritis and a systemic necrotising vasculitis, affecting small-to-medium-sized vessels. Neurological involvement has been reported, with the most common symptoms being mononeuritis multiplex, followed by distal symmetric sensorimotor neuropathy. Less common is involvement of the brain and meninges that can present as intracerebral or subarachnoid haemorrhage, and cerebral arterial or venous thrombosis. Typical CNS findings such as diffuse linear or focal dural thickening and enhancement, infarcts, non-specific white matter changes, an enlarged pituitary gland with infundibular thickening and enhancement, granulomatous lesions and atrophy are well presented on MRI.[30]

Polyathritis Nodosa. A classic systemic necrotising vasculitis that affects medium-sized and small vessels is polyarteritis nodosa (PAN). Neurologically, both CNS and PNS occur in PAN. CNS involvement is seen in up to 40% of patients and may occur as diffuse encephalopathy with cognitive decline and seizures secondary to the involvement of small arteries. Stroke-like symptoms with focal or multifocal findings are seen secondary to involvement of medium-sized arteries. Other uncommon findings are cranial nerve palsies, intracerebral or subarachnoid haemorrhages or spinal cord involvement secondary to vasculitis of the spinal arteries.

NEUROSARCOIDOSIS

Sarcoidosis is a multisystem disease process of unknown aetiology whose pathogenesis involves formation of an inflammatory lesion known as a granuloma. The lungs are affected most frequently, but other organs like the eyes, the CNS, heart, kidneys, bones and joints may also be affected. CNS involvement—neurosarcoidosis—is seen in approximately 25% of patients with systemic sarcoidosis, although it is subclinical in most of these cases. In over 80% of established cases of neurosarcoidosis the chest radiograph is abnormal. Neurosarcoidosis is slightly more common in women than men. Cranial neuropathy, particularly facial nerve palsy, often multifocal with other neuropathies, is the most common clinical presentation. Other clinical presentations of neurosarcoidosis include encephalopathy, peripheral neuropathy with muscle weakness and sensory loss, meningitis, seizure, cerebellar ataxia, psychiatric disorders, spinal cord dysfunction and myopathy. MRI is the method of choice in the diagnostic evaluation and follow-up of patients with neurosarcoidosis and both FLAIR images and images after administration of gadolinium are recommended to increase sensitivity. The most frequent finding is meningeal disease with dural thickening and masses that can mimic meningioma and enhancement of the basal and suprasellar meninges. Other common MRI findings include non-enhancing lesions with high signal on T_2-weighted images in the periventricular white matter and brainstem that might mimic MS lesions, multiple small contrast-enhancing granulomas often located superficially in brain parenchyma bordering the basal cisterns (Fig. 5-27), enhancement of the optic nerve and other cranial nerves, and intramedullary spinal cord lesions[31] (Fig. 5-28). Less often, subependymal granulomatous infiltration causes hydrocephalus (Fig. 5-29). There is no known cure for sarcoidiosis. Treatment is indicated if symptoms are severe or progressive and might include prednisone to reduce inflammation, hormone replacement and immunosuppressive treatment if needed. The goal of treatment is to reduce symptoms.

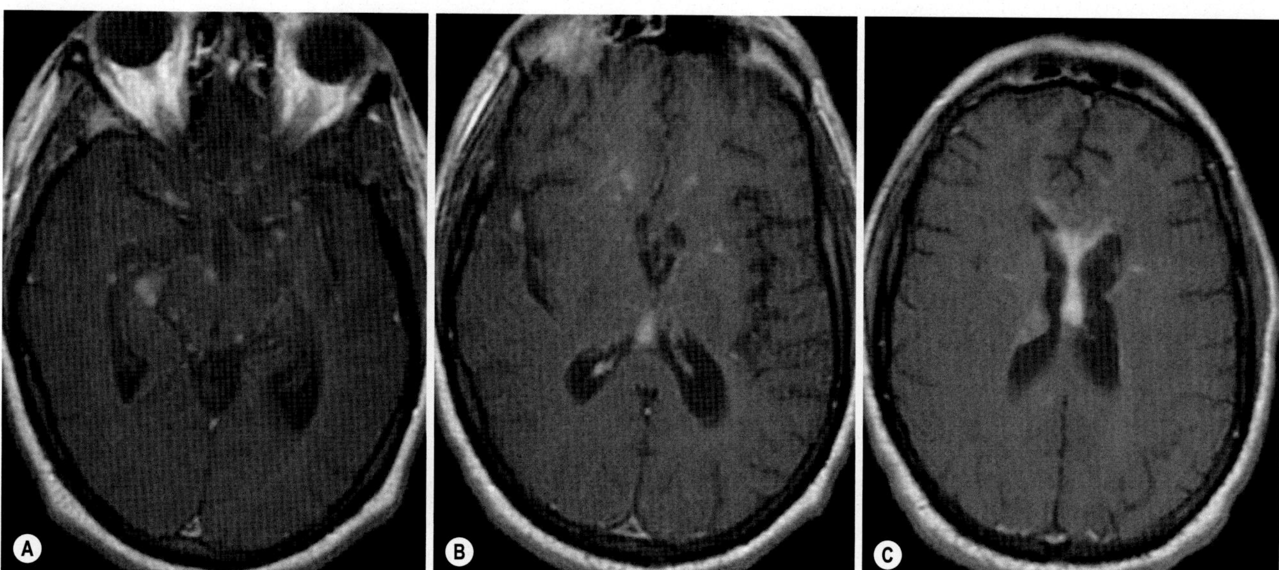

FIGURE 5-27 ■ Axial post-contrast-enhanced T_1-weighted images of the brain in a 40-year-old woman with neurosarcoidosis demonstrate multiple contrast-enhancing lesions on the leptomenginal surfaces (A), and subependymal lesions (B, C) with slight enlargement of the lateral ventricles (C).

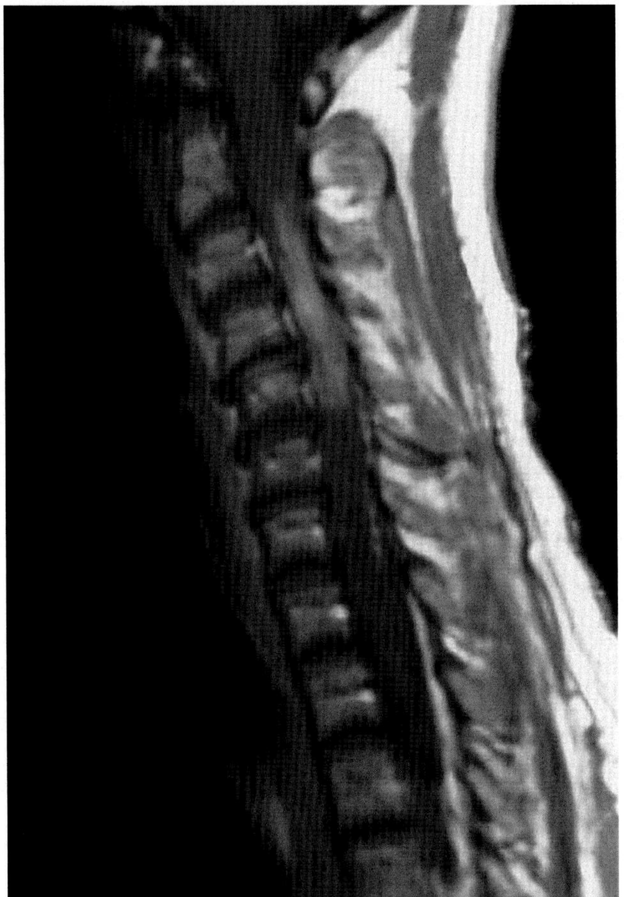

FIGURE 5-28 ■ Sagittal post-contrast-enhanced T_1-weighted image in a patient with known neurosarcoidosis demonstrates en focal pathological enhancing intramedullary lesion in the cervical cord.

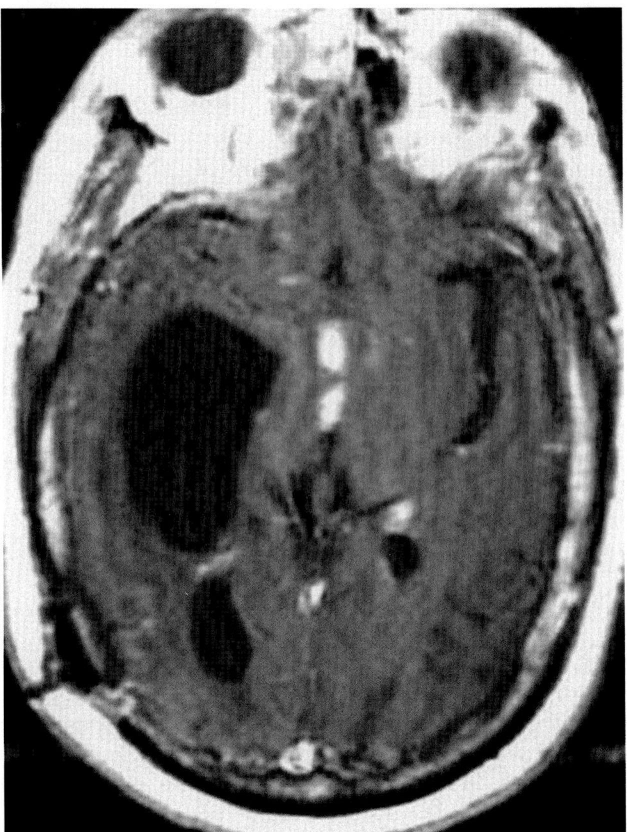

FIGURE 5-29 ■ Transverse contrast-enhanced T_1-weighted image demonstrates multiple enhancing subependymal granulomatous infiltrative lesions causing obstructing hydrocephalus with enlargement of the temporal horn of the right lateral ventricle.

BEHÇET'S DISEASE

Behçet's disease (BD) is a multisystemic, vascular inflammatory disease of unknown origin involving the larger vessels that may present with a classic triad of oral and genital ulcerations with uveitis. Patients present with different focal or multifocal neurological problems. The most common neurological symptom is severe headache; other common symptoms are weakness, and different cognitive and behavioural changes. Isolated optic neuritis, aseptic meningitis and intracranial haemorrhage secondary to ruptured aneurysms are rare manifestations of the disease. Neurological involvement in BD is a cause of major morbidity, and approximately 50% of the patients are moderate-to-severely disable after 10 years of disease.[32] CNS involvement most often occurs as a chronic meningoencephalitis.[9] MRI is very sensitive to demonstrate the typical reversible inflammatory parenchymal lesions generally located within the brainstem, occasionally with extension to the diencephalon, or within the basal ganglia, the periventricular and subcortical white matter[33,34] (Fig. 5-30). Rarely, the lesions may resemble those seen in MS. Brainstem atrophy is seen in chronic cases. Neuro-BD is treated with either oral or intravenous prednisolone until improvement.

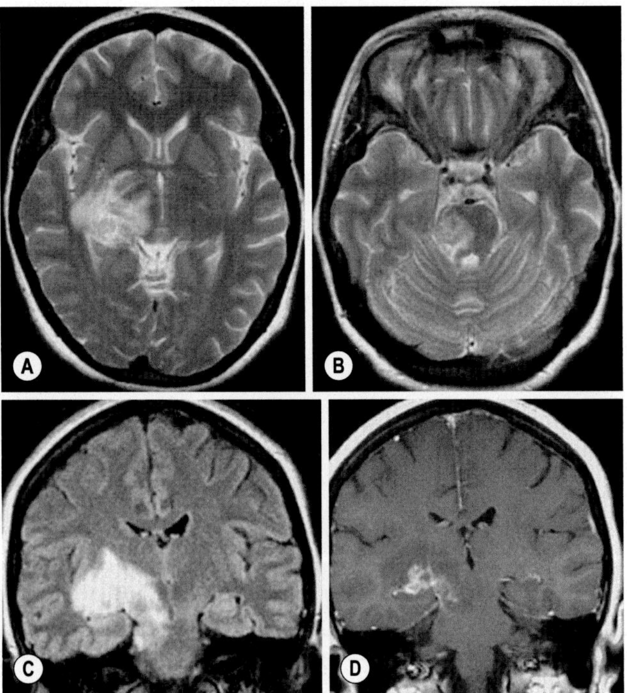

FIGURE 5-30 ■ **Neuro-Behçet's disease.** Transverse T_2-weighted images (A, B) and coronal T_2 FLAIR and contrast-enhanced T_1-weighted images (C, D). Observe the contrast-enhancing right pontomesencephalic lesion that extends to the basal ganglia. (Courtesy of Dr. A. Rovira-Gols, UDIAT-Parc Tauli, Sabadell. Spain.)

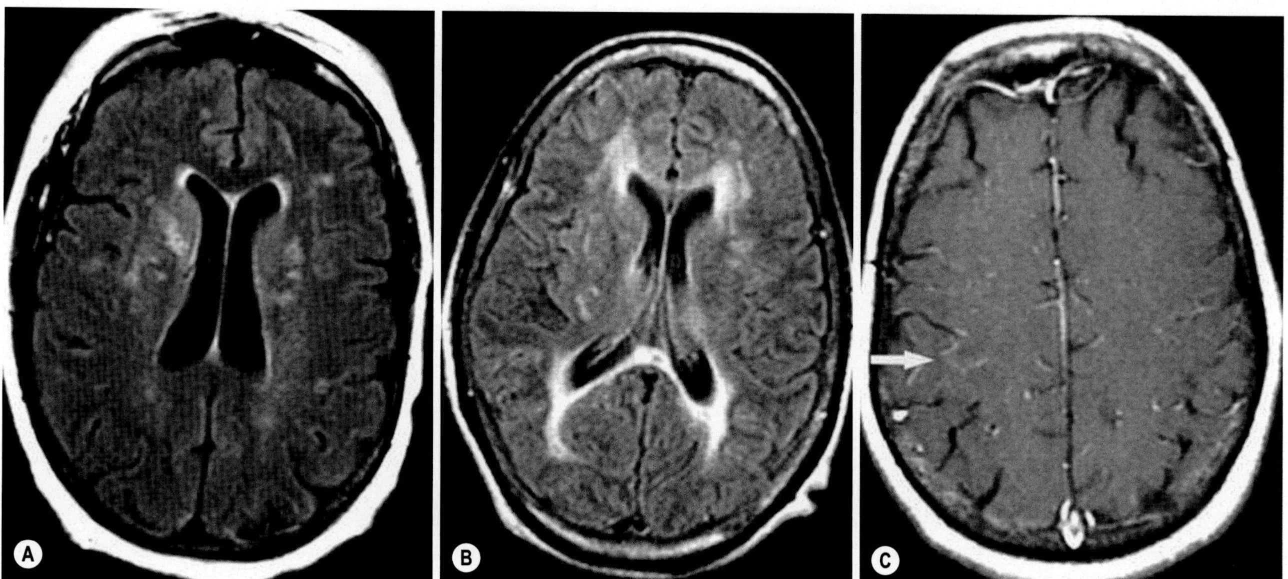

FIGURE 5-31 ■ Brain MRI in a 45-year-old woman with SLE. Axial fluid-attenuated inversion recovery (FLAIR) demonstrates small foci of increased signal in the periventricular and deep white matter (A) and more confluent areas of increased signal in the periventricular white matter (B). Axial post-contrast-enhanced image demonstrates diffuse faint pathological contrast enhancement (arrow) in a systemic lupus erythematosus female patient with vasculitis (C).

SYSTEMIC LUPUS ERYTHEMATOSUS

Systemic lupus erythematosus (SLE) is an autoimmune disorder with an annual incidence of 2.0–7.6 per 100,000 and with myriad manifestations. One of those manifestations is neuropsychiatric systemic lupus erythematosus (NPSLE), which occurs in 25–70% of patients with SLE and is associated with increased morbidity and mortality. Unfortunately, NPSLE patients have a worse prognosis and more cumulative damage than patients with SLE alone. Currently, the underlying causes as to why patients develop NPSLE are still unknown and unclear. Investigators speculate that CNS damage is secondary to autoantibody production, microangiopathy, atherosclerosis, or intrathecal production of proinflammatory cytokines.[35] Histopathologically, patients with NPSLE might show multifocal microinfarcts, cortical atrophy, gross infarcts, haemorrhage, ischaemic demyelination and patchy multiple sclerosis-like areas of demyelination. The clinical manifestations of NPSLE include psychosis, stroke and epilepsy, in addition to more subtle symptoms such as headache and neurocognitive dysfunction.[36] Patients with concomitant antiphospholipid antibodies (APL-ab) are at additional risk for neuropsychiatric events. Lupus patients are also at increased risk for a wide range of CNS events related to immunosuppressive therapy, including infection and drug toxicity, hypercoagulability and accelerated atherosclerosis. CNS vasculitis and/or cerebritis represent a potentially severe form of NPSLE and may present with seizures, movements disorders, altered consciousness, stroke and coma.[37] While CNS inflammation is uncommon in SLE, this diagnosis must be entertained any time a lupus patient presents with CNS signs or symptoms. Although clinical assessment is the keystone in the diagnosis of NPSLE, the diagnosis is often difficult and remains presumptive in some patients. MR findings are variable and in some cases the MRI is unremarkable. However, abnormal conventional MRI findings are common in both SLE and NPSLE patients and range from non-specific small punctate focal lesions in white matter (present in the majority of NPSLE patients, but not specific) (Fig. 5-31) to more severe findings such as cortical atrophy, ventricular dilation, cerebral oedema, cerebral infarctions, intracranial haemorrhage and signs of vasculitis[38–40] (Fig. 5-32). These findings are attributed to different mechanisms, including thrombosis, vasculitis and antibody-mediated neuronal injury imaging. Several MR spectroscopy studies have demonstrated a decrease in *N*-acetylaspartate (NAA), known as a neuronal marker, and an increase in the choline peak, a marker for cell membrane turnover and activity.[40] These changes in metabolic activity are suggestive of neuronal loss and axonal damage that, based on recent studies, might be in part reversible after treatment. Another metabolite, *myo*-inositol (mI), has been found to be elevated early in the course of an active flare of NPSLE prior to changes on MRI. Studies using diffusion-weighted imaging and magnetic transfer have demonstrated that NPSLE patients have increased whole-brain diffusivity as well as differences in grey and white matter compared to healthy individuals.[41,42] Altogether, these findings are suggestive of the presence of subtle and widespread damage in the brain parenchyma. Reduced structural integrity in the brain, such as axonal loss and/or demyelination, is a possible aetiology for this widespread damage.

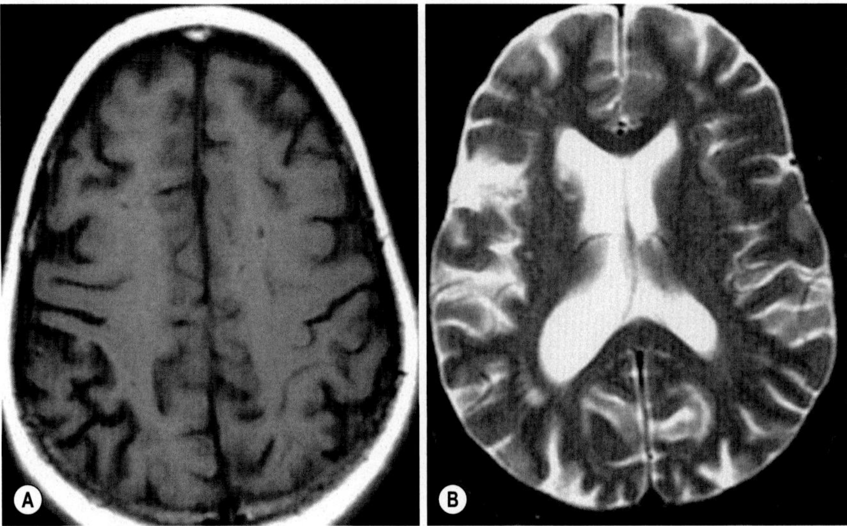

FIGURE 5-32 ■ Axial T_1-weighted (A) and T_2-weighted (B) MR images demonstrate mild-to-moderate cortical atrophy in a 35-year-old woman with long-standing systemic lupus erythematosus.

METABOLIC AND TOXIC DISORDERS IN THE ADULT

While in childhood metabolic diseases are in most cases congenital on inherited bases, toxic and metabolic diseases are usually acquired disorders in adults. CNS exposure to toxic factors can be endogenous or exogenous, and happens when metabolic toxins or exogenous toxic substances circulate in high concentrations in the blood and accumulate in the CNS, causing intoxication. Structures with high metabolic activity are mainly involved. This may be the reason of the predominant involvement of basal ganglia and brainstem, without or with cortical involvement. White matter involvement may be present, but is usually less noticeable than in hereditary metabolic diseases.

Ethanol Intoxication

Brain abnormalities in alcoholics include atrophy, Marchiafava–Bignami disease, Wernicke's encephalopathy, osmotic myelinolysis, and consequences of liver cirrhosis such as hepatic encephalopathy and coagulopathy.[43,44] All the reported entities are not specific to alcohol and can be found in many other toxic or metabolic conditions. Ethanol direct brain toxicity is caused by under-regulation of receptors of *N*-methyl-D-aspartate, abnormal catabolism of homocysteine, resulting in an increased susceptibility to glutamate excitatory and toxic effects. Moreover, immune response occurs mediated by lipid peroxidation products that bind to neurons, resulting in neurotoxicity.[45] Neuroimaging studies show a characteristic distribution of loss of volume: initially there is infratentorial predominance with atrophy of the vermis and the cerebellum. Frontal and temporal atrophy is subsequently evident, followed by diffuse atrophy of the brain. The possibility of partial reversibility of these alterations is also observed. In pregnancy, ethanol determines inhibition of maturation of Bergmann's fibres of cerebellum, with consequential marked cerebellar atrophy (Fig. 5-33).

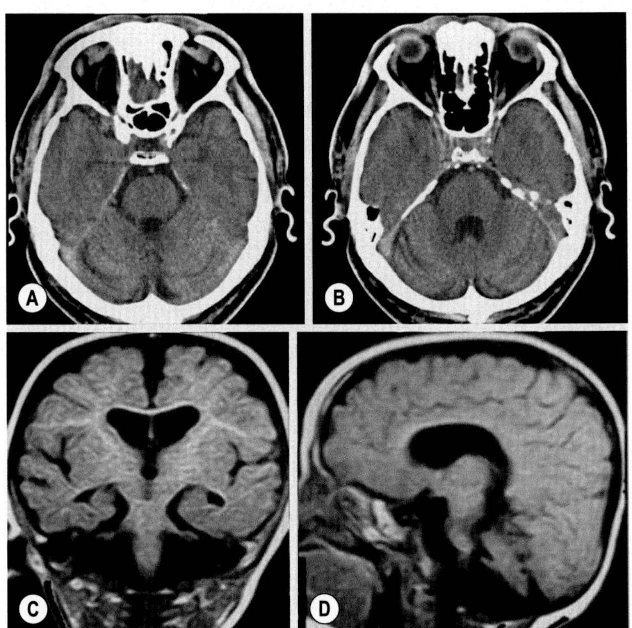

FIGURE 5-33 ■ (A, B) CT demonstrates atrophic changes selectively involving the cerebellum in a chronic alcoholic subject. In the initial stages, volume reduction is caused by water loss and brain tissue shrinkage, and is therefore reversible. (C, D) T_1-weighted MRI images show global cerebellar hypotrophy in a baby born from an alcoholic. Alcohol inhibits development of Bergmann's fibres and consequently impairs processes of neuroblastic migration and normal cerebellar development.

Marchiafava–Bignami Disease

Marchiafava–Bignami disease is a rare complication of chronic alcoholism, characterised by demyelination and

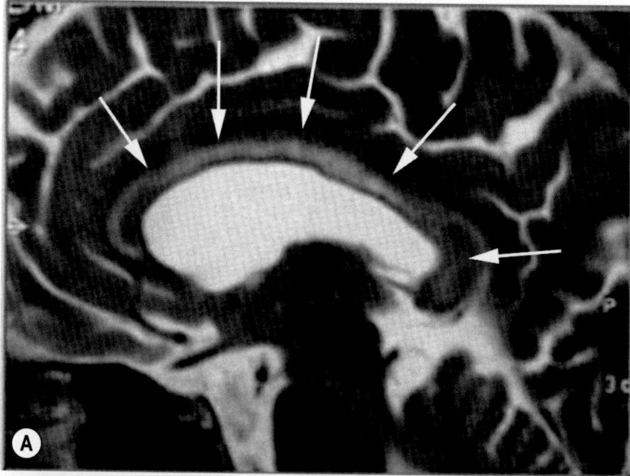

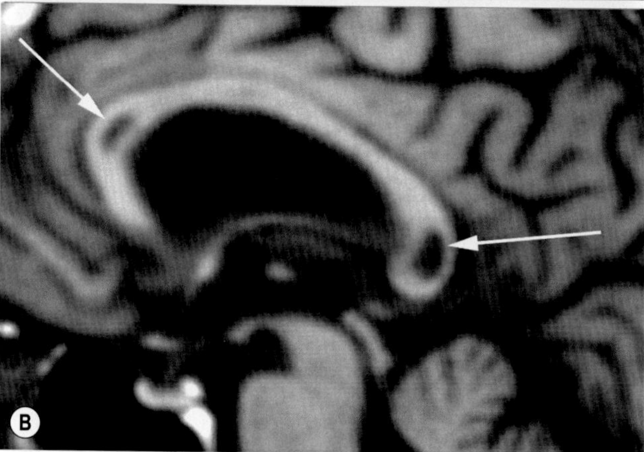

FIGURE 5-34 ■ Two cases of Marchiafava–Bignami disease. (A) Sagittal T_2-weighted image shows typical acute–subacute aspect of the disease, characterised by diffuse oedema of the corpus callosum without significant mass effect. (B) T_1-weighted image obtained in chronic phase, showing typical necrotic cavities selectively involving the genu and splenium.

necrosis of the corpus callosum, with rare involvement of extracallosal regions. Aetiology remains unknown but is believed to be caused by toxic agents in low-quality red wine and deficiency of Group B vitamins. Rarely, it has also been reported in non-alcoholic patients. Symptoms are mainly represented by cognitive deficits, psychosis, hypertonia and interhemispheric disconnection, until coma and death. Typical features at MRI in the acute phase are corpus callosum hyperintensity on T_2-weighted sequences and FLAIR, without significant mass effect, with peripheral enhancement. Diffusion is restricted due to cytotoxic oedema. In chronic forms, necrosis of the genu and splenium can be detected[46] (Fig. 5-34).

Wernicke's Encephalopathy

Wernicke's encephalopathy (WE) is an acute condition first described by the French ophthalmologist Gayet in 1875, and later by the German neurologist Wernike in 1881, caused by a deficiency of vitamin B_1 (thiamine). WE develops frequently but not exclusively in alcoholics. Other potential causes include extended fasting, malabsorption, digitalis poisoning and massive infusion of glucose without vitamin B_1 in weak patients. The autoptic incidence is reported to be 0.8–2% in random autopsies, and 20% in chronic alcoholics.[47] The classic clinical triad of ocular dysfunctions (nystagmus, conjugate gaze palsy, ophthalmoplegia), ataxia and confusion is observed only in 30% of cases. Treatment consists of thiamine infusion, and avoids irreversible consequences like Korsakoff's dementia or death. Memory impairment and dementia are related to damage of the mamillary bodies, anterior thalamic nuclei and interruption of the diencephalic-hippocampal circuits. Depletion of thiamine leads to failure of conversion of pyruvate to acetyl-CoA and α-ketoglutarate to succinate, altered pentose monophosphate shunt and the lack of Krebs cycle, with cerebral lactic acidosis, intra- and extracellular oedema, swelling of astrocytes, oligodendrocytes, myelin fibres and neuronal dendrites. Neuropathological aspects include neuronal degeneration, demyelination, haemorrhagic petechiae, proliferation of capillaries and astrocytes in periacqueduct grey substance, mamillary bodies, thalami, pulvinar, III cranial nerves nuclei and cerebellum.[47,48] At MRI, bilateral and symmetrical hyperintensities on T_2-weighted sequences and FLAIR are evident at the level of the already-mentioned structures, mainly mamillary bodies and thalami[49,50] (Fig. 5-35). Rarely, cortex of the forebrain can be involved.[50] DWI shows areas of high signal with ADC signal reduced due to cytotoxic oedema (Fig. 5-35), although the ADC can sometimes be high due to the presence of vasogenic component.[50] Rarely T_1-weighted images show bleeding ecchymotic haemorrhages in the thalami and mamillary bodies, a sign considered clinically unfavourable (Fig. 5-35). In 50% of cases, contrast enhancement is present in periacqueductal regions. Marked contrast enhancement of mamillary bodies is evident in 80% of cases, even prior to the development of visible changes in T_2-weighted sequences, and is considered highly specific for WE[51] (Fig. 5-35). In chronic forms, change of signal in T_2-weighted sequences becomes less prominent due to the diffuse brain atrophy, more pronounced at the level of mesencephalon and mamillary bodies.

Subacute Combined Degeneration

This disorder of the spinal cord, also known as funicular myelitis or Putnam–Dana syndrome, occurs in patients with vitamin B_{12} deficiency, and is characterised by a slight-to-moderate degree of gliosis in association with spongiform degeneration of the posterior and lateral columns. Clinical presentation consists in spastic paraparesis and spinal ataxia. At MRI, T_2-weighted hyperintensities are detected in the spinal cord posterior and lateral columns.[52] These lesions can be reversible after adequate vitamin B_{12} administration, or evolve towards atrophy. In some cases hyperintensity can be also detected along the spinothalamic tracts and lemnisci mediali (Fig. 5-36).

Osmotic Myelinolysis

Osmotic myelinolysis (OM) usually occurs in patients with hyponatremia that is too quickly corrected. This causes destruction of the blood–brain barrier with

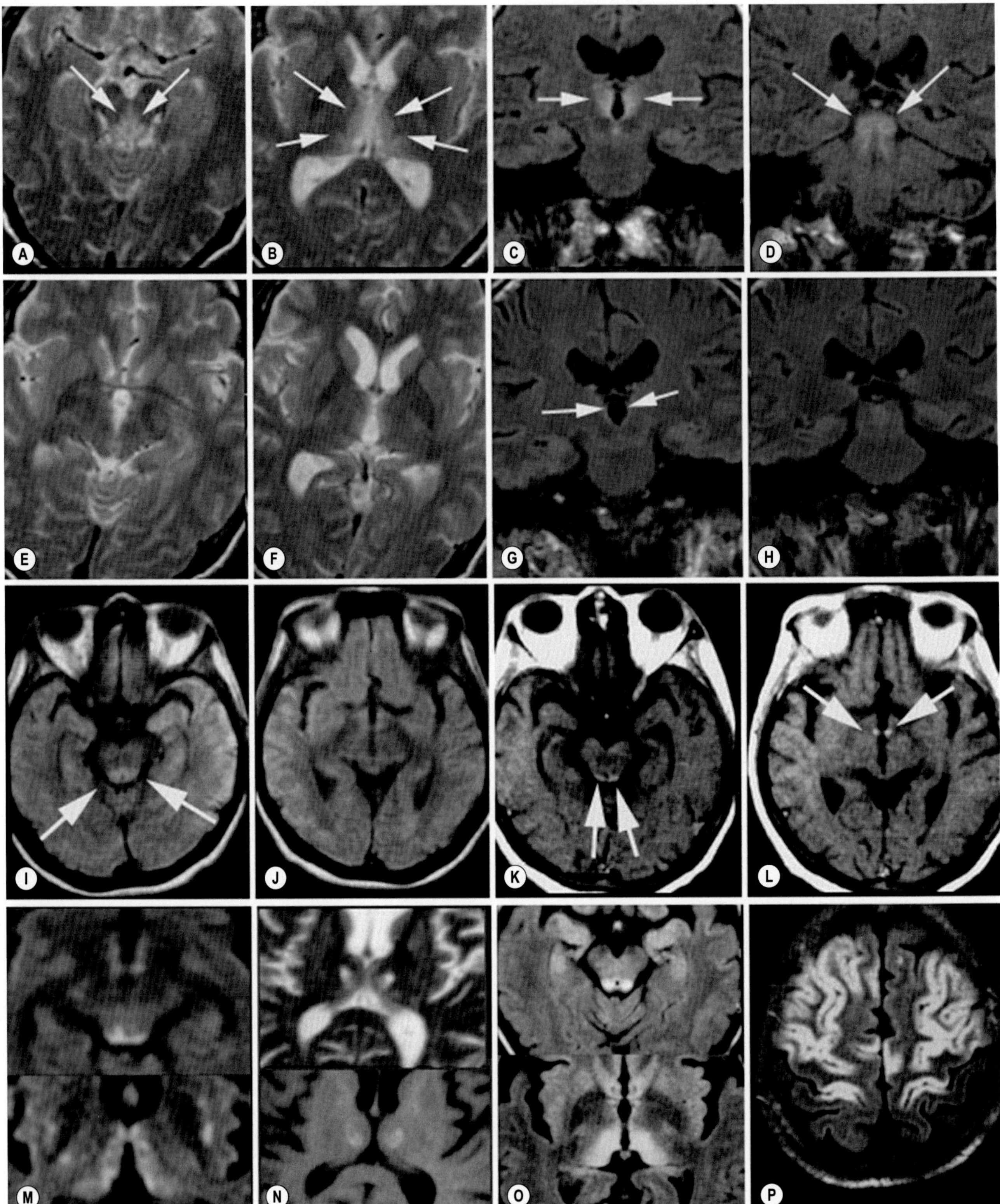

FIGURE 5-35 ■ Different cases of Wernicke's encephalopathy. (A–D) Typical case studied in the acute phase: prolongation of T_2 involves periacqueductal grey matter, colliculi, mid-thalamic and pulvinar regions. (E–H) Same case after therapy: normalisation of signal with mild atrophic changes (III ventricle dilatation). (I–L) Colliculi and mamillary bodies are involved and there is a clear contrast enhancement in both structures. (M) DWI of a different case with restricted diffusion in mamillary bodies, mesencephalic roof and thalami. (N) Lethal case with petechial haemorrhages in thalami. (O, P) Typical lesions associated with diffuse cortical involvement.

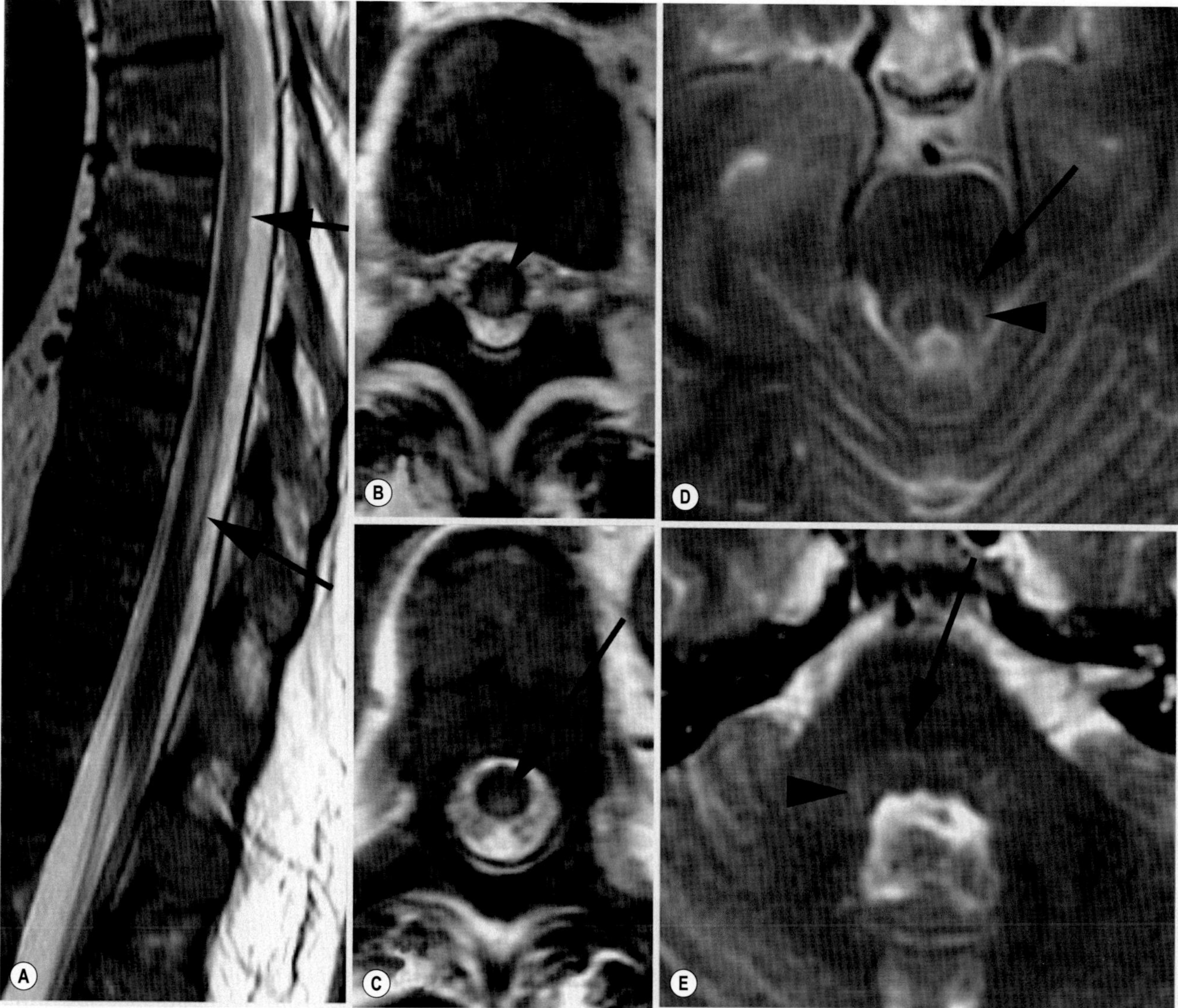

FIGURE 5-36 ■ **Two cases of combined sclerosis.** (A–C) Sagittal and axial T_2-weighted sequences show hyperintensities selectively involving the posterior columns in a young vegan female patient suffering from progressive spinal ataxia. (D, E) A different case in which hyperintensities extended to ascending sensitive pathways: lemniscus medialis (arrows) and spinothalamic tracts (arrowheads).

hypertonic fluid accumulation in extracellular space, resulting in a non-inflammatory demyelination. The most common damage is in the pontine fibres.[53,54] OM is observed in alcoholics with nutritional deficiency. The most common symptoms include paralysis, dysphagia, dysarthria and pseudobulbar palsy. Death is frequent. Rarely, OM affects other regions, especially basal ganglia, thalami and deep white matter. MRI usually shows an area of high signal on T_2-weighted sequences and FLAIR in the central part of the pons, sparing ventrolateral portions and corticospinal tracts.[53] The lesion is moderately hypointense in T_1 and may show positive contrast enhancement (Fig. 5-37). If the patient survives, the acute phase can evolve in a cavitated pontine lesion.

Methanol Poisoning

Acute methanol poisoning usually occurs after drinking counterfeit alcoholic beverages or following accidental ingestion of solvents and coolants. Toxic effects are due to formic acid, the main metabolite of methanol, which causes metabolic acidosis; the more susceptible structures are putamen, and symptoms occur within hours after ingestion and are characterised by headache, visual disturbances, nausea and vomiting. Coma, respiratory arrest and death can occur typically 6–36 hours after the poisoning.

Putaminal necrosis appears hypodense on CT and hyperintense on T_2-weighted sequences[55] (Fig. 5-38). More than 10% of cases are associated with putaminal ecchymotic haemorrhages, appearing hyperintense on T_1-weighted sequences. Alterations may also involve pallidum and centrum ovale.

Diethylene Glycol

Diethylene glycol is commonly used as a solvent for paints, antifreeze and other chemicals. About 12 hours

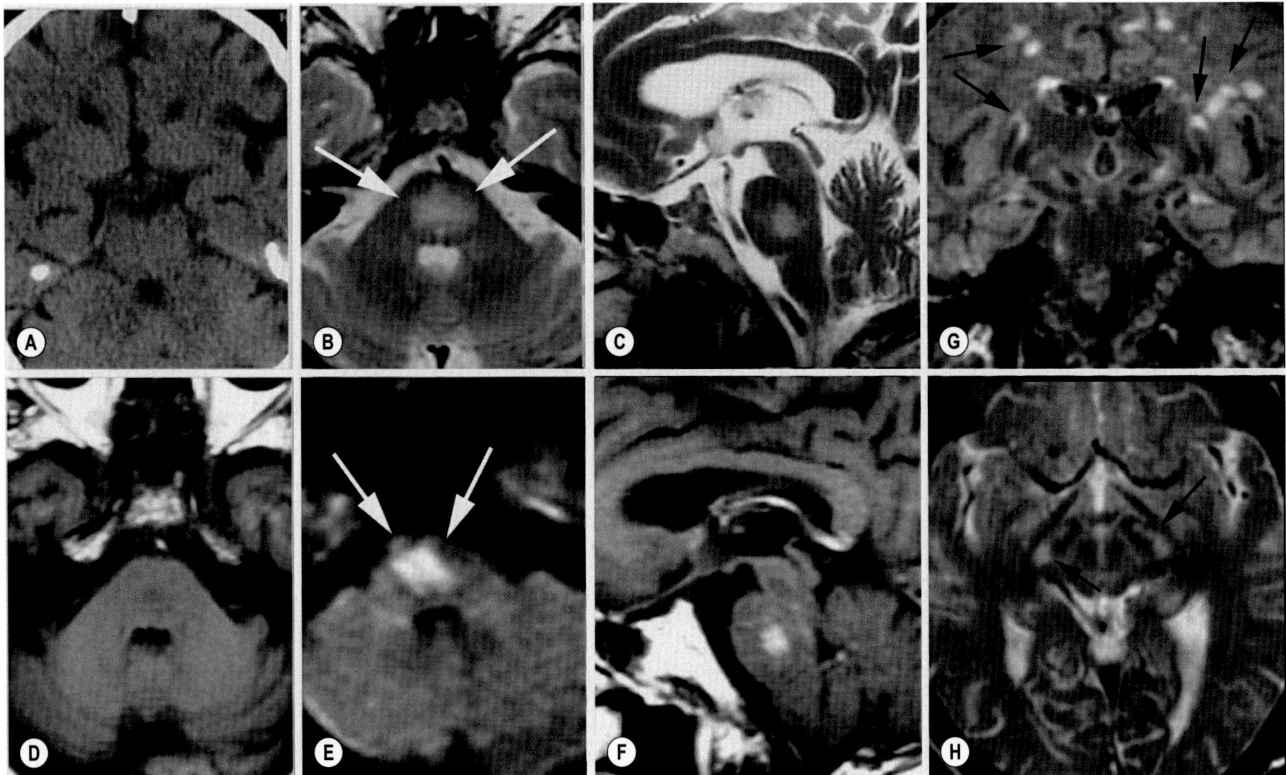

FIGURE 5-37 ■ **Osmotic myelinolysis.** (A–F) Typical pontine localisation in an alcoholic patient (central pontine myelinolysis, CPM). CT does not show any abnormality. MR shows a tegmental pontine lesion, hyperintense on T_2-weighted images, central, with restricted diffusivity (E), and positive contrast enhancement (F). (G, H) Different case affected by post-dyalitic extrapontine osmotic myelinolysis. Lesions are located in the basal ganglia (putamina and substantia nigra) and supratentorial white matter.

after ingestion patients develop fulminant hepatorenal insufficiency, coma and seizures. MRI shows brain oedema initially widespread; then after 24–48 hours frontal white matter necrosis, basal ganglia, thalami and brainstem involvement appear[56] (Fig. 5-38).

Hepatic Encephalopathy

The term *hepatic encephalopathy* (HE) includes a spectrum of neuropsychiatric abnormalities occurring in patients with liver dysfunction. Most cases are associated with cirrhosis and portal hypertension or portal-systemic shunts, but the condition can also be seen in patients with acute liver failure and, rarely, in those with portal-systemic bypass and no associated intrinsic hepatocellular disease. Although HE is a clinical condition, several neuroimaging techniques, particularly MR imaging, may eventually be useful for the diagnosis because they can identify and measure the consequences of CNS increase in substances, which, under normal circumstances, are efficiently metabolised by the liver. Classical MR abnormalities in chronic HE include high signal intensity in the globus pallidum on T_1-weighted images, likely a reflection of increased tissue concentrations of manganese (Fig. 5-39), and an elevated glutamine/glutamate peak coupled with decreased *myo*-inositol and choline signals on proton MR spectroscopy, representing disturbances in cell-volume homeostasis secondary to brain hyperammoniemia.[57] Recent data have shown that white matter abnormalities, also related to increased CNS ammonia concentration, can also be detected with several MR imaging techniques: magnetisation transfer ratio measurements show significantly low values in otherwise normal-appearing brain white matter, fast-FLAIR sequences reveal diffuse and focal high signal intensity lesions in the hemispheric white matter and diffusion-weighted images disclose increased white matter diffusivity. All these MR abnormalities, which return to normal with restoration of liver function, probably reflect the presence of mild diffuse interstitial brain oedema, which seems to play an essential role in the pathogenesis of HE.

In acute HE, bilateral symmetric signal-intensity abnormalities on T_2-weighted images, often with associated restricted diffusion involving the cortical grey matter, are commonly identified (Fig. 5-40). Involvement of the subcortical white matter and the basal ganglia, thalami and midbrain may also be seen. These abnormalities, which can lead to intracranial hypertension and severe brain injury, reflect the development of cytotoxic oedema secondary to the acute increase of brain hyperammoniemia.[58]

Carbon Monoxide

Carbon monoxide (CO) is a source of accidental acute intoxication with relatively frequent high mortality. CO

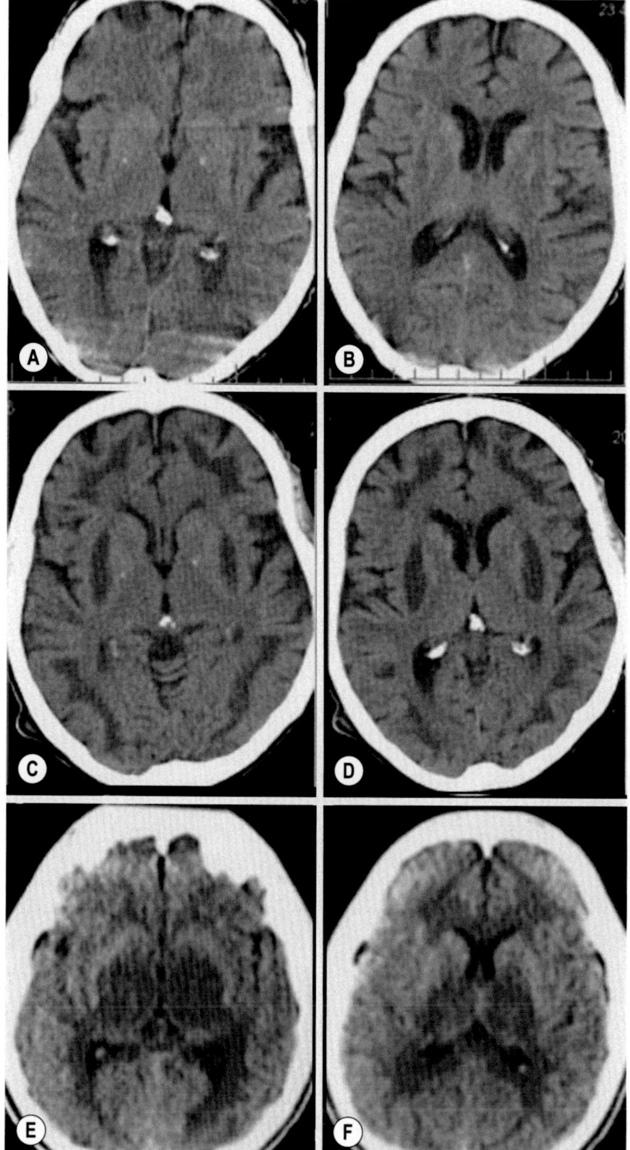

FIGURE 5-38 ■ (A, B) Methanol intoxication: CT examination performed in the acute phase. Oedema of the putamen and external capsule is becoming evident. (C, D) Same case after 24 hours: clear hypodense lesions in both putamen extended in the subcortical white matter with prevalence in frontal and occipital regions. (E, F) Diethylene glycol intoxication in subacute phase. Oedema is mostly localised in thalami, internal capsules and pallidi.

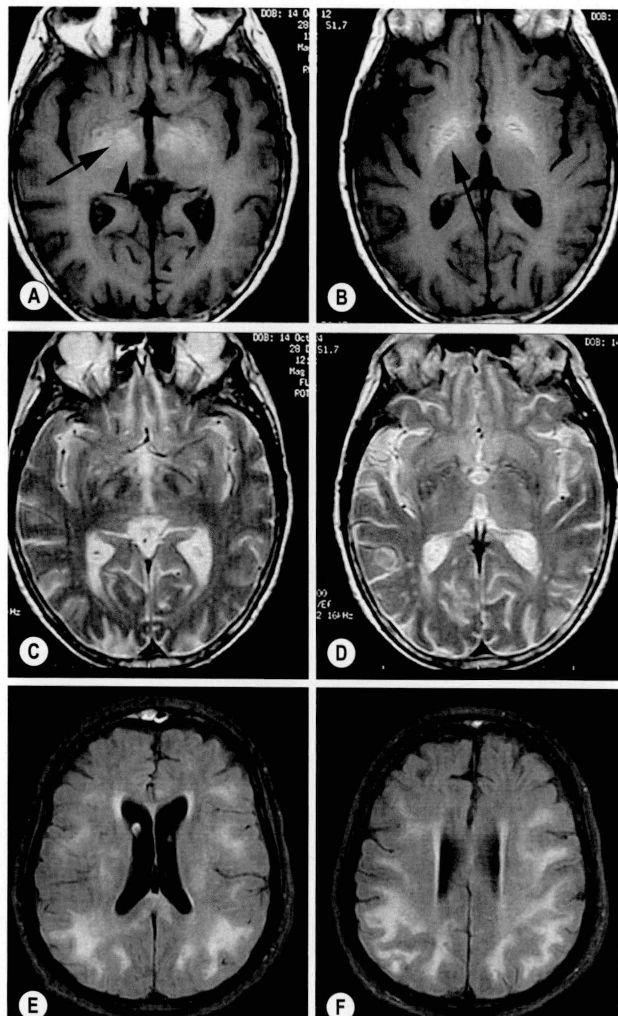

FIGURE 5-39 ■ **Hepatic encephalopathy.** Typical hyperintense signal on T_1-weighted sequences involves substantia nigra (arrow in A), red nucleus (arrowhead in A), and pallidum (arrow in B). These alterations are visible even though less prominent on T_2-weighted sequences (C, D). (E, F) A different case with diffuse white matter oedema. ((E, F) Courtesy of Dr. T. Krings, Toronto Western Hospital, Canada.)

determines a neurological hypoxic damage. In fact, CO has an affinity for haemoglobin 250 times greater than oxygen, with whom it competes. CO attaches to haemoglobin, resulting in the formation of carboxyhaemoglobin, and thereby reducing the ability of haemoglobin to transport oxygen. Clinically, CO poisoning causes headache, tinnitus, dizziness and nausea, then progressive disorders of consciousness arise until death; the survivors often have severe extrapyramidal disorder or dementia.

CO poisoning causes bilateral globus pallidus necrosis, sometimes extended to lenticular nuclei and caudate; more rarely involved are thalami and hippocampus. Sometimes distal frontal white matter involvement is also evident. Selective damage of pallidi is probably not only from hypoxia but also from specific toxic phenomena. At MRI, bilateral signal alteration of the pallidi is evident. The basal ganglia affected usually have low signal on T_1 and high on T_2. Sometimes, the presence of microbleeding determines inhomogeneous signal. Hyperintensity in the subcortical white matter can be present in most severe cases.[59] Temporal involvement is rare. In the acute phase, diffusion-weighted imaging shows diffusion restriction in the basal ganglia, and may also show reduced diffusivity in areas with normal signal at the conventional sequences (Fig. 5-41). The lesions tend gradually to evolve towards cavitation and atrophy.

Heavy Metal Poisoning

Some heavy metals are rare due to acute or chronic intoxication, usually professionally exposed workers are

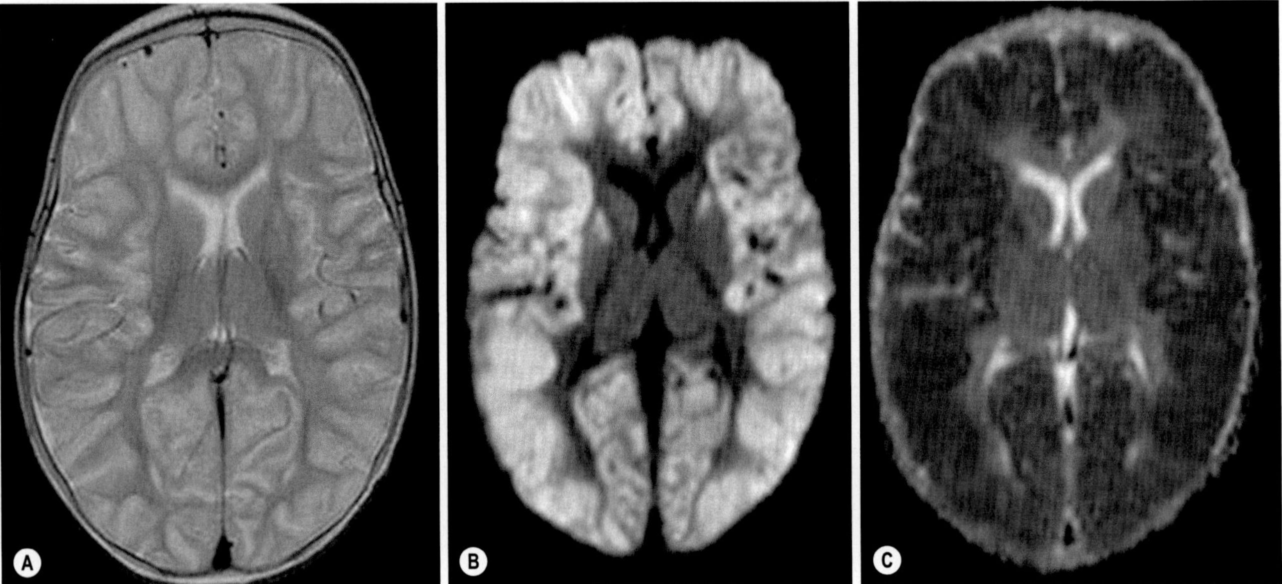

FIGURE 5-40 ■ **Acute hepatic encephalopathy.** A 7-month-old boy with acute hepatic failure. Brain MRI imaging shows symmetric and diffuse abnormal high signal intensity on T_2-weighted images involving the cortical grey matter (A). This abnormality showed increased signal intensity on the isotropic diffusion-weighted image (B) and low signal on the apparent diffusion coefficient map (C) which corresponds to cytotoxic oedema.

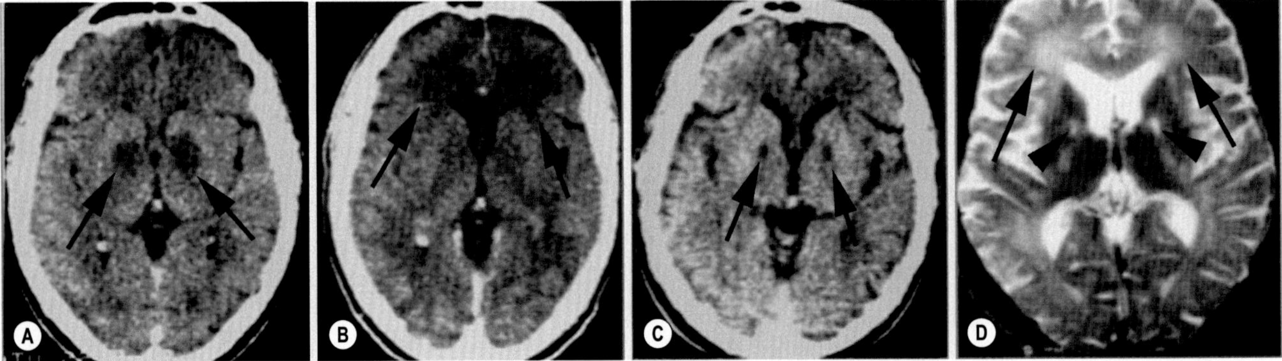

FIGURE 5-41 ■ **Carbon monoxide intoxication.** (A, B) CT imaging performed in acute phase; oedema of both pallidi and frontal deep and subcortical white matter. In chronic phase, CT (C) shows necrotic degeneration of pallidi and hypodensity of the frontal white matter. T_2-weighted sequences (D) confirm diffuse hyperintensity of the frontal white matter and both pallidi.

victims. Manganese poisoning can affect workers in the mining industry, patients in chronic parenteral nutrition and, rarely, patients who abuse ephedrine. Chronic poisoning causes accumulation of manganese and neuronal loss in the basal ganglia; the main symptoms include dementia, hallucinations and extrapyrimidal disorders. The accumulation of manganese appears at MRI as bilateral hyperintensity on T_1-weighted sequence of pallidi nuclei, sometimes extended to other nuclei and cerebral peduncles.[59] T_2 signal is usually normal. Mercury poisoning mainly affects miners or consumers of fish caught in contaminated water. The metal accumulates mainly in the cerebellar vermis and visual cortex, and manifests as a signal hypointense on T_1, iso- and hypointense on T_2 and hypointense on T_2*-weighted sequences.

Lead intoxication can cause alteration of the signal in subcortical and thalamic regions. Aluminium can intoxicate patients undergoing dialysis and is characterised by elective involvement of the limbic system.

Organic Solvent Poisoning

This particular poisoning occurs among people who inhale glue. Toluene and other organic solvents are readily transported by air to the blood, cross the blood–brain barrier and enter the central nervous system. This poisoning manifests as neurological impairment and cognitive decline. Pathological studies reveal axonal loss with diffuse cerebral white matter demyelination and cerebellar degeneration and gliosis. At MRI, diffuse T_2 increase in cerebellar and cerebral white matter is registered, often with a slight shortening of T_2 in the putamen. In some cases it may be a shortening of T_2, also in the thalamus and in the cerebral cortex.[60]

Cocaine

Cocaine acts by blocking reuptake of catecholamines. This causes a short-lived intense feeling of euphoria, increased energy and alertness. Acute neurotoxic effects include agitation and convulsions. Most commonly, cocaine is inhaled in the form of cocaine hydrochloride; its alkaline base (crack) can be smoked.

Most of the central nervous system complications induced by cocaine are ischaemic and haemorrhagic strokes. Bleeding related to cocaine can be localised in the subarachnoid space or intracerebral, and is twice more frequent than infarctions. Approximately 50% of patients are bearers of a concomitant pathology as cerebral arteriovenous malformations or aneurysms, which break consequently to increased blood pressure and heart rate caused by cocaine-induced sympathetic effects. In cases where it is not possible to document the presence of concomitant vascular pathology, intraparenchymal bleedings are most commonly located in the basal ganglia and thalami; the risk of bleeding increases with alcohol abuse.

While the pathogenetic mechanisms of haemorrhagic stroke are clear, the causes of ischaemic stroke are diverse and include vasoconstriction induced by cocaine and vasculitis (by additives/contaminants added to cocaine) (Fig. 5-42). Cocaine increases the platelet response to arachidonic acid with a increased level of thromboxane that increases platelet aggregation, resulting in thrombosis and heart and/or brain infarcts. Brain lesions are mostly located in the subcortical white matter or in the middle cerebral artery territory (Fig. 5-42). Mesencephalic infarcts seem to be more frequent when cocaine is used in conjunction with amphetamine. Angiography may show focal constrictions of the main arteries, while contrast enhancement of the vessel wall indicates the presence of vasculitis. Cerebral atrophy is observed in patients who are chronic abusers of cocaine. The frontal lobe is typically more severely involved, followed by the temporal. Chronic ischaemia may be the causative mechanism of the atrophy.[61]

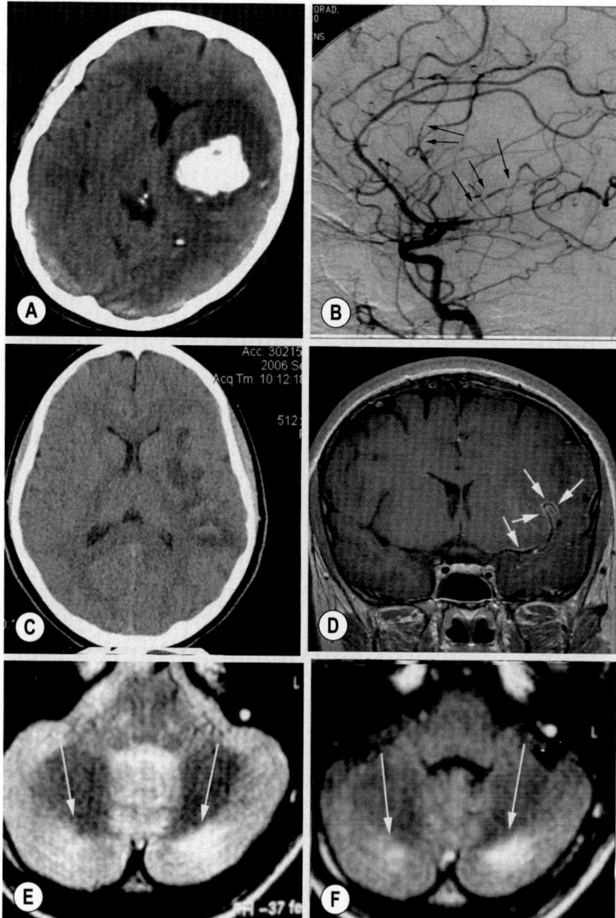

FIGURE 5-42 Different cases of vascular disease: consequences of illegal drugs administration. (A, B) Capsulolenticular haemorrhage in a cocaine abuser with clear angiographic 'pearl and string signs' along different branches of middle cerebral artery, suggesting vasculitis. (C, D) A different case of vasculitis in a cocaine user, with ischaemic stroke in the territory of the left middle cerebral artery. (D) Contrast-enhanced T_1-weighted image shows positive enhancement of the perivascular leptomeninges, and the vessel walls, indicating active inflammation. (E, F) Acute bilateral cerebellar infarction in a cocaine consumer. ((A–D) Courtesy of Dr. T. Krings, Toronto Western Hospital, Canada.)

Ecstasy

Ecstasy or 3,4-methylenedioxymethamphetamine (MDMA), a drug derived from methamphetamine, is known as a party drug that has stimulatory and moderately hallucinatory effects. In the acute phase the subject experiences euphoria, increased self-esteem and sensory perceptions and hyperthermia, tachycardia, and sometimes acute psychosis and lockjaw. These effects disappear in 24–48 hours and are accompanied by muscle aches, depression, fatigue and decreased concentration. MDMA causes a sharp and quick release of 5-hydroxytryptamine (5-HT), a serotonin receptor, with a powerful vasoconstriction, and determines an increase of synaptic dopamine in different brain areas. Although the permanent neurotoxicity is still a matter of debate, there is evidence that the stimulation of the 5-HT 2A receptors in the small vessels results in prolonged vasospasm and necrosis of brain regions is involved. The occipital cortex and the globus pallidus are the most vulnerable areas to high levels of 5-HT.[61]

Opioids and Derivatives

Heroin is the most common drug among those in this group, and is also the one responsible for more neurological side effects. Other derivatives include morphine, hydrocodone, oxycodone, hydromorphine, codeine and other opiates (i.e. fentanyl, pethidine and methadone). Both acute and chronic effects of heroin on the brain have been reported. These include neurovascular disorders, leucoencephalopathy and atrophy. Moreover, beyond the direct effects of heroin, complications secondary to the addition of additives should be considered, as lipophilic substances (cutting of heroin) or crystalline impurities. Ischaemic strokes are the most frequent

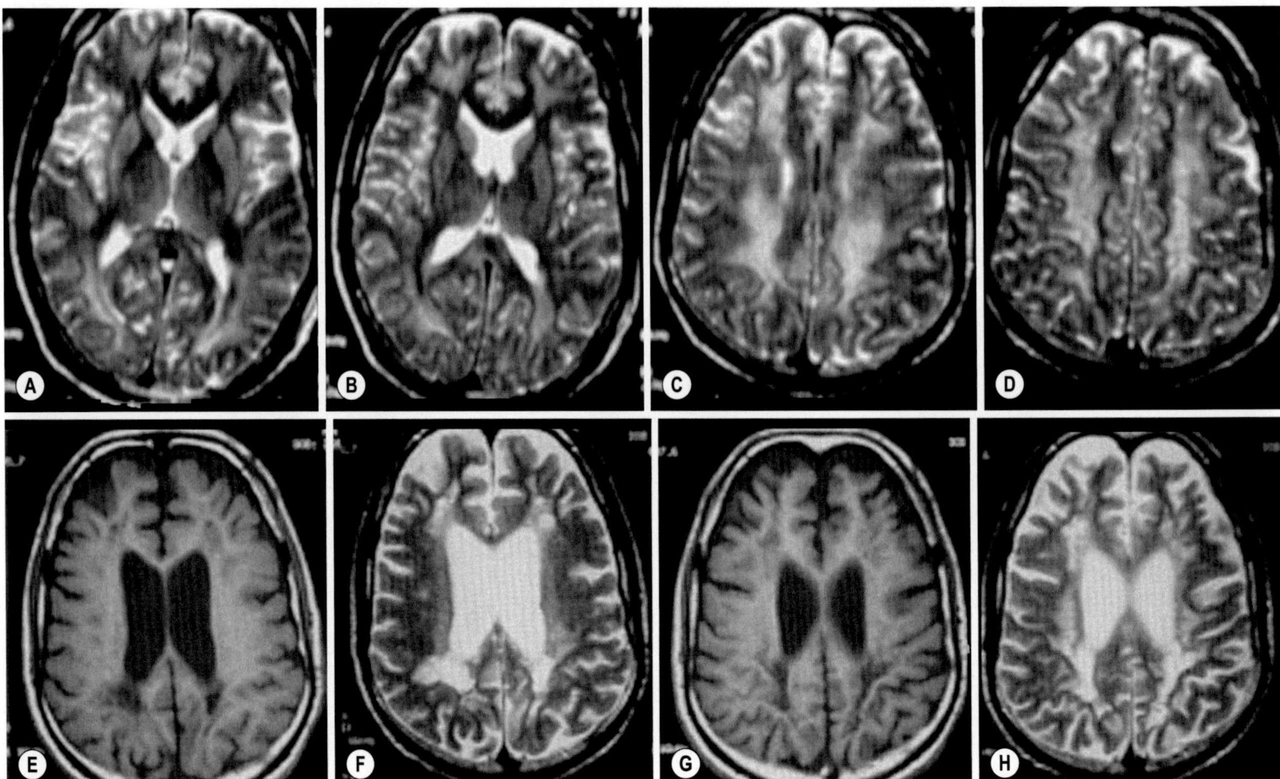

FIGURE 5-43 ■ (A–H) Delayed post-hypoxic leucoencephalopathy (DPHL) in a 29-year-old heroin user. In the upper row, T_2-weighted images show diffuse oedema of the supratentorial white matter 4 hours after prolonged cardiac arrest following intravenous drug injection. In the lower row, a follow-up brain MR obtained 1 year later. Extensive necrotic degeneration of the white matter is evident, while the cortex is spared.

heroin complication. The pathogenetic mechanisms proposed are similar to those for cocaine, and can be reversible: vasospasm, immune-mediated vasculitis, embolic events for crystalline additives. Ischaemia is more frequently observed in patients who take heroin intravenously than by oral ingestion or inhalation. Globus pallidus is most frequently involved (5–10% of subjects chronically abusing heroin). In chronic abuse, white matter changes from microvascular pathology can be seen. These aspects are, however, generally less severe than in cocaine chronic abuse. Haemodynamic cerebral infarcts are also possible in consequence of cardiac arrest (Fig. 5-43). A major heroin-induced complication is the leucoencephalopathy. It occurs in the process of inhalation, when the drug is heated on a piece of tin, and the fumes inhaled. Presumably, leucoencephalopathy associated with generalised oedema is the consequence of activation of a substance not yet known.[61]

The chronic form of subacute encephalopathy is characterised by spongiform degeneration of the corticospinal tracts associated with vacuolar degeneration of oligodendrocytes. Symptoms progress from cerebellar and extrapyramidal, to diffuse spasms and palsy, which ultimately can lead to death. Radiological aspects on MRI are quite specific and consist of hyperintense lesions on T_2, mainly localised in the supratentorial white matter, the cerebellar hemispheres and the posterior limb of the internal capsule, sparing the anterior one and the subcortical white matter. In the acute phases, diffusion is restricted by cytotoxic oedema, while subacute phases are associated with an increased prevalence of myelin damage (Fig. 5-44).

The most common secondary complications from heroin abuse are infections. Up to 45–58% of patients with localised endocarditis develop neurological sequelae from septic embolism (mycotic aneurysms, brain abscesses).

Excytotoxic Oedema

Among the category of toxic encephalopathies, the so-called 'excytotoxic' forms are also considered. These are due to altered metabolism of glutamate related to various aetiology, resulting in an altered 'uptake' of this metabolite that accumulates in the synaptic region, thus determining an increase of post-synaptic excitatory activity followed by cytotoxic oedema, in most cases reversible. These conditions are detectable in hepatic insufficiency and in some forms of status epilepticus, particularly in cases associated with the use of opiates.[62] In those cases, the epileptogenic effect of an additive, acetylcodeine, is considered responsible (Fig. 5-45). Similar conditions can be also detected as a consequence of pharmacological intoxication (valproate) or sudden

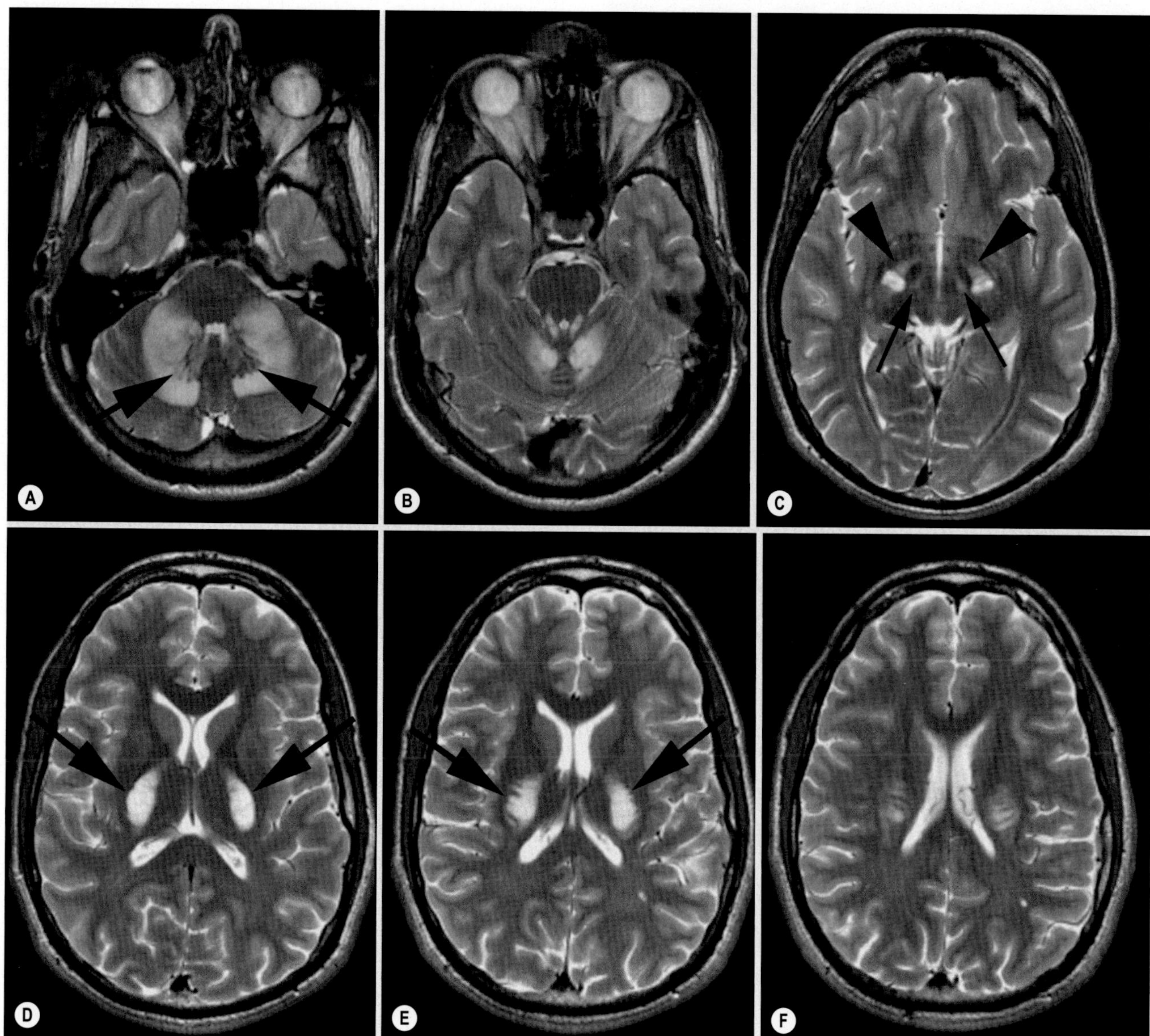

FIGURE 5-44 ■ **Extensive myelin degeneration after inhalation of heroin (so-called 'chasing the dragon').** Diffuse white matter changes are present, involving the posterior limb of the internal capsule (arrows in D, E), with sparing of the dentate nuclei (arrows in A) and the cerebellar cortex, and involvement of the corticospinal tracts (arrowheads in C) and medial lemnisci (arrows in C). (Courtesy of Dr. T. Krings, Toronto Western Hospital, Canada.)

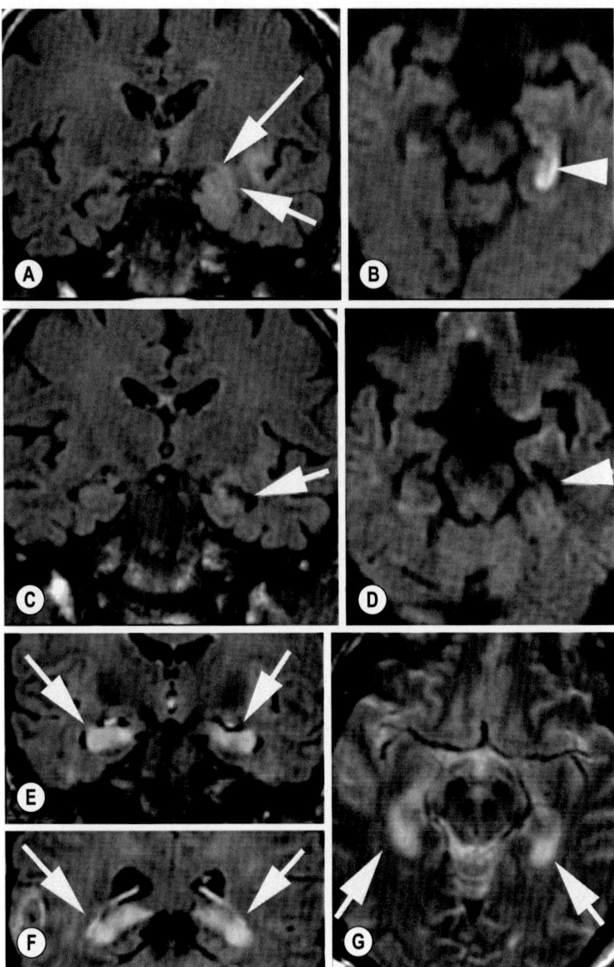

FIGURE 5-45 ■ **Two different examples of hippocampal excytotoxic oedema as a consequence of exogenous intoxication.** (A, B) A case of delirium tremens in alcohol withdrawal. (C, D) Same case in the chronic phase. Hippocampal signal is normalised and atrophic changes are evident with dilatation of the temporal horns. (E, F) Status epilepticus after heroin injection. This condition is probably related to epileptogenic addictives (such as acetylcodeine). Bilateral hippocampal oedema is clearly evident on both FLAIR (E, F) and T_2-weighted sequences (G).

withdrawal of alcohol or antiepileptic drugs. In this last case, the splenium of the corpus callosum can be selectively involved.[63]

REFERENCES

1. Lublin FD, Reingold SC. Defining the clinical course of multiple sclerosis: results of an international survey. National Multiple Sclerosis Society (USA) Advisory Committee on Clinical Trials of New Agents in Multiple Sclerosis. Neurology 1996;46:907–11.
2. Rovira Cañellas A, Rovira Gols A, Río J, et al. Idiopathic inflammatory-demyelinating diseases of the central nervous system. Neuroradiology 2007;49:393–409.
3. Ascherio A, Munger KL. Environmental risk factors for multiple sclerosis. Part I: the role of infection. Ann Neurol 2007;61:288–99.
4. Rovira A, León A. MR in the diagnosis and monitoring of multiple sclerosis: an overview. Eur J Radiol 2008;67:409–14.
5. Filippi M, Rocca MA. MR imaging of multiple sclerosis. Radiology 2011;259:659–81.
6. McFarland HF, Stone LA, Calabresi PA, et al. MRI studies of multiple sclerosis: implications for the natural history of the disease and for monitoring effectiveness of experimental therapies. Mult Scler 1996;2:198–205.
7. Calabrese M, Filippi M, Gallo P. Cortical lesions in multiple sclerosis. Nat Rev Neurol 2010;6:438–44.
8. Bagnato F, Jeffries N, Richert ND, et al. Evolution of T1 black holes in patients with multiple sclerosis imaged monthly for 4 years. Brain 2003;126:1782–9.
9. Lycklama G, Thompson A, Filippi M, et al. Spinal-cord MRI in multiple sclerosis. Lancet Neurol 2003;2:555–62.
10. Cotton F, Weiner HL, Jolesz FA, Guttmann CR. MRI contrast uptake in new lesions in relapsing-remitting MS followed at weekly intervals. Neurology 2003;60:50–6.
11. Masdeu JC, Quinto C, Olivera C, et al. Open-ring imaging sign: highly specific for atypical brain demyelination. Neurology 2000;54:1427–33.
12. Montalban X. Primary progressive multiple sclerosis. Curr Opin Neurol 2005;18:261–6.
13. Rocca MA, Hickman SJ, Bö L, et al. Imaging the optic nerve in multiple sclerosis. Mult Scler 2005;11:537–41.
14. Bermel RA, Bakshi R. The measurement and clinical relevance of brain atrophy in multiple sclerosis. Lancet Neurol 2006;5:158–70.
15. Stadelmann C, Ludwin S, Tabira T, et al. Tissue preconditioning may explain concentric lesions in Baló's type of multiple sclerosis. Brain 2005;128:979–87.
16. Given CA, Stevens BS. The MRI appearance of tumefactive demyelinating lesions. Am J Roentgenol 2004;182:195–9.
17. Wingerchuk DM, Weinshenker BG. Neuromyelitis optica: clinical predictors of a relapsing course and survival. Neurology 2003;60:848–53.
18. Wingerchuk DM, Lennon VA, Pittock SJ, et al. Revised diagnostic criteria for neuromyelitis optica. Neurology 2006;66:1485–9.
19. Ghezzi A, Bergamaschi R, Martinelli V, et al. Clinical characteristics, course and prognosis of relapsing Devic's Neuromyelitis Optica. J Neurol 2004;251:47–52.
20. Pittock SJ, Lennon VA, Krecke K, et al. Brain abnormalities in neuromyelitis optica. Arch Neurol 2006;63:390–6.
21. Menge T, Hemmer B, Nessler S, et al. Acute disseminated encephalomyelitis: an update. Arch Neurol 2005;62:1673–80.
22. Krupp LB, Tardieu M, Amato MP, et al. International Pediatric Multiple Sclerosis Study Group criteria for pediatric multiple sclerosis and immune-mediated central nervous system demyelinating disorders: revisions to the 2007 definitions. Mult Scler 2013;19:1261–7.
23. Tenembaum S, Chamoles N, Fejerman N. Acute disseminated encephalomyelitis: a long-term follow-up study of 84 pediatric patients. Neurology 2002;59:1224–31.
24. Mondejar RR, Santos JMG, Villalba EF. MRI findings in a remitting-relapsing case of Bickerstaff encephalitis. Neuroradiology 2002;44:411–14.
25. Siva A. Vasculitis of the nervous system. J Neurol 2001;248:451–68.
26. Birnbaum J, Hellmann DB. Primary angiitis of the central nervous system. Arch Neurol 2009;66:704–9.
27. Salvarani C, Brown RD Jr, Calamia KT, et al. Primary central nervous system vasculitis: analysis of 101 patients. Ann Neurol 2007;62:442–51.
28. Lie JT. Classification and histopathologic spectrum of central nervous system vasculitis. Neurol Clin 1997;15:805–19.
29. Goodwin J. Temporal arteritis. In: Gilman S, editor. Neurobase. 4th ed. Ann Arbor, MI: Ann Arbor Publishing; 2000.
30. Provenzale JM, Allen NB. Wegener granulomatosis: CT and MR findings. Am J Neuroradiol 1996;1996;17:785–92.
31. Christoforidis GA, Spickler EM, Recio MV, et al. MR of CNS sarcoidosis: correlation of imaging features to clinical symptoms and response to treatment. Am J Neuroradiol 1999;20:655–69.
32. Siva A, Kantarci OH, Saip S, et al. Behçet's disease: diagnostic and prognostic aspects of neurological involvement. J Neurol 2001;248:95–103.
33. Akman-Demir G, Bahar S, Coban O, et al. Cranial MRI in Behçet's disease: 134 examinations of 98 patients. Neuroradiology 2003;45:851–9.
34. Koçer N, Islak C, Siva A, et al. CNS involvement in neuro-Behcet's syndrome: an MR study. Am J Neuroradiol 1999;20:1015–24.

35. Hanly JG. Neuropsychiatric lupus. Rheum Dis Clin North Am 2005;31:273–98.
36. Sibley JT, Olszynski WP, Decoteau WE, Sundaram MB. The incidence and prognosis of central nervous system disease in systemic lupus erythematosus. J Rheumatol 1992;19:47–52.
37. Brey RL. Neuropsychiatric syndromes in lupus: prevalence using standardized definitions. Neurology 2002;58:1214–20.
38. Appenzeller, S, Pike GB, Clarke AE. Magnetic resonance imaging in the evaluation of central nervous system manifestations in systemic lupus erythematosus. Clin Rev Allergy Immunol 2008;34: 361–6.
39. Sibbitt WL Jr, Brooks WM, Kornfeld M, et al. Magnetic resonance imaging and brain histopathology in neuropsychiatric systemic lupus erythematosus. Semin Arthritis Rheum 2010;40:32–52.
40. Sundgren PC, Jennings J, Attwood TJ, et al. MRI and 2D-MR CSI spectroscopy of the brain in the evaluation of patients with acute onset of neuropsychiatric systemic lupus erythematosus. Neuroradiology 2005;47:576–85.
41. Steens SCA, Admiraal-Behloul F, Bosma GP, et al. Selective gray damage in neuropsychiatric lupus. A magnetisation transfer study. Arthritis Rheum 2004;50:2877–81.
42. Welsh RC, Rahbar H, Foerster B, et al. Brain diffusivity in patients with neuropsychiatric systemic lupus erythematosus with new acute neurological symptoms. J Magn Reson Imagn 2007;26:541–51.
43. Geibprasert S, Gallucci M, Krings T. Alcohol-induced changes in the brain as assessed by MRI and CT. Eur Radiol 2010;20: 1492–501.
44. Torvik A, Lindboe CF, Rogde S. Brain lesions in alcoholics. A neuropathological study with clinical correlations. J Neurol Sci 1982;56:233–48.
45. Harper C. The neurotoxicity of alcohol. Hum Exp Toxicol 2007; 26:251–7.
46. Arbelaez A, Pajon A, Castillo M. Acute Marchiafava-Bignami disease: MR findings in two patients. Am J Neuroradiol 2003;24: 1955–7.
47. Harper C. Wernicke's encephalopathy: a more common disease than realised. A neuropathologicalstudy of 51 cases. J Neurol Neurosurg Psychiatry 1979;42:226–31.
48. Victor M, Adams RD, Collins GH. The Wernicke-Korsakoff syndrome: a clinical and pathological study of 245 patients, 82 with post-mortem examinations. Contemp Neurol Ser 1991;7:1–206.
49. Gallucci M, Bozzao A, Splendiani A, et al. Wernicke encephalopathy: MR findings in five patients. Am J Roentgenol 1990;155: 1309–14.
50. Zuccoli G, Santa Cruz D, Bertolini M, et al. MR imaging findings in 56 patients with Wernicke encephalopathy: nonalcoholics may differ from alcoholics. Am J Neuroradiol 2009;30:171–6.
51. Shogry ME, Curnes JT. Mamillary body enhancement on MR as the only sign of acute Wernicke encephalopathy. Am J Neuroradiol 1994;15:172–4.
52. Larner AJ, Zeman AZ, Allen CM, Antoun NM. MRI appearances in subacute combined degeneration of the spinal cord due to vitamin B_{12} deficiency. J Neurol Neurosurg Psychiatry 1997;62: 99–100.
53. Hagiwara K, Okada Y, Shida N, Yamashita Y. Extensive central and extrapontine myelinolysis in a case of chronic alcoholism without hyponatremia: a case report with analysis of serial MR findings. Intern Med 2008;47:431–5.
54. Ruzek KA, Campeau NG, Miller GM. Early diagnosis of central pontine myelinolysis with diffusion-weighted imaging. Am J Neuroradiol 2004;25:210–13.
55. Blanco M, Casado R, Vazquez F, Pumar JM. CT and MR imaging findings in methanol intoxication. Am J Neuroradiol 2006;27: 452–4.
56. Daubert GP, Katiyar A, Wilson J, Baltarowich L. Encephalopathy and peripheral neuropathy following diethylene glycol ingestion. Neurology 2006;66:782–3.
57. Rovira A, Alonso J, Cordoba J. MR imaging findings in hepatic encephalopathy. Am J Neuroradiol 2008;29:1612–21.
58. O'Donnell P, Buxton PJ, Pitkin A, Jarvis LJ. The magnetic resonance imaging appearances of the brain in acute carbon monoxide poisoning. Clin Radiol 2000;55:273–80.
59. Aydin K, Sencer S, Demir T, et al. Cranial MR findings in chronic toluene abuse by inhalation. Am J Neuroradiol 2002;23:1173–9.
60. Josephs KA, Ahlskog JE, Klos KJ, et al. Neurologic manifestations in welders with pallidal MRI T1 hyperintensity. Neurology 2005;5:2033–9.
61. Geibprasert S, Gallucci M, Krings T. Addictive illegal drugs: structural neuroimaging. Am J Neuroradiol 2010;31:803–8.
62. Brennan FN, Lyttle JA. Alcohol and seizures: a review. J R Soc Med 1987;80:571–3.
63. Gallucci M, Limbucci N, Paonessa A, Caranci F. Reversible focal splenial lesions. Neuroradiology 2007;49:541–4.

CHAPTER 6

Neurodegenerative Diseases and Epilepsy

Beatriz Gomez Anson • Frederik Barkhof

CHAPTER OUTLINE

AGEING AND DEMENTIA—INTRODUCTION AND CLINICAL

With the rising age of the population, both normal ageing phenomena in the brain and neurodegenerative disorders become more prevalent. While exceptionally the brain may not be affected by age (successful ageing), the more typical or unusual ageing involves general involutionary alterations, which may mimic or herald neurodegenerative disease. Clinically, mild memory loss and reduced processing speed are considered normal for age, and can only be objectively established with extensive neuropsychological testing.

Dementia is a clinical syndrome that is defined as an acquired condition involving multiple cognitive impairments that are sufficient to interfere with activities of daily living, and often is progressive. Alzheimer's disease (AD) is the most common cause of dementia and often presents with memory impairment, but in other diseases like frontotemporal dementia (FTD), behavioural or language problems may prevail. Diagnosis is critically dependent on careful history taking from patient and informant, followed by clinical and cognitive examination supported by ancillary investigations, of which neuroimaging is one of the most important.

The a priori chance of a particular disease being present is dependent on age. In younger patients, more rare disease may occur and FTD is relatively common, although AD is still the most prevalent disorder. In the older patients, AD, dementia with Lewy bodies (DLB) and vascular disease are the most common. Mixed AD and vascular disease is the most frequent pathology in the elderly (>85 years). Genetic causes of dementia are important in FTD, but only explain 1–2% of (presenile) AD cases. Neoplasms rarely present with cognitive decline.

Ancillary investigations in the work-up of suspected dementia are quite important, since clinical diagnosis has a relatively low accuracy compared to histopathology. Cerebrospinal fluid (CSF) analysis plays an important role by examining levels of β-amyloid and (phosphorylated) tau. Neuroimaging is the most important ancillary investigation in the work-up of suspected dementia, and should be combined with clinical, neuropsychological and laboratory data in a multidisciplinary conference to enhance diagnostic accuracy. Despite the absence of definitive treatment for most disorders, establishing a correct nosological disorder is important in terms of counselling and planning, and identifying relevant (vascular) comorbidity.

NORMAL AGEING PHENOMENA IN THE BRAIN

Normal ageing may be subdivided into successful ageing (without any discernible changes) and the more commonly observed typical (usual) ageing. Typical ageing includes a variety of changes, including overall brain shrinkage, but also local alterations, such as white matter changes. Many of these 'normal' ageing phenomena have been linked to risk factors (e.g. vascular) and although cognitive function may seem intact, subtle abnormalities may be detected on detailed neuropsychological testing.

TABLE 6-1 Brain Alterations Observable during Typical/Usual Ageing

Mild-to-moderate brain volume loss:
- Ventricular enlargement, including third ventricle
- Sulcal enlargement mostly affecting frontal and parietal lobes
- Mild medial temporal lobe atrophy and hippocampal sulcus cavities

Enlarged perivascular (Virchow–Robin) spaces on/in the:
- Basal ganglia region, near the anterior commissure (large ones seen on CT)
- White matter of centrum semiovale, near the vertex (MRI only)
- Mesencephalon (MRI only)

Changes of the vascular wall:
- Elongation and tortuosity (e.g. basilar artery)
- Wall-thickening and calcification (e.g. carotid siphon or vertebral artery)

Vascular changes (better visible on MRI than CT):
- Punctiform or early confluent ischaemic white matter changes
- Lacunar infarcts and microbleeds

Iron accumulation on MRI in the:
- Globus pallidus, putamen, dentate nucleus

Calcifications on CT in the:
- Globus pallidus, pineal gland, choroid plexus (esp. foramen of Luschka)
- Cerebral falx, sometimes with bony transformation

Such relationships are often only discernible on a group level, and predictions in individual subjects are difficult to provide.

Table 6-1 lists the alterations observable in typical/usual ageing.

DEMENTIA—IMAGING APPROACH

Indications for Imaging

The focus of imaging in suspected dementia has shifted from an exclusionary to an inclusionary approach.[1] Exclusion of a (surgically) treatable cause of dementia (e.g. tumour or subdural haematoma) can be ascertained by using computed tomography (CT), but demonstration of positive disease markers (e.g. hippocampal atrophy for AD) becomes increasingly more relevant and magnetic resonance imaging (MRI) adds positive predictive value to the diagnosis in dementia. Catheter angiography (DSA) is hardly ever indicated, except perhaps for suspicion of vasculitis. While MRI is the modality of choice for investigating dementia, multislice CT offers a reasonable alternative, with coronally reformatted images enabling examination of the medial temporal lobe. However, CT is still clearly inferior to MRI, for example, in subjects suspected of having some rare disorders causing dementia, such as encephalitis or Creutzfeldt–Jakob disease (CJD).

When structural imaging is equivocal or does not lead to the diagnosis, functional imaging may add diagnostic value.[2] Second-line investigations include metabolic information obtained by using single-photon emission computed tomography (SPECT) or positron emission

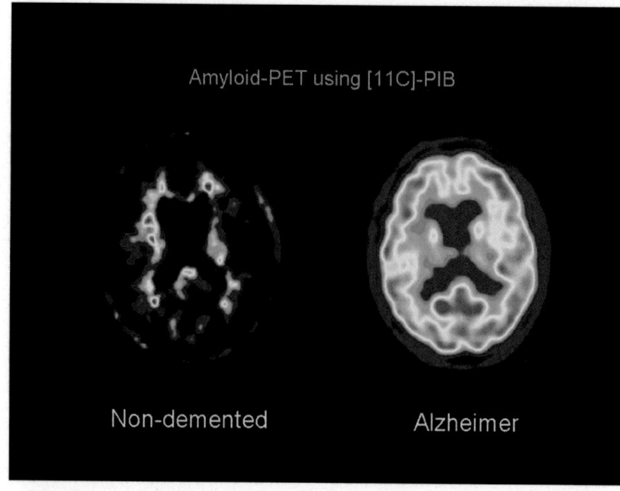

FIGURE 6-1 ■ Amyloid-PET using [^{11}C]-PIB in a healthy control (left) and patient with Alzheimer's disease (right). Note low physiological binding to the white matter only in the control and widespread cortical tracer uptake in AD. (Image courtesy of Bart van Berckel.)

tomography (PET), or physiological information obtained by using diffusion or perfusion MRI. For example, in the early stages of frontotemporal lobar degeneration (FTLD) without discernible atrophy, fluorodeoxyglucose PET (FDG-PET) or hexamethylpropyleneamine oxime SPECT (HMPAO-SPECT) may already demonstrate decreased metabolism or hypoperfusion. Molecular imaging provides even more early and specific information, e.g. amyloid-PET in Alzheimer's disease (Fig. 6-1) and dopaminergic tracers in Lewy-body dementia.

Protocol for CT and MRI

Sructured reporting is essential in dementia[3] and should consider:

- Exclusion of mass lesion, haematoma or hydrocephalus.
- Vascular pathology: territorial infarcts, lacunes, thalamic lesions, white matter lesions.
- Focal atrophy:
  - Medial temporal lobe and hippocampus or precuneus (AD)
  - Frontal lobe and temporal pole (FTLD)
  - Mesencephalon (progressive supranuclear palsy)
  - Pons (multisystem atrophy).

ALZHEIMER'S DISEASE AND OTHER PRIMARY NEURODEGENERATIVE DEMENTIAS

Alzheimer's Disease

The disease is named after Aloïs Alzheimer, who first described senile plaques and neurofibrillary tangles in a 51-year-old woman in 1906. Although the aetiology of AD is uncertain, the amyloid cascade predicts that

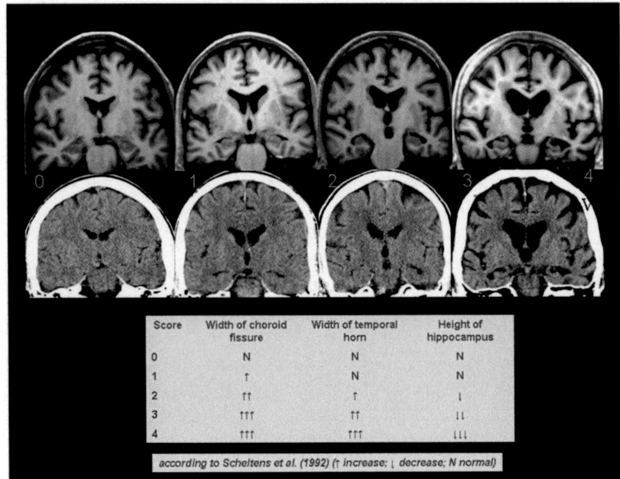

Score	Width of choroid fissure	Width of temporal horn	Height of hippocampus
0	N	N	N
1	↑	N	N
2	↑↑	↑	↓
3	↑↑↑	↑↑	↓↓
4	↑↑↑	↑↑↑	↓↓↓

according to Scheltens et al. (1992) (↑ increase; ↓ decrease; N normal)

FIGURE 6-2 ■ Visual rating of medial temporal lobe atrophy (MTA). In these same-day studies a perfect similarity between MRI and CT is noted for assessment of the medial temporal lobe for visual rating of MTA. (Modified with permission from Radiology 2009;253:174–183.)

FIGURE 6-3 ■ In this patient with onset of Alzheimer's disease at the age of 62, there is little hippocampal atrophy (green circle) but more severe atrophy of the precuneus, including the posterior cingulate (red circle).

abnormal aggregation of amyloid leads to impaired nerve function, formation of extracellular amyloid (neuritic) plaques and subsequent formation of intracellular neurofibrillary tangles, leading to neuronal loss and atrophy. The process usually starts in the medial temporal lobe (entorhinal cortex and hippocampus) or the posterior cingulate, and then spreads to the tempoparietal cortex. In <1% of cases, a mutation in genes encoding for amyloid-processing enzymes is found; however, most cases are sporadic, with APOE4 genotype increasing the risk of AD moderately. Age and cardiovascular risk factors are important predictors as well.

The clinical manifestations of AD are episodic memory impairment, but in younger patients visuospatial disturbances may prevail, and even language problems can be seen. While a clinically probable AD diagnosis requires interference in at least two separate domains, biomarkers such as CSF amyloid, PET and MRI can be useful in the prodromal stage of mild cognitive impairment (MCI) by providing evidence of amyloid pathology and subsequent neurodegeneration. The conversion rate from MCI to AD is 10–15% per year and this risk increases markedly when MRI shows atrophy suggestive of AD, e.g. hippocampal atrophy.

MRI and CT are both useful for excluding surgically treatable disorders and demonstrate focal atrophy suggestive of AD.[4] Coronal images perpendicular to the long axis of the temporal horn should be used to determine the amount of hippocampal and medial temporal lobe atrophy (MTA). Since volumetric analysis of the hippocampus is quite time-consuming, MTA can best be analysed using a visual rating scale depicted in Fig. 6-2.

A score of 2 is considered abnormal under the age of 75, and a score of 3 above that age. Strong asymmetry between left and right side should trigger a suspicion of FTD, which can be recognised by concomitant atrophy of the temporal poles and frontal lobes. In younger subjects with AD, the hippocampus may be spared, with pathology dominating in the precuneus (including posterior cingulate) and parietal cortex (Fig. 6-3).

Vascular changes and AD are common and therefore coexisting pathologies in the elderly. The combination of infarcts and Alzheimer pathology is the strongest predictor of dementia in population-based autopsy studies. Atherosclerosis may lead to ischaemic brain damage and probably also accelerates the formation of Alzheimer pathology. In individual patients, it may be difficult to pinpoint their respective relevance, but vascular alterations, especially white matter lesions on MRI, provide an independent target for treatment. Treatment of vascular risk factors may not only prevent further vascular pathology but also benefit progress of AD.

FRONTOTEMPORAL LOBAR DEGENERATION

The term FTLD describes a group of disorders with tau pathology presenting with language and behavioural symptoms. FTLD is the third most common degenerative cause of dementia after AD and dementia with Lewy bodies, accounting for about 5–10% of all cases of dementia and, in younger patients, it is second in frequency after AD. Arnold Pick first described patients with focal atrophy of the frontal and temporal lobes in 1892, including patients with both personality change and language impairment.

The Lund-Manchester criteria recognise three main subtypes of FTLD:

- behavioural variant frontotemporal dementia (bvFTD);
- progressive non-fluent aphasia (PNFA); and
- semantic dementia (SD).

Less commonly, patients with right-sided FTLD present with difficulty recognising faces. It should be noted that language and behavioural disturbances can also be seen

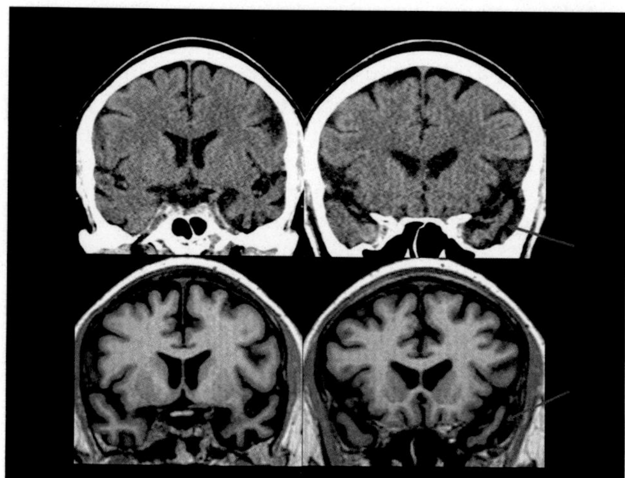

FIGURE 6-4 ■ **Coronal CT and MR in a patient with semantic dementia, part of the FTLD spectrum.** Note that the coronal reformats of the multidetector CT (top) are quite comparable to the coronal MR (bottom) images in showing left more than right anterior temporal atrophy in the same patient. (Images courtesy of Mike Wattjes.)

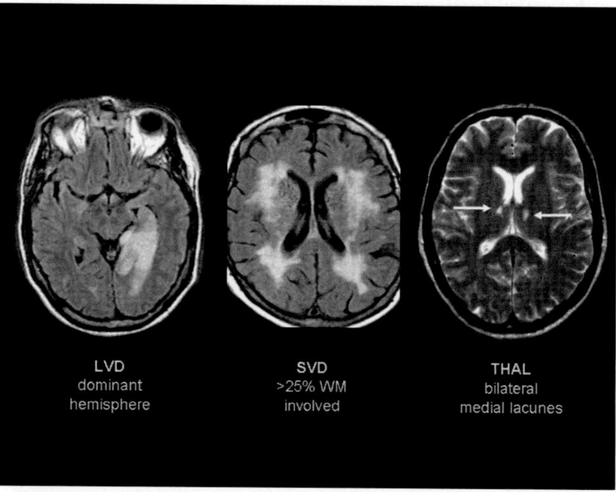

FIGURE 6-5 ■ Vascular dementia is a heterogeneous group of disorders that can be caused by large-vessel infarcts in strategic locations (mostly in the dominant hemisphere), by extensive small-vessel disease and/or by bilateral thalamic lesions. Large-vessel vascular disease (LVD), small-vessel vascular disease (SVD), thalamic disease (THAL).

in (atypical) AD cases and corticobasal degenration (CBD) and progressive supranuclear palsy (PSP).

In contrast to AD, a significant proportion of patients with FTLD have an autosomal dominant family history, sometimes linked to chromosome 17, which can be due to mutations in the microtubule-associated protein tau (MAPT) or progranulin. Other mutations can be found as well, especially in patients with increasingly recognised overlap syndromes with motor neuron disease and amyotrophic lateral sclerosis (ALS).

The hallmark imaging finding in FTLD is atrophy of the temporal and frontal lobes, often (initially) asymmetrical (Fig. 6-4). The patients presenting with the language variant SD often have marked left temporal lobe atrophy (temporal pole more than hippocampus), but in patients with bvFTD, atrophy of the frontal lobes can be mild at the time of presentation. In particular, in these patients, FDG-PET and perfusion MRI can be useful detect functional changes, although care should be taken to exclude depression, which may be similar clinically and on imaging.

VASCULAR DEMENTIA

Vascular dementia (VaD) is the second most common type of dementia after AD, especially in the elderly (where they often coexist and even reinforce one another). The term VaD implies the existence of dementia; however, it is often hard to prove dementia is indeed secondary to cerebrovascular disease (only). Furthermore, VaD is a heterogeneous entity and comprises various conditions due to small- or large-vessel involvement:

- Diffuse confluent age-related white matter changes (ARWMC):
  - also referred to as subcortical arteriosclerotic encephalopathy (SAE).
- Multilacunar state ('état lacunaire').
- Multiple (territorial) infarcts.
- Strategic cortical–subcortical or borderzone infarcts.
- Cortical laminar necrosis (granular cortical atrophy).
- Delayed post-ischaemic demyelination.
- Hippocampal sclerosis.

Clearly, not every vascular pathological finding seen on brain MRI or CT is sufficient to associate with occurrence of dementia in a given patient.[5] The NINDS-AIREN (National Institute of Neurological Disorders and Stroke and Association Internationale pour la Recherché et l'Enseignement en Neurosciences) criteria are the most strict ones for VaD and detail various causes of small- and large-vessel pathology that are likely to cause dementia (Fig. 6-5), which we will discuss in the following sections.

Large-Vessel VaD

Dementia may result from multiple or single cortical–subcortical or subcortical (e.g. borderzone) cerebrovascular lesions (infarcts) involving strategic regions of the brain, such as the hippocampus, paramedian thalamus and the thalamocortical networks, especially if they occur in the dominant hemisphere.

Small-Vessel VaD

Also referred to as leukoaraïosis or subcortical arteriosclerotic encephalopathy, extensive small-vessel disease due to microangiopathy is the most common form of VaD. Most of these cases are idiopathic or sporadic; i.e. there is no proven or specific/genetic cause that can be identified, although many patients will have a history of cardiovascular risk factors. Within the group of small-vessel VaD, the following subtypes exist:

- extensive white matter lesions—confluent hyperintensities involving >25% of WM;

- multiple lacunes—at least two lacunes in basal ganglia and centrum semiovale each; and
- bilateral thalamic lesions—small infarcts in both medial thalami.

Fluid-attenuated inversion recovery (FLAIR) is most suited for detecting small-vessel disease and is able to differentiate (hyperintense) white matter lesions from (hypointense) lacunes. Thalamic lesions, however, are better seen on T2 than FLAIR images. Recent white matter lesions can be bright on diffusion-weighted imaging (DWI), suggesting recent 'lacunar' infarction (i.e. involving a single perforating arteriolar territory). White matter lesions with more severe tissue destruction become T1 hypointense and are better appreciated on CT and tend to correlate better with clinical severity. The white matter lesions in small-vessel VaD involve most of the deep white matter of frontal and parietal lobes, but tend to spare the U-fibres (in contrast to multiple sclerosis) and the temporal lobes (in contrast to multiple sclerosis and CADASIL; see below). The basal ganglia and the central pons are also frequently affected.

CADASIL, Fabry's Disease and CAA

While no specific cause can be identified in most cases of small-vessel VaD, there are few examples of inherited/genetic diseases that can be identified readily using MRI:

- cerebral autosomal dominant arteriopathy with subcortical infarcts and leukoencephalopathy (CADASIL);
- Fabry's disease; and
- cerebral amyloid angiopathy (CAA).

CADASIL is caused by a mutation in the gene *notch-3* and may present with headache and presenile dementia. In presymptomatic mutation carriers, the white matter of the temporal poles is often affected in mid-life, and by the time patients become symptomatic, very extensive white matter changes extending into the U-fibres at the convexity are present (Fig. 6-6). Lacunes and microbleeds are common.

Fabry's disease is an X-linked recessive vasculopathy resulting from α-galactosidase A deficiency. Since it accounts for ~1% of male strokes, there should be screening for it in young male patients. The imaging findings are mostly non-specific small- and large-vessel pathology on CT or MRI. A relatively specific MRI finding is hyperintensity of the pulvinar on T1-weighted images, with hypointensity on T2*-weighted images in the more severe cases, related to calcification on CT.

Several rare genetic causes of CAA exist in small genetic clusters. Most CAA cases, however, are sporadic and present with lobar haemorrhaging and extensive white matter lesions and (silent) infarcts. Less advanced cases may present with multiple cerebral microbleeds (MBs) only, which can be visualised with T2* gradient-echo images or susceptibility-weighted images (Fig. 6-7). Such MBs are a risk factor for subsequent bleeding and stroke in CAA, but also in more typical cases of stroke. CAA is due to β-amyloid deposition in the media and adventitia of small- to medium-sized cerebral arteries and is linked to Alzheimer pathology in a substantial number of cases.

Systemic Causes of VaD

In addition to ischaemia caused by vascular wall changes, as discussed in the preceding sections, systemic disorders can also cause ischaemia and lead to cognitive dysfunction and ultimately dementia. Systemic causes of ischaemia include cellular dysfunction (mitochondrial disease), but also clotting disorders (e.g. sickle-cell disease) and anaemia/hypotension.

Differential Diagnosis of WM Disorders in Dementia

While most white matter lesions in ageing and dementia are of vascular origin, there is a long differential diagnosis that might be considered, especially in young-onset cases.

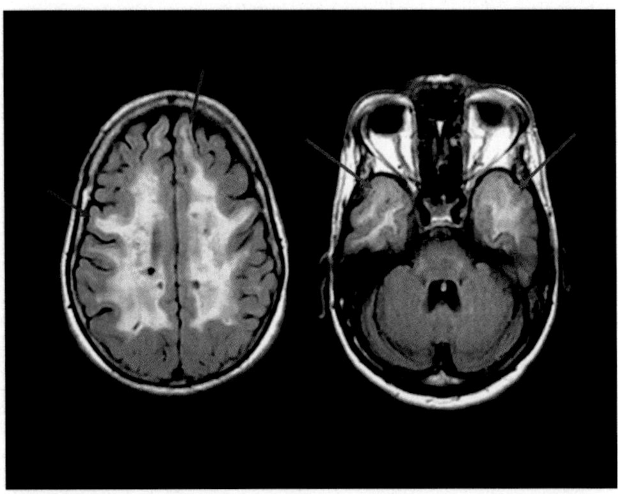

FIGURE 6-6 ■ White matter lesions in CADASIL differ from those in common small-vessel disease by involving the temporal poles (red arrows) and U-fibres at the convexity (blue arrows).

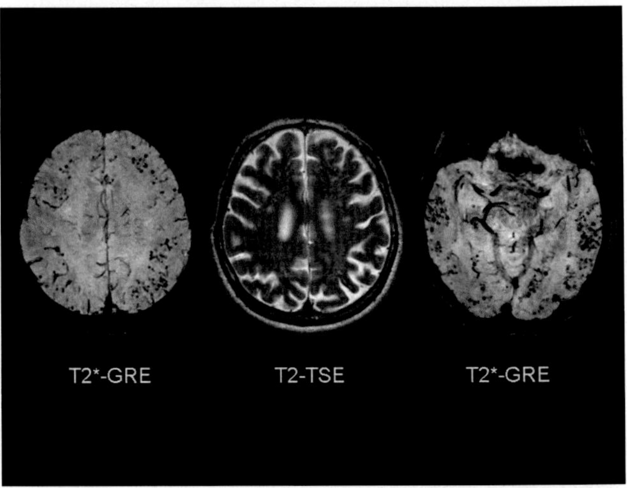

FIGURE 6-7 ■ Gradient-echo (GRE) T2*-weighted images reveal hundreds of small lobar microbleeds not seen on routine T2 spin-echo (TSE) images due to the blooming effect caused by haemosiderin in vessel walls, which became fragile due to amyloid deposition in this patient with Alzheimer's disease.

For example, multiple sclerosis may first present with cognitive impairment, especially when juxtacortical lesions are abundant. Other autoimmune disorders that tend to impair cognition include SLE. Several metabolic disorders may first present in adulthood, e.g. vanishing white matter disease and adult polyglucosan body disease. These typically present with symmetric confluent white matter abnormalties and should be differentiated from toxic disorders. Finally, several infections can manifest with dementia, e.g. HIV encephalitis and progressive multifocal leukoencephalopathy (PML), which will be discussed in the next section.

RAPIDLY PROGRESSIVE AND OTHER ATYPICAL DEMENTIAS

Infectious and Inflammatory Disease

HIV and PML

HIV may affect the brain in several ways. First, direct infection may lead to HIV encephalitis. Secondly, opportunistic infections, such as toxoplasmosis, CMV and PML, may occur. HIV encephalitis is best demonstrated on FLAIR images that may show an ill-defined and often symmetrical hyperintensity in the cerebral white matter, with no typical predilection—the subcortical U-fibres are characteristically spared. PML is an opportunistic infection that occurs in up to 5% of AIDS patients, and has a very poor prognosis, even with treatment. PML is caused by the JC papovavirus, a ubiquitous DNA virus that infects oligodendrocytes in immunocompromised patients and leads to massive demyelination with rapidly progressive clinical presentation. CT may reveal multifocal lesions with swelling and marked hypodensity with little contrast enhancement. MRI is more sensitive and shows multiple focal T2 hyperintense and markedly T1 hypointense lesions, located in the subcortical white matter, with gyral swelling mostly sparing the cortical ribbon—so-called 'scalloping out' of the grey–white border. Gadolinium enhancement is rare and, if it occurs, is patchy.

Prion Disease

Prions are protein-like structues that may cause disease in an infectious manner, especially in those that are genetically susceptible. Prion diseases include:

- Creutzfeldt–Jakob disease (CJD)—sporadic, familial and iatrogenic forms;
- variant CJD (vCJD)—sporadic (and possibly iatrogenic);
- Gerstmann–Sträussler–Scheinker (GSS) syndrome—only familial;
- fatal familial insomnia (FFI)—familial and sporadic; and
- kuru—only sporadic.

CJD usually presents in the fifth to seventh decade, and is sporadic in the vast majority of cases. Presentation typically is with a triad of subacute dementia, myoclonus and motor disturbances (extrapyramidal or cerebellar)

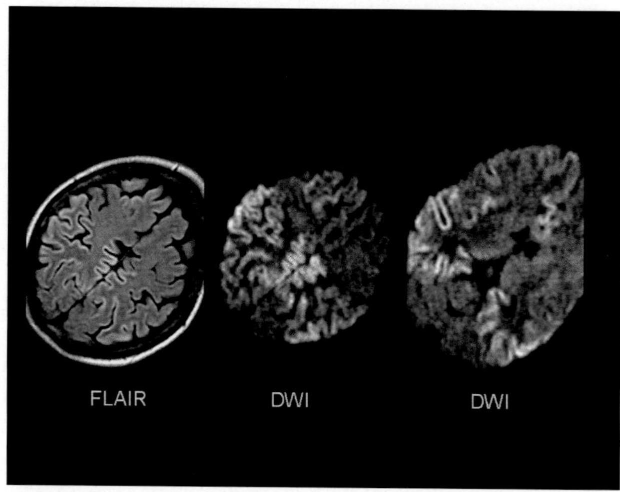

FIGURE 6-8 ■ In this patient with rapid cognitive decline due to CJD, FLAIR images show mildly increased signal intensity in multiple areas of the neocortex, which are much more prominent on DWI.

with a characteristic EEG pattern consisting of triphasic waves and CSF abnormalities (increased tau and/or 14-3-3 protein).

MRI should include DWI; images after contrast material administration are useful for ruling out alternative disorders. FLAIR sequences may show increased signal in the striatum, especially the putamen, or discontinous involvement of the neocortex (Fig. 6-8). Abnormal DWI may be especially prominent in early phases of the disease when vacuoles are small, leading to restricted diffusion (which may disappear in late stages). Sometimes there is a combination of neocortical and subcortical involvement. Usually the pattern of involvement is bilateral, but it may be unilateral as well (initially).

Autoimmune Limbic Encephalitis

Non-infectious limbic encephalitis occurs in patients presenting with a subacute onset of memory impairment and confusion, focal, usually medial temporal lobe seizures. Classically, this occurs in the context of a distant malignancy (mostly lung cancer) through a variety of antibodies. However, non-neoplastic variants exist as well, with a similar autoimmune basis. These include antibodies against voltage-gated potassium channels or the NMDA-receptor, but may also involve antibodies that are gluten-sensitivity or thyroid-related (Hashimoto's encephalitis). Typically, the hippocampus is involved with hyperintensity and swelling on coronal FLAIR images, but more extensive abnormalities may involve the basal ganglia as well (e.g. in Hashimoto's encephalitis). The differential diagnosis includes herpes simplex encephalitis, which is often unilateral and involves the insula as well.

Toxic/Metabolic Disorders

Toxic encephalopathies include vitamin B deficiencies, dialysis dementia, CO intoxication, delayed post-hypoxic demyelination, organic solvents (including toluene) and heroin intoxication. Wernicke's encephalopathy mostly occurs in alcoholics due to vitamin B_1 deficiency and typical MRI findings comprise T2/FLAIR hyperintensity in the medial thalamus, mamillary bodies, periaqueductal grey matter and colliculi. Increased signal on T1 may occur due to microhaemorrhages and diffusion can be restricted in the acute phase. In vitamin B_{12} deficiency, brain MRI may show diffuse supratentorial areas of T2 hyperintensity in the periventriclular and deep white matter, while brainstem and the cerebellar white matter are relatively spared. Spinal cord MRI may show a mild swelling and signal abnormalities in the dorsal and lateral columns. Contrast enhancement is not observed.

Most leukodystrophies are genetically determined and present early in life and lead to dementia in a later phase. However, some leukodystrophies present later in life and do have cognitive decline as a characteristic feature, e.g vanishing white matter, mitochondrial disease and cerebro-tendinous xanthomatosis. The cardinal imaging feature of the leukodystophies is involvement of the white matter, with hyperintensity on T2-weighted and FLAIR images. Involvement usually occurs in a strictly symmetric fashion, except in mitochondrial disorders such as mitochondrial encephalomyopathy, lactic acidosis and stroke-like episodes (MELAS). The corticospinal tracts and cerebellum are frequently involved structures. Important diagnostic clues can be obtained from the family history, and from involvement of the peripheral nervous system, the eyes, adrenal glands, tendons or other organs. The most common genetic disorder is fragile X associated tremor/ataxia syndrome (FXTAS), which presents mostly in men after the age of 50 with intention tremor or gait ataxia; bilateral hyperintensity of the middle cerebellar peduncles is one of the diagnostic criteria.

PARKINSON'S DISEASE AND RELATED DISORDERS

Idiopathic Parkinson's Disease and Differential Diagnosis

Idiopathic Parkinson's disease is caused by abnormal accumulation of α-synuclein protein in grey matter of the brainstem and basal ganglia. The symptoms include bradykinesia, rigidity, tremor and loss of postural reflexes. The disease process starts in the substantia nigra in the mesencephalon and by the time patients become symptomatic, 90% of neurons have disappeared. The dopaminergic deficit itself can be demonstrated using PET or SPECT.

Since parkinsonism can be caused by other pathological features leading to the same dopaminergic deficit, structural imaging should aim to rule out:

- Secondary parkinsonism caused by focal pathological features in the basal ganglia:
  - especially vasculoischaemic lesions (Fig. 6-9).
- Parkinson-plus syndromes: progressive supranuclear palsy (PSP) and multiple system atrophy (MSA):
  - selective atrophy in the mesencephalon (PSP) and pons (MSA).

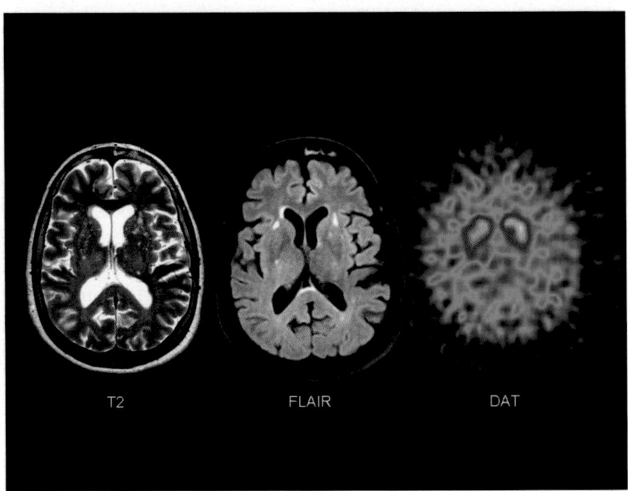

FIGURE 6-9 ■ This case of parkinsonism was secondary to vascular lesions in the basal ganglia seen on MRI, while a DAT-SPECT revealed normal striatal tracer uptake, which rules out primary Parkinson's disease.

  - Typical hyperintensities on MRI in the middle cerebellar peduncles and midpons in the cerebellar form of MSA (MSA-C), and along the lateral aspects of the putamina in the parkinsonian form of MSA (MSA-P).

Dementia with Parkinsonism

A number of neurodegenerative diseases present with a combination of cognitive impairment and parkinsonism. In many of these conditions additional phenotypic features such as dysautonomia, gaze palsies, cerebellar and pyramidal signs may suggest one pathological process over another, but none are pathognomonic for PSP, MSA or corticobasal degeneration (CBD).

Lewy body disease is the most common cause of progressive cognitive decline with parkinsonism. DLB and Parkinson's disease dementia (PDD) are regarded as ends of a continuous spectrum—the former with an initial presentation with dementia, the latter presenting with parkinsonism followed by dementia after more than a year, but ultimately both have widely distributed Lewy bodies in the cerebral cortex.

Imaging findings in dementia with parkinsonism (Fig. 6-10) include:

- DLB—normal hippocampi on MRI, abnormal dopamine SPECT;
- PSP—mesencephalic atrophy on MRI ('humming-bird' sign); and
- MSA—pontine atrophy and 'hot-cross bun' sign.

Neurodegeneration and Other Movement Disorders

Non-parkinsonian movement disorders can be found in a rare number of other neurodegenerative disorders. For example, amyotrophic lateral sclerosis (ALS)-like phenotypes can be seen in FTD.

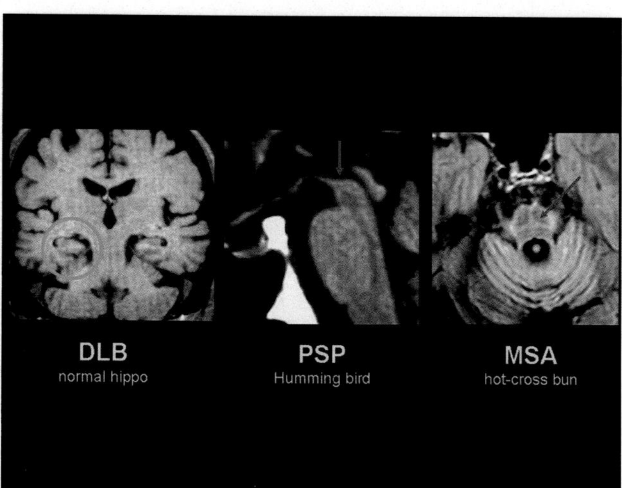

FIGURE 6-10 ■ MRI findings in patients with dementia and parkinsonian features. In DLB, a normal hippocampus helps to rule out Alzheimer's disease. In progressive supranuclear palsy (PSP), severe mesencephalic atrophy occurs, giving the appearance of a hummingbird on mid-sagittal images. In multisystem atrophy (MSA), there is severe atrophy of the pons, sometimes with a hot cross bun-like pattern on FLAIR and T2-weighted images.

Neuroimaging can help in the following diseases:

- Neurodegeneration with brain iron accumulation (NBIA, formerly Hallervorden–Spatz disease):
  - low signal on T2* images in the basal ganglia.
- Huntington's disease: atrophy of the caudate nucleus; and
- Wilson's disease: T2 hyperintensity in the mesencephalon.

EPILEPSY—INTRODUCTION AND CLINICAL

Epilepsy is defined as a chronic neurological condition of patients having spontaneous, recurrent seizures as a result of increased neuronal discharges. It has a prevalence of 0.4 to 1% in the population.[6] Epilepsy syndromes can be divided into two groups: generalised and focal (partial). In generalised syndromes seizures originate simultaneously from both cerebral hemispheres, which can either occur primarily or as a consequence of focal seizures extending to the rest of the brain (secondary generalisation).

Focal seizures/epilepsy syndromes start in a localised area of the brain and are classified as simple partial seizures, if the patient does not suffer any loss of consciousness during the seizure, or complex partial seizures, which are always associated with loss of consciousness.

Classification of Seizures

- Generalised
  - Primary generalised
  - Secondarily generalised
- Focal (partial)
  - Simple partial
  - Complex partial

Initial treatment of epilepsy is medical, with a large variety of antiepileptic drugs currently available in clinical practice. Most patients with generalised seizures respond to antiepileptic drug treatment. Although about 30% of patients with partial seizures are resistant to medical treatment,[7] further treatment options are available, the most effective being surgical resection of the brain region/lesion causing the seizures.

Appropriate classification of patients with seizures, and especially those having medically refractory epilepsy, is crucial for improving management and care of patients. Imaging tools, especially MRI, play a substantial role in detecting pathological features underlying the seizure origin. However, the ability of MRI to detect underlying brain lesions/abnormalities in patients with epilepsy varies and depends on the patient groups studied. In general, MRI has a greater sensitivity for lesion detection in patients with intractable epilepsy, amounting to about 85%.[8] The value of MRI in patients with idiopathic, generalised epilepsy is very little. However, with advances in technology, improved knowledge of neuroradiologists and more dedicated epilepsy clinics, the value of imaging will certainly increase, especially when MRI is combined with functional imaging techniques, including nuclear medicine (PET and SPECT).

EPILEPSY—IMAGING APPROACH

Indications for Imaging

Current published guidelines for management of patients with epilepsy include that MRI should always be performed in a non-urgent setting, excluding those patients with idiopathic, generalised seizures. In the urgent setting, especially if there are focal neurological signs, or associated fever or trauma, CT remains the examination of choice.

The main role of MRI in a patient with epilepsy is to identify an underlying brain abnormality that relates to the patient's symptoms and that helps to define the clinical syndrome. MRI helps in characterising underlying pathological substrates, and in defining their relationship to functional brain areas, such as those related to motor or language tasks. Concordance of the lesion seen on imaging with either clinical or electrophysiological data, indicating a possible origin of the seizures (lateralisation to one cerebral hemisphere), is crucial for appropriate patient assessment. Finally, MRI also helps in defining surgical treatment options in patients with intractable epilepsy, and in the postsurgical setting. In this regard, MRI, either alone or combined with other functional imaging techniques, such as PET, may provide further insight in patients having poor response to surgery, identifying remaining epileptogenic areas.[9]

Imaging Protocol

Appropriate MRI of the brain in patients with epilepsy should include high-resolution volumetric T1, high-resolution T2 (Fig. 6-11) and FLAIR images covering the entire brain. Coronal images are very helpful in depicting

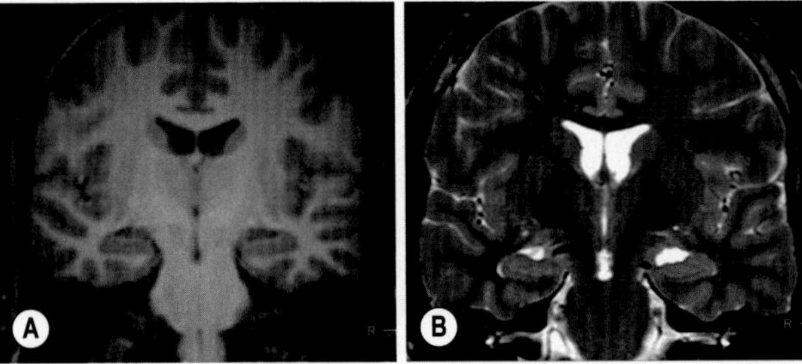

FIGURE 6-11 ■ Dedicated MRI to study patients with epilepsy. High-resolution T1 coronal (A) and T2 (B) images, covering the entire brain, and allowing detailed assessment ot the medial temporal lobes, should be obtained.

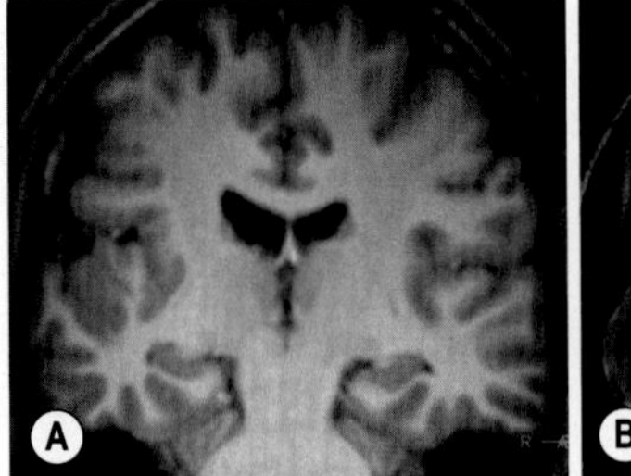

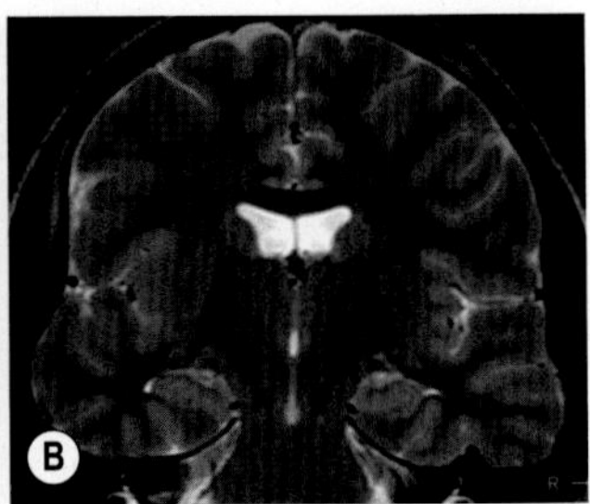

FIGURE 6-12 ■ MRI findings in a patient with an abnormality of cortical development. There is abnormal cortex, with abnormal gyri, around the right sylvian fissure (A), faint cortical T2 hyperintensity and blurring of the normal grey–white matter differentiation in the right insula (B).

the anatomical details of the temporal lobe structures, and especially of the hippocampus, as well as the cortex, where most epileptogenic lesions are encountered. As the search for asymmetries between both cerebral hemispheres is an important aspect of the neuroradiological assessment, adequate patient positioning is crucial. As a general rule, both internal auditory meati should be identified on the same MR image.

Most common causes for epilepsy identified on MRI include post-traumatic brain lesions, tumours, vascular malformations and infections. Additionally, MRI is particularly helpful in identifying further entities, more commonly seen in patients with intractable epilepsy, such as hippocampal sclerosis, abnormalities of cortical development, syndromes associating with several intracranial abnormalities, such as the phacomatoses, and other less common abnormalities, including non-specific areas of gliosis.

EPILEPSY—CONGENITAL DISORDERS

Migration and Gyration Disorders

Developmental disorders have been increasingly recognised on MRI in children and young adults with epilepsy, accounting for up to 50% of paediatric cases of intractable epilepsy, and about 25% of those in young adults.[10] Disorders altering neuronal and glial proliferation, migration or organisation of the cortical layers are now grouped together as abnormalities of cortical development and further subclassified, depending on the most relevant underlying pathogenesis.

These abnormalities include the following entities, which may also coexist in the same patient, and involve different brain regions simultaneously:

- cortical dysplasia
- focal cortical dysplasia (FCD)
- agyria/pachygyria
- polymicrogyria
- heterotopias
- schizencephaly
- hamartomas, or cavernous malformations (according to some authors).

Typical MRI findings are the presence of abnormal cortex, which may be thickened, or have few or too many, abnormal gyri. There may also be abnormal sulci, cortical signal abnormalities and abnormalities in the underlying white matter, with blurring and loss of the normal cortical–subcortical differentiation on MRI (Fig. 6-12).

Abnormalities of cortical development, especially in focal cortical dysplasia, are characterised by areas of abnormal lamination of the cortex, and abnormal 'balloon neurons' on histology. MRI features include thickened cortex, which may be slightly hyperintense on T2 images, and blurring of the cortical–subcortical boundaries. The patients may have further abnormalities in the ipsilateral, or even contralateral medial temporal lobe structures on MRI, including changes in the hippocampi with loss of hippocampal volume and T2 signal change, reflecting neuronal loss and gliosis, as shown on epilepsy surgery specimens.[11] Abnormalities of cortical metabolism on FDG-PET may be larger than the abnormal area on structural MRI, indicating that abnormalities in the brain of patients with FCD are more extensive than previously thought. The significance of these findings with respect to patients' symptoms is unclear, but they may potentially indicate additional areas of epileptogenesis.[12,13]

Heterotopias are characterised by the presence of normal neurons in abnormal locations, and they are usually divided into three types based on clinical and imaging features: subependymal/periventricular, subcortical and band/laminar. Heterotopias typically show the same signal as cortical grey matter on all sequences, and they may be associated with other abnormalities of cortical development, such as schizencephaly. Band heterotopias (Fig. 6-13) are considered as a mild form of lissencephaly (smooth brain) by some authors, and have recently been associated with several different genes.[14]

In general, many abnormalities of cortical development are indeed epileptogenic, but the extent of the epileptogenic area may be greater than the lesion seen on MRI, or the epileptogenic area may not precisely correlate with the malformation itself. As mentioned already, FDG-PET can show more widespread areas of abnormal metabolism in the brain than those seen on structural MRI.[15] For these reasons imaging information always needs to be considered within the context of all patient investigations, taking into account clinical and electrophysiological data, especially if patients are being considered as surgical candidates.

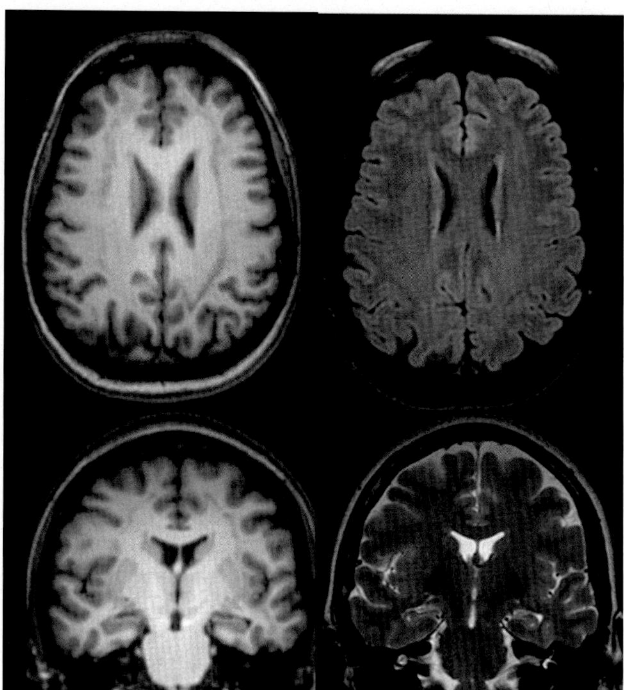

FIGURE 6-13 ■ MRI findings in a patient with band heterotopias in both cerebral hemispheres. Axial and coronal T1 (left top and bottom, respectively), axial FLAIR (right top) and coronal T2 (right bottom) images. There are band-like appearances of grey matter signal on all sequences within the white matter of both cerebral hemispheres which are most conspicuous on the T1 images.

Genetic Syndromes

Several genetic and congenital syndromes are associated with epilepsy, including some of the better known neurocutaneous syndromes, such as tuberous sclerosis and Sturge–Weber syndrome.

Tuberous sclerosis complex is a multisystem congenital syndrome with widespread CNS anomalies. Neurological manifestations include epilepsy and cognitive impairment, and approximately 90% of patients have seizures, with intractable epilepsy developing in 25–30% of patients. Typical imaging findings include cortical or subcortical tubers, subependymal nodules, subependymal giant cell astrocytomas and white matter radial migration lines (Fig. 6-14). On T2-weighted and FLAIR MR images, tubers typically appear as areas of increased signal intensity in the cortical and subcortical regions. Subependymal nodules are found on the walls of the lateral ventricles. Subependymal giant cell astrocytomas can grow, eventually resulting in ventricular obstruction and hydrocephalus. Radial migration lines are believed to represent heterotopic glia and neurons along the expected path of cortical migration. Radial migration lines are primarily located in the subcortical white matter and are occasionally seen in relation to tubers.

Patients with the Sturge–Weber neurocutaneous syndrome present typically with a facial angioma in the trigeminal nerve distribution and ipsilateral meningeal angiomatosis. Clinically, patients have intractable seizures, hemiparesis, hemianopsia and mental retardation.

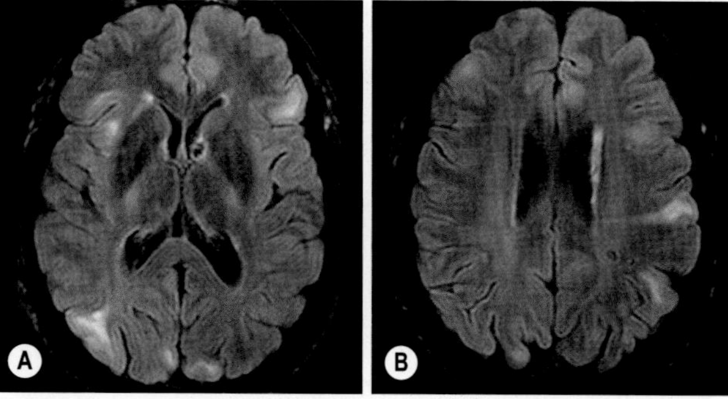

FIGURE 6-14 ■ MRI findings in a patient with tuberous sclerosis. Axial FLAIR image (A) shows several hyperintense cortical–subcortical tubers in both cerebral hemispheres, a subependymal tumour at the level of the foramen of Monroe on the left and signal change areas in the white matter representing radial migration lines, reaching the left lateral ventricle (B).

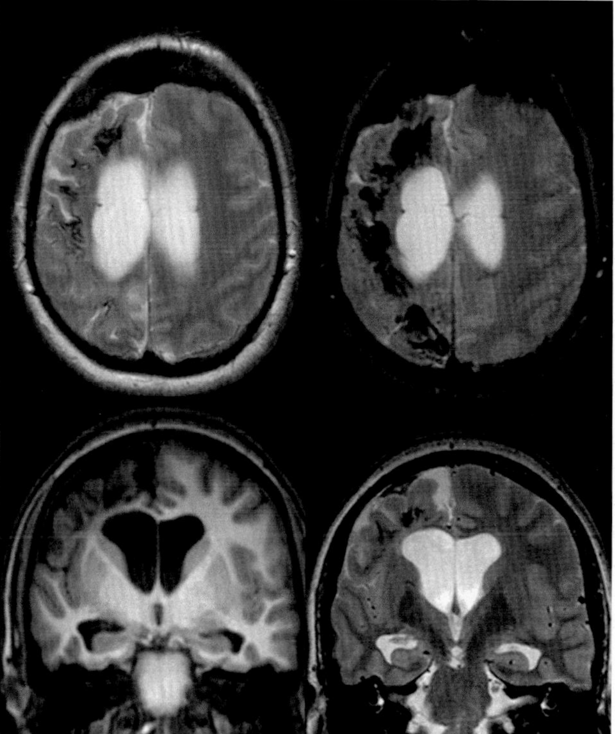

FIGURE 6-15 ■ Typical MRI findings in a patient with Sturge–Weber syndrome. The predominantly hypointense pial angioma is seen in the right cerebral hemisphere, which has a smaller volume. T2* gradient-echo images show the signal change associated with the pial angiomata more clearly (above right side).

MRI findings in these patients may include (Fig. 6-15):

- pial angiomata in the parieto-occipital regions;
- cortical calcifications subjacent to the cortex and white matter, typically in the parieto-occipital region;
- enlarged choroid plexus;
- atrophy of the ipsilateral cerebral hemisphere (angioma side);
- enlarged and elongated globe of the eye; and

- prominent enlarged subependymal and medullary veins, and secondary signs of cerebral atrophy involving the paranasal sinuses, mastoid cells and calvarium.

EPILEPSY—ACQUIRED DISEASES

Hippocampal Sclerosis

This is the most common abnormality found in temporal lobe resections of patients with intractable epilepsy undergoing surgery. On pathology, this entity is defined by the presence of neuronal loss and gliosis. Typical MRI findings[16] are hippocampal volume loss and increased T2 signal within the abnormally small hippocampus (Fig. 6-16).

Further imaging findings on MRI in patients with hippocampal sclerosis include:

- loss of the internal architecture of the hippocampus;
- atrophy of the ipsilateral mamillary body and fornix; and
- dilatation of the adjacent temporal horn.

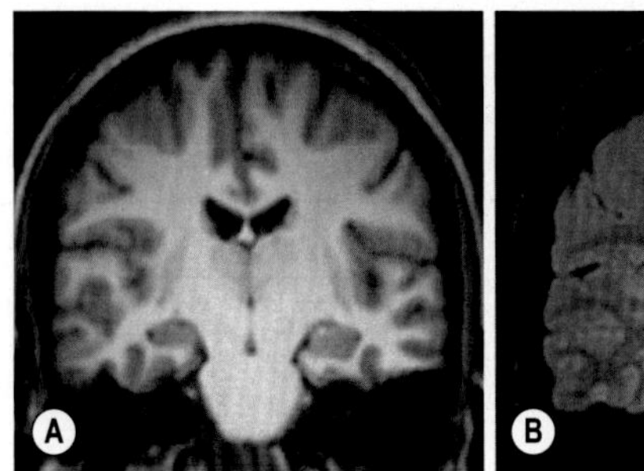

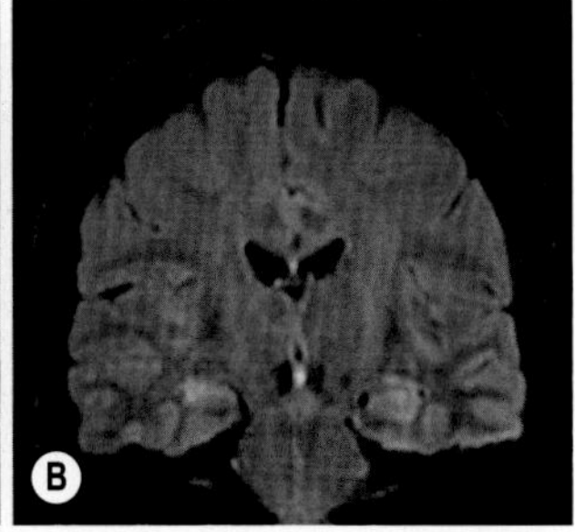

FIGURE 6-16 ■ MRI findings in hippocampal sclerosis. There is loss of volume of the right hippocampus seen on high-resolution T1-weighted images (A), as well as increased T2 signal within it on coronal FLAIR images (B), reflecting neuronal loss and gliosis, respectively.

MRI identifies up to 90% of the cases of hippocampal sclerosis. Hippocampal sclerosis may also occur bilaterally in up to 20% of the cases. Some patients may have an additional epileptogenic area, either temporal extra-hippocampal or even extratemporal, which is referred as 'dual pathology'. The most common association occurs between cortical dysplasia and hippocampal sclerosis. Surgery is curative in up to 70% of patients with hippocampal sclerosis, especially in those not having dual pathology, and where there is a concordance in lateralisation among clinical, electrophysiological and MRI information.[17]

Neoplasms

A tumour is found in about 4% of patients having epilepsy. About 70% of those tumours causing epilepsy are found in the temporal lobes and in most cases near the cortex. MRI is particularly helpful in defining the relationship of tumours to functionally eloquent areas of the brain, as complete resection of the tumour and overlying cortex results in complete control of seizures in many cases, and improves the patient's outcome.

In patients with seizures, the tumours most frequently found include low-grade astrocytomas, gangliogliomas, dysembryoplastic neuroepithelial tumour (DNET), oligodendroglioma, pleomorphic xanthoastrocytoma and metastasis.[16] The precise characterisation of these tumour types is not always straightforward. Gangiogliomas are usually found in the temporal lobes in young adults, are partly solid and partly cystic and are located in the cortex. They may show calcification and contrast enhancement. DNETs are low-grade, multicystic tumours, also located in the cortex, or middle temporal lobe structures, usually occurring in children and young adults. Their radiological appearance is variable, and there may be calcification, bleeding and contrast enhancement in up to a third of cases (Fig. 6-17).

In patients with tumours, functional MRI techniques have proven to be useful for surgical planning. Using different paradigms, such as a motor or verbal task, eloquent areas of the brain and their relationship to the

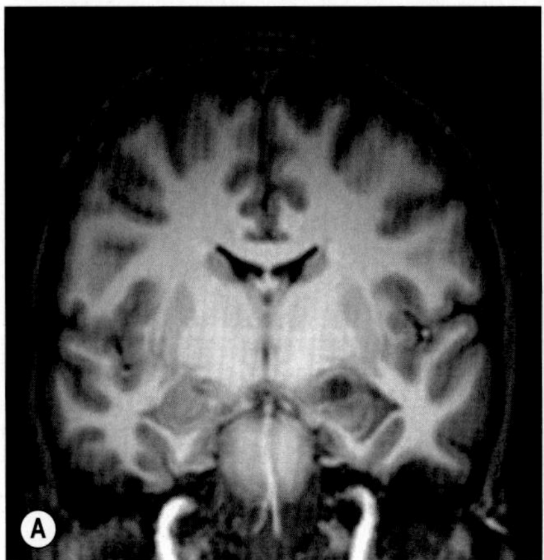

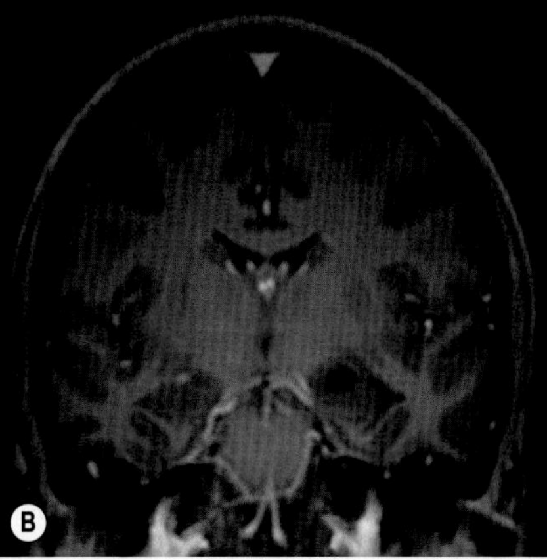

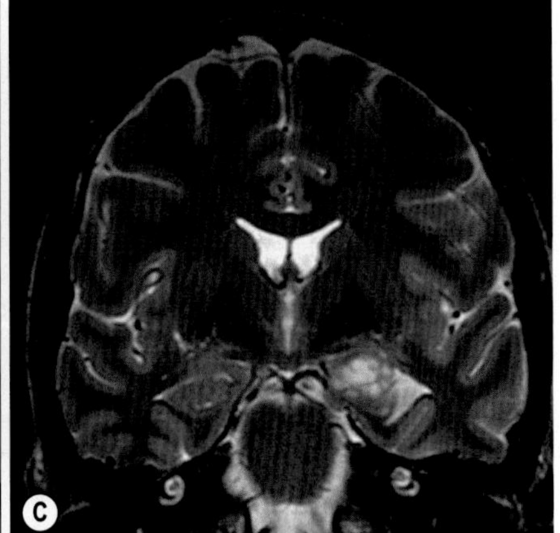

FIGURE 6-17 ■ MRI findings in a patient with a DNET in the left medial temporal lobe, involving the hippocampus. The mass appears heterogenously T1 hypointense with a cystic component (A), and no contrast enhancement (B), as well as heterogeneous T2 hyperintense (C).

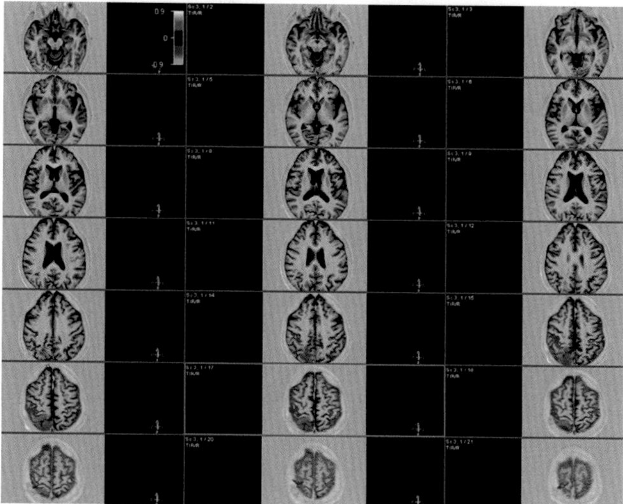

FIGURE 6-18 ■ fMRI using a motor task (opposition of all digits, alternating both hands). The primary motor cortex of both cerebral hemispheres is shown. The right hemisphere tumour lies posterior to the right-sided primary motor area, being adjacent to it, but not in close contact. The risk for motor-deficit postsurgically exists, but is less than with a tumour attached to or involving the functional area.

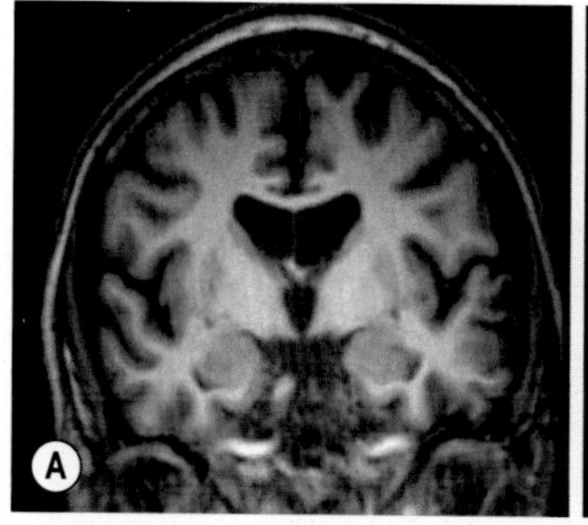

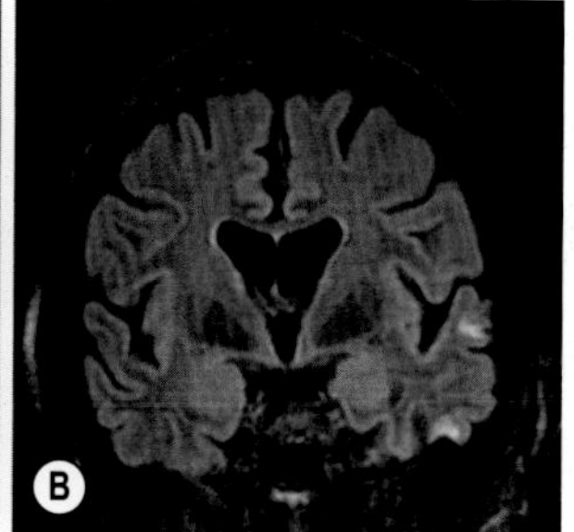

FIGURE 6-19 ■ MRI findings in a patient with post-traumatic epilepsy. There is an abnormal left superior temporal gyrus, showing cortical thinning and signal change, which is hypointense on T1 images (A), and hyperintense on FLAIR images (B), in keeping with mature damage (encephalomalacia).

tumour can be identified, allowing a better assessment of potential for focal deficits after surgery (Fig. 6-18).

Post-Traumatic Epilepsy

This is not an uncommon condition. Head injuries can cause damage to the cortex, most frequently in the frontal lobes or in the temporal regions, due to the underlying, adjacent bony structures. Cerebral contusions at these sites may leave haemosiderin deposits and gliosis, which are known to be involved in seizure generation and propagation. Several risk factors have been identified for late post-traumatic epilepsy, such as early seizures, severe brain injury, depressed skull fractures, penetrating injuries or brain contusions. MRI is very helpful in showing acute and chronic haemorrhage, diffuse axonal injury and gliosis (Fig. 6-19).

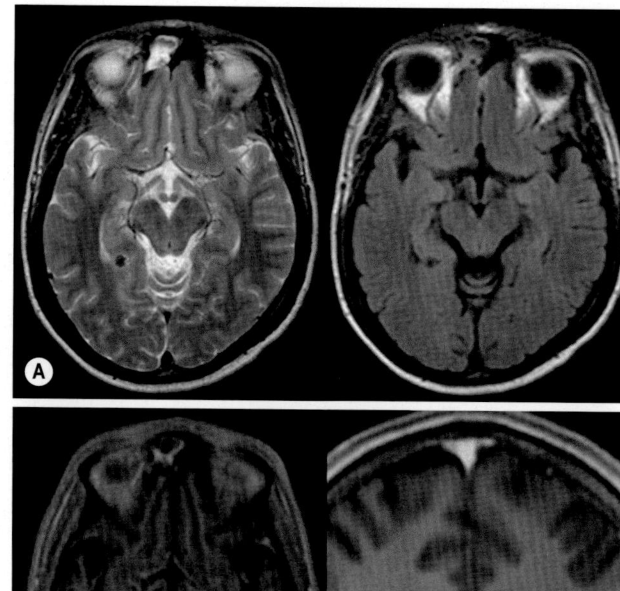

FIGURE 6-20 ■ MRI findings in a patient with cysticercosis. There is a small, rounded lesion in the right posterior part of the medial temporal lobe, of low signal on T2 and FLAIR images (A) region, which enhances only very minimally (B). The appearances are consistent with a partially calcified nodular stage of cysticercosis.

Infections

Bacterial, viral, fungal, mycobacterial or parasitic infections may cause seizures, both in the acute phase (being the early clinical presentation), as well as in the chronic stage, as a result of gliosis. Among these, cysticercosis frequently presents with seizures, and can be identified on imaging studies. In the active phase, cysticercosis appears as thin-walled, non-enhancing cysts that may have an eccentrically located nodule (scolex) within them. Death of the parasite causes inflammatory changes in the adjacent brain, with vasogenic oedema and enhancement. In the final stages, calcification occurs (Fig. 6-20).

Rasmussen encephalitis is a chronic encephalitis characterised by partial motor seizures and progressive neurological and cognitive deterioration, mostly seen in children. MRI demontrates involvement of one cerebral hemisphere, with increased T2 signal in the cortex and subcortical white matter, progressing to atrophy in the late stages.

REFERENCES

1. Scheltens P, Fox N, Barkhof F, De Carli C. Structural magnetic resonance imaging in the practical assessment of dementia: beyond exclusion. Lancet Neurol 2002;1(1):13–21.
2. Filippi M, Agosta F, Barkhof F, et al. EFNS task force: the use of neuroimaging in the diagnosis of dementia. Eur J Neurol 2012; 19(12):e131–40, 1487–501.

3. Barkhof F, Fox NC, Bastos-Leite A, Scheltens P. Neuroimaging in Dementia. Berlin: Springer-Verlag; 2011.
4. Wattjes MP, Henneman WJ, van der Flier WM, et al. Diagnostic imaging of patients in a memory clinic: comparison of MR imaging and 64-detector row CT. Radiology 2009;253(1):174–83.
5. van Straaten EC, Scheltens P, Knol DL, et al. Operational definitions for the NINDS-AIREN criteria for vascular dementia: an interobserver study. Stroke 2003;34(8):1907–12.
6. Bell GS, Sander JW. The epidemiology of epilepsy: the size of the problem. Seizure 2001;16:165–70.
7. Arroyo S. Evaluation of drug-resistant epilepsy. Rev Neurol 2000; 30:881–9.
8. Bronen RA, Fulbright RK, Spencer DD, et al. Refractory epilepsy: comparison of MR imaging, CT, and histopathologic findings in 117 patients. Radiology 1996;201:97–105.
9. Duncan J. The current status of neuroimaging for epilepsy. Curr Opin Neurol 2009;22(2):179–84.
10. Raymond AA, Fish DR, Sisodiya SM, et al. Abnormalities of gyration, heterotopias, tuberous sclerosis, focal cortical dysplasia, microdysgenesis, dysembryoplastic neuroepitheliala tumour and dysgenesis of the archicortex in epilepsy. Clinical, EEG and neuroimaging features in 100 adult patients. Brain 1995;118:629–60.
11. Gomez-Anson B, Thom M, Moran N, et al. Imaging and radiological-pathological correlation in histologically proven cases of focal cortical dysplasia and other glial and neuronoglial malformative lesions in adults. Neuroradiology 2000;42(3):157–67.
12. Palmini A, Gambardella A, Andermann F, et al. Operative strategies for patients with cortical dysplastic lesions and intractable epilepsy. Epilepsia 1994;35:57–71.
13. Sisodiya SM, Free SL, Stevens JM, et al. Widespread cerebral structural changes in patients with cortical dysgenesis and epilepsy. Brain 1995;118:1039–50.
14. Barkovich AJ, Raybaud CA. Malformations of cortical development. Neuroimag Clin N Am 2004;14:401–23.
15. Engel J Jr, Henry TR, Risinger MW, et al. Presurgical evaluation for partial epilepsy: relative contributions of chronic depth-electrode recordings versus FDG-PET and scalp-sphenoidal ictal EEG. Neurology 1990;40(11):1670–7.
16. Vatipally VR, Bronen RA. MR imaging of epilepsy: strategies for successful interpretation. Neuroimag Clin N Am 2004;14:349–72.
17. Spencer SS. When should temporal lobe epilepsy be treated surgically? Lancet Neurol 2002;1:375–82.

CHAPTER 7

Orbit

Stefanie C. Thust • Katherine Miszkiel • Indran Davagnanam

CHAPTER OUTLINE

THE ORBIT

INTRODUCTION

The orbit represents a key element of the visual pathway. Diseases of the orbit, particularly those affecting vision, may be severely debilitating and impact on many aspects of the affected individual's life. Owing to its complex structure and specialised function, there are several pathologies, which are specific to the orbit. Alternatively, the orbit may be involved in a variety of systemic processes including diseases of the retro-orbital visual pathway.

ORBITAL ANATOMY

The shape of the orbit can be likened to that of an elongated pyramid, whereby the base lies anteriorly and the apex posteriorly. The orbit has four walls: a roof, floor, medial and lateral wall, all of which converge posteriorly at the orbital apex. The medial orbital walls run virtually parallel, but due to the shape of the orbits, their long axes diverge at approximately 45°.[1] The roof of the orbit is composed of the frontal bone anteriorly and the lesser wing of sphenoid posteriorly. The orbital roof forms the floor of the frontal sinus and part of the anterior cranial fossa. At the anterior margin of the orbital roof, a small notch or sometimes a complete foramen can be found, which transmits the supraorbital nerve, a branch of the ophthalmic division (V1) of the trigeminal nerve. The floor of the orbit is made up of the zygomatic bone laterally and the maxilla medially, with a small contribution from the orbital process of the palatine bone; it contains a small canal for the infraorbital nerve, a branch of the maxillary division of the trigeminal nerve. The orbital floor forms the roof of the maxillary sinus and is relatively thin, thus susceptible to blow-out fracture or spread of severe sinus infection. The medial orbital wall is composed of several bones (maxilla, frontal, ethmoid, lacrimal and sphenoid) and separates the orbit from the ethmoid air cells. It is a very thin wall, also referred to as the lamina papyracea, and can easily be injured. The lateral wall of the orbit is formed by the frontal and zygomatic bones. It runs obliquely from lateral to medial posteriorly, separating the orbit from the temporal fossa anteriorly and from the middle cranial fossa posteriorly.

The following apertures can be found in the orbit posteriorly: the superior orbital fissure lies between the lateral orbital wall and roof and contains the cranial nerves (CN) III, IV and VI and the ophthalmic veins, which drain into the cavernous sinus; the optic nerve canal lies at the junction of the roof and medial wall and contains the optic nerve and ophthalmic artery; the inferior orbital fissure lies between the lateral wall and floor of the orbital and contains the infraorbital nerve.

There are six extraocular muscles: namely, four rectus muscles and two oblique muscles. The four rectus muscles arise from the annulus of Zinn, a fibrous tendon ring which surrounds the optic nerve at the orbital apex, and inserts into the globe. The superior oblique muscle runs from the orbital apex to the superior orbital border, where it loops around the trochlea and then passes posteriorly to insert in the globe. The inferior oblique muscle originates anteriorly from the orbital floor and inserts on the back of the globe. The lateral rectus muscle is innervated by the abducens nerve (CN VI) and the superior oblique muscle by the trochlear nerve (CN IV). All other extraocular muscles and also the levator palpebrae are supplied by the oculomotor nerve (CN III). The rectus muscles with their fascial layers form the *orbital cone*, a landmark which can be used to divide the orbit into three compartments: the *extraconal* compartment, which comprises all structures *peripheral* to the cone, the *conal* compartment and the *intraconal* compartment, which comprises all structures central to muscle. A compartmental approach is very useful when defining the anatomical location of orbital pathology, as this may significantly narrow the list of potential differentials. Even in cases of a multi-compartmental lesion, defining the epicentre of an abnormality may still be useful.

The orbital septum is an important anatomical boundary, which can be found anterior to the globe. It is an incomplete fibrous membrane continuous with the levator palpebrae superioris superiorly and the tarsus inferiorly and forms a barrier between the orbit and subcutaneous tissues. This can be relevant for the spread of infection.

The globe is divided into three major tissue layers. These are:

- the sclera and cornea, which constitute the outer layer;
- the middle layer representing the uvea, which consists of the choroid, the iris and ciliary body; and
- the inner layer, the retina.

The globe is divided by the lens and iris into an anterior chamber filled with aqueous humour and a posterior chamber filled with vitreous humour.

The optic nerve (CN II) consists of four segments: a very short intraocular portion, an intraorbital, intracanalicular and intracranial segment. Embryologically, it is not a true cranial nerve, but rather an extension of brain parenchyma; it is myelinated by oligodendrocytes and not Schwann cells. This explains why pathologies such as gliomas and meningiomas affect the optic nerve, whereas schwannomas and neurofibromas occur in other cranial nerves. Arterial supply to the optic nerve is via the retinal artery (a branch of the ophthalmic artery), which runs inside the nerve to the globe. Further branches of the ophthalmic artery which supply the orbit are the frontal, lacrimal and nasociliary branches. The superior and inferior ophthalmic veins represent the main venous drainage pathways of the orbit.

IMAGING OF THE ORBIT

Plain film radiography was historically performed as an initial assessment in suspected bony trauma, but had limited sensitivity and does not reliably assess the intraorbital soft tissues. Ultrasound, including colour Doppler sonography, can be very useful in evaluation of the globe, particularly of the retina and anterior chamber but is also useful in assessing vascularity in ocular tumours and directional flow through the superior ophthalmic veins. However, it has only limited benefit in assessing structures beyond the globe itself.

Computed tomography (CT) is readily available at most institutions and offers quick multiplanar orbital imaging. The different densities of orbital structures (bone, fat, muscles and vitreous humour) provide good natural contrast resolution. CT is useful in trauma to identify orbital and periorbital injuries, especially fractures, which are best identified on thin-section multiplanar bone reconstructions. The main role of contrast-enhanced CT of the orbits lies in evaluation of suspected infiltrative, inflammatory and neoplastic disease. Reconstruction is usually performed in the axial, coronal and sagittal planes, both with a soft-tissue and a bone reconstruction algorithm and a slice thickness of 1–3 mm (depending on equipment and local protocol) or less depending on equipment and the clinical question. Axial imaging should be acquired parallel to the orbital axis to allow visualisation of the optic nerve, medial and lateral rectus muscle on a single image. Coronal imaging must be perpendicular to the optic axis.[1]

Magnetic resonance imaging (MRI) has superior soft-tissue contrast to CT and is the most accurate technique in characterising orbital mass lesions. Like CT, MRI is capable of multiplanar imaging; however, these require usually separate acquisitions rather than reconstructions in at least two planes (usually axial and coronal). A typical orbital MRI protocol includes pre-contrast T1 and T2 fat-suppressed imaging and post-contrast imaging with at least one fat-suppressed sequence, all at a slice thickness of 3 mm or less. At minimum, a T2 sequence of the whole brain should also be performed to not miss coexisting intracranial pathology.

ORBITAL PATHOLOGY

Congenital Disease

Coats' Disease

Coats' disease is a congenital vascular malformation of the retina, which results in telangiectasis and aneurysm formation. Due to endothelial damage, leakage of exudative lipoproteniaceous fluid and blood product into the subretinal space occurs and results in progressive thickening of the retina and subsequent retinal detachment. The disease is usually unilateral and presents in childhood age. The most common presenting feature is leukocoria, but visual impairment, pain, secondary glaucoma and strabismus may occur.[2] The nature of the disease is progressive, with loss of vision over a variable length of time. CT findings include increased attenuation along the subretinal space or even filling the entire vitreous. MR imaging may demonstrate increased T1 and T2 signal due to presence of lipoproteinaceous material (Fig. 7-1). There is typically no contrast enhancement.

Persistent Hypertrophic Primary Vitreous (PHPV)

In embryogenesis, the primary vitreous connects the posterior aspect of the lens with the retina. As it is gradually being replaced by the definitive vitreous, the primary vitreous regresses into a band-like fibrovascular structure between the posterior lens surface and retina. A central hyaloid artery can remain present within this. There may

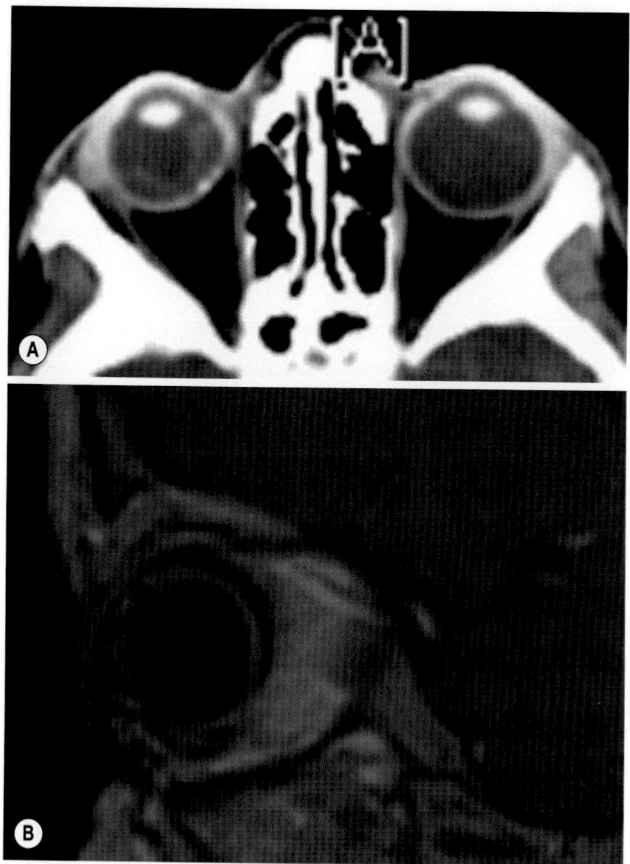

FIGURE 7-1 ■ **Coats' disease.** Axial CT of the orbits (A) demonstrates a right posterior hyloid detachment and filling of the posterior hyloid space which appears T1W hyperintense on the sagittal MRI of the orbits (B) representing accumulation of lipoproteniaceous fluid. Note that the right globe is small.

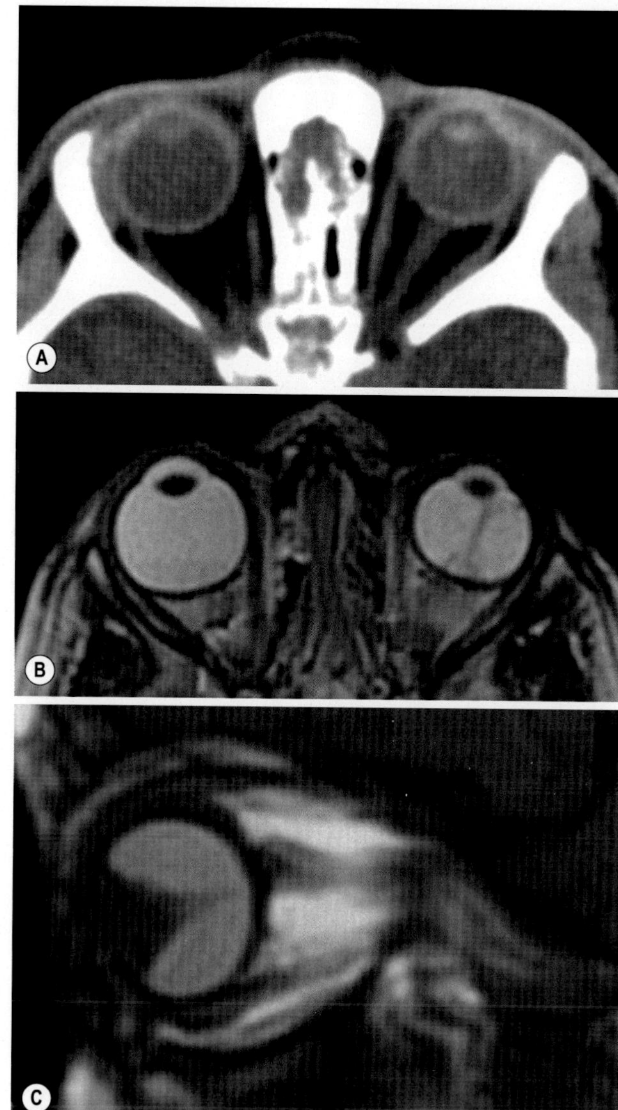

FIGURE 7-2 ■ **Persistent hypertrophic primary vitreous.** Axial CT of the orbits demonstrates a small left globe with a V-shaped retrolental density (A). On the MRI of the orbits on the axial T2W this confirms the presence of a retrolental hypointense fibrovascular band (B). The sagittal T1W (C) shows retinal detachment with T1W hyperintense subretinal haemorrhage.

be an associated defect in the posterior lens capsule resulting in complications such as lens swelling and destruction or cataract formation. Secondary retinal detachment is common and may appear as a V-shaped structure within the globe on axial imaging (owing to the retina being relatively fixed bilaterally at the ora serrata and posteriorly at the optic disc). Recurrent haemorrhage or glaucoma are indications for enucleation surgery.[2] On imaging, PHPV demonstrates a cone or band-shaped structure at the posterior aspect of the lens and is usually associated with microphthalmia. Blood product including fluid–fluid levels within the globe can be present if there has been recent haemorrhage. The presence of a linear septum extending from the lens to the retina is diagnostic (Fig. 7-2). The primary vitreous may demonstrate contrast enhancement. Surgical intervention with preservation of the eye is an option in patients with disease confined to the anterior portion of the globe, but not infrequently PHPV progresses to phthisis bulbi or requires enucleation.

Retinopathy of Prematurity

This has also been termed *retrolental fibroplasia* and represents a condition which occurs secondary to excessive oxygen therapy to treat premature lungs. This results in the arrested development of the retinal vasculature, which then recommences in a disorganised fashion with the growth of new vessels and fibrous tissue that may contract to cause retinal detachment. With the introduction of surfactant therapy to aid lung maturation, retinopathy of prematurity is becoming less common. Simultaneous periventricular leukomalacia may be encountered on brain imaging.

Coloboma

Congenital coloboma represents an anomaly of the optic nerve head, occurring during development of the eye. This may take the form of small optic pits to colobomas

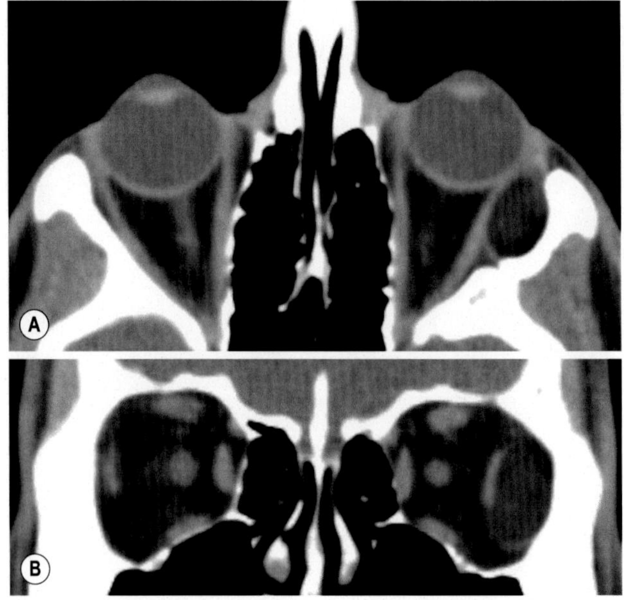

FIGURE 7-3 ■ **Dermoid tumour.** Axial (A) and coronal (B) CT reconstructions of the orbits demonstrating a well-circumscribed fatty density mass occupying the temporal aspect of the extraconal space of the left orbit. Note the scalloping of the overlying bone.

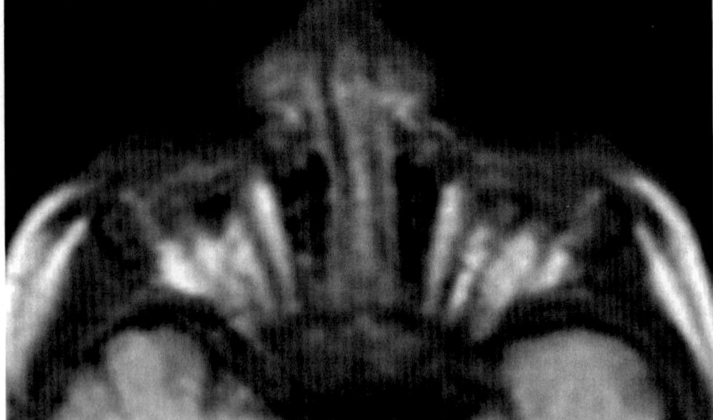

FIGURE 7-4 ■ **Anophthalmia.** The T1W MRI examination demonstrates an infant with no recognisable ocular structures in either orbit.

which involve the entire optic disc, the latter known as 'morning-glory papilla', and may involve the retina, the choroid/iris and the lids. Diagnostic imaging plays no direct role in the assessment of optic nerve coloboma; however, it may represent an associated finding in CHARGE, Patau's, Joubert's or Warburg's syndrome.

Dermoid

Dermoid cysts are the most common congenital mass lesion of the orbit[3] and are usually situated within the extraconal space. They result from inclusion of ectodermal components within the developing orbit and demonstrate slow growth over time with associated bony remodelling or focal erosion. Dermoids are most commonly found at the superolateral orbital margin in the region of the frontozygomatic suture and medially near the frontoethmoidal suture.[3,4] They may be an incidental imaging finding; however, symptomatic presentation occurs particularly following rupture. Fatty elements are a useful diagnostic feature on CT and MR imaging; fat-fluid levels or calcification may also be observed (Fig. 7-3).

Disorders of Globe Size or Shape

When assessing ocular size, it is necessary to determine which is the abnormal side taking into account the possibility of bilateral pathology. Macrophthalmia is defined as generalised enlargement of the globe, which can be congenital or acquired. This is most commonly due to myopia, i.e. axial elongation of the globe resulting in convergence of light anterior to the retina with the patient being shortsighted. Macrophthalmia also occurs in collagen vascular disorders such as Marfan's, Ehlers-Danlos syndrome and homocystinuria.

Microphthalmia is defined as a small globe; if this is congenital or acquired in early childhood an associated small bony orbit will be evident on imaging. Causes include PHPV, Coats' disease, coloboma, previous infection, trauma or radiotherapy and syndromes associated with hemifacial hypoplasia. Anophthalmia refers to complete absence of the embryological formation of an optic vesicle globe in the presence of ocular adnexae, although 'clinical anophthalmia' refers to the absence of a clinically identifiable globe on examination or imaging (Fig. 7-4). In some cases, there may be remnants of globe tissue in the orbit only detectable on histological examination.

Buphthalmos (*bous* = Greek for ox, cow) refers to generalised globe enlargement due to increased intraocular pressure, which is typically seen in children rather than adults as the infantile sclera is relatively elastic, allowing the globe to expand under pressure.[5] Buphthalmos occurs in paediatric glaucoma and is also seen in association with neurofibromatosis 1 (NF1). Apparent globe enlargement may also be due to exophthalmos secondary to an intraorbital mass; therefore imaging should be mandatory, especially if symptoms are rapidly progressive. Staphyloma is a term used to describe a focal protrusion in the sclera, which can occur anywhere along the globe surface, but is most commonly seen posteriorly on the temporal side of the optic disc.[5] The latter is frequently associated with myopia, but staphyloma can also be idiopathic, caused by previous infection, trauma or surgery (Fig. 7-5).

Degenerative Disease

Drusen

Drusen are deposits of lipoproteinaceous material between the basal lamina of the retinal pigment epithelium and the inner collagenous layer of Bruch's membrane. They are commonly asymptomatic and found as a normal feature in aging eyes but also in association with age-related macular degeneration.[6] On funduscopy, drusen can be a cause of blurring of the optic disc margin

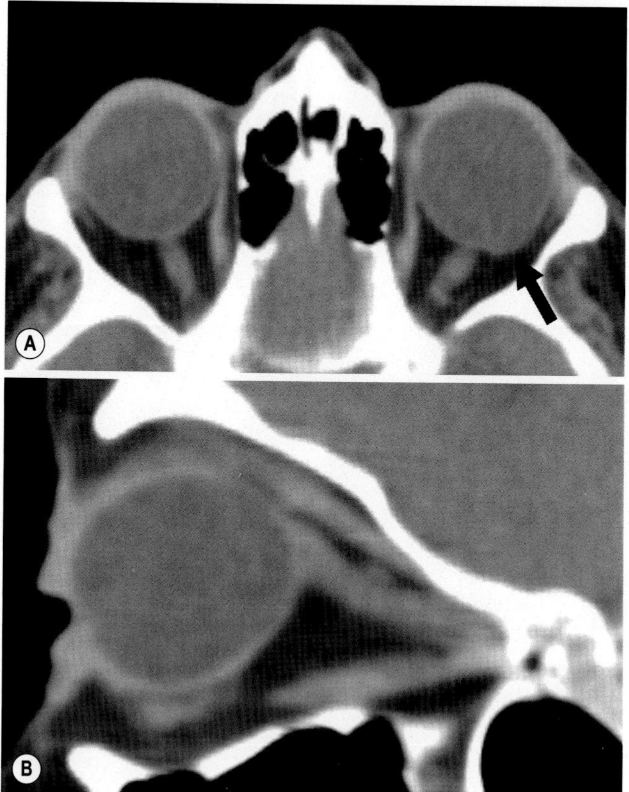

FIGURE 7-5 ■ **Staphyloma in myopia.** Axial (A) and sagittal (B) CT reconstructions of the orbit demonstrating axial elongation of the left globe with a focal outpouching of the posterior sclera just lateral to the optic nerve head (black arrow).

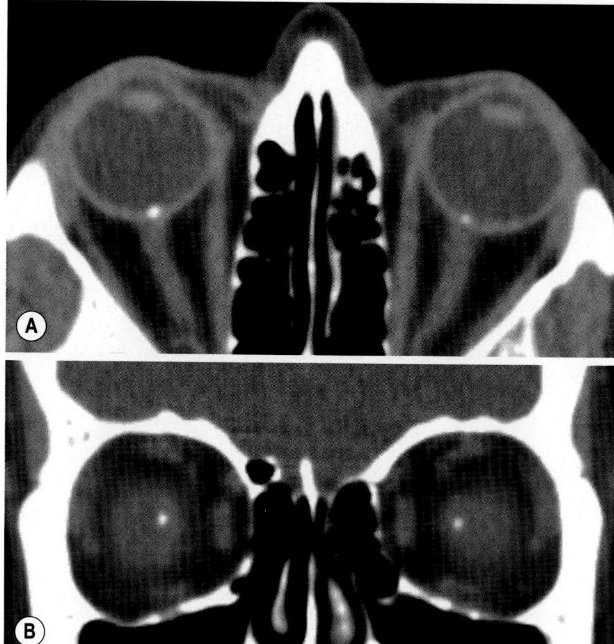

FIGURE 7-6 ■ **Drusen.** Axial (A) and coronal (B) CT reconstructions of the orbits demonstrating bilateral calcific foci at the optic nerve heads.

and hence may be mistaken for papilloedema. The classic CT appearances are those of small punctate and often bilateral calcific foci at the optic nerve heads (Fig. 7-6).

Orbital Inflammatory Disease

Idiopathic Orbital Inflammation

Idiopathic orbital inflammation (also known as *idiopathic orbital pseudotumour*) is a non-infective disease of unknown cause. Pseudotumour can affect individuals of any age with no clear sex predilection, but most commonly occurs around the fifth decade. It is the most common cause of a painful orbital mass in adults and represents approximately 10% of all orbital mass lesions.[7,8] An immune-modulated aetiology has been postulated, and although orbital pseudotumour mostly occurs in isolation, it can be associated with systemic autoimmune inflammatory conditions such as vasculitis and collagen-vascular disorders. Pseudotumour is usually a diagnosis of exclusion, which relies on a combination of clinical and radiological findings. Patients may present with proptosis, chemosis, painful restricted eye movements, diplopia and occasionally associated cranial nerve palsy. The disease often presents acutely, but can be more insidious. Approximately 80% of patients show good response to first-line treatment with steroids.[9] Recurrent or chronic pseudotumour may result in fibrosis, which has a worse prognosis.

Radiotherapy may be useful in patients who poorly respond to steroids or in those with rapidly progressive disease. Methotrexate is an option in patients who are refractory to conventional treatment.

The anatomical pattern of orbital pseudotumour may vary significantly between individuals. Any orbital structure can be affected; however, the lacrimal gland is most frequently involved.[3] A classic feature is tubular enlargement of the extraocular muscles, including the tendon, an important distinction from thyroid orbitopathy, in which the tendon is spared. Unilateral involvement of a single muscle is most common (Fig. 7-7) and in order of frequency this typically affects the medial rectus, superior rectus, lateral rectus and inferior rectus. Manifestation of pseudotumour at the orbital apex and in the cavernous sinus may be indistinguishable on imaging from *Tolosa–Hunt syndrome*.

CT is mostly sufficient in demonstrating features of orbital pseudotumour such as muscle enlargement, lacrimal gland involvement and infiltration of the orbital fat. However, MRI may be useful in complex cases, particularly if there is concern regarding intracranial extension and to delineate fibrosis, which is characterised by reduced T1 and T2 signal.[7]

Thyroid Orbitopathy

Thyroid eye disease is an immune-mediated disorder, which most commonly presents in association with hyperthyroidism in Graves' disease. However, it may be seen in euthyroid or even hypothyroid individuals. Importantly, orbitopathy may precede the actual thyroid disease. Thyroid orbitopathy occurs with a female-to-male ratio of 4:1 and a peak in the fourth to fifth decade.[4]

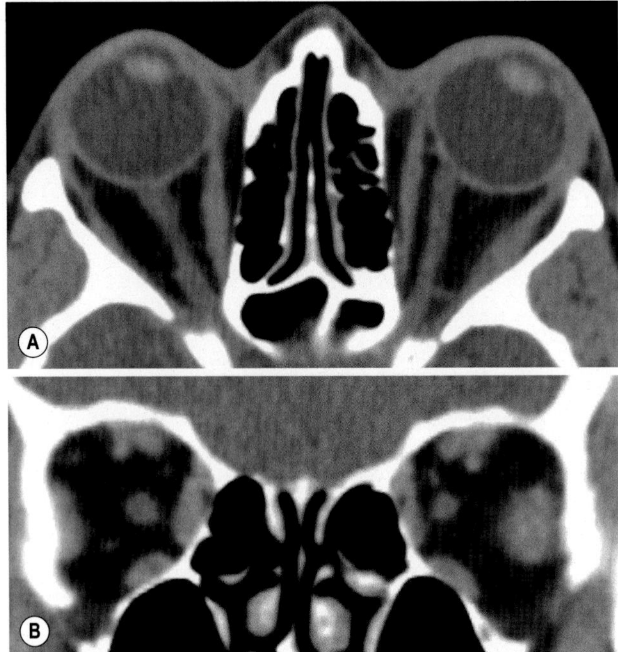

FIGURE 7-7 ■ Idiopathic orbital inflammation (orbital pseudotumour). Axial (A) and coronal (B) CT reconstructions of the orbits demonstrating asymmetrical swelling of the left lateral rectus muscle and tendon. Note the stranding of the adjacent orbital fat indicative of an active inflammatory process.

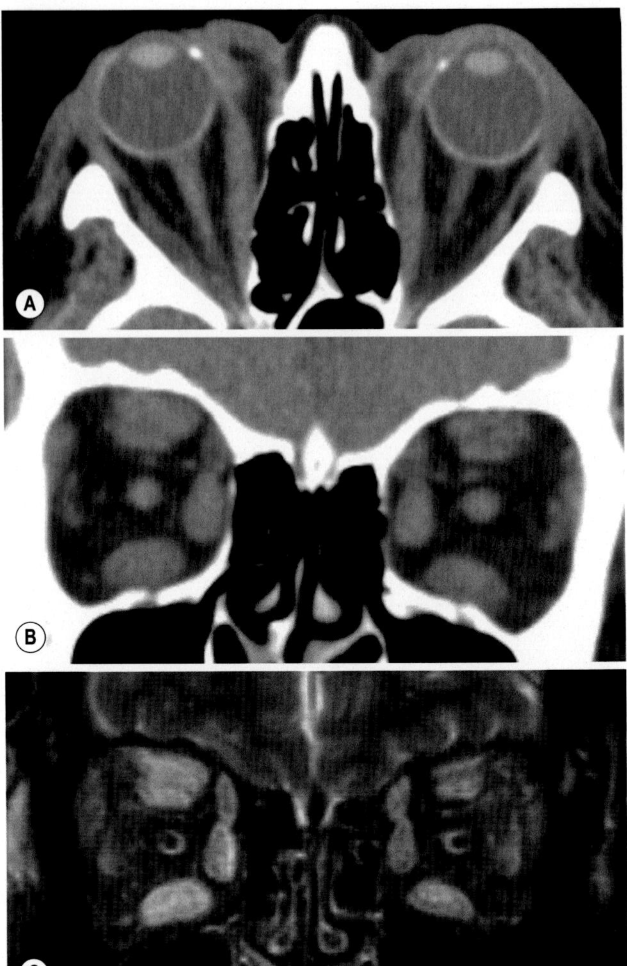

FIGURE 7-8 ■ Thyroid orbitopathy. Axial (A) and coronal (B) CT reconstructions of the orbits as well as a corresponding coronal STIR MRI (C). There is bilateral proptosis, extraocular muscle enlargement, intraorbital fat stranding and expansion as well as thickening of the eyelids.

It is the most common cause of bilateral or unilateral proptosis. Bilateral involvement is the most frequent presentation; in fact in some individuals, 'unilateral' proptosis may represent bilateral asymmetrical disease. Histologically, there is deposition of mucopolysaccharides, namely hyaluronic acid, within the extraocular muscles. This results in a classic imaging appearance of fusiform muscle enlargement with sparing of the muscular tendon. In descending order of frequency, the inferior, medial, superior and lateral recti are most commonly affected. Isolated lateral rectus involvement is rare and should prompt consideration of an alternative diagnosis.[3] There may be an increase of intraorbital fat, and fat stranding with a 'dirty' appearance on imaging (Fig. 7-8).

Systemic Inflammatory Diseases with Orbital Involvement

A variety of systemic autoimmune conditions such as vasculitides, sarcoidosis, connective tissue disorders and inflammatory bowel disease may show associated ocular inflammation. Episcleritis is a benign idiopathic condition which represents inflammation of the superficial sclera layer only. This is usually self-limiting and does not require imaging.[10] Scleritis, however, is more serious and can occur either in isolation or associated with a host of autoimmune conditions as listed above. Posterior scleritis may be evident on imaging as scleral thickening (Fig. 7-9) and can result in complications such as necrosis, retinal or choroidal detachment. Uveitis represents inflammation of the vascular layer of the globe and can be seen in both autoimmune disease, for example rheumatoid, seronegative arthropathies and sarcoid but also in infection.[10] Retinal vasculitis may result in ischaemia, microaneurysm formation and haemorrhages.[11] The majority of pathologies confined to the globe may be more readily appreciated on ophthalmological examination rather than cross-sectional imaging. However, there may be imaging evidence of inflammation in the form of fat infiltration, necrotising features or inflammatory masses.

Sjögren's syndrome, either in isolation or on a background of rheumatoid arthritis, involves the lacrimal gland and clinically results in dry eyes. Sarcoidosis is a disorder of multisystemic inflammation which commonly affects the respiratory tract, skin and eyes. Ocular involvement occurs in as many as 50–80% of patients and may present as non-caseating granulomas of the conjunctiva, uveitis or lacrimal gland infiltration.[12,13] Orbital sarcoid is typically bilateral and tends to respond to steroid treatment. Imaging features may be non-specific, ranging from diffuse infiltration to mass-like appearances

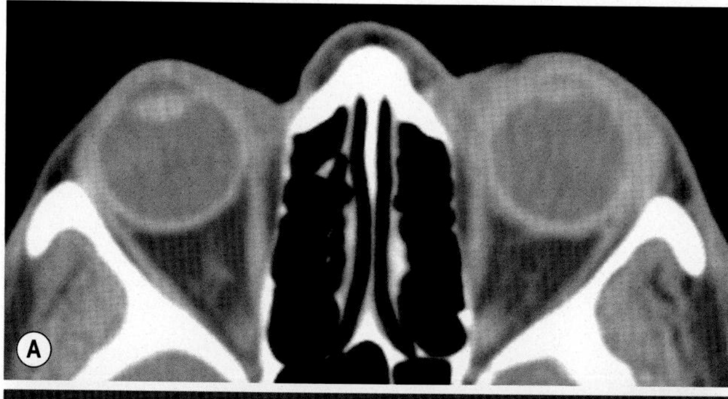

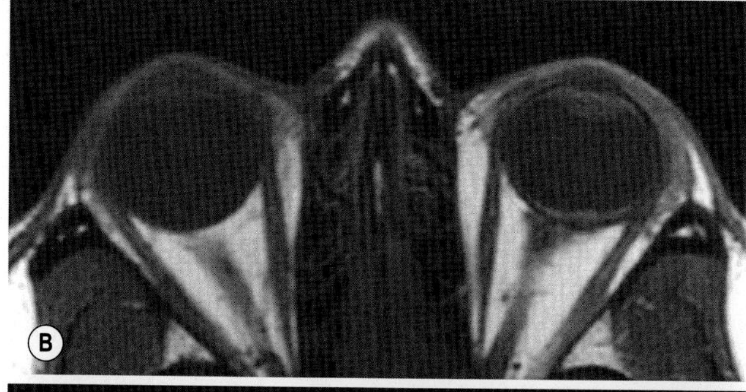

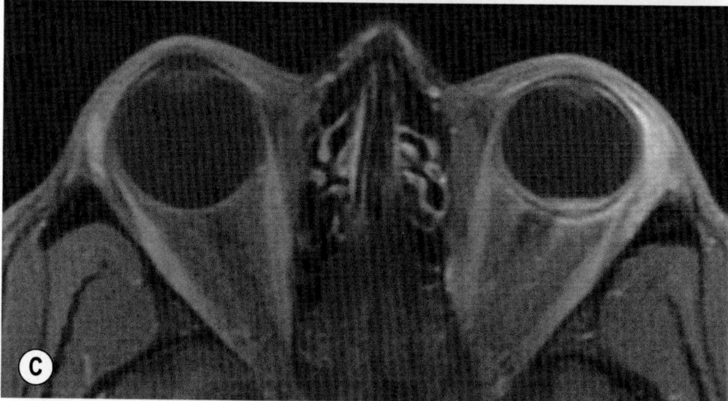

FIGURE 7-9 ■ Posterior scleritis. Axial (A) CT of the orbits demonstrating thickening of the left posterior sclera and associated subtle stranding of the retrobulbar fat suggestive of inflammation. Axial pre- (B) and post-gadolinium (C) fat-saturated contrast MRI of the orbits demonstrating thickening and enhancement of the left posterior sclera and retrobulbar fat.

(Fig. 7-10). Lacrimal gland enlargement with enhancement is a typical feature.[13] Chest imaging may provide a hint to the underlying sarcoidosis, but not infrequently histological sampling is required to conclusively establish the diagnosis.

Wegener's granulomatosis (now known as *granulomatosis with polyangiitis)* is a multisystem small-vessel necrotising granulomatous vasculitis. This most commonly involves the respiratory tract and the renal system of patients. Involvement of ocular and orbital structures may be present 40–50% of patients.[14] Orbital disease is commonly associated with sinus disease with bony erosions (Fig. 7-11). As with other granulomatous disease, orbital disease may appear hypointense on T2 MRI.

Orbital Infection

Toxocara endophthalmitis (also known as *ocular larva migrans*) results from infection with the nematode *Toxocara cani* or *T. cati* via ingestion of eggs in faecally contaminated soil or sandboxes. The source is from domestic dogs or cats. Larvae hatch from the ingested eggs and transgress the human intestinal wall into the bloodstream, whereby they reach various end organs such as the liver, lungs, brain and eyes.[15] Infection typically occurs in childhood and ocular disease tends to present between the ages of 5 and 10 years. *Toxocara* endophthalmitis is the result of a granulomatous immune response to retinal infiltration with larvae. Loss of vision due to retinal detachment is the most common presenting complaint; other non-specific signs include pain, leukocoria and a red eye. Imaging features are mostly non-specific, but the absence of calcification can be a helpful distinguishing feature from retinoblastoma. CT may demonstrate increased attenuation within the vitreous, representing protein leakage from retinal and choroidal vessels.[10] MRI signal is variable, especially on T2 sequences, where both hyper- and hypointensity can occur depending on the degree of fibrosis with contrast enhancement usually present.[16] Untreated, *Toxocara* invariably leads to blindness.

Endophthalmitis can also be fungal (*Candida* sp.) or bacterial in aetiology with *Staphylococcus aureus*, *Staphylococcus epidermidis*, *Streptococcus* sp. representing the most common pathogens.[10] Infectious uveitis may be bacterial, viral, fungal or parasitic (e.g. toxoplasmosis, Lyme disease, leptospirosis) in nature. Orbital tuberculosis is rare, even in endemic areas, and most commonly occurs in children. Clinically, the disease may be indolent with non-specific symptoms, only mild pain and proptosis. The lacrimal gland and orbital walls are most commonly affected, extending from adjacent paranasal sinus inflammatory/infective disease, and can be associated with simultaneous intracranial disease.[17] Imaging features include inflammatory soft-tissue masses and retrobulbar or subperiosteal abscess formation (Fig. 7-12).

A serious complication of intraorbital infection spread usually via paranasal sinus infection is superior ophthalmic vein thrombosis, which can be further complicated by cavernous sinus thrombosis (Fig. 7-13).

Benign Neoplasms and Mass-Like Lesions

Pleomorphic Adenoma

Pleomorphic adenoma is the most common tumour of the lacrimal gland, comprising over half of all epithelial gland tumours.[18] Imaging findings may vary from a homogeneous mass to a more heterogeneous appearance with cystic or necrotic elements. On MRI, small lesions tend to be of relatively uniform low T1 and high T2 signal, whereas larger lesions typically show heterogeneous signal, sometimes also containing haemorrhagic elements (Fig. 7-14). Similar to its behaviour in the parotid gland, lacrimal pleomorphic adenoma has a propensity for malignant transformation, making excision desirable.

Nerve Sheath Tumour

Schwannoma is the most common nerve sheath tumour in the orbit. It is a slow-growing benign peripheral nerve

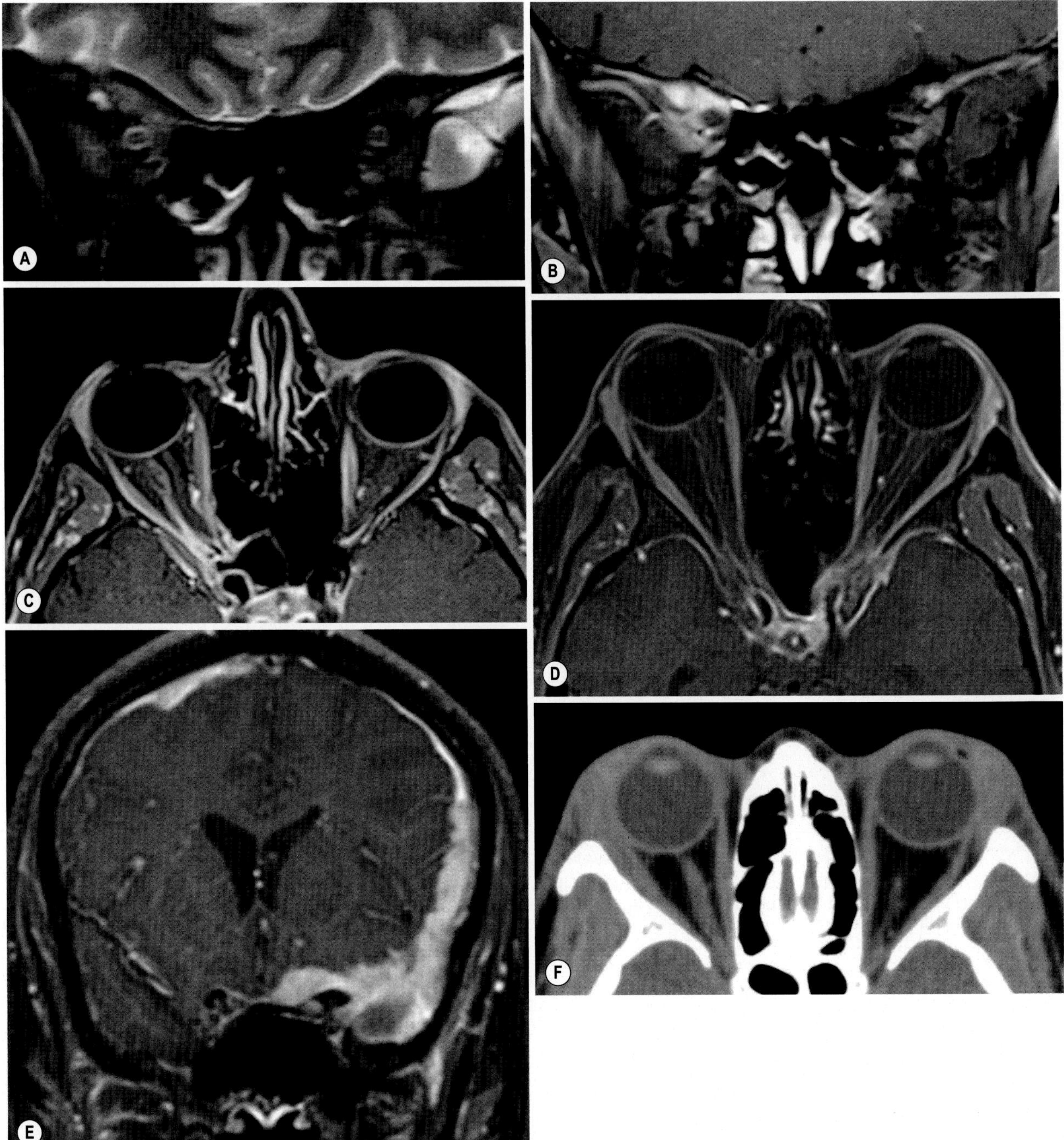

FIGURE 7-10 ■ Orbital sarcoid. Coronal STIR (A), coronal (B) and axial (C) T1-weighted post-gadolinium fat-suppressed MRI of the orbits demonstrating T2-weighted hyperintensity and enhancement at the right orbital apex. Axial T1-weighted post-gadolinium fat-suppressed MRI of the orbits (D) in another patient demonstrating thickening and enhancement of both optic nerve sheaths in a sarcoid perineuritis resembling the 'tram-track sign'. The corresponding T1-weighted post-gadolinium fat-suppressed MRI of the brain (E) demonstrates extensive convexity dural thickening and enhancement, predominantly on the left. Note the extension through the left optic canal and superior orbital fissure. CT of the orbits (F) in a patient with proptosis and bilateral lacrimal gland enlargement.

sheath tumour and is mostly seen in adults. Painless progressive proptosis is a classic, although not specific, presentation. Schwannomas frequently arise from sensory branches of the ophthalmic nerve (V1), namely the supraorbital, supratrochlear or lacrimal nerve, which explains their sometimes extraconal position within the superior portion of the orbit.[19] On MRI, these tumours tend to be hypointense on T1- and hyperintense on T2-weighted sequences (Fig. 7-15). Imaging features also depend on the histological tumour composition, whereby so-called Antoni A lesions with densely packed cells demonstrate more homogeneous enhancement than

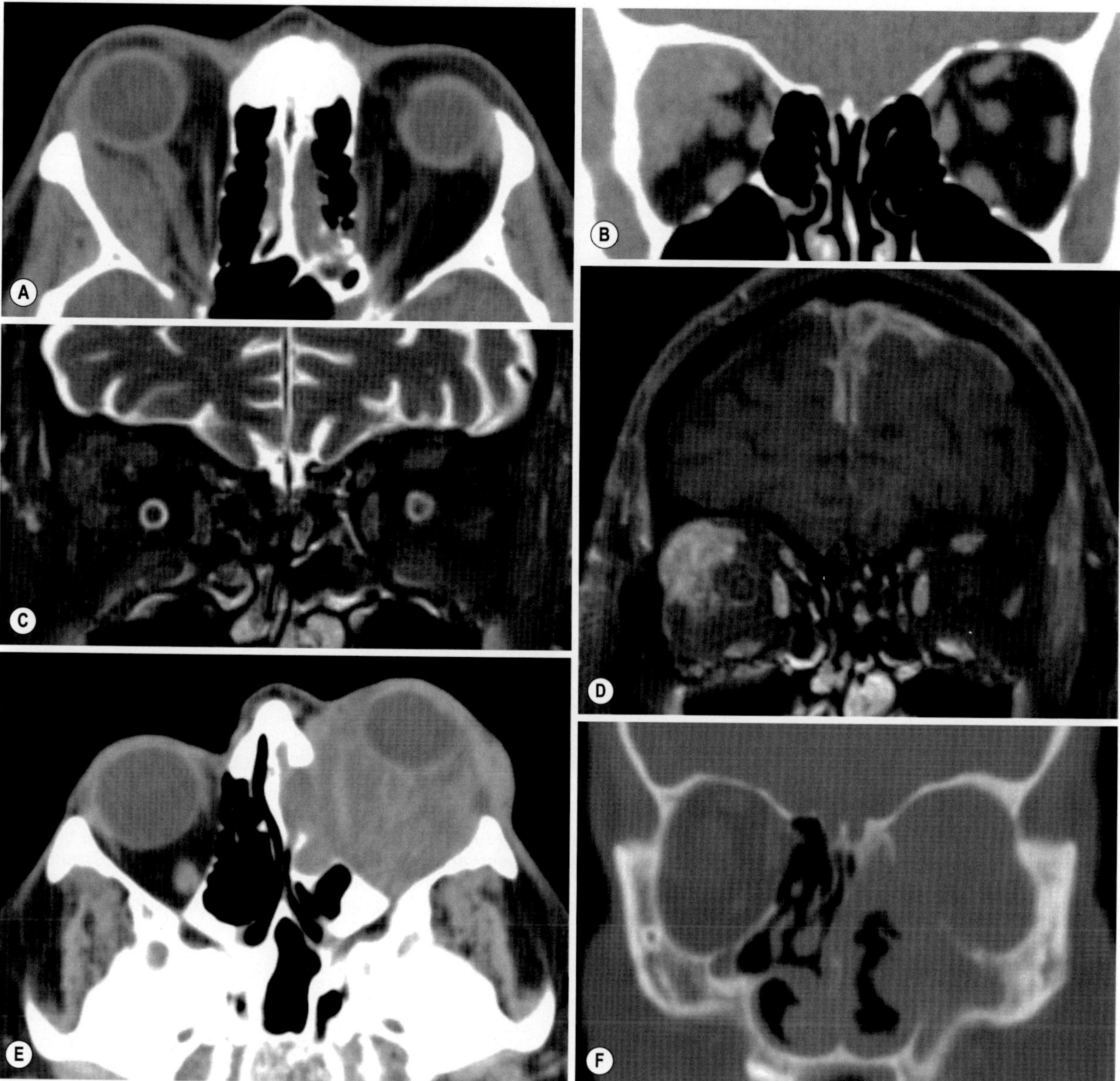

FIGURE 7-11 ■ **Wegener's granulomatosis (granulomatosis with polyangiitis).** Axial (A) and coronal (B) CT of an inflammatory mass occupying the upper temporal quadrant of the right orbit causing right proptosis. The corresponding coronal STIR (C) and T1-weighted post-gadolinium fat-suppressed MRI (D) of the orbits demonstrates T2-weighted intermediate signal inflammatory mass with enhancement in that location. Note the dural involvement along the falx cerebri. CT of another patient with a large inflammatory mass occupying the left orbit causing left proptosis on the soft-tissue windows (E) as well as bony erosion with extension of the inflammatory mass through the lamina papyracea and nasal septum on the coronal reformats on bone windows (F).

Antoni B lesions.[3] Neurofibroma may also occur in the orbit and can have similar imaging features to schwannoma. It can arise either in isolation or in the context of neurofibromatosis 1 (NF1). Plexiform neurofibroma is associated with hypoplasia of the greater wing of sphenoid in NF1 patients. Calcification may be present in some neurofibromata and can help distinguish this from schwannoma, which rarely calcifies.

Optic Nerve Glioma

This intrinsic tumour predominantly presents in young patients, with a peak in the first decade. Bilateral optic nerve glioma is virtually diagnostic of NF1. Histologically, pilocytic astrocytoma (WHO grade 1) is the most common and may show little or no progression over time. Visual loss is more common in non-NF patients than in neurofibromatosis.[20] The rarer adult form of optic nerve glioma can be more aggressive when of a corresponding histology of anaplastic glioma (WHO grade 3) or glioblastoma multiforme (WHO grade 4) and has a rapidly progressive clinical course. On imaging, there may be fusiform enlargement of the optic nerve, with associated expansion of the optic canal. MRI is the most accurate at demonstrating optic nerve glioma, which appears isointense to hypointense on T1 and

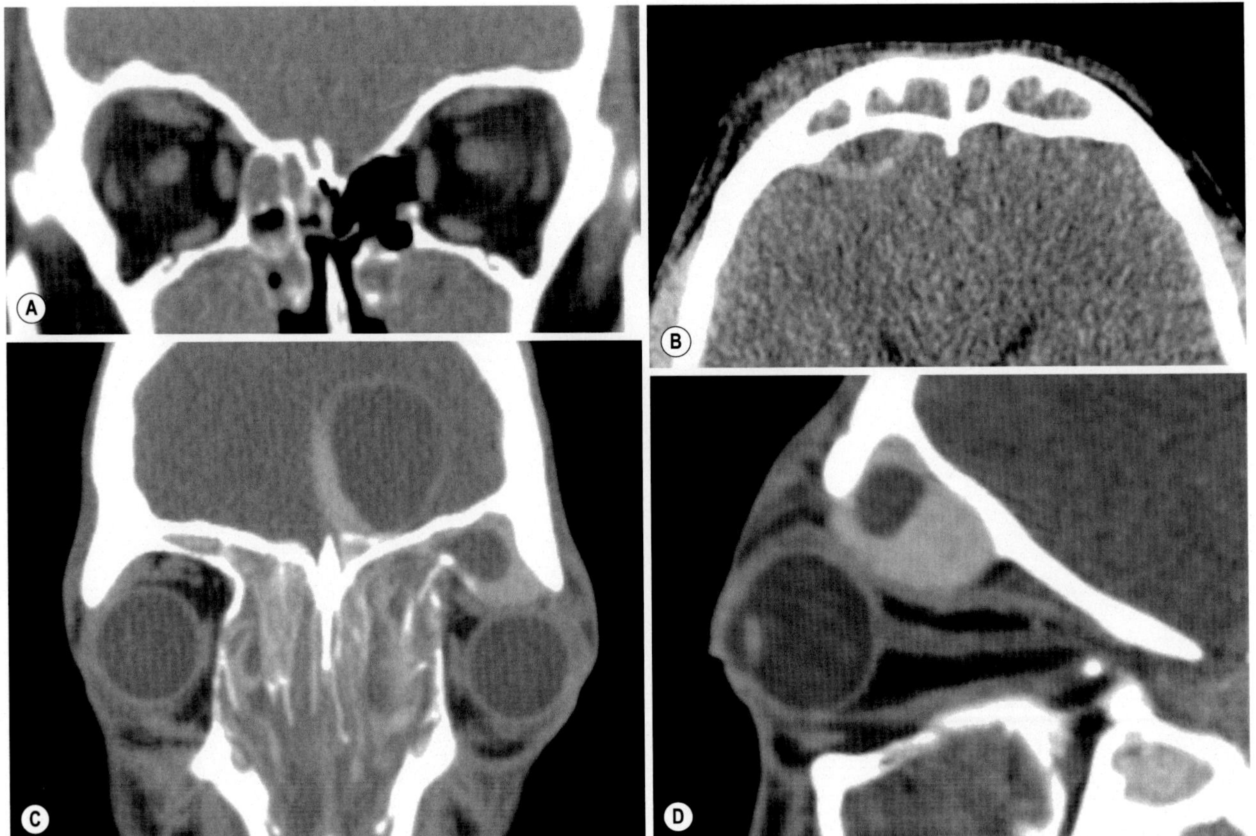

FIGURE 7-12 ■ **Orbital infection.** Coronal CT of the orbits (A) in a patient with right orbital cellulitis, demonstrating subtle stranding of the intraorbital fat on the right with asymmetric swelling of the superior-rectus levator complex and a soft-tissue inflammatory mass superior to it. Note the extensive opacification of the maxillary antra and right ethmoidal air cells. Axial CT of the brain in this patient (B) revealed an empyema subjacent to opacified frontal sinuses and right forehead cellulitis. Coronal (C) and sagittal (D) reformatted post-contrast CT of a patient with severe chronic fungal sinusitis. Proptosis and hypoglobus on the left is seen secondary to displacement of the left frontal sinus pyocele. Note the left frontal cerebral abscess and the gross expansion and opacification of the paranasal sinuses.

hyperintense on T2 sequences with variable contrast enhancement (Fig. 7-16).

Optic Nerve Sheath Meningioma

Primary optic nerve sheath meningioma arises from the arachnoid sheath of the optic nerve and should be distinguished from secondary meningioma, which has spread from an intracranial tumour either centred on the anterior clinoid process or sphenoid wing to involve the orbit via the optic canal or the orbital fissure (Fig. 7-17). Both occur most frequently in middle-aged women. Bilateral optic nerve sheath meningiomas are a feature of neurofibromatosis 2 (NF2). On imaging, generalised circumferential or fusiform enlargement of the optic nerve-sheath complex are the most common, but focal eccentric masses can also occur. CT may be useful for demonstrating calcification within the meningioma, a relatively specific finding, which occurs in 20–50% of cases and is not observed in optic nerve glioma. Another feature of optic nerve meningioma is the so-called tram-track sign, which is defined as relative hypoattenuation of the optic nerve on CT or reduced signal on fat-suppressed post-gadolinium MRI due to peripheral enhancement of the tumour around the nerve. This is not a specific appearance, however, and can be seen in other pathologies, including pseudotumour, optic neuritis, sarcoid (e.g. Fig. 7-10D), lymphoma and metastatic disease.[21]

Vascular Lesions of the Orbit

Cavernous Haemangioma

Cavernous haemangioma is the most common primary orbital tumour in adults, representing approximately 6% of all orbital masses.[22] The classification as a tumour is actually a misnomer; in fact, this lesion type represents an angiographically silent venous malformation consisting of endothelial-lined vascular spaces with a fibrous pseudocapsule. It is usually centred on the intraconal compartment and may contain phleboliths on imaging (Fig. 7-18). Frank haemorrhage is atypical, but haemosiderin staining may occur. Rarely, cavernous haemangiomas can be intraosseous and therefore extraconal. The

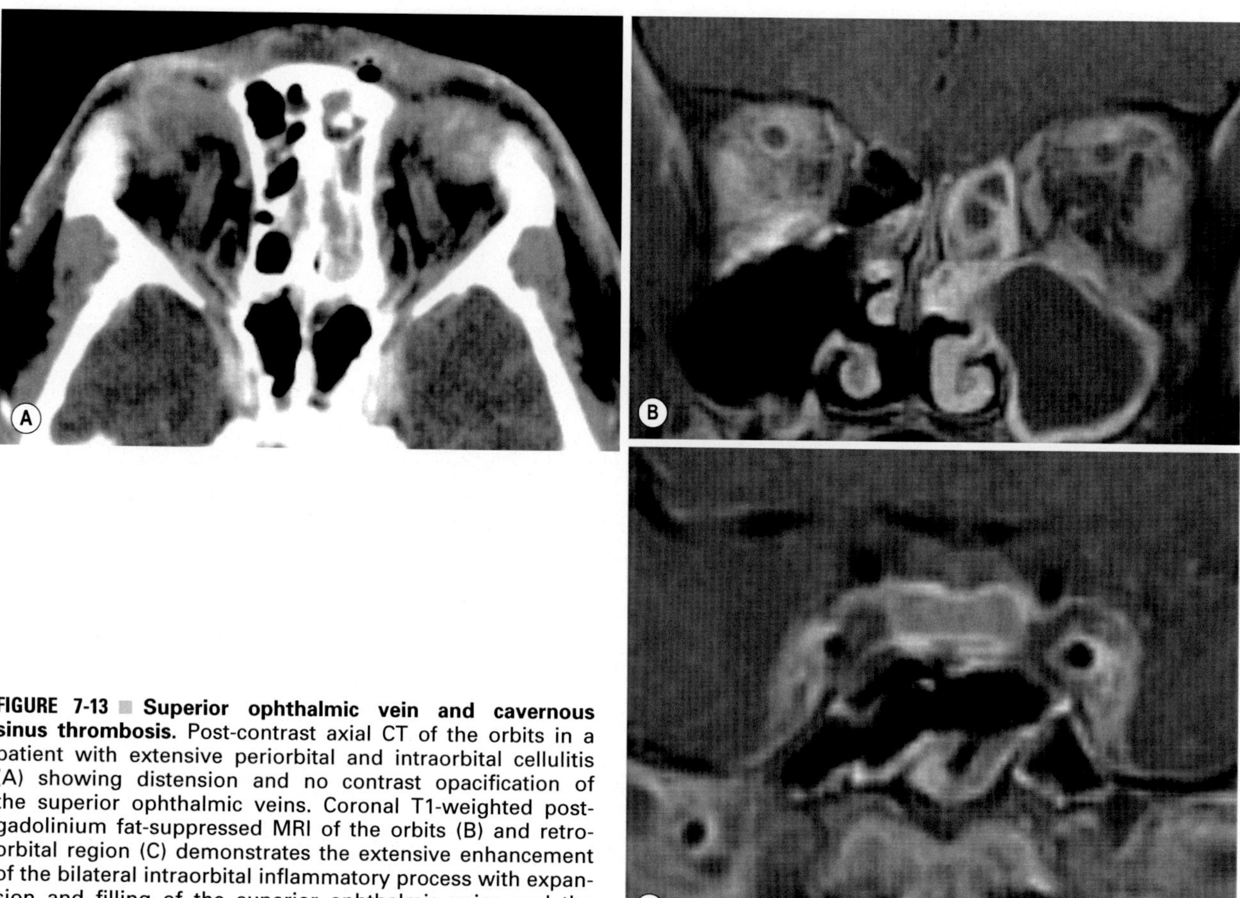

FIGURE 7-13 ■ **Superior ophthalmic vein and cavernous sinus thrombosis.** Post-contrast axial CT of the orbits in a patient with extensive periorbital and intraorbital cellulitis (A) showing distension and no contrast opacification of the superior ophthalmic veins. Coronal T1-weighted post-gadolinium fat-suppressed MRI of the orbits (B) and retro-orbital region (C) demonstrates the extensive enhancement of the bilateral intraorbital inflammatory process with expansion and filling of the superior ophthalmic veins and the cavernous sinuses with intermediate signal thrombus.

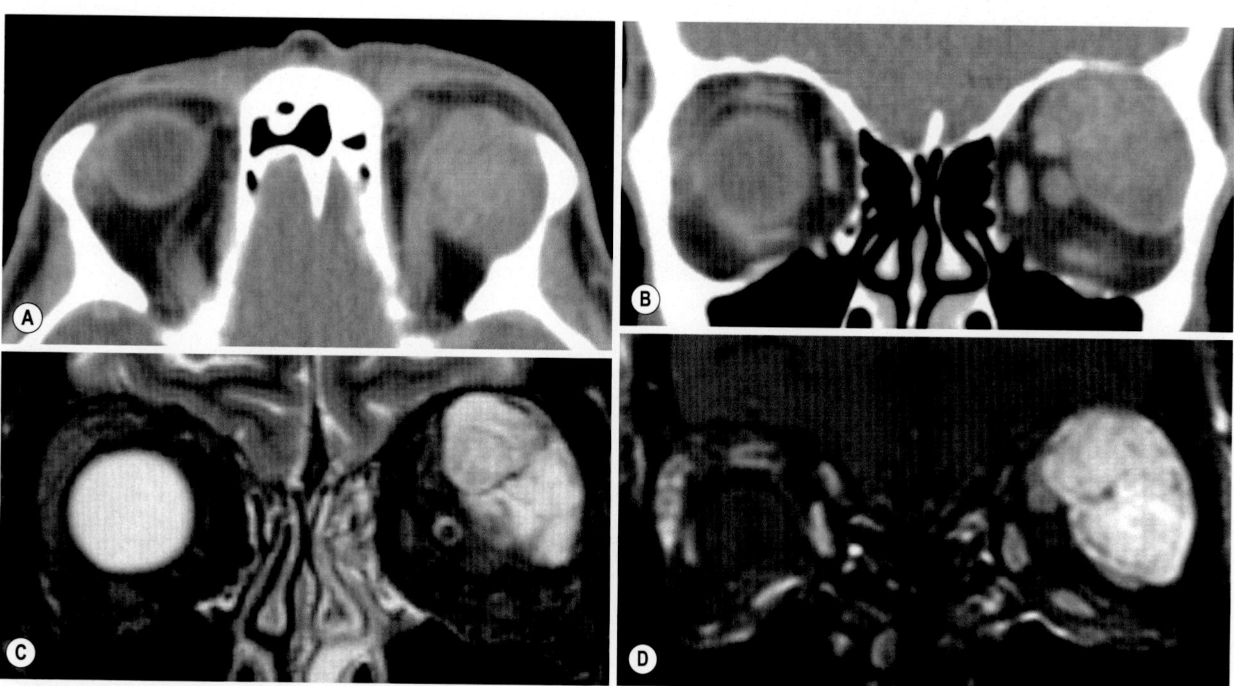

FIGURE 7-14 ■ **Pleomorphic adenoma.** Axial (A) and coronal (B) CT of the orbits demonstrating a well-circumscribed soft-tissue mass in the superior-temporal quadrant of the left orbit, causing remodelling of the overlying sphenoid bone. The coronal STIR (C) and T1-weighted post-gadolinium fat-suppressed (D) MRI of the mass reveals avid and homogeneous enhancement.

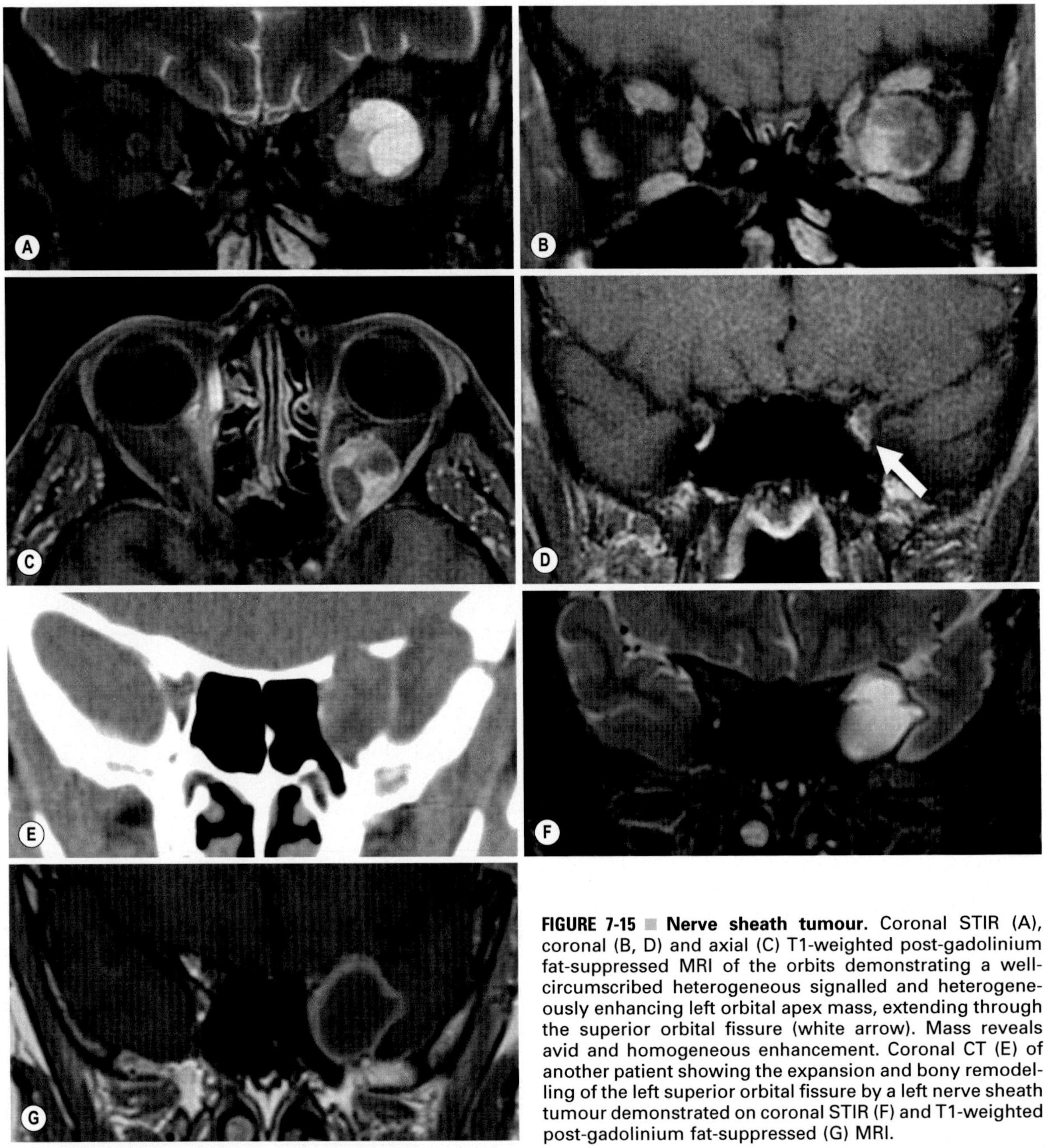

FIGURE 7-15 ■ **Nerve sheath tumour.** Coronal STIR (A), coronal (B, D) and axial (C) T1-weighted post-gadolinium fat-suppressed MRI of the orbits demonstrating a well-circumscribed heterogeneous signalled and heterogeneously enhancing left orbital apex mass, extending through the superior orbital fissure (white arrow). Mass reveals avid and homogeneous enhancement. Coronal CT (E) of another patient showing the expansion and bony remodelling of the left superior orbital fissure by a left nerve sheath tumour demonstrated on coronal STIR (F) and T1-weighted post-gadolinium fat-suppressed (G) MRI.

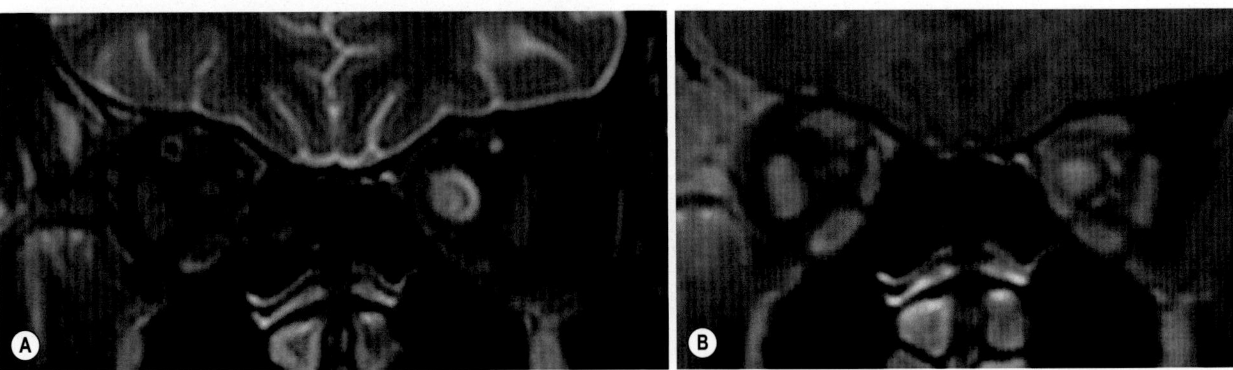

FIGURE 7-16 ■ **Optic nerve glioma.** Coronal STIR (A), coronal (B) and axial (D) T1-weighted post-gadolinium fat-suppressed and axial T2-weighted (C) MRI of the orbits demonstrating expansion and enhancement of the intraorbtial and canalicular segments of the left optic nerve through an expanded left optic canal (white arrow). The retro-orbital intracranial segment and optic chiasm are also involved.

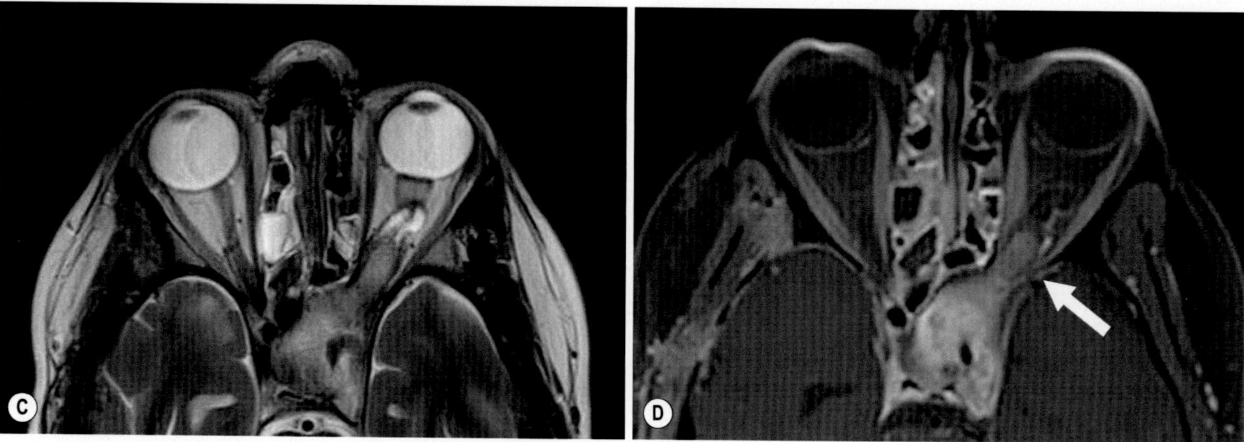

FIGURE 7-16, Continued

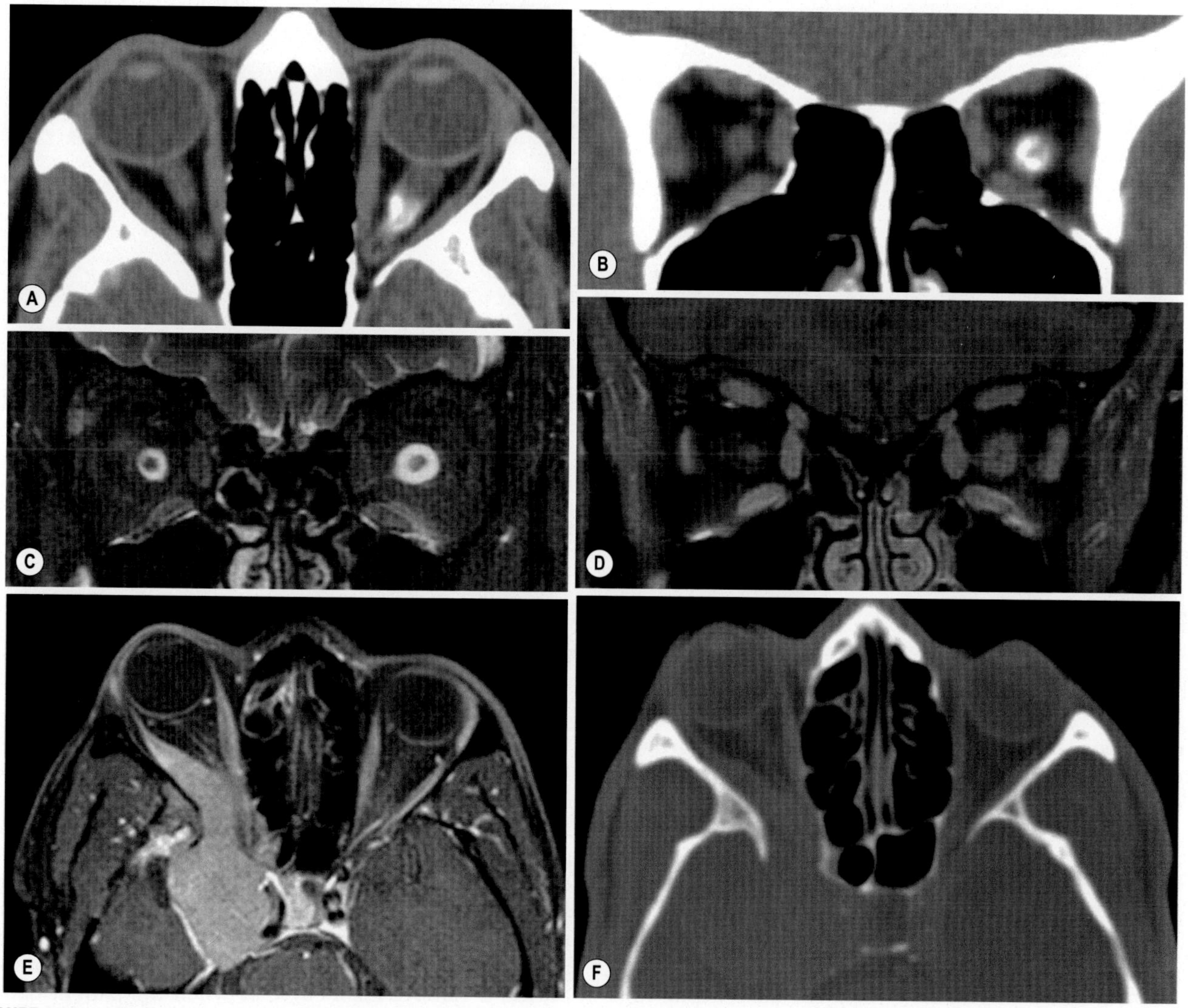

FIGURE 7-17 ■ **Optic nerve sheath and sphenoid wing meningioma.** Axial (A) and coronal (B) CT of the orbits showing enlargement of the left optic nerve-sheath complex with segmental circumferential calcification. The corresponding coronal STIR (C) and coronal T1-weighted post-gadolinium fat-suppressed (D) MRI of the orbits demonstrates expansion and enhancement of the intraorbital of the left optic nerve-sheath complex. Axial T1-weighted post-gadolinium fat-suppressed MRI (E) and axial CT on bone windows (F) showing a right sphenoid wing meningioma causing proptosis and expanding the superior orbital fissure.

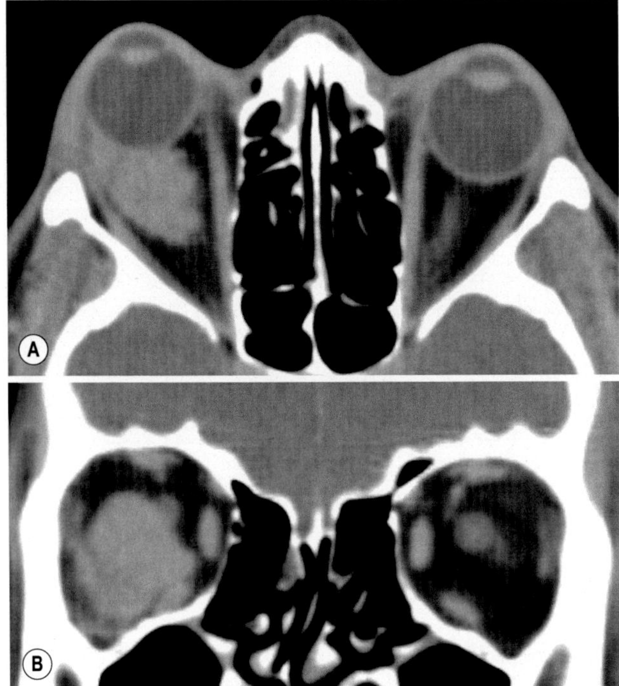

FIGURE 7-18 ■ Cavernous haemangioma. Post-contrast axial (A) and coronal (B) CT examination of a well-circumscribed retrobulbar enhancing mass causing right proptosis.

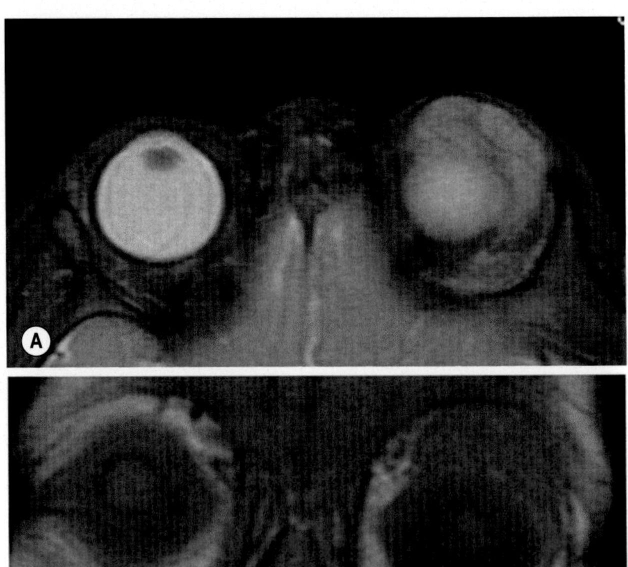

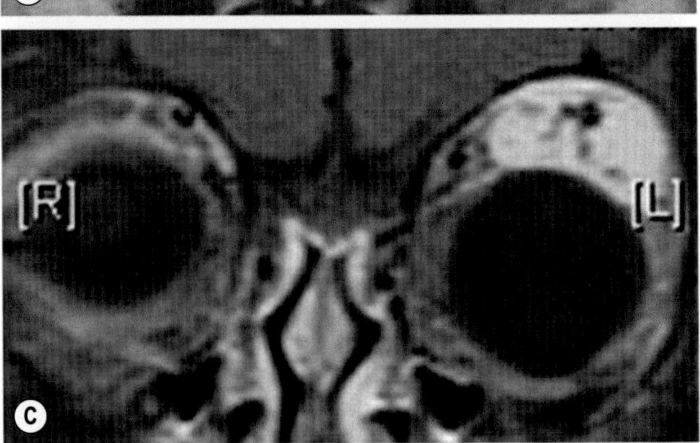

FIGURE 7-19 ■ Capillary haemangioma. Axial STIR (A), coronal pre- (B) and fat-suppressed post-gadolinium (C) T1-weighted orbital MRI of a child demonstrating a left anterior and superior lobulated enhancing orbital mass causing proptosis and hypoglobus.

clinical presentation is that of painless slowly progressive proptosis and diplopia. Increased growth may occur in pregnancy or following trauma.[3] On MR, cavernous haemangioma mostly demonstrates low T1 signal and high T2 signal with variable enhancement and progressive spread of enhancement from a single point or small component of the mass on dynamic post-gadolinium MRI; the latter is a characteristic feature of cavernous haemangioma, similar to progressive 'filling-in' of cavernous haemangioma in the liver.[22–24] This is relevant as, in some of these lesions, a conservative approach and monitoring may be favoured over surgical resection.

Capillary Haemangioma

This is a different entity of vascular malformation, which should not be confused with cavernous haemangioma. Capillary haemangioma presents in the paediatric population soon after birth and demonstrates rapid growth during the first year of life with often subsequent involution approximately by the age of 10.[4] There is an association with cutaneous facial malformations, the presence of which may aid the diagnosis. Capillary haemangioma is most commonly found in the extraconal compartment anteriorly and within the superomedial orbital quadrant[3] (Fig. 7-19). Irregularity of the mass and spread to the intraconal compartment can mimic malignancy. On T2 MR imaging, low signal flow voids can be a helpful differentiating feature. These result from arterial flow supply via the external or internal carotid branches. Retinal haemangioblastoma (also termed retinal capillary haemangioma) is a further lesion category and occurs in association with von Hippel–Lindau disease (VHL) and familial cancer syndromes.

Venous Varix

A varix is defined as an abnormally dilated vein or cluster of veins. Although sometimes cited as part of the orbital lymphovascular malformation spectrum, orbital varices are now thought to represent a discrete entity.[3] Varices can occur at any age, but are most common in the second and third decade with no gender predilection.[25] The hallmark of an orbital varix is enlargement under pressure, resulting in a sometimes dramatic proptosis, for example during a Valsalva manoeuvre or when the patient bends forward. Importantly, varices may not always be evident on standard supine cross-sectional imaging and therefore may require a provocation manoeuvre during imaging (Fig. 7-20). On CT, varices may demonstrate increased

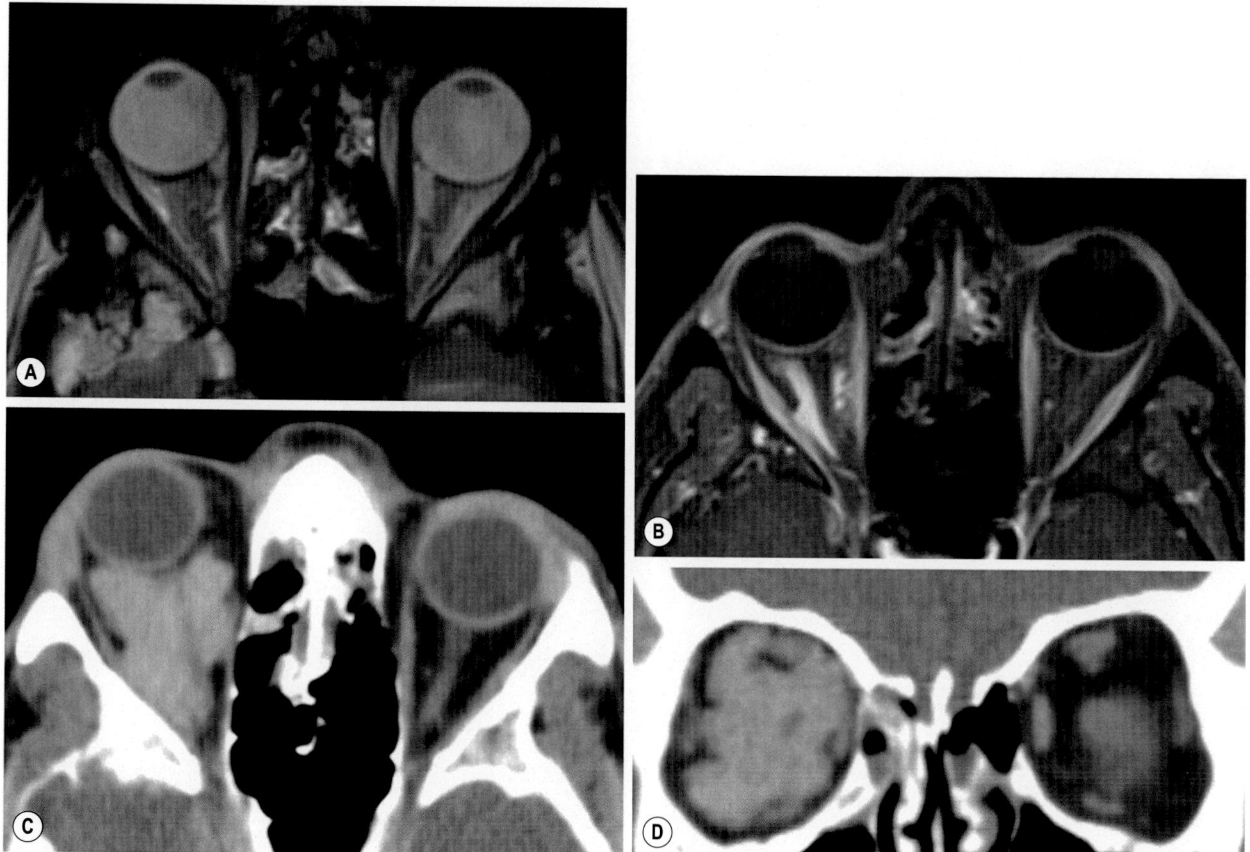

FIGURE 7-20 ■ **Orbital varices.** Axial T2-weighted (A) and fat-suppressed post-gadolinium T1-weighted (B) orbital MRI demonstrating a right proptosis from a left retrobulbar enhancing lesion surrounding the optic nerve-sheath complex. A subsequent post-contrast axial (C) and coronal (D) CT examination with the patient performing a Valsalva manoeuvre illustrates the characteristic enlargement of the mass and worsening proptosis due to venous engorgement.

attenuation due to blood product and, if present, calcified phleboliths are pathognomonic. T2-weighted MRI may reveal flow voids, but these can be absent, especially if there is variceal thrombosis. Haemorrhage is also a potential complication and may result in acute painful proptosis.

Venous Lymphatic Malformation

This type of lesion is sometimes referred to as *lymphangioma*, but it does not represent a neoplasm. Venous lymphatic malformations may manifest at birth or in early childhood and typically demonstrate slow growth or no growth at all. Clinically, they can result in proptosis, restriction of ocular movements and occasional haemorrhage. Unlike a varix, a venous lymphatic malformation does not enlarge under Valsalva-type stress. MRI (Fig. 7-21) is the most sensitive method of characterising these lesions, which may show proteinaceous and haemorrhagic components with fluid–fluid levels and typically enhance poorly.[25]

Arteriovenous Malformations (AVMs)

Congenital arteriovenous malformations purely involving the orbit are extremely rare, resulting in visible cutaneous stigmata due to congestive changes within the periorbital soft tissues and orbit. They may also involve the bony orbit. The arterial supply of these AVMs is typically from the anterior ethmoidal rami off the ophthalmic artery or the internal and external maxillary arteries (Fig. 7-22). When these AVMs involve the retina and midbrain (Fig. 7-23), the terms *congenital unilateral retinocephalic vascular malformation syndrome* or *Bonnet–Dechaume–Blanc syndrome* or *Wyburn-Mason syndrome* describe a neurocutaneous syndrome characterised by these AVMs.[1,26]

Carotid-Cavernous Fistula

A carotid-cavernous fistula represents an abnormal direct or indirect connection between one or more branches of the internal or external carotid artery and the cavernous sinus. This can occur spontaneously, most frequently in the context of a collagen vascular disorder, but more commonly is the result of trauma, surgery, previous thrombosis or aneurysm rupture.[4,25] Middle-aged to elderly women are most frequently affected. The clinical findings are those of pulsatile exophthalmos, conjunctival injection and there may be an auscultatory bruit. Imaging features (Fig. 7-24) include dilatation of the superior ophthalmic vein, proptosis, fullness of the cavernous sinus and extraocular muscle congestion.[25]

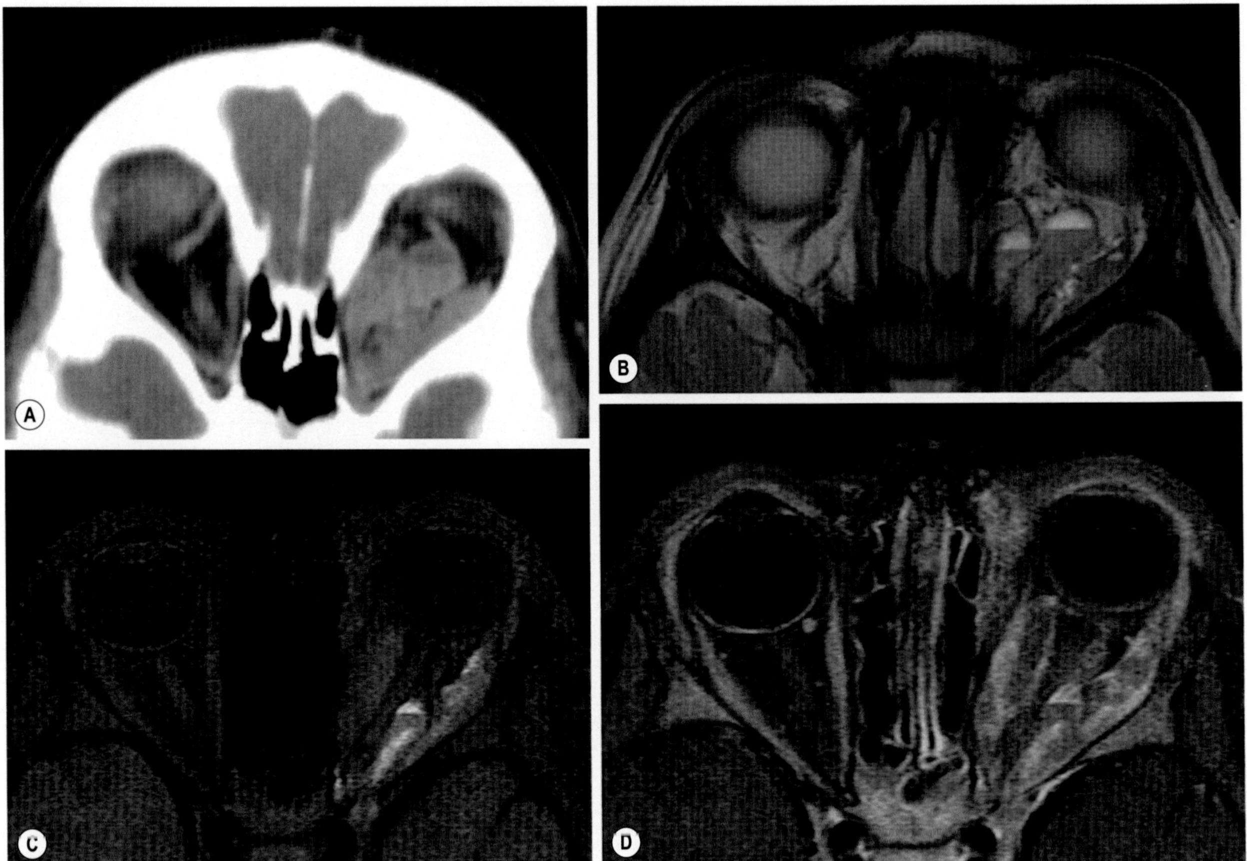

FIGURE 7-21 ■ Orbital venous lymphatic malformation. Post-contrast axial CT (A), axial T2-weighted (B) and pre- (C) and post- (D) fat-suppressed T1-weighted orbital MRI demonstrating a left superior orbital complex heterogeneously enhancing mass causing left proptosis and containing multiple fluid–fluid levels representing proteinaceous and haemorrhagic components.

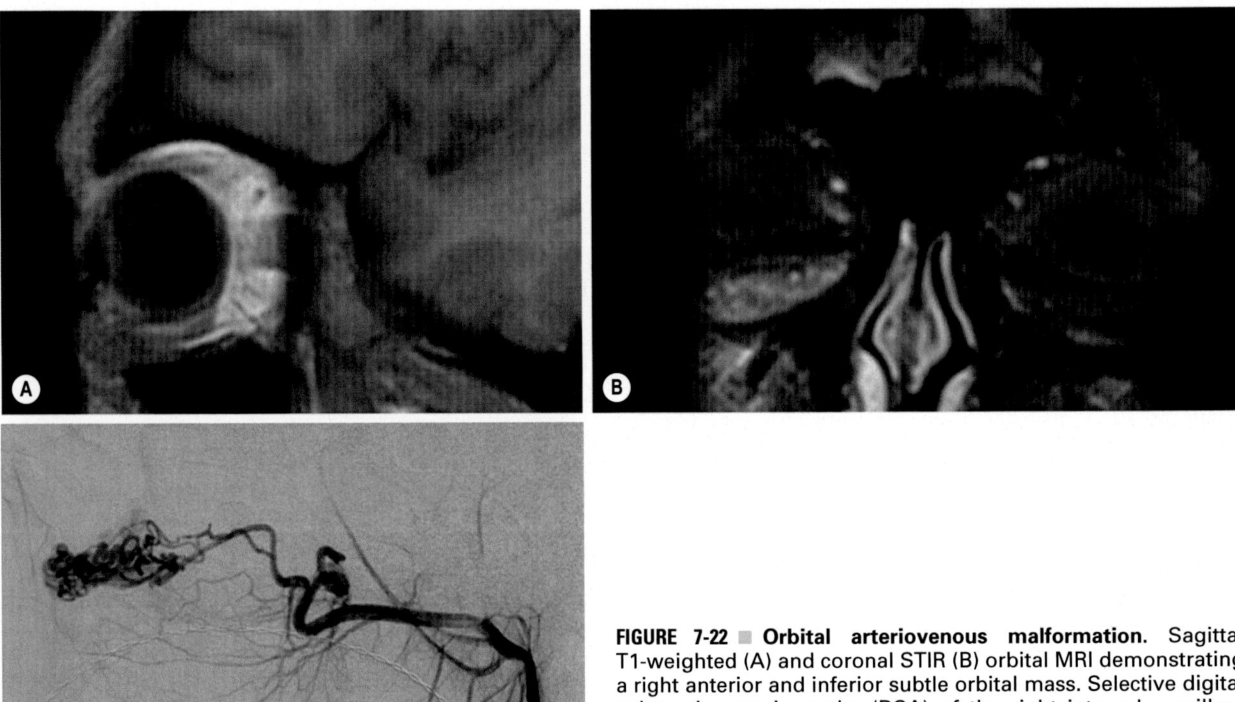

FIGURE 7-22 ■ Orbital arteriovenous malformation. Sagittal T1-weighted (A) and coronal STIR (B) orbital MRI demonstrating a right anterior and inferior subtle orbital mass. Selective digital subtraction angiography (DSA) of the right internal maxillary artery (C) demonstrates arteriovenous shunting through the mass through a tangle of abnormal vessels representing the nidus of an AVM.

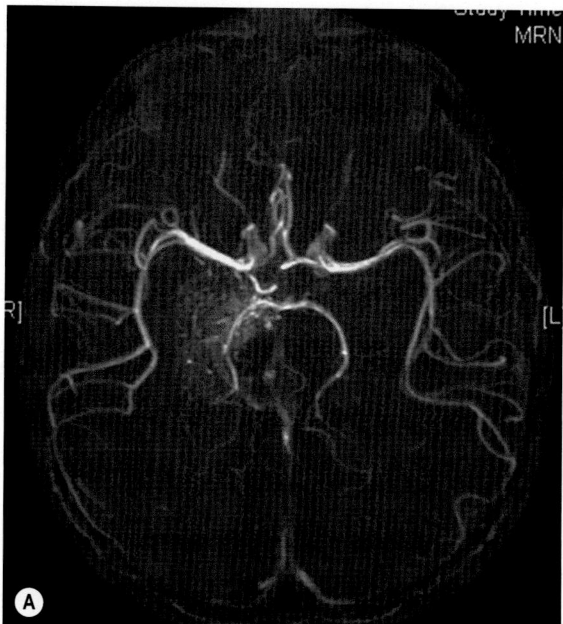

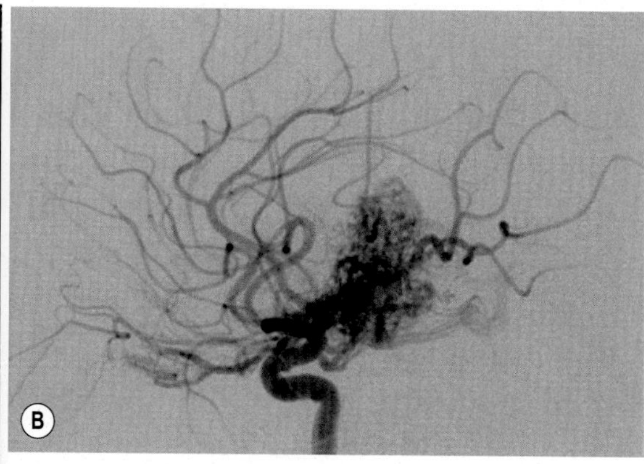

FIGURE 7-23 ■ Congenital unilateral retinocephalic vascular malformation syndrome (Wyburn-Mason syndrome). Time-of-flight MR angiography (A) and selective digital subtraction angiography of the right internal carotid artery (B) demonstrating a right mesencephalic AVM in a patient with a known right retinal AVM.

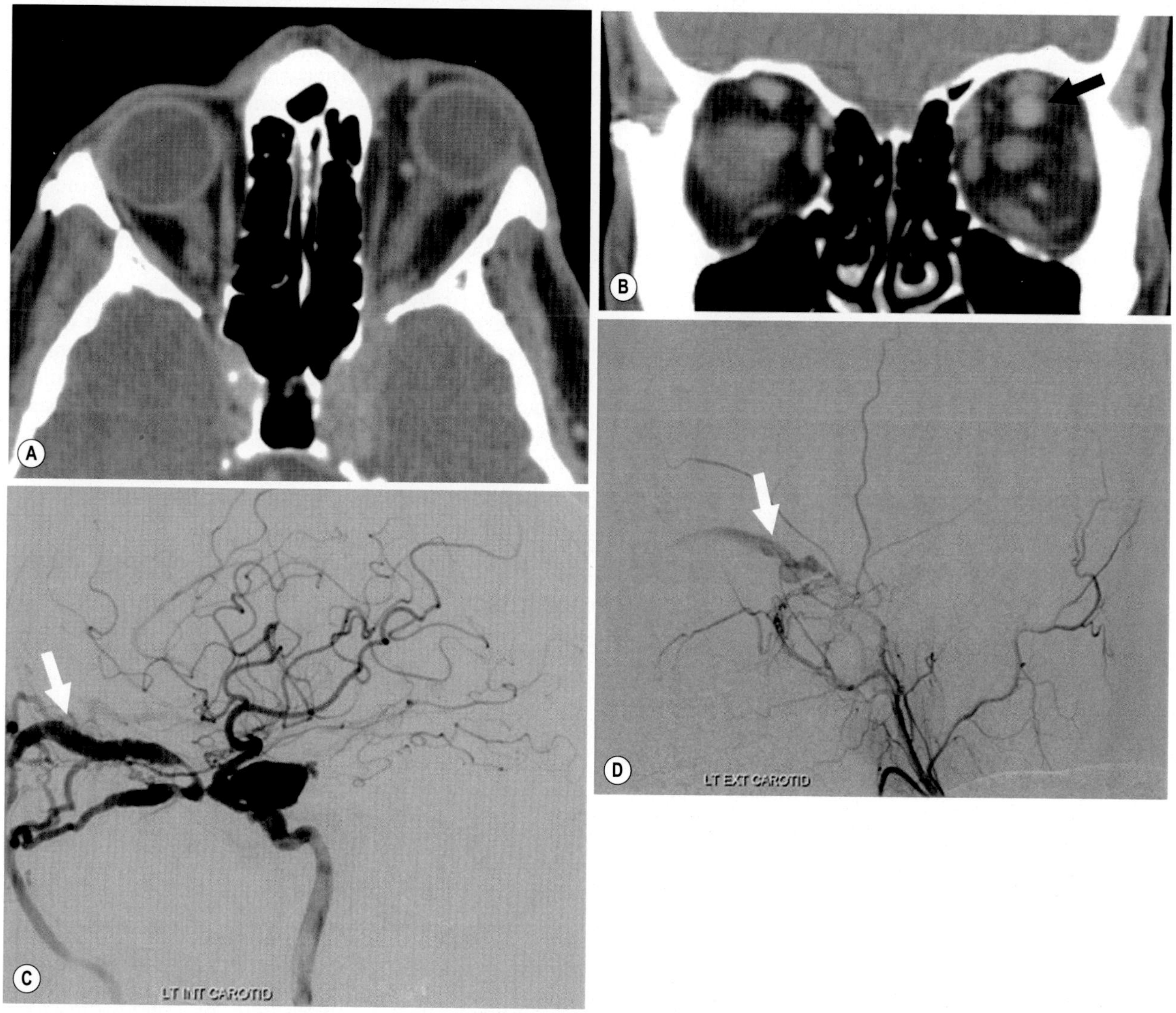

FIGURE 7-24 ■ Carotid-cavernous fistula. Post-contrast axial (A) and coronal (B) CT examination demonstrating left proptosis, stranding of the intraorbital, swelling of the extraocular muscles as well as asymmetric bulkiness of the left cavernous sinus and dilatation of the left superior ophthalmic vein (black arrow). Selective digital subtraction angiography of the left (C) internal and (D) external carotid arteries in two different patients demonstrating a direct and indirect arteriovenous fistula with early filling and retrograde flow through the superior ophthalmic vein (white arrows).

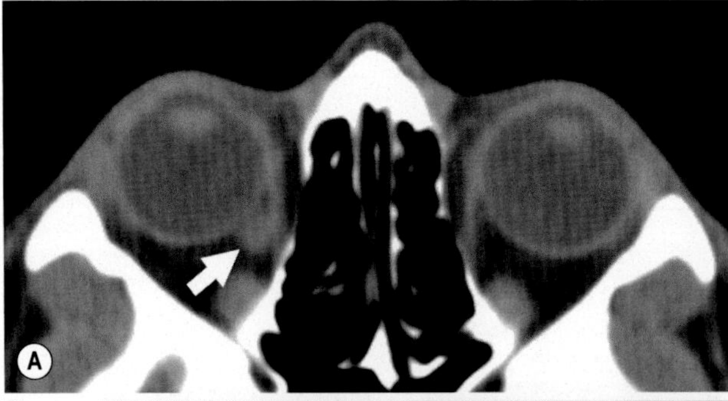

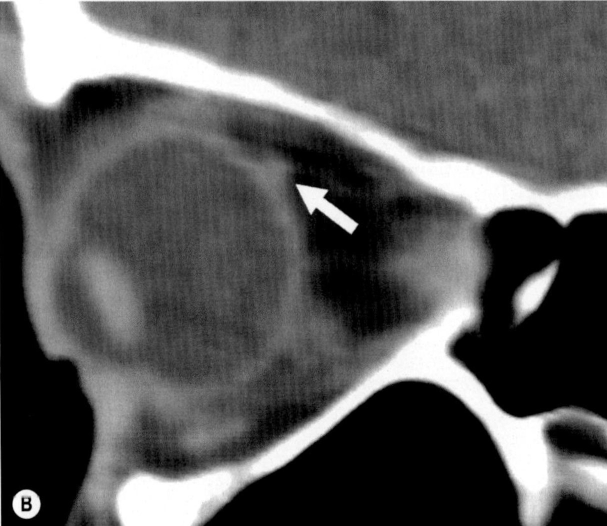

FIGURE 7-25 ■ **Uveal exophytic melanoma.** Post-contrast axial (A) and right sagittal (B) reformats of a CT examination of the orbits demonstrating a small enhancing nodule on the posterior nasal aspect of the right globe (white arrows).

Malignant Neoplasms

Uveal Melanoma

Uveal melanoma is the commonest intraocular primary malignancy in adults[10,20] and commonly presents with progressive visual loss. Extensive spread beyond the globe is common, even in the presence of only a small ocular lesion,[10] resulting in the typical *'collar button'* lesion. Tumour morphology can vary from nodular (Fig. 7-25) to plaque-like lesions and diffuse infiltration. Ophthalmological examination and ultrasound typically form part of the initial work-up. Cross-sectional imaging, particularly MRI, is useful to evaluate for optic nerve involvement and extraocular spread. Increased attenuation on CT as well as T1 shortening (paramagnetic effect) on MRI may be observed due to the presence of melanin. There may also be avid lesional contrast enhancement.

Metastatic Disease

Metastases from extraorbital cancers are most frequently located within the uveal layer, but can involve any intraorbital or adexal structure (Fig. 7-26). Breast, lung cancers and cutaneous melanoma are the most common primaries.[10,27] Prostate cancer is also relatively common, with a propensity for the bony orbit. Rapidly worsening proptosis and globe displacement, diplopia and pain are typical clinical presentations. In children, neuroblastoma commonly metastasises to the orbit. Of note, metastases from sclerosing carcinoma types such as scirrhous breast cancer or gastric carcinoma can result in enophthalmos. Simultaneous brain metastases may provide an important clue on imaging and can be present in up to two-thirds of patients with orbital metastatic disease.[3]

Lymphoproliferative Malignancy

Orbital lymphoma and leukaemia constitute a large share of orbital malignant neoplasms.[28] Orbital involvement can occur in the context of spread from systemic non-Hodgkin's lymphoma (NHL), although only a minority (<2%) of patients with systemic lymphoma demonstrate secondary orbital involvement.[29] Primary orbital lymphoma most frequently represents low-grade mucosa-associated lymphoid tissue (MALT) lymphoma. This commonly affects the lacrimal gland or orbital adnexa and occurs in the absence of systemic disease. Alternatively, orbital involvement may be the initial presentation of systemic lymphoma; therefore, supplementary body imaging as well as appropriate follow-up should be considered in patients with apparently isolated orbital disease. Orbital lymphoma predominantly affects the older population, with a peak of 50–70 years, but can occur at a younger age, especially in immunosuppressed individuals.[30] Clinical symptoms are often insidious, including painless proptosis, diplopia or visual disturbances. Malignant lymphoma may demonstrate hyperdensity on CT both pre- and post-contrast[31] (Fig. 7-27). Decreased signal on T1 and variable signal on T2 MR imaging may be observed. Bone destruction is rare, but can occur in high-grade lesions. Imaging can be non-specific or even negative in early disease, if there is isolated ocular or adnexal involvement.[29,31] Intermediate T1 and T2 signal, post-contrast gadolinium enhancement on MRI and, importantly, PET positivity can be features of adnexal lymphoma.[32]

Orbital involvement in leukaemia is rare but has been described in both in myeloid and lymphoblastic leukaemias. Any orbital structure can be involved, whereby leukaemic infiltration of the optic nerve constitutes an oncological emergency because of the threat to vision. Leukaemia may present as a diffuse infiltrate or mass. In particular, acute myeloid leukaemia (AML) can be associated with mass formation, which is referred to as *chloroma* or *granulocytic sarcoma*. The most common eye complication of leukaemia is retinal haemorrhage secondary to thrombocytopenia.[28]

Adenoid Cystic Carcinoma

This represents the most common malignant epithelial neoplasm of the lacrimal gland and most commonly is the result of malignant transformation of a benign mass, i.e. carcinoma ex pleomorphic adenoma rather than a de novo malignancy.[18] Unless there are convincing aggressive features (Fig. 7-28), this type of lesion may be difficult to distinguish from other lacrimal gland pathologies

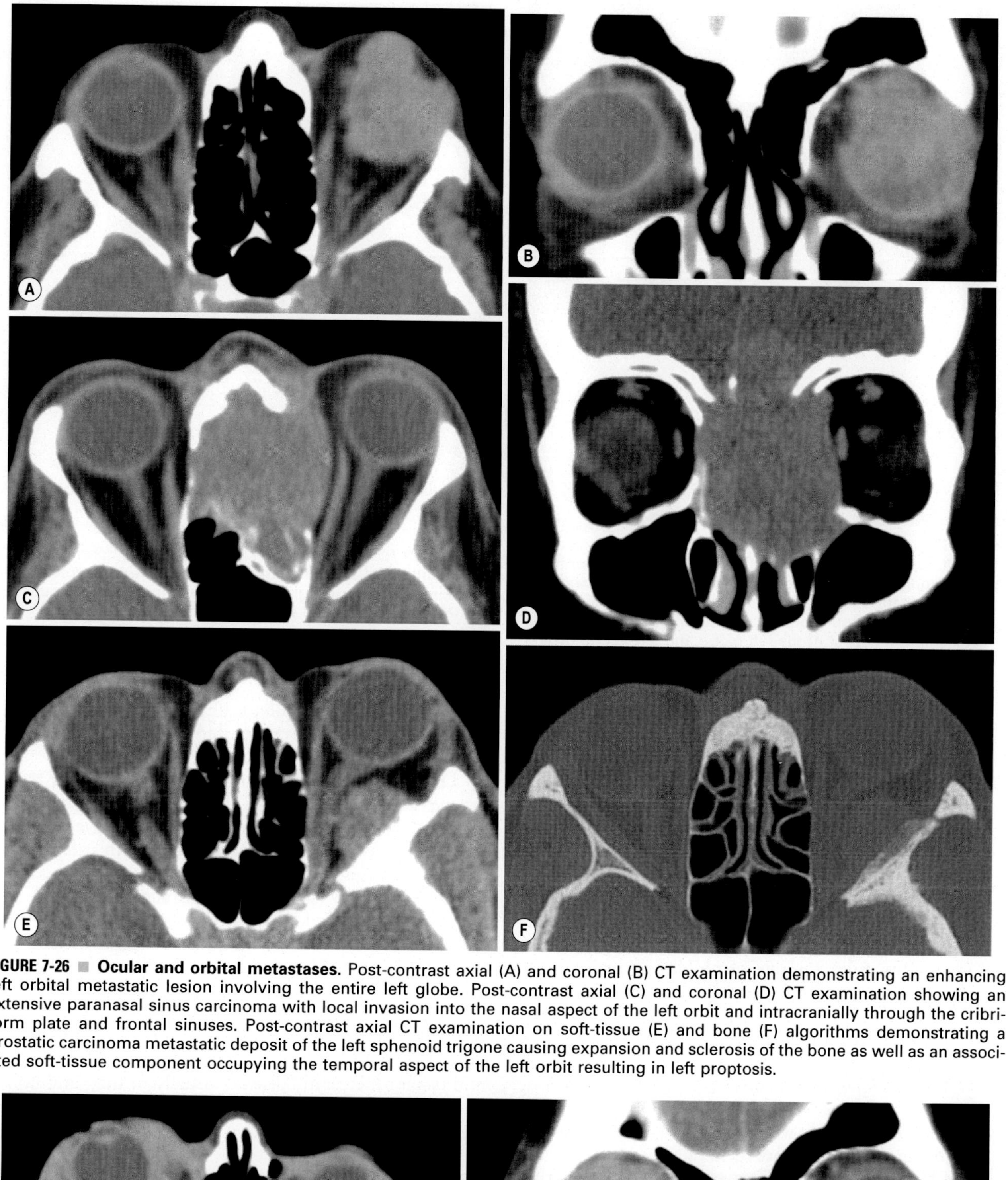

FIGURE 7-26 ■ **Ocular and orbital metastases.** Post-contrast axial (A) and coronal (B) CT examination demonstrating an enhancing left orbital metastatic lesion involving the entire left globe. Post-contrast axial (C) and coronal (D) CT examination showing an extensive paranasal sinus carcinoma with local invasion into the nasal aspect of the left orbit and intracranially through the cribriform plate and frontal sinuses. Post-contrast axial CT examination on soft-tissue (E) and bone (F) algorithms demonstrating a prostatic carcinoma metastatic deposit of the left sphenoid trigone causing expansion and sclerosis of the bone as well as an associated soft-tissue component occupying the temporal aspect of the left orbit resulting in left proptosis.

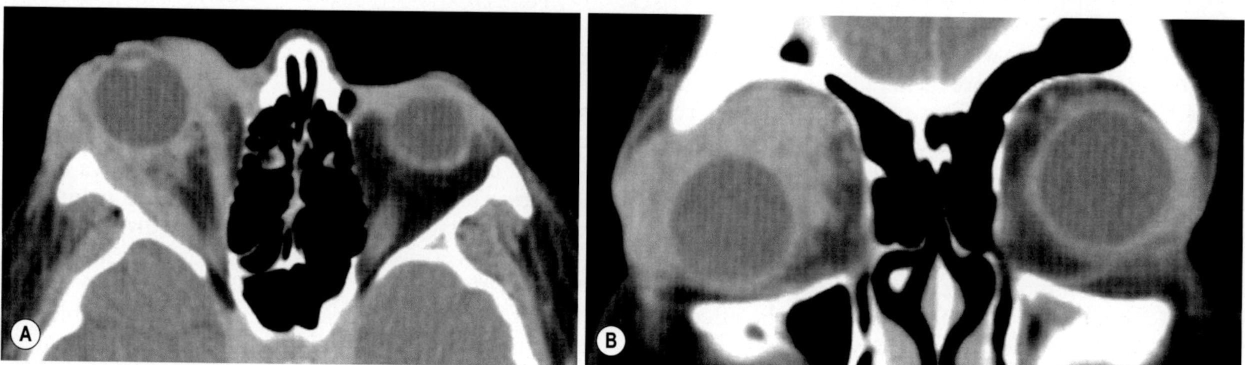

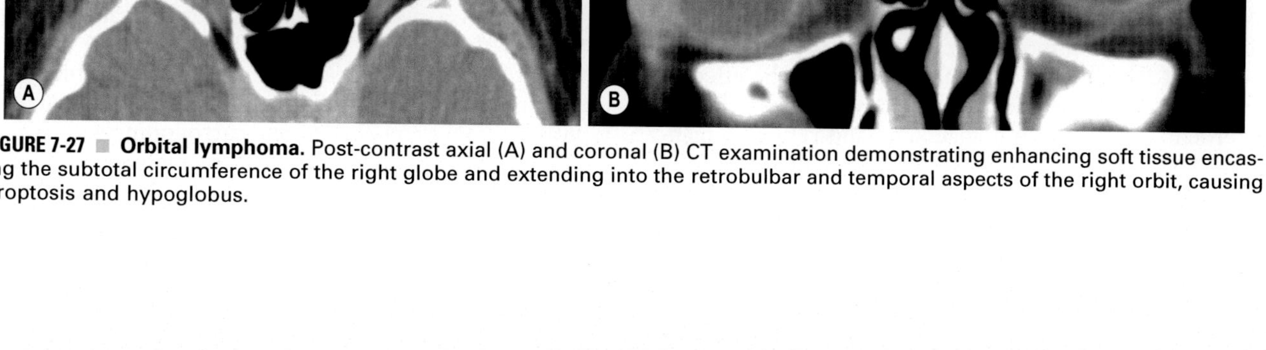

FIGURE 7-27 ■ **Orbital lymphoma.** Post-contrast axial (A) and coronal (B) CT examination demonstrating enhancing soft tissue encasing the subtotal circumference of the right globe and extending into the retrobulbar and temporal aspects of the right orbit, causing proptosis and hypoglobus.

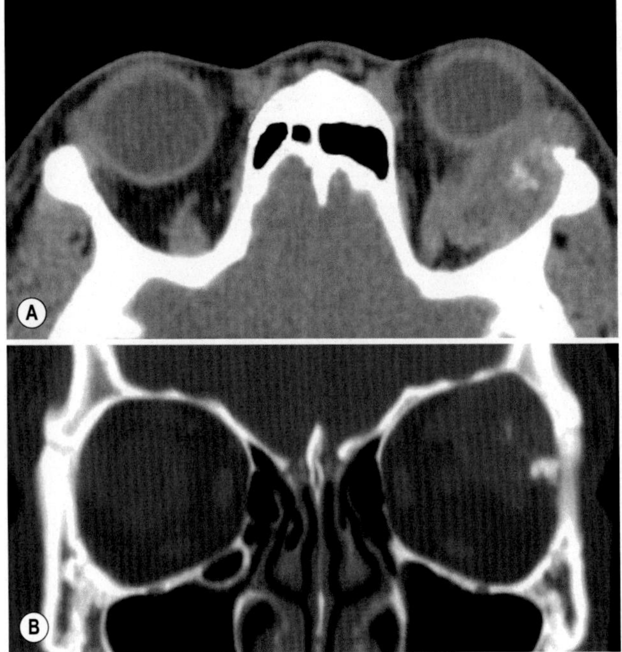

FIGURE 7-28 ■ **Adenoid cystic carcinoma.** Post-contrast axial CT on a soft tissue (A) and coronal CT on a bone (B) algorithms demonstrating a heterogeneous, peripherally enhancing left orbital mass with central coarse calcification indistinguishable from the lacrimal gland. Note the proptosis, deformation of the posterotemporal aspect of the left globe and left lateral orbital wall erosion and bony remodelling by the mass.

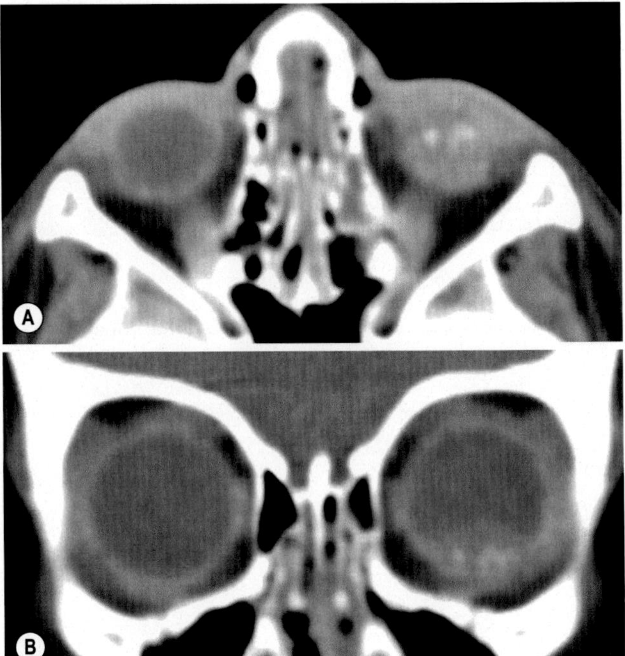

FIGURE 7-29 ■ **Retinoblastoma.** Axial (A) and coronal (B) CT examination in a child demonstrating a lesion involving the inferior aspect of the globe, extending into the vitreous and containing areas of fine punctate calcification.

such as dacryoadenitis, adenoma or lymphoma on imaging alone.

Paediatric Neoplasms

Retinoblastoma

Retinoblastoma is an aggressive malignant neoplasm, which arises from the immature retina. It is the most common intraocular tumour of childhood and usually manifests by the age of 5. Sporadic cases, heritable de novo mutations and familial cases have been reported. The underlying pathomechanism is damage to the RB1 tumour suppressor gene on the long arm of chromosome 13 with subsequent uncontrolled cell proliferation. Patients with inherited retinoblastoma tend to present at a younger age than those with sporadic tumours. Multifocal or bilateral tumours are generally associated with inherited disease. These patients are also at increased risk of associated neuroblastic tumours of the sellar or pineal region, a constellation which is referred to as *trilateral retinoblastoma*. Additionally, patients with inherited retinoblastoma demonstrate an increased incidence of somatic tumours such as osteosarcoma, melanoma and carcinomas. The most common clinical presentation is with leukocoria, i.e. loss of the normal red reflex of the affected eye. Secondary signs include pain, visual disturbance, heterochromia of the iris, glaucoma and retinal detachment. Some retinoblastomas elicit a periocular inflammatory response, which may simulate orbital cellulitis and delay diagnosis.[15] Histologically, endophytic, exophytic and mixed forms are recognised and may demonstrate varying imaging appearances.

The most common finding is that of a nodular lesion arising from the retina. CT is the initial imaging technique of choice and typically demonstrates a hyperattenuating mass in the posterior globe with calcification in 95% of cases[33] (Fig. 7-29). MR imaging is the most sensitive method to delineate intracranial spread and should always include dedicated orbital and whole-brain sequences. Retinoblastoma follows the signal intensity of grey matter on MRI and generally demonstrates contrast enhancement. Prognosis has much improved over the years, resulting in a shift from preservation of life to preservation of sight. However, decreased survival is associated with delayed diagnosis, extraocular extension and distant metastatic disease, usually to lung and bone.

Rhabdomyosarcoma

Rhabdomyosarcoma is the most prevalent extraocular malignancy in children, accounting for approximately 5% of all childhood cancers.[2,34] Approximately a third of paediatric rhabdomyosarcomas arise in the orbit, most often in the first decade, with a peak age around 7 years. It presents as a rapidly progressive unilateral proptosis with or without globe displacement and there may be periorbital swelling, particularly lid swelling, which can lead to misdiagnosis as cellulitis. An aggressive course is typical, with invasion of bone and surrounding soft tissues including the paranasal sinuses. Intracranial spread does occur but is less common.

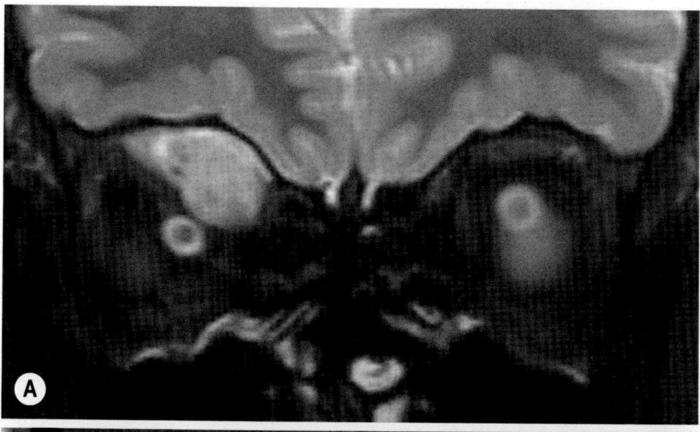

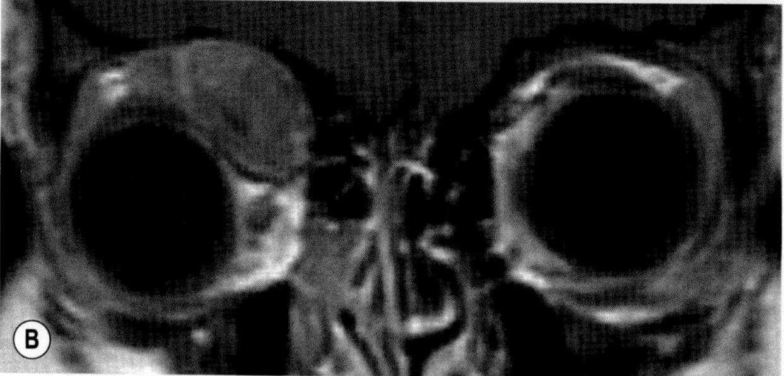

FIGURE 7-30 ■ **Rhabdomyosarcoma.** Coronal STIR (A) and post-contrast T1-weighted (B) orbital MRI in a child demonstrating a superonasal enhancing mass and inferotemporal displacement and some distortion of the right globe.

Metastases are typically haematogenous, with lung and bone involvement being the most common. Cross-sectional imaging is used both for staging and follow-up, whereby CT is most useful to identify bony invasion and MRI is very sensitive at delineating intracranial spread. On CT, the neoplasm may show attenuation similar to muscle or brain, with relatively homogeneous contrast enhancement. The tumour itself does not calcify, but occasionally may contain hyperdense foci if it had infiltrated through bone. On MRI, rhabdomyosarcoma tends to be isoattenuating to muscle on T1 and mildy hyperattenuating on T2 sequences[2,4,34] (Fig. 7-30).

Medulloepithelioma

This is a rare embryonal tumour, which arises from the medullary epithelium of the ciliary body and usually occurs around the age of 5 years, although it can occasionally manifest later, even in adulthood. Benign and malignant variants have been described. On CT imaging, the tumour may demonstrate increased attenuation, sometimes with dystrophic calcifications or cartilaginous components. Localisation of the neoplasm within the ciliary body may be an important clue; however, medulloepithelioma may also arise from or spread to the retina, thus becoming indistinguishable from retinoblastoma on imaging alone.

Ischaemia

Ischaemia of the retina or optic nerve may result in transient (*amaurosis fugax*) or permanent loss of vision. This is commonly caused by a stenosis or occlusion of the ipsilateral internal carotid artery with secondary retinal emboli.[20] Anterior ischaemic optic neuropathy (AION) as the term implies results in ischaemia damage of the optic nerve and constitutes one of the major causes of seriously impaired vision among the middle-aged and elderly, particularly the non-arteritic form (NAION).[35] Arteritic AION is secondary to temporal (giant cell) arteritis, a medium-vessel inflammatory vasculopathy.

Retinal vein occlusion may occur in patients with hypercoaguability; for example, systemic lupus erythematosus and antiphospholipid syndrome.[36] Migraine is also a differential for transient loss of vision, particularly in young patients with a relevant history.

ORBITAL TRAUMA

Injury to the orbital region represents a significant proportion of emergency department attendances and is common in patients with multisystem trauma: for example, following motor vehicle accidents. To date, trauma remains a leading cause of monocular blindness. Certain eye injuries, such as superficial lacerations and a proportion of globe ruptures, may be evident on clinical examination. However, imaging plays a major role in assessing for occult injuries, evaluation of the bony orbit, deep orbital structures and in identifying foreign bodies.

Plain radiography has limited sensitivity in identifying orbital fractures and cannot reliably assess the intraorbital soft tissues. Ultrasound (US) may be of value when there is concern regarding intraocular injury such as traumatic retinal detachment, but it is contraindicated in suspected globe rupture. The technique of choice for the evaluation of suspected orbital injury is thin-section (0.625–1.25 mm slice thickness) CT with multiplanar bone and soft-tissue reconstructions. MR imaging is less commonly employed in acute trauma and is inferior to CT in identifying fractures. Owing to its soft-tissue contrast, it can be useful in complex cases. It must be borne in mind that MR is contraindicated whenever a metallic foreign body is present.

Within the bony orbit, an orbital floor fracture may be a cause of ophthalmoplegia as a result of herniation of fat or muscle into a defect and para/anaesthesia of the maxillary division of the trigeminal nerve when involving the infraorbital canal/nerve. The lamina papyracea is another common site for fractures, as it consists of very thin bone. In addition to a functional deficit, orbital wall fractures may have cosmetic impact: for example, when there is hypoglobus. Care should be taken to review the orbital apex, where a small fracture can be associated with optic nerve injury and require urgent surgical intervention.[37] Evaluation of the orbital soft tissues may reveal fat stranding, haematoma or gas as signs of significant injury (Fig. 7-31).

Metallic and glass orbital foreign bodies are of increased attenuation and best delineated on CT. The appearance of wood on CT can be of similar attenuation to air, thus mimicking intraorbital gas (Fig. 7-32). A wood or organic foreign body should be suspected when there is a low attenuation collection with a geometric margin.[38]

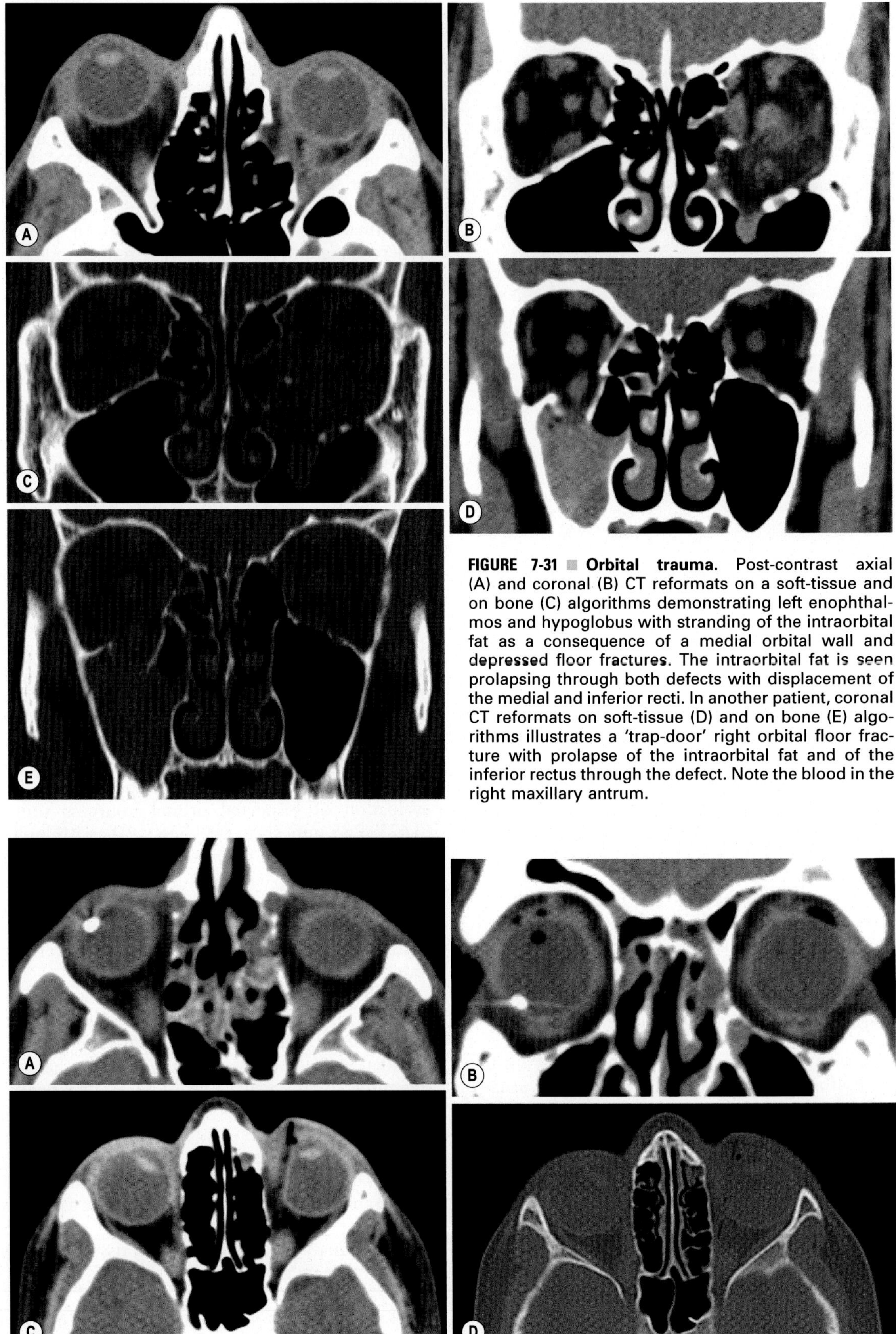

FIGURE 7-31 ■ **Orbital trauma.** Post-contrast axial (A) and coronal (B) CT reformats on a soft-tissue and on bone (C) algorithms demonstrating left enophthalmos and hypoglobus with stranding of the intraorbital fat as a consequence of a medial orbital wall and depressed floor fractures. The intraorbital fat is seen prolapsing through both defects with displacement of the medial and inferior recti. In another patient, coronal CT reformats on soft-tissue (D) and on bone (E) algorithms illustrates a 'trap-door' right orbital floor fracture with prolapse of the intraorbital fat and of the inferior rectus through the defect. Note the blood in the right maxillary antrum.

FIGURE 7-32 ■ **Ocular foreign bodies.** Axial (A) and coronal (B) CT showing a metallic radiodense intraocular penetrating foreign body and vitreal air. Axial CT on soft-tissue (C) and bone (D) algorithms demonstrating a linear hypodensity, resembling air, traversing the nasal aspect of the left globe in a patient with penetrating injury from a wooden splinter. A small locule of air is also seen in the anterior chamber of the eye.

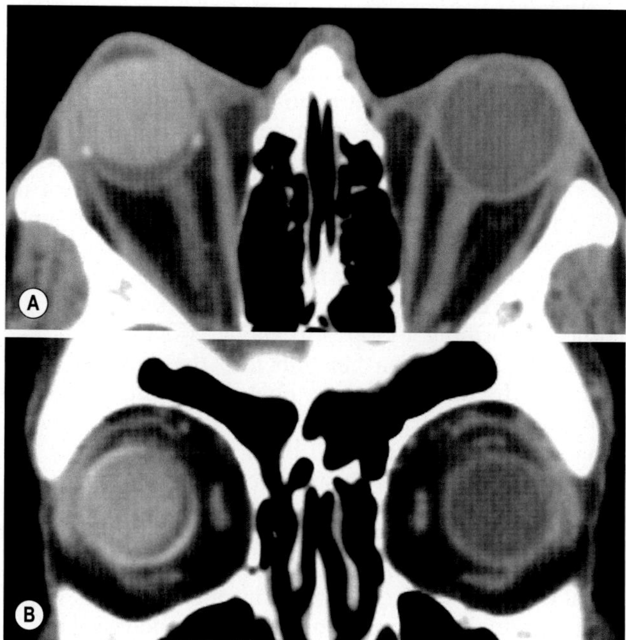

FIGURE 7-33 ■ Axial (A) and coronal (B) CT of a right scleral banding and silicone tamponade as treatment of retinal detachment.

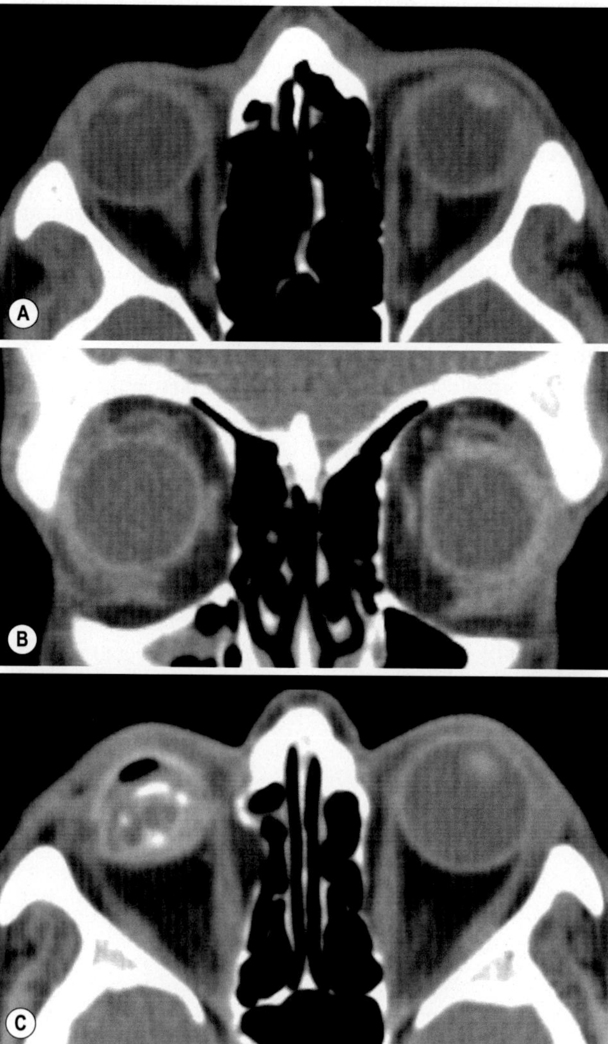

FIGURE 7-34 ■ **Globe rupture.** Axial (A) and coronal (B) CT demonstrating some vitreal haemorrhage in a relatively smaller left globe in a patient with a penetrating injury of the left globe. Note the flattening of the nasal aspect of the globe resembling a 'flat tyre' reflecting globe hypotonia. Axial CT (C) in a patient with previous traumatic injury to the right eye illustrating a small non-functioning calcific right globe or phthisis bulbi.

Within days of the injury, the attenuation of a wooden foreign body may increase, approaching that of water.[39] In challenging cases, T2-weighted and post-contrast fat-suppressed MR imaging can be a potential aid in delineating an inflammatory reaction around the foreign body.[37] Potential mimics of penetrating injury with presence of gas include previous gas injections and placement of low-attenuation silicone sponges for the treatment of retinal detachment. A high-attenuation scleral band around the globe, also a treatment for retinal detachment, can be mistaken for a foreign body; therefore correlation with any previous history of orbital intervention is mandatory (Fig. 7-33).

Signs of globe rupture include loss of globe volume and contour (excluding non-traumatic causes such as coloboma or staphyloma), the *flat tyre* sign and intraocular gas. Retinal detachment shows as a characteristic V-shape structure within the globe, because the retina is relatively fixed at the optic disc posteriorly and at the ora serrata anteriorly. Choroidal detachment can occur as a result of ocular pressure loss: for example, in globe perforation (Figs. 7-34A, B). Increased depth of the anterior chamber is a more subtle sign of open globe injury. *Hyphaema* is defined as blood within the anterior chamber; this may be seen as a blood–fluid level on clinical inspection or as increased attenuation on CT. Decreased depth of the anterior chamber may occur due to corneal laceration or anterior lens subluxation. Posterior lens dislocation is more common, however. Bilateral lens subluxation or dislocation is rare and should raise suspicion of a collagen disorder such as Marfan's, Ehlers-Danlos syndrome or homocystinuria.

Phthisis bulbi refers to a shrunken calcified globe as long-term sequelae of (penetrating) injury (Fig. 7-34C).

THE RETRO-ORBITAL VISUAL PATHWAY

INTRODUCTION

Various diseases have potential to affect the retro-orbital visual pathway, whereby the clinical deficit is usually determined by the anatomical location of the abnormality more than its histological nature. Because the optic nerve is a fibre tract of the brain rather than a true cranial nerve, it may be affected by the same disease processes as the brain and meninges.[40] We provide a brief overview of retro-orbital visual pathway anatomy and pathology according to the respective lesion location.

ANATOMY

Where the intracanalicular optic nerve exits intracranially from its canal, it becomes the intracranial optic nerve. This prechiasmatic segment is approximately 10 mm long, lies below the A1 segment of the anterior cerebral artery and above the internal carotid artery.[40] The optic chiasm is located in the midline at the floor of the third ventricle in close relation to the pituitary stalk and diaphragm sellae. At the optic chiasm, nerve fibres from the nasal aspect of both retinas (carrying information from the temporal visual fields) decussate, whereas fibres from the lateral retina (carrying information from the nasal visual fields) do not decussate. The partially decussated fibre tracts, which emerge dorsally from the chiasm, are termed optic tracts, each containing axons from the ipsilateral temporal and contralateral nasal retina, respectively.

From the chiasm, the optic tracts run dorsolaterally and slightly upwards on each side, passing anterolateral to the tuber cinereum of the hypothalamus towards the lateral geniculate nucleus (LGN) of the thalalmus. Most of the axons from the optic tracts terminate in the LGN, with a few fibres terminating in the superior colliculus of the midbrain. Additional neural connections exist between the LGN and the superior colliculus.[1,41] From the LGN, the optic radiation arises with approximately half of its fibres running posterolaterally, forming part of the superolateral wall of the lateral ventricles. The other half of the optic radiation passes first forward and then backwards along the lateral aspect of the temporal and occipital horns, forming a loop, also known as *Meyer's loop*.

The optic radiation fans out into the primary visual cortex of the occipital lobes. This is sometimes referred to as the striate cortex (named after the *stria of Gennari*, a relatively thick myelinated band within layer 4 of the visual cortex) or V1. The striate cortex is located in the occipital lobe along the banks of the calcarine fissure and at the occipital pole. As a result of the partial decussation and anatomical distribution of nerve fibres, the primary visual cortex of each cerebral hemisphere receives information from the contralateral visual field and visual information is projected upside down; i.e. visual signals from the caudal retina are projected into the cranial aspect of the visual cortex and vice versa (Fig. 7-35). The primary

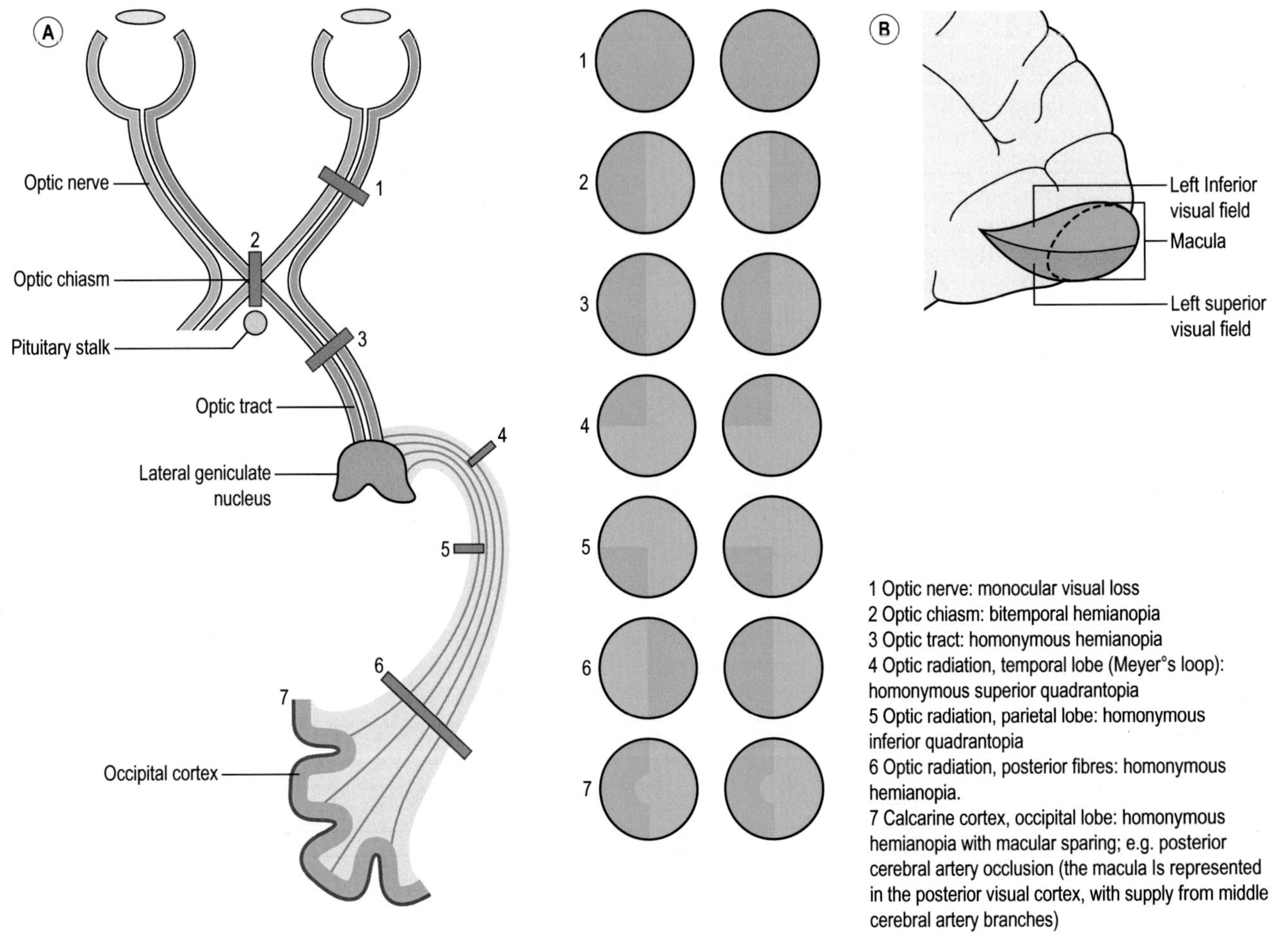

FIGURE 7-35 ■ **Schematic diagram of the visual pathway and the associated field defects with its disruption at different points on the pathway.** (Reproduced from Butler P, Mitchell A, Healy J 2012 Applied Radiological Anatomy 2nd edn. Cambridge University Press, Cambridge, UK.)

visual cortex (V1) is surrounded by several areas of visual association cortex (V2, V3, etc.). Fundamentally, some functions of the associate visual cortical regions overlap with those of the striate cortex, whereas others are involved in higher visual processing such as complex pattern recognition and visual memory formation. To deal with higher visual function in detail would be beyond the scope of this chapter, but for further reading see references 1 and 42.

Vascular supply to the primary visual cortex is predominantly via the posterior cerebral artery, which gives rise to the calcarine artery. Small medial and lateral choroidal branches arise from the P2 segment. Rarely, when these are occluded in isolation, this can result in specific deficits of the central post-chiasmatic visual pathway such as sector anopsia.[43]

PATHOLOGIES OF THE ANTERIOR VISUAL PATHWAY (OPTIC NERVES, CHIASM AND OPTIC TRACTS)

Congenital

Hypoplasia, or in severe cases aplasia, of the optic nerve can occur for several reasons. Examples are chromosomal abnormalities, sporadic mutations, intrauterine insult such as maternal drug intake, but also advanced maternal age.[44] The imaging findings are those of a reduced-calibre nerve without pathological enhancement, usually best appreciated on coronal T2W and STIR MR images (Figs. 7-36A–D).

Septo-optic dysplasia represents a symptom complex featuring a variable combination of midline defects.

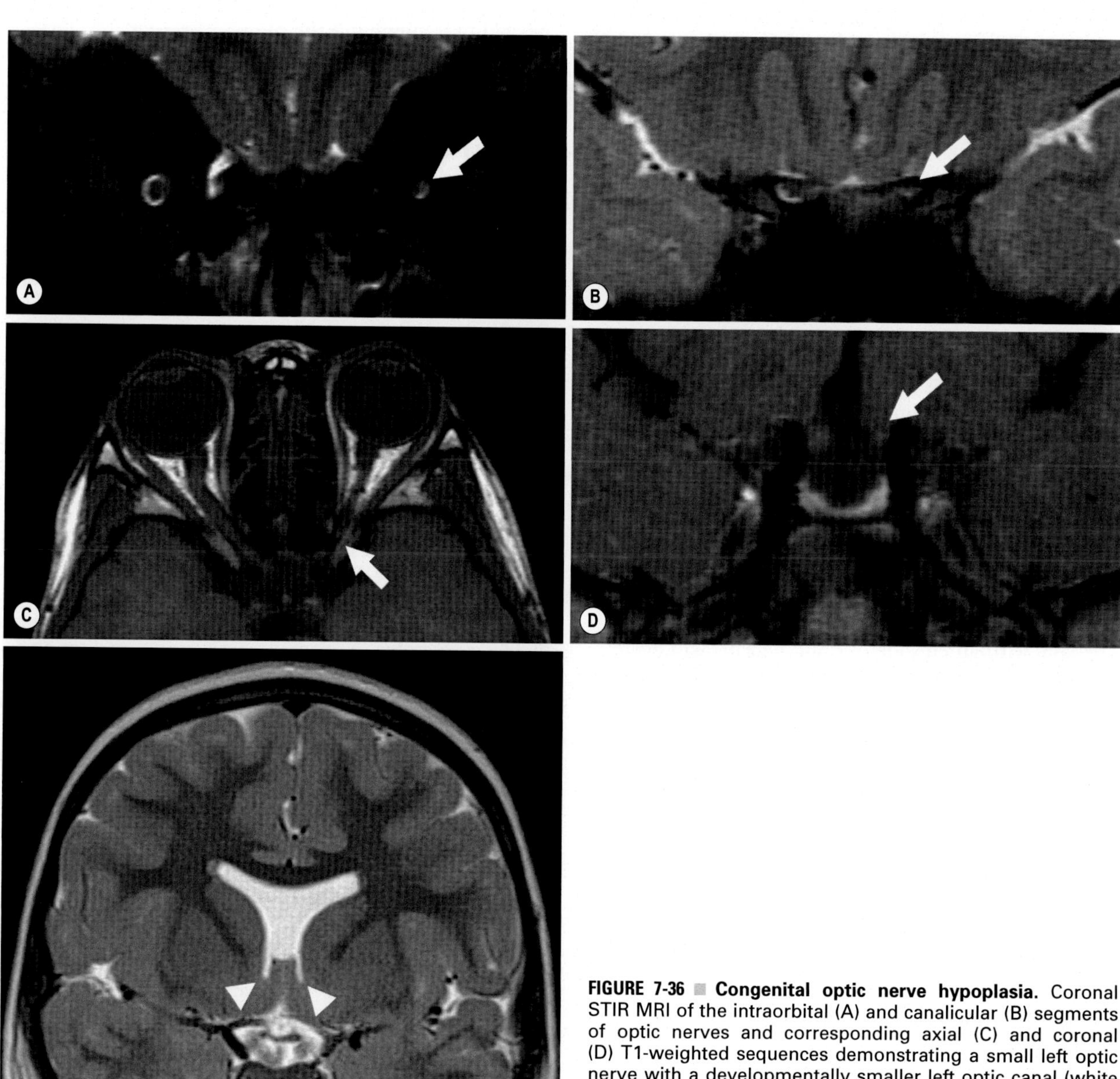

FIGURE 7-36 ■ **Congenital optic nerve hypoplasia.** Coronal STIR MRI of the intraorbital (A) and canalicular (B) segments of optic nerves and corresponding axial (C) and coronal (D) T1-weighted sequences demonstrating a small left optic nerve with a developmentally smaller left optic canal (white arrows). Coronal T2-weighted MRI (E) in a child with septo-optic dysplasia. Note the right optic nerve hypoplasia, absence of the septum pellucidum and 'point-down' appearance of the frontal horns of the lateral ventricles (white arrowheads).

These typically include hypoplasia of the optic nerves, hypoplasia or absence of the septum pellucidum and dysplasia/dysfunction of the hypothalamus–pituitary axis (Fig. 7-36E). Clinical signs consist of visual dysfunction, hormonal abnormalities and varying degrees of learning impairment. Septo-optic dysplasia can be associated with other brain abnormalities such as corpus callosum dysplasia, schizencephaly or cortical dysplasia. In a recent study, 75% of children with septo-optic dysplasia showed associated brain malformations on imaging.[45] Cross-sectional coronal MRI is particularly useful for depicting abnormal optic nerves and sagittal images may demonstrate low-lying fornices if the septum pellucidum is absent.[33]

Intrinsic Tumours

As described in 'The Orbit' section, most intrinsic gliomas are of low grade (pilocytic astrocytoma) and involve the optic nerve in young patients, with a peak in the first decade. Some of these tumours extend to involve the optic chiasm (Fig. 7-18) and approximately 7% of gliomas are confined to the chiasm exclusively.[46] Mortality increases if there is additional hypothalamic involvement. High-grade optic pathway glioma occurs in adult patients and is universally fatal.

Cavernoma is an angiographically occult venous malformation and can occur in any brain parenchymal structure, including the anterior visual pathway. This may be discovered incidentally or present due to slow expansion or haemorrhage, although the latter is rarely clinically apparent.[46] MRI appearances are often diagnostic with the classic 'popcorn' appearance and blooming artefact due to haemosiderin staining and/or calcification visible on gradient-echo and susceptibility-weighted imaging (Fig. 7-37).

Inflammatory/Demyelinating Lesions

Retrobulbar optic neuritis is the initial manifestation of multiple sclerosis in 15–20% of patients and up to half of patients with an episode of optic neuritis will eventually develop MS.[40] Although optic neuritis can be asymptomatic, painful loss of vision with a relatively acute onset over days is more common. MRI is the most sensitive imaging technique for assessing suspected optic neuritis. There may be swelling of the optic nerve with associated signal increase of the nerve on T2 and STIR imaging and post-gadolinium enhancement (Fig. 7-38). Neuromyelitis optica (NMO, also known as *Devic's disease*) should be considered as a differential for bilateral optic neuritis, both on imaging and clinically. NMO may be associated with spinal cord abnormality, which typically affects a longer cord segment (three or more vertebral segments) than MS-type demyelination. Of note, positivity for aquaporin-4 antibodies is a specific finding associated with NMO.

Less commonly, granulomatous inflammation in TB or sarcoidosis (Fig. 7-39) may involve the anterior visual pathway. Imaging abnormalities include nodular or smooth enhancement along the optic nerve or chiasm, and occasionally nerve swelling may be observed.[40] However, these features are not specific and may be difficult to distinguish from a neoplasm on imaging alone. Metastatic disease is also a differential to be considered in this imaging scenario.

Extrinsic Compression

Extrinsic compression of the optic chiasm is more common than intrinsic lesions of this region. Compressive symptoms can occur secondary to a host of different intracranial pathologies such as pituitary macroadenoma, craniopharyngioma, Rathke's cleft cyst, meningioma, germinoma, chordoma, metastases and aneurysms (Fig. 7-40). The classic deficit arising from midline chiasmatic compression is a bitemporal hemianopia. In contrast, a lesion compressing the chiasm laterally is more likely to cause a nasal visual field defect due to compression of nerve fibres supplying the temporal retina.

PATHOLOGIES OF THE POSTERIOR VISUAL PATHWAY (LATERAL GENICULATE NUCLEUS, OPTIC RADIATION AND VISUAL CORTEX)

Although there are no diseases which specifically target the LGN, this may be involved by intracranial pathology in its proximity. Isolated LGN pathology is rare, but this is known to produce a specific visual deficit of homonymous sector defects on the horizontal meridian.[47]

Equally, the optic radiation and visual cortex can be compromised by intracranial pathology of any nature nearby. The clinical picture and visual deficit will be dictated predominantly by the lesion location. Posterior cerebral artery (PCA) infarction is a common central cause for acute-onset visual impairment, with the field defect being determined by location and extent of ischaemia. If involving the entire primary visual cortex, bilateral PCA infarction may lead to 'cortical blindness' or *Anton–Babinski syndrome*. A large infarct may be evident on CT within hours of onset, but generally MRI, including diffusion-weighted imaging, is the most sensitive method, particularly for the detection of small infarcts, and MR is able to demonstrate imaging abnormality earlier than CT (Fig. 7-41).

Space-occupying masses may produce symptoms either due to direct infiltration or secondary to compression of neural structures. Intrinsic primary brain tumours, but also intracranial metastases (commonly breast, lung or melanoma) or lymphoma, are typical examples. Infection, including abscess formation, can involve any intracranial structure and should be considered particularly in immunosuppressed patients. Other aetiologies, which may be encountered along the posterior visual pathway, include encephalitis, abscesses, posterior reversible encephalopathy syndrome (PRES), progressive multifocal leukencephalopathy (PML) and arteriovenous malformations (Fig. 7-42). For a more detailed description of intracranial pathologies, please see Chapter 2.

Text continued on p. 208

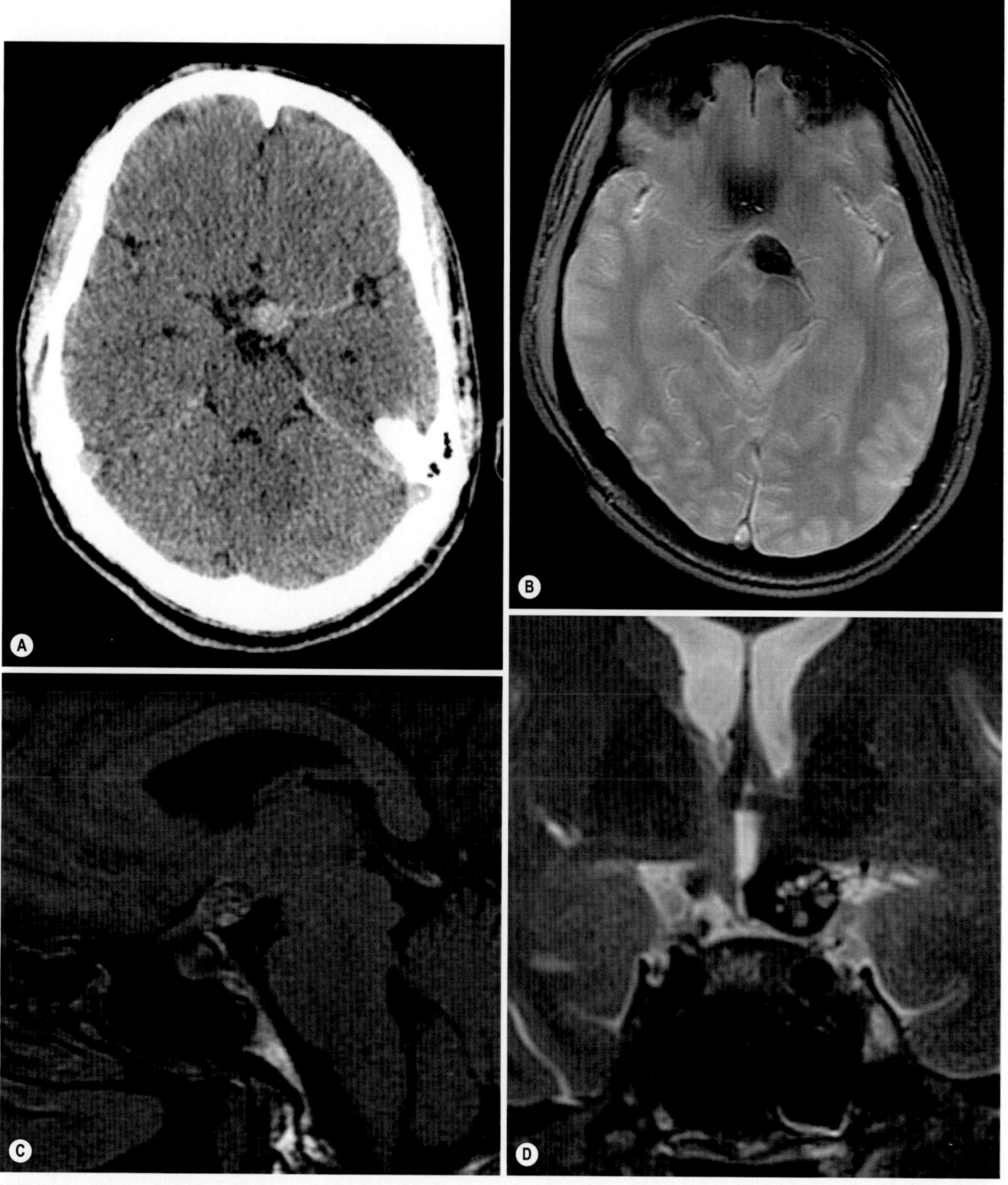

FIGURE 7-37 ■ **Optic pathway cavernoma.** Post-contrast axial CT (A) showing a hyperattenuating mass in the left suprasellar cistern, thought initially to be an aneurysm. Corresponding axial T2*- (B), sagittal T1- (C) and coronal T2-weighted (D) MRI demonstrating the classic 'popcorn' appearance of a cavernoma intrinsic to the left optic chiasm and tract.

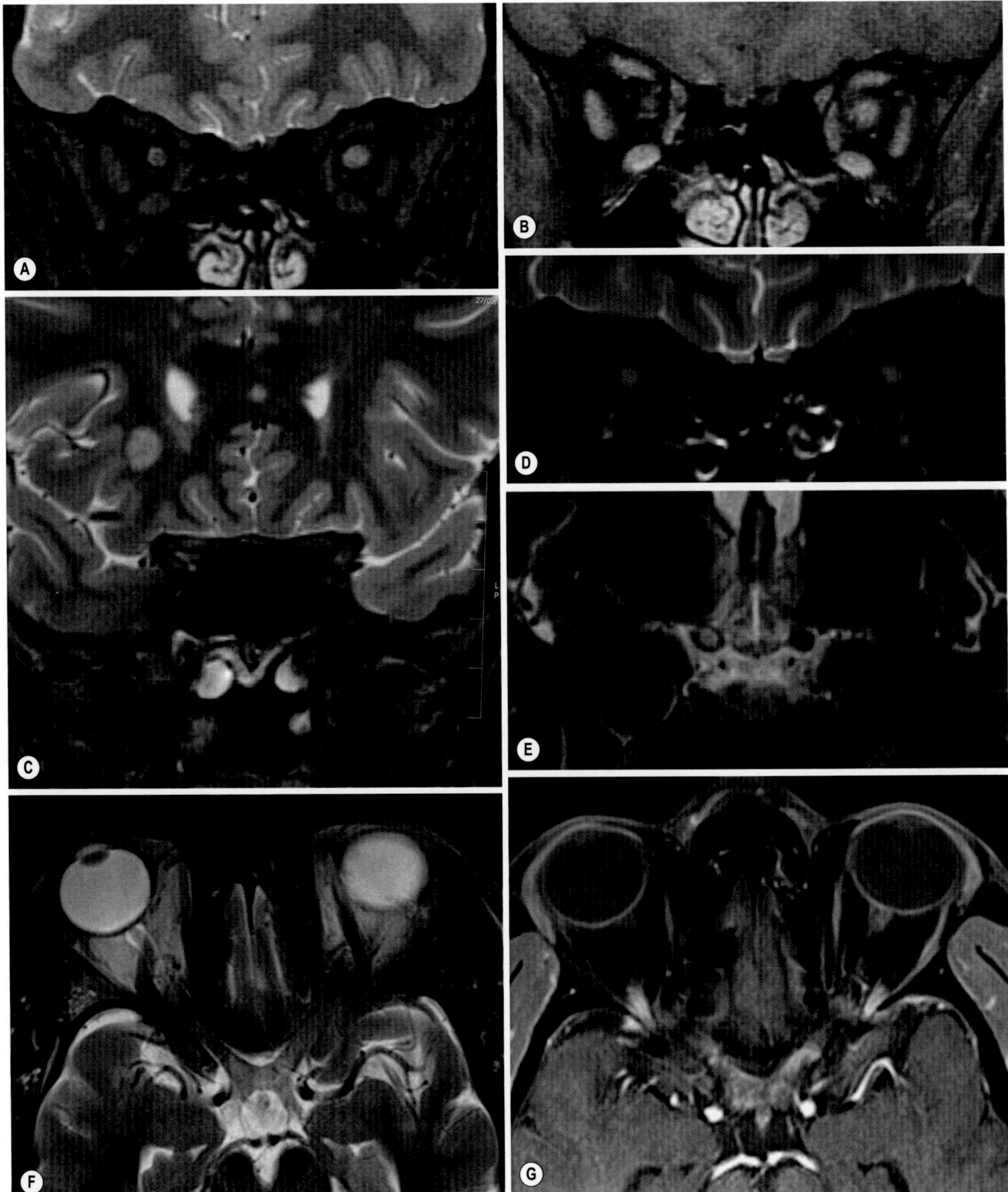

FIGURE 7-38 ■ Optic neuritis in multiple sclerosis. Coronal STIR (A) and post-contrast fat-suppressed T1-weighted (B) MRI of the orbits demonstrating hyperintensity, swelling and enhancement of the intraorbital segment of the left optic nerve in a patient presenting with left optic neuritis. Coronal STIR images through the canalicular (C) and intraorbital (D) segment of the optic nerves and of the optic tracts (E) in two other patients. In (C), there is hyperintensity and swelling of the canalicular right optic nerve and demyelinating lesions in the white matter of the frontal lobes. Neuromyelitis optica: In (D, E), bilateral inflammation involving the intraorbital segment of the optic nerves and the right optic tract. Note the associated hypothalamic inflammation. The axial T2- (F) and post-contrast fat-suppressed T1-weighted (G) MRI of the orbits as well as a sagittal T2-weighted image of the upper spinal cord (H) demonstrate inflammation and enhancement of the optic chiasm as well as a contiguous segmental myelitis of the upper thoracic spinal cord.

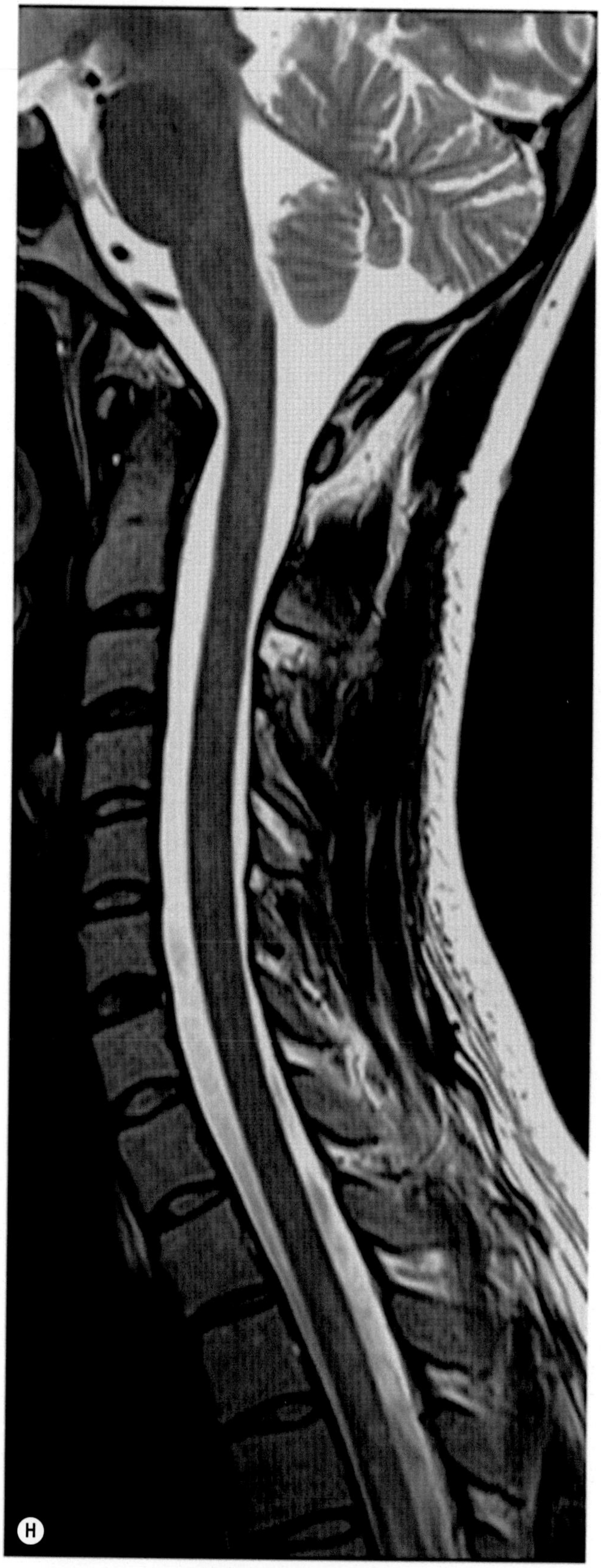

FIGURE 7-38, Continued

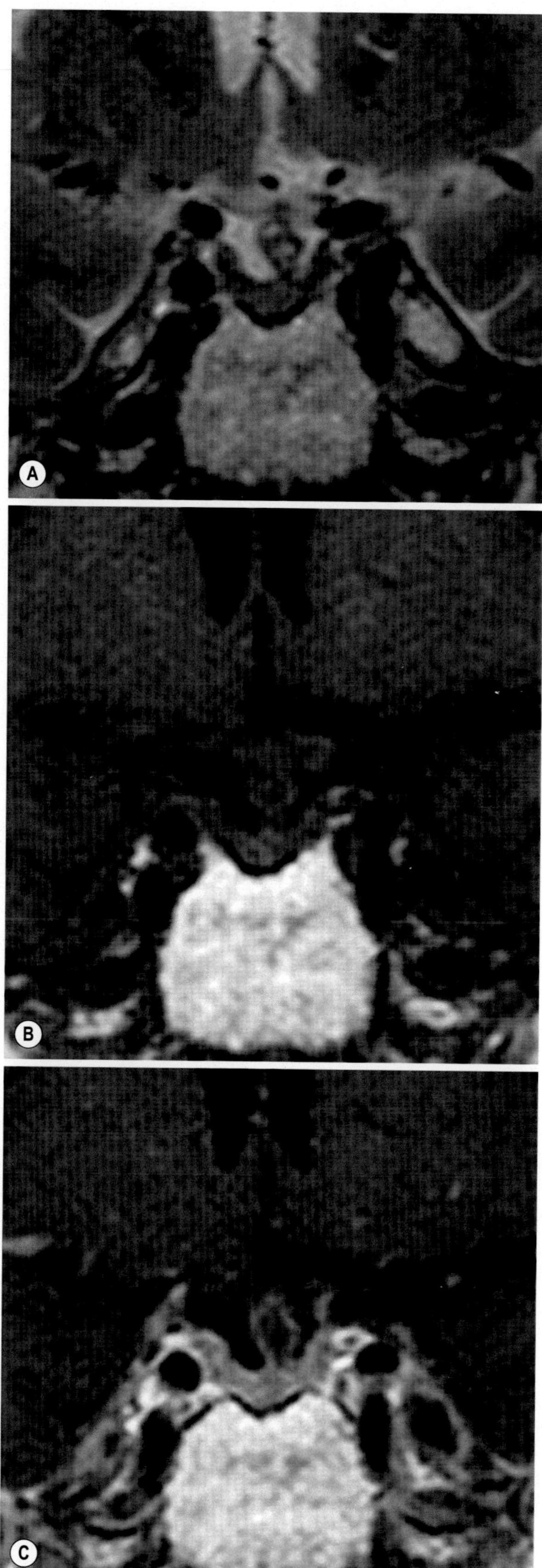

FIGURE 7-39 ■ Optic pathway granulomatous inflammation. Coronal T2- (A), T1- (B) and post-contrast coronal (C) and sagittal (D) T1- weighted MRI of an enhancing inflammatory process of the pituitary infundibulum and the optic chiasm in a patient with sarcoidosis. *Continued on following page*

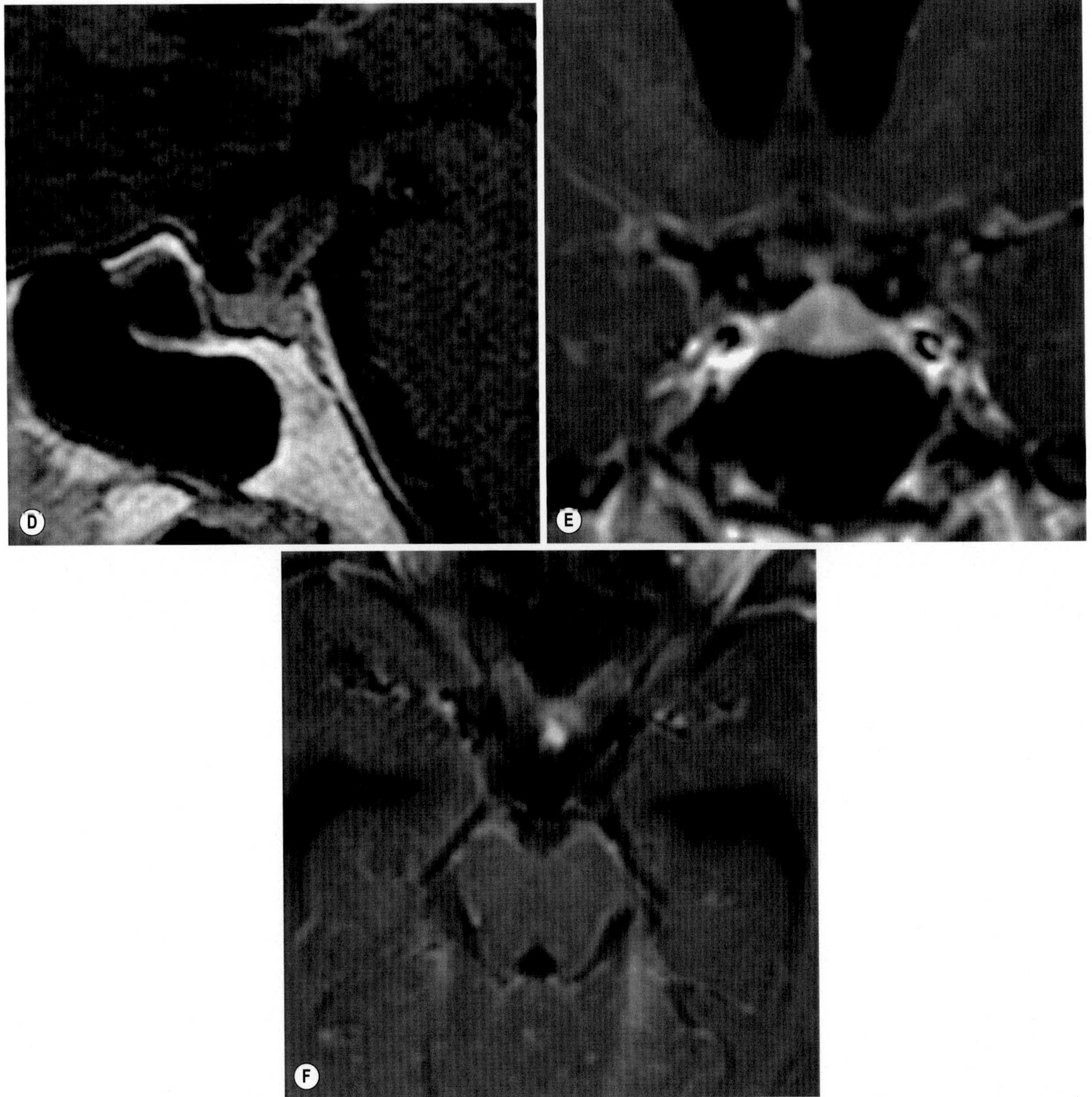

FIGURE 7-39, Continued ■ Post-contrast coronal (E) and axial (F) T1-weighted MRI demonstrating a diffuse enhancing leptomeningeal process affecting the intracranial optic nerves and optic chiasm in a patient with tuberculous basal meningitis.

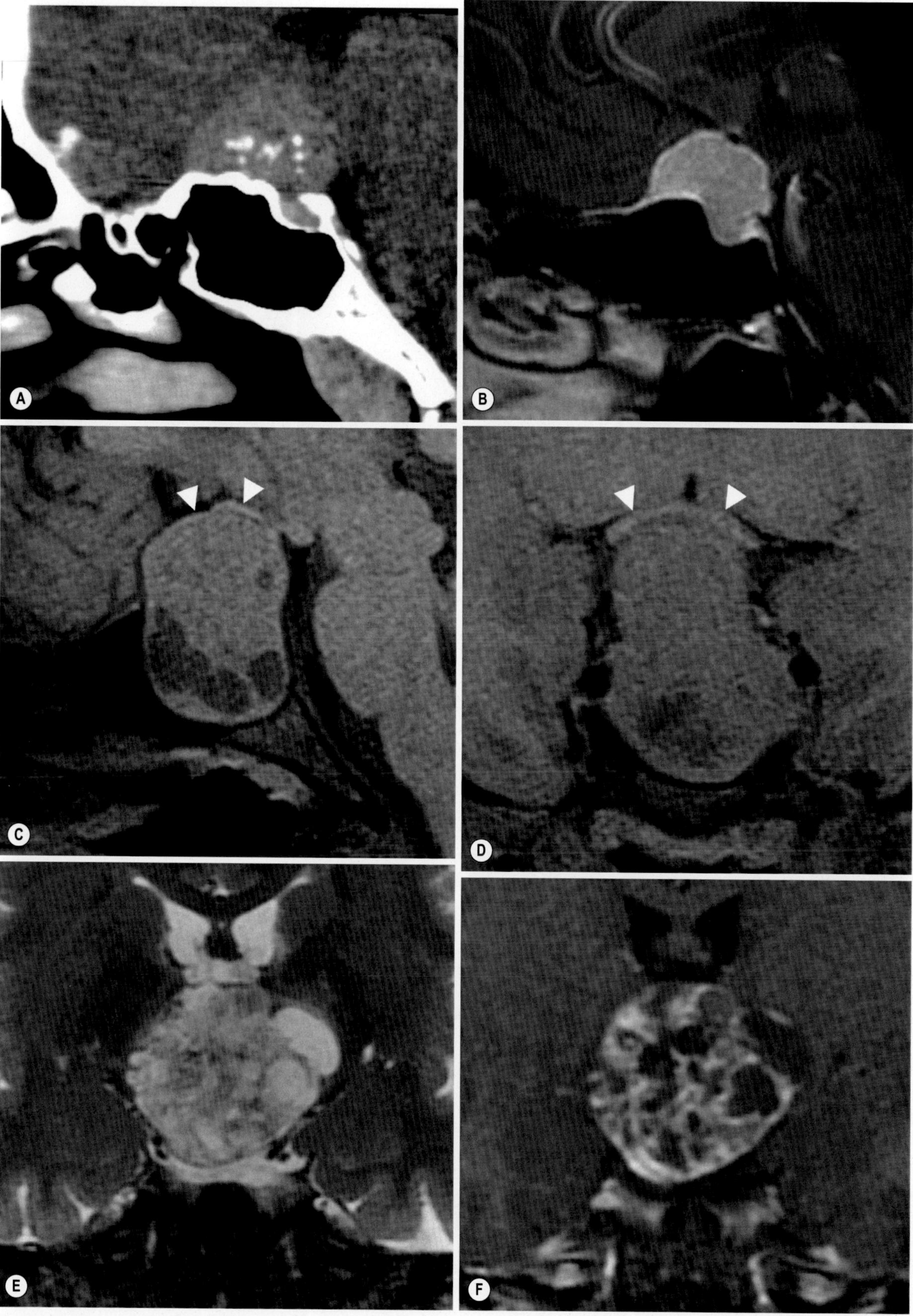

FIGURE 7-40 ■ Optic pathway compressive tumours. Sagittal reformatted post-contrast CT (A) and post-contrast sagittal T1-weighted MRI (B) of an enhancing calcific meningioma of the planum sphenoidale, compressing the optic chiasm. Sagittal (C) and coronal (D) T1-weighted MRI of a pituitary macroadenoma compressing the optic chiasm. Note the optic chiasm draped over the suprasellar component of the tumour (white arrowheads). Coronal T2- (E) and post-contrast T1-weighted (F) MRI of a craniopharyngioma causing similar compression.

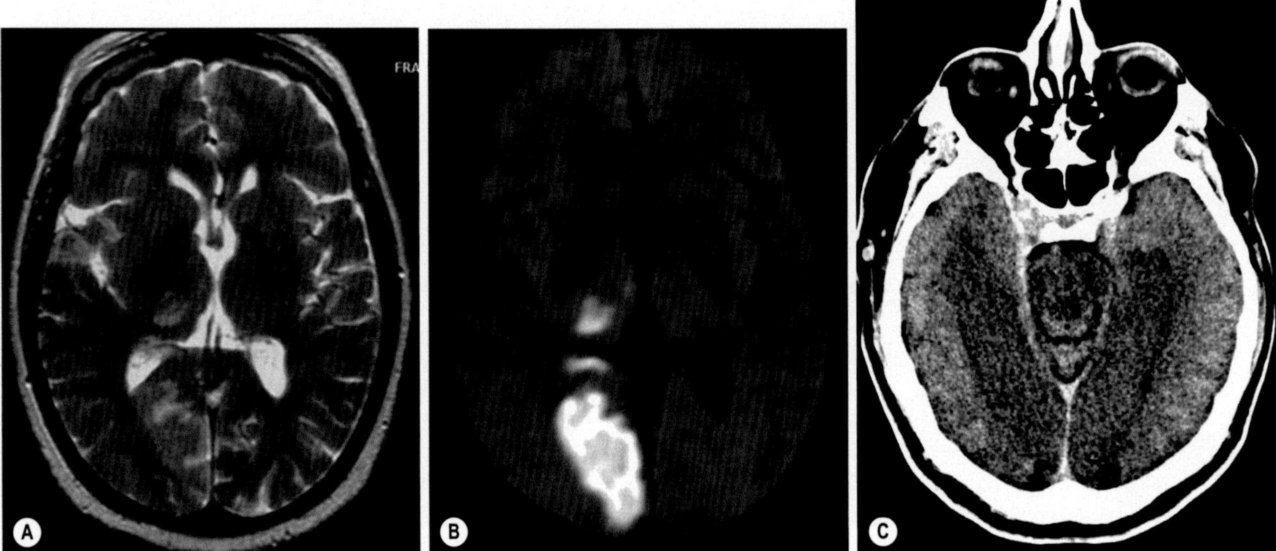

FIGURE 7-41 ■ Posterior cerebral artery (PCA) infarction. Axial T2- (A) and diffusion-weighted (B) MRI illustrating an acute right occipital and thalamic infarct with restriction on DWI. Axial CT (C) of a basilar artery thrombosis with pontine and bilateral PCA territory hypodense infarcts.

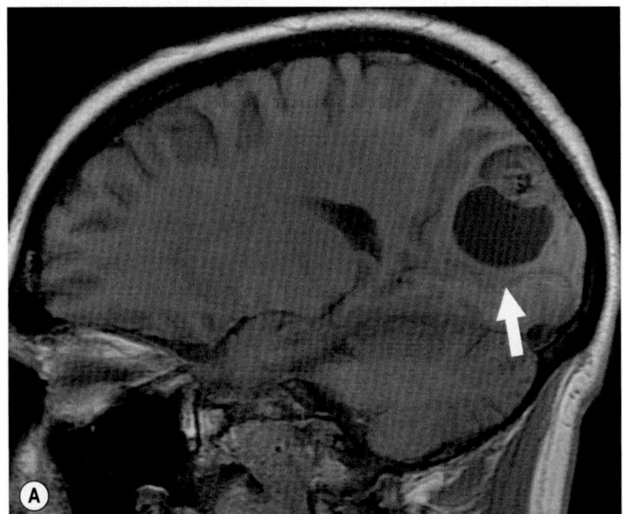

FIGURE 7-42 ■ Lesions of the posterior visual pathway. Sagittal T1-weighted MRI (A) of an intrinsic glioma of the cuneus of the occipital lobe. Note the displaced calcarine sulcus (white arrow). Axial T2- (B) and post-contrast T1-weighted (C) MRI of enhancing primary CNS lymphoma in a periventricular distribution. Axial T2- (D) and post-contrast T1-weighted (E) MRI of enhancing metastases from a lung primary.

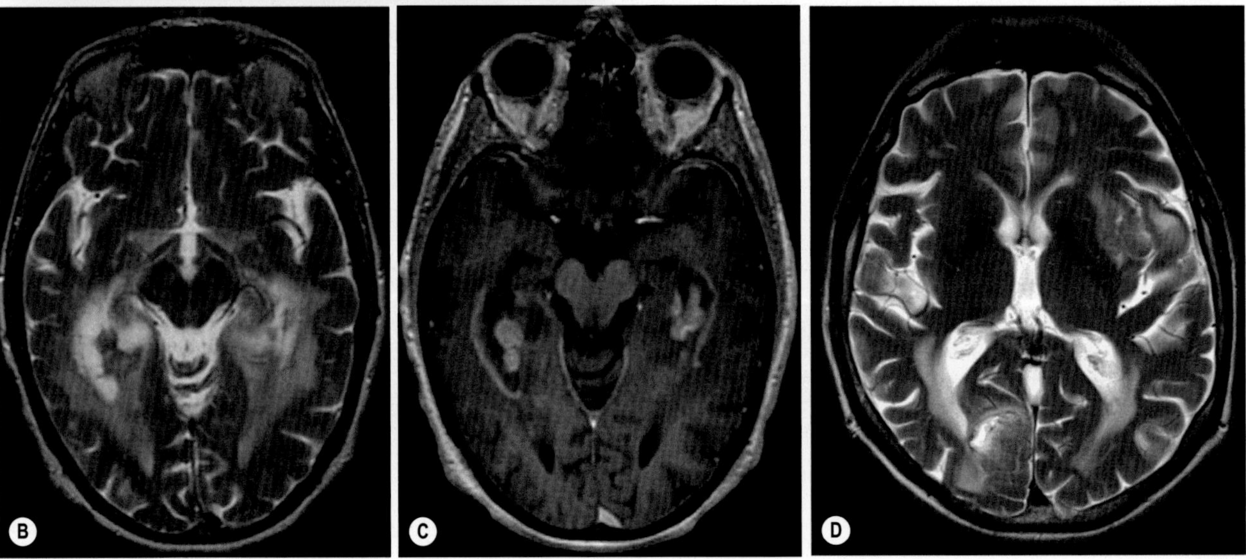

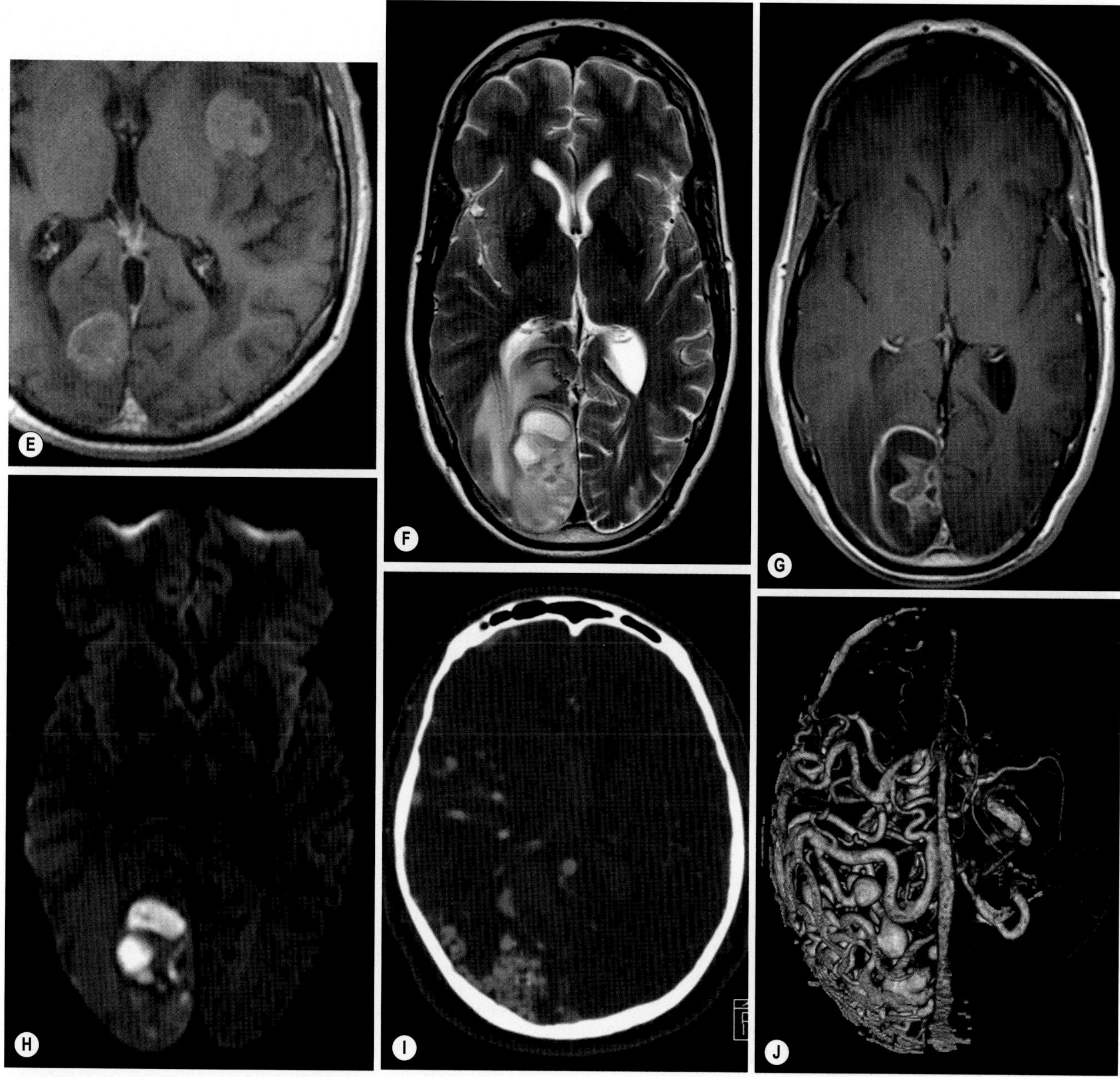

FIGURE 7-42, Continued ■ Axial T2- (F), post-contrast T1- (G) and diffusion-weighted (H) MRI of a right occipital lobe abscess. Axial CT angiogram (I) and 3D surface-rendered reconstruction (J) of a large right occipital lobe arterio-venous malformation.

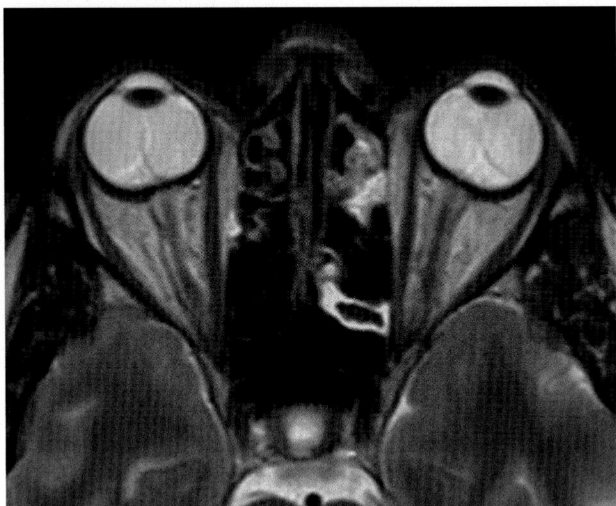

FIGURE 7-43 ■ Papilloedema in idiopathic intracranial hypertension. Axial T2-weighted MRI of the orbits demonstrating ectasia of the optic nerve sheaths, posterior globe flattening and protrusion of the optic nerve heads into the globes.

OTHER NEURO-OPHTHALMOLOGICAL CONDITIONS

Idiopathic Intracranial Hypertension

Idiopathic intracranial hypertension (previously known as *pseudotumour cerebri*) is a disease of unknown aetiology, typically affecting young obese women and producing a syndrome of raised intracranial pressure that is not related to an intracranial disorder, a meningeal process or cerebral venous thrombosis.[48] Associated imaging findings include tortuosity and ectasia of the optic nerve sheaths, flattening of the posterior globes (Fig. 7-43), which correlate with the clinical observation of papilloedema, an expanded empty sella turcica and narrowing of the distal transverse venous sinuses.

Recurrent Ophthalmoplegic Cranial Neuropathy

Recurrent ophthalmoplegic cranial neuropathy (*ophthalmoplegic migraine*) is a rare and poorly understood neurological syndrome which usually presents in children, but can persist in adulthood. It is characterised by recurrent bouts of head pain and ophthalmoplegia which recovers in most patients within days to weeks, but a small proportion of patients affected are left with persistent neurological deficits. The oculomotor nerve is most commonly affected, at times associated with mydriasis and ptosis. This can be associated with thickening and enhancement of the third (in approximately 75%) or rarely the fourth and/or sixth cranial nerve on contrast-enhanced MRI.[49]

REFERENCES

1. Baert AL, Sartor K, Mueller-Forell WS, editors. Imaging of the Orbital and Visual Pathway. Springer; 2002.
2. Chung EM, Specht CS, Schroeder JW. Pediatric orbit tumours and tumourlike lesions: neuroepithelial lesions of the ocular globe and optic nerve. Radiographics 2007;27:1159–86.
3. Aviv RI, Miszkiel K. Orbital imaging: Part 2. Intraorbital pathology. Clin Radiol 2005;60:288–307.
4. Goh PS, Gi MT, Charlton A, et al. Review of orbital imaging. Eur J Radiol 2008;66:387–95.
5. Smith M, Castillo M. Imaging and differential diagnosis of the large eye. Radiographics 1994;14:721–8.
6. Spaide RF, Curcio CA. Drusen characterization with multimodal imaging. Retina 2010;30(9):1441–54.
7. Ding ZX, Lip G, Chong V. Idiopathic orbital pseudotumour. Clin Radiol 2011;886–92.
8. Swamy BN, McCluskey P, Nemet A, et al. Idiopathic orbital inflammatory syndrome: clinical features and treatment outcomes. Br J Ophthalmol 2007;91:1667–70.
9. Mendenhall WM, Lessner AM. Orbital pseudotumour. Am J Clin Oncol 2010;33:304–6.
10. Mafee MF, Karimi A, Shah J, et al. Anatomy and pathology of the eye: role of MR imaging and CT. Radiol Clin North Am 2006;44:135–57.
11. McCluskey P, Powel RJ. The eye in systemic inflammatory diseases. Lancet 2004;364:2125–33.
12. Gordon LK. Orbital inflammatory disease: a diagnostic and therapeutic challenge. Eye 2006;20:1196–206.
13. Koyama T, Ueda H, Togashi K, et al. Radiologic manifestation of sarcoid in various organs. Radiographics 2004;24:87–104.
14. Provenzale JM, Mukherji S, Allen NB, et al. Orbital involvement by Wegener's granulomatosis: imaging findings. Am J Roentgenol 1996;166(4):929–34.
15. Chung EM, Smirniotopoulos JG, Specht CS, Schroeder JW. Pediatric orbit tumours and tumourlike lesions: Nonosseous lesions of the extraocular orbit. Radiographics 2007;27:1777–99.
16. Smirniotopoulos JG, Bargallo N, Mafee MF. Differential diagnosis of leukokoria: radiologic-pathologic correlation. Radiographics 1994;14:1059–79.
17. Narula MK, Chaudhary V, Baruah D, et al. Pictorial essay: Orbital tuberculosis. Indian J Radiol Imaging 2010;20(1):6–10.
18. Jung WS, Ahn KJ, Park MR, et al. The radiological spectrum of orbital pathologies that involve the lacrimal gland and the lacrimal fossa. Korean J Radiol 2007;8:336–42.
19. Rootman J, Goldberg C, Robertson W. Primary orbital schwannomas. Br J Ophthalmol 1982;66:192–204.
20. Jaeger HR. Loss of vision: Imaging the visual pathways. Eur Radiol 2005;15(3):501–10.
21. Kanamalla US. The optic nerve tram-track sign. Radiology 2003;227(3):718–19.
22. Xian J, Zhang Z, Wang Z, et al. Evaluation of MR imaging findings differentiating cavernous haemangiomas from schwannomas in the orbit. Eur Radiol 2010;20:2221–8.
23. Thorn-Kany M, Delisle MB, Lacroix F, et al. Cavernous haemangiomas of the orbit: MR imaging. J Neuroradiol 1999;26:79–86.
24. Tanaka A, Mihara F, Yoshiura T, et al. Differentiation of cavernous haemangioma from schwannoma of the orbit: a dynamic MRI study. Am J Roentgenol 2004;183:1799–804.
25. Smoker W R K, Gentry LR, Yee NK, et al. Vascular lesions of the orbit: More than meets the eye. Radiographics 2008;28:185–204.
26. Schmidt D, Pache M, Schumacher M. The congenital unilateral retinocephalic vascular malformation syndrome (Bonnet–Dechaume–Blanc syndrome or Wyburn-Mason syndrome): review of the literature. Surv Ophthalmol 2008;53(3):227–49.
27. Ahmad SM, Esmaeli B. Metastatic tumours of the orbit and ocular adnexa. Curr Opin Ophthalmol 2007;18:405–13.
28. Valvassori GE, Sabnis SS, Mafee RF, et al. Imaging of orbital lymphoproliferative disorders. Radiol Clin North Am 1999;37(1):135–50.
29. Haque S, Law M, Abrey LE, Young RJ. Imaging of lymphoma of the central nervous system, spine and orbit. Radiol Clin North Am 2008;46:339–61.
30. Vohra ST, Escott EJ, Stevens D, Branstetter BF. Categorisation and characterisation of lesions of the orbital apex. Neuroradiology 2011;53:89–107.
31. Akansel G, Hendrix L, Erickson BA, et al. MRI patterns in orbital malignant lymphoma and atypical lymphocytic infiltrates. Eur J Radiol 2005;53:175–81.
32. O'Sullivan TJ, Valenzuela AA. Imaging features of ocular adnexal lymphoproliferative disease. Eye 2006;20:1189–95.
33. Barkovich AJ. Pediatric Neuroimaging. 4th ed. Philadelphia: Lippincott & Williams; 2005.

34. Chung EM, Murphey MD, Specht CS, et al. From the Archives of the AFIP. Pediatric orbit tumors and tumorlike lesions: osseous lesions of the orbit. Radiographics 2008;28(4):1193–214.
35. Hayreh SS. Vascular disorders in neuro-ophthalmology. Curr Opin Neurol 2011;24(1):6–11.
36. Au A, O'Day J. Review of severe vaso-occlusive retinopathy in systemic lupus erythematosus and the antiphospholipid syndrome: associations, visual outcomes, complications and treatment. Clin Experiment Ophthalmol 2004;32:87–100.
37. Kubal WS. Imaging of orbital trauma. Radiographics 2008;28: 1729–39.
38. Go JL, Vu VN, Lee KJ, Becker TS. Orbital trauma. Neuroimaging Clin North Am 2002;12:311–24.
39. Yamashita K, Noguchi T, Mihara F, et al. An intraorbital wooden foreign body: description of a case and a variety of CT appearances. Emerg Radiol 2007;14:41–3.
40. Smith MM, Strothmann JM. Imaging of the optic nerve and visual pathways. Semin Ultrasound CT MRI 2001;22:473–87.
41. Wichmann W, Mueller-Forell W. Anatomy of the visual system. Eur J Radiol 2004;49:8–30.
42. Aminoff M, Boller F, Swaab D, editors. Handbook of Clinical Neurology, vol. 102. Neuro-ophthalmology. Elsevier; 2011.
43. Neau JP, Bogousslavsky J. The syndrome of posterior choroidal artery territory infarction. Ann Neurol 1996;39(6):779–88.
44. Becker M, Masterson K, Delavelle J, et al. Imaging of the optic nerve. Eur J Radiol 2010;74:299–313.
45. Polizzi A, Pavone P, Manfre L, Ruggieri M. Septo-optic dysplasia complex: a heterogenous malformation syndrome. Pediatr Neurol 2006;34:66–71.
46. Mueller-Forell W. Intracranial pathology of the visual pathway. Eur J Radiol 2004;49:143–78.
47. Levin LA. Clinical signs and symptoms requiring computed tomography and magnetic resonance imaging evaluation. Neuroimaging Clin North Am 1996;6:1–14.
48. Biousse V, Bruce BB, Newman NJ. Update on the pathophysiology and management of idiopathic intracranial hypertension. J Neurol Neurosurg Psychiatry 2012;83(5):488–94.
49. Gelfand AA, Gelfand JM, Prabakhar P, Goadsby PJ. Ophthalmoplegic 'migraine' or recurrent ophthalmoplegic cranial neuropathy: new cases and a systematic review. J Child Neurol 2012;27(6): 759–66.

CHAPTER 8

ENT, Neck and Dental Radiology

Timothy Beale • Jackie Brown • John Rout

CHAPTER OUTLINE

INTRODUCTION

The anatomy of the head, neck and dental regions is complex. The continued advances in imaging (in particular computed tomography (CT), cone beam computed tomography (CBCT) and magnetic resonance imaging (MRI)) with ever faster imaging times and higher resolution studies have resulted in more anatomical detail revealing itself, none more so than in the head, neck and dental region where identifying subtle changes in the normal anatomy such as middle ear ossicular erosion in cholesteatoma, widening of the cranial nerve foramina in perineural/intracranial extension of disease and subtle erosion of the laryngeal cartilages in squamous cell carcinoma (SCC) of the larynx is crucial in the accurate diagnosis and staging of head and neck pathology and the planning of appropriate treatment. Knowledge of the normal anatomy and anatomical variants is the essential foundation required to support the recognition and accurate assessment of pathology in this complex region, even more so with the advent of more targeted treatment such as intensity-modulated radiotherapy (IMRT), brachytherapy or proton beam therapy.

THE EAR, PARANASAL SINUSES AND NASAL CAVITY

THE AURICLE AND EXTERNAL AUDITORY CANAL

Anatomy

The auricle and external auditory canal (EAC) funnel the sound to the tympanic membrane. The EAC is approximately 25 mm in length, lined by squamous epithelium, has an S-shaped course and consists of a fibrocartilaginous lateral third and an osseous medial two-thirds (Fig. 8-1). In cross-section the canal has an oval configuration. The fibrocartilaginous portion is deficient inferiorly (fissures of Santorini) that act as conduits for infection and malignancy (see below).

Pathology

High-resolution axial CT (HRCT) or cone beam CT CBCT with multiplanar reformats (MPR) in the coronal and sagittal planes is essential for assessing the bony EAC.

Chronic Stenosing Otitis Externa

Recurrent otitis externa (Fig. 8-2) may result in a fibrotic band of soft tissue occluding the medial EAC. It is important for the radiologist to answer the following questions: Is there any erosion of the adjacent bony walls to suggest a more aggressive process? What is the depth of the occluding soft tissue? Does the fibrotic tissue extend to involve the tympanic membrane (TM)? Is there a normally pneumatised middle ear cleft deep to the occluding soft tissue? Always review the contralateral side as this pathology is commonly bilateral.

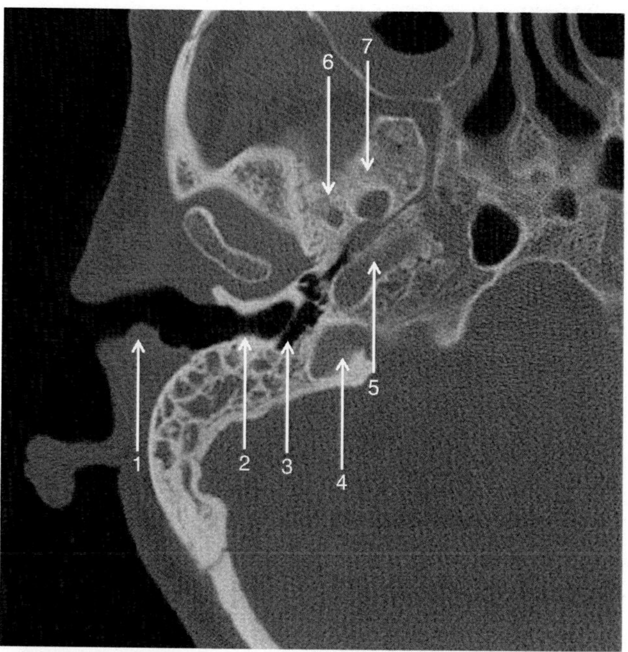

FIGURE 8-1 ■ **Axial CT of right petrous temporal bone.** 1 = fibrocartilaginous EAC; 2 = isthmus bony EAC; 3 = tympanic membrane (TM); 4 = jugular bulb; 5 = intrapetrous ICA (horizontal segment); 6 = foramen spinosum; 7 = foramen ovale.

Exostoses and Osteoma of the External Auditory Canal

The EAC osteoma usually arises spontaneously, but exostoses are associated with repeated exposure to cold water and are also known as 'surfer's ear'. The two pathologies (Fig. 8-3) cannot be distinguished histopathologically; however, exostoses are usually broad-based and bilateral, whereas osteoma are pedunculated, unilateral and lateral to the bony isthmus of the canal. They may cause sufficient narrowing of the EAC to require surgery. It is important when assessing EAC exostoses and osteoma to answer the following questions: What is the maximum depth and transverse diameter of the exostosis? What is the exact site of origin of the osteoma? What is the distance between the medial aspect of the exostosis and the TM and the deep aspect of the exostosis and the descending facial nerve canal? Are there any associated obstructed secretions in the medial EAC and is the middle ear cleft normally pneumatised?

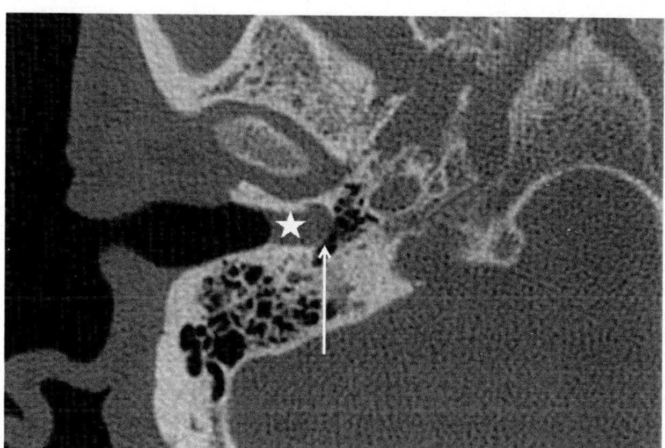

FIGURE 8-2 ■ **Axial CT of right petrous temporal bone.** Star = fibrotic band occluding EAC; arrow = tympanic membrane.

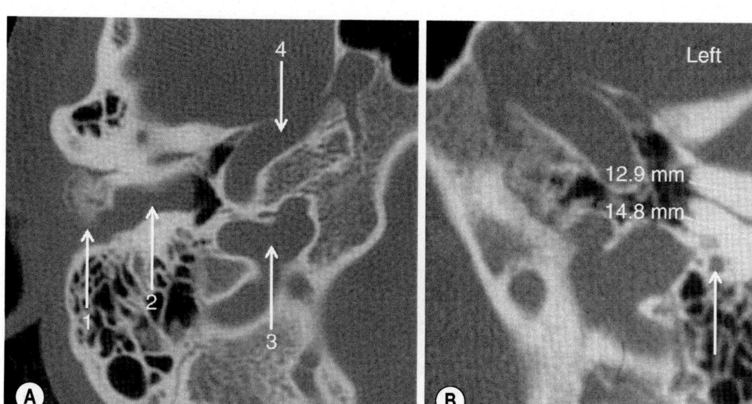

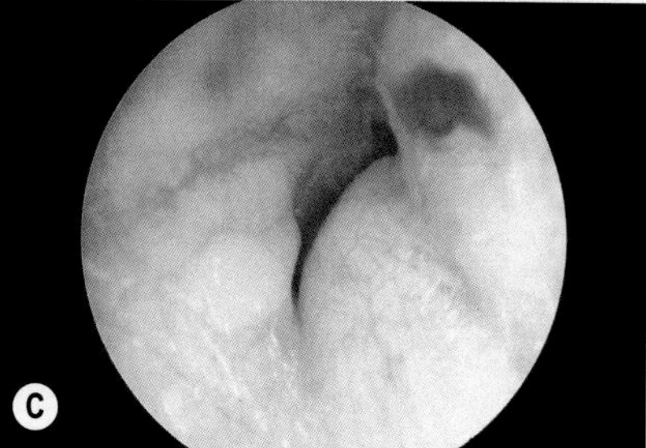

FIGURE 8-3 ■ (A) Axial CT of right petrous temporal bone: 1 = pedunculated osteoma; 2 = soft tissue filling bony EAC medial to obstructing osteoma; 3 = jugular foramen; 4 = intrapetrous ICA (horizontal segment). (B) Axial CT of left petrous temporal bone: arrow = descending (mastoid) segment facial nerve canal. The measurements are of the transverse distance of the broad-based exostoses. (C) Otoscopic view of exostoses narrowing the EAC.

Keratosis Obturans

Keratosis obturans (Fig. 8-4) is usually a bilateral accumulation of keratin within the EAC. The CT appearances are of soft tissue filling the EAC that may be associated with expansion of the canal and remodelling but not erosion of the bony canal walls. Keratosis obturans is associated with otalgia and conductive hearing loss and most frequently occurs in young men.

External Auditory Canal Cholesteatoma

An EAC cholesteatoma (Fig. 8-5) can be differentiated from keratosis obturans as it is associated with erosion of the floor/posterior wall of the bony EAC and is usually seen in an older population (>40 years).

It may be indistinguishable on CT from SCC and otoscopy ± biopsy is suggested.

Necrotising Otitis Externa (NOE)

Also known as malignant otitis externa, a misleading term used because of what used to be the high mortality associated with this condition. The pathology is a necrosis usually of the walls and in particular floor of the EAC at the bony cartilaginous junction typically in the elderly diabetic patient who presents with severe otalgia. *Pseudomonas* is the usual organism. The infection commonly extends inferiorly via the fissures of Santorini (see the section 'Anatomy', above), causing a skull base osteomyelitis, and involves the soft tissues inferior to the skull base where the lower cranial nerves (VII to XII) may be affected (Fig. 8-6). Anterior extension into the temporomandibular joint may cause destruction of the mandibular condyle.

HRCT of temporal bone is the usual initial imaging technique. MR will more clearly assess any soft-tissue involvement, meningeal enhancement or oedema of the bone marrow. Nuclear medicine (gallium 67) is helpful in confirming the location of the infection and monitoring its response to treatment.

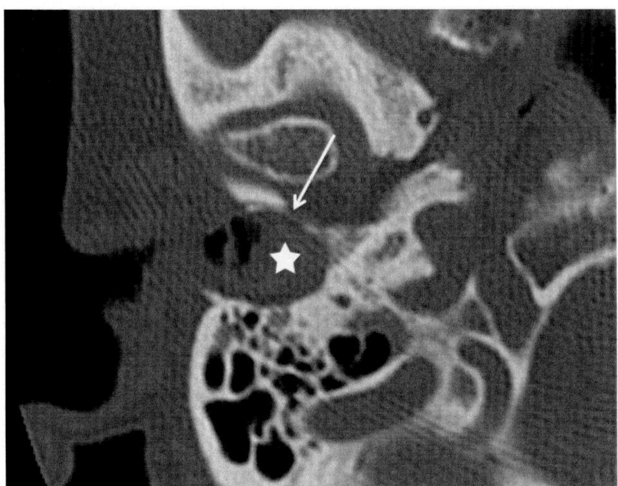

FIGURE 8-4 ■ Axial CT of right petrous temporal bone. Star = soft tissue expanding and remodelling walls of bony EAC; arrow = focal dehiscence of anterior wall of bony EAC.

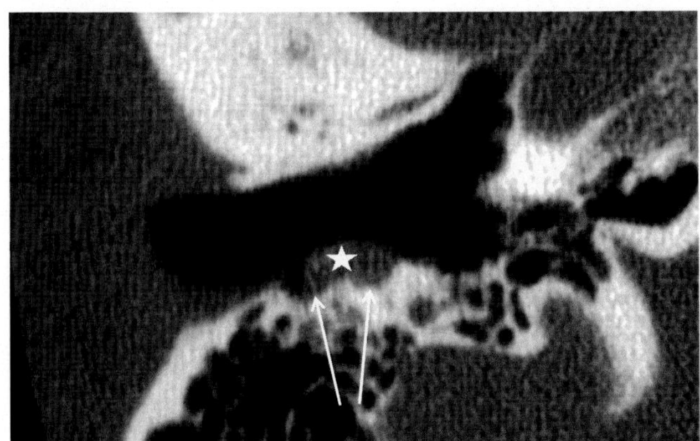

FIGURE 8-5 ■ Axial CT of right petrous temporal bone. Star = lobulated cholesteatoma eroding underlying posterior wall; arrows = highlight areas of focal erosion.

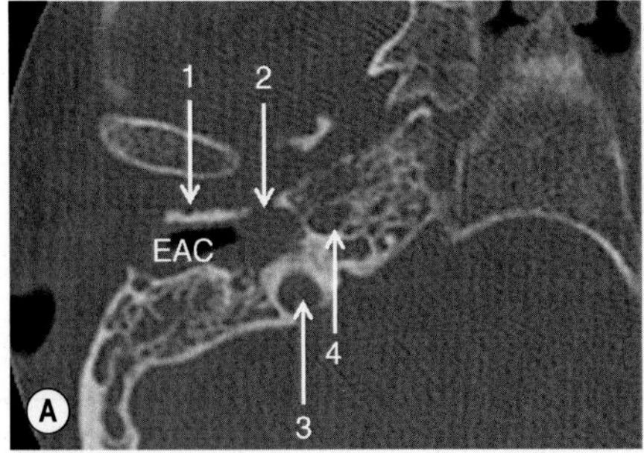

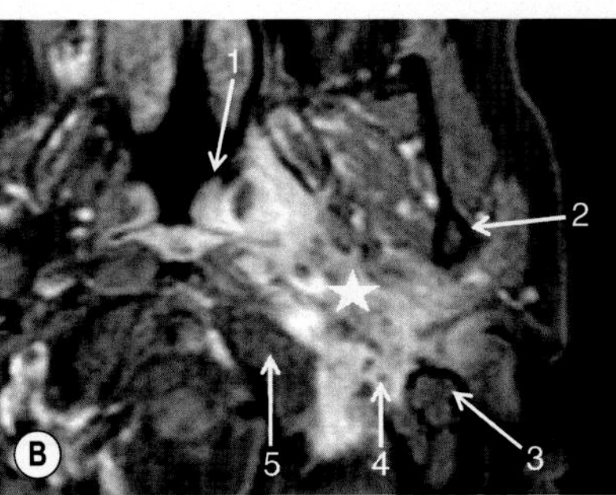

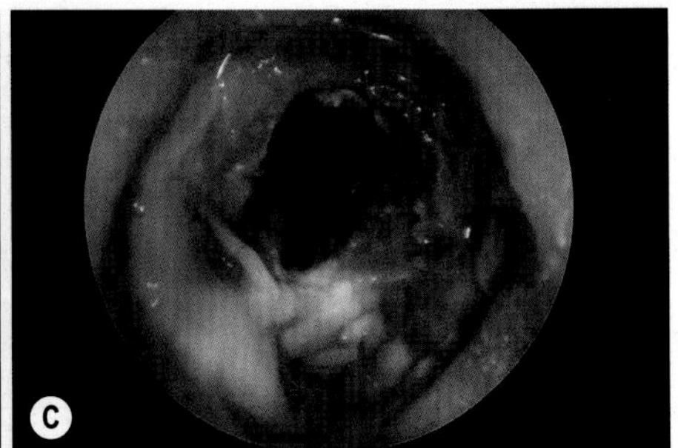

FIGURE 8-6 ■ (A) Axial CT of right petrous temporal bone: Note soft-tissue lining the EAC and the opacified middle ear cleft. 1 & 2 = Eroded anterior wall of bony EAC; 3 = jugular bulb; 4 = posterior genu intrapetrous ICA. (B) Axial T1W fat-saturated post gadolium MR of the soft tissues just inferior to the left EAC. Star = centre of ill-defined enhancing soft tissue extending from the stylomastoid foramen and facial nerve posteriorly to the nasopharynx medially. 1 = torus of nasopharynx; 2 = neck of condyle; 3 = opacified mastoid process; 4 = facial nerve in stylomastoid foramen; 5 = occipital condyle. (C) Otoscopic view of necrotising otitis externa. Note necrotic slough replacing the normal mucosa.

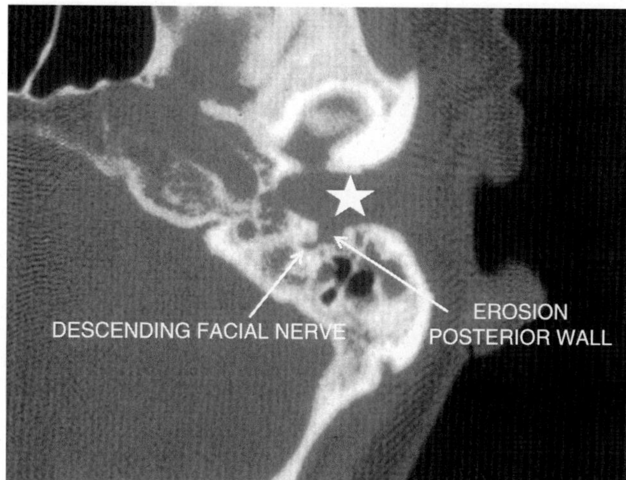

FIGURE 8-7 ■ **Axial CT of left petrous temporal bone.** Star = soft tissue filling the EAC. Note the bony erosion of the posterior wall extending up to the mastoid (descending) segment of the facial nerve canal.

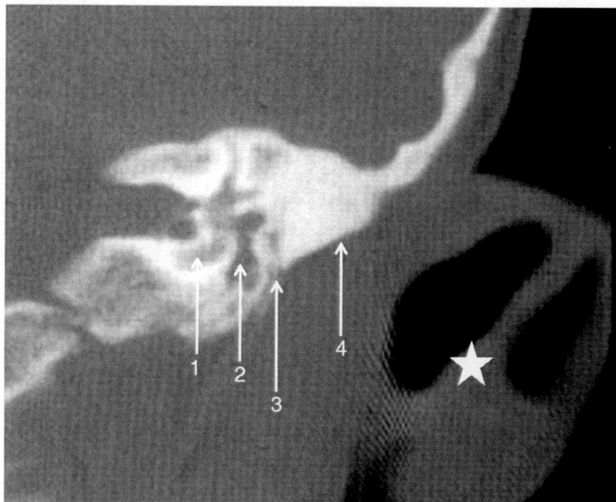

FIGURE 8-8 ■ **Coronal CT of left petrous temporal bone.** Patient with Treacher Collins syndrome: star = deformed auricle; 1 = basal turn of cochlea; 2 = small opacified middle ear cleft; 3 = displaced (anterior and laterally positioned) mastoid segment of the facial nerve canal; 4 = atretic bony plate.

It is important to answer the following questions when assessing patients with NOE: Is there any erosion of the bony walls of the EAC? Is there any inflammatory change in the soft tissues inferior to the skull base, in particular around the stylomastoid opening of the facial nerve, and is there involvement/effacement of the normal parapharyngeal fat? Is there erosion of the skull base (look for loss of the normal dense line of the bony cortex of the clivus, petroclival region and petrous apex)? Is there anterior extension to involve the mandibular condyle or involvement of the contralateral side via the prevertebral and retropharyngeal soft tissues anterior to the clivus? Has the differential of an SCC of the EAC or a nasopharyngeal tumour with extension to the skull base been excluded?

Squamous Cell Carcinoma of the Auricle and External Auditory Canal

These are rare tumours presenting in the elderly (F > M) with a painful, discharging ulcerative lesion of the EAC that most frequently extends inferiorly. CT is the usual imaging technique (Fig. 8-7), but MRI is recommended if there is suspected superior extension into the middle cranial fossa or medial extension into the middle ear cleft (both are rare).

It is important to answer the following questions: As with all soft tissue noted within the bony EAC, is there any associated bony erosion? Is there extension outside of the EAC? Is there any nodal involvement (in particular, review the intraparotid and upper deep cervical nodes)?

Congenital Atresia/Stenosis of the External Auditory Canal

The EAC may be stenosed or completely atretic (absent). The atresia may be membranous, bony or a mixture of the two. The atresia is usually unilateral in non-syndromic and bilateral in syndromic patients (Fig. 8-8). The rule of thumb is the more severe the EAC abnormality, the greater the auricular deformity (microtia/anotia). The inner ear structures are usually not affected unless there is severe EAC atresia with an absent auricle, small middle ear cleft and absent ossicles. If surgery is being considered it is important to assess the following on CT:

- The severity and type of the atresia.
- The size and degree of pneumatisation of the middle ear cleft.
- The appearance of the ossicles, in particular:
  - Is a stapes superstructure present?
  - Is the oval window atretic?
- The course of the tympanic segment of the intrapetrous facial nerve as the posterior genu (junction of tympanic and descending segments) is often more anteriorly and laterally positioned than normal and therefore at risk during surgery.

THE MIDDLE EAR

Anatomy and Physiology

The tympanic membrane (TM) is inclined at an angle of 140° in relation to the superior border of the EAC, measures 9–10 mm in diameter and separates the middle ear from the external ear (Fig. 8-9). The lateral (short) process of the malleus is attached to the TM at the malleal prominence and the handle at the umbo. Extending both anterior and posterior from the malleal prominence are folds separating the TM into a superior, thinner and more flexible pars flaccida and the more inferior pars tensa. The middle ear cleft is divided from superior to inferior into epitympanum (attic), mesotympanum and hypotympanum and contains three ossicles (the malleus, incus and stapes), two muscles (tensor tympani attached to the neck of the malleus and stapedius to the head of

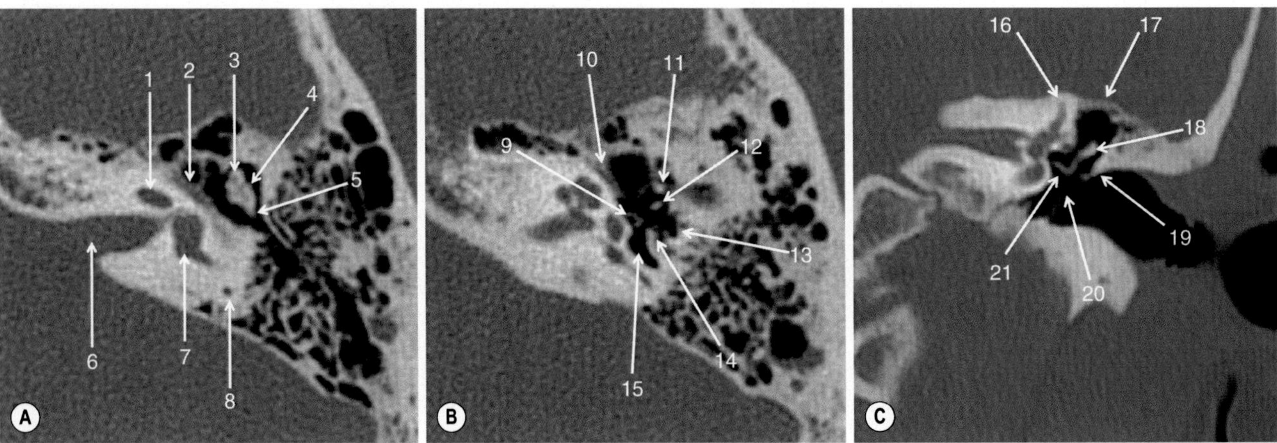

FIGURE 8-9 ■ **(A, B) Axial and (C) coronal CT of left petrous temporal bone.** 1 = cochlea (middle turn); 2 = facial nerve (tympanic segment); 3 = malleus (head); 4 = incus (body); 5 = incus (short process); 6 = IAC; 7 = vestibule; 8 = posterior SCC; 9 = stapes superstructure; 10 = tensor tympani muscle; 11 = malleus (neck); 12 = incus (long process); 13 = facial recess; 14 = pyramidal eminence; 15 = sinus tympani; 16 = superior SCC; 17 = tegmen tympani; 18 = incus (body); 19 = scutum; 20 = tympanic membrane; 21 = incus (lenticular process).

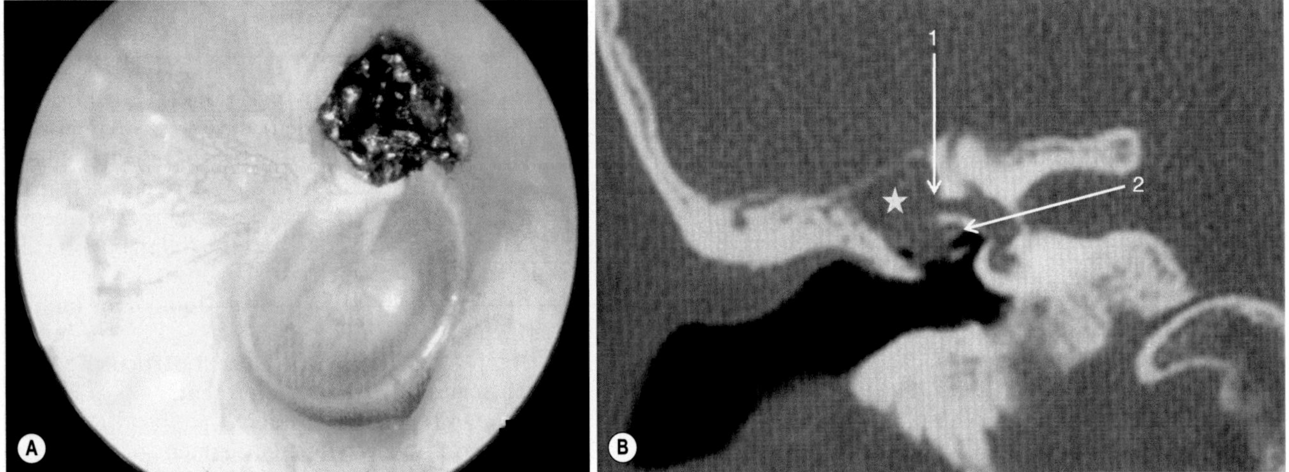

FIGURE 8-10 ■ (A) Otoscopic view showing a retraction pocket in pars flaccida of TM. (B) Coronal CT of right petrous temporal bone. Star = cholesteatoma in attic; 1 = eroded otic capsule over lateral SCC; 2 = facial nerve (tympanic segment).

the stapes). Part of the intrapetrous course of the facial nerve and one of its branches (the chorda tympani) also pass through the middle ear cleft.

HRCT including CBCT is the most common technique used for assessing the middle ear cleft usually in the clinical setting of conductive or mixed hearing loss. MRI is a complementary investigation used to assess possible intracranial complications arising from middle ear pathology, the rare middle ear tumours such as glomus tympanicum or where a recurrence of cholesteatoma is suspected (see below).

Pathology

Cholesteatoma

Cholesteatoma is a poor term for this pathology as it neither is a tumour nor does it contain cholesterol. It is actually skin in the wrong place. There are two types: the common acquired (98%) and the rarer congenital (2%) cholesteatoma. In acquired cholesteatoma, as a consequence of negative middle ear pressure, a retraction pocket develops usually in the more flexible pars flaccida (superior aspect) of the TM (Fig. 8-10A), but occasionally in the pars tensa (inferior aspect). Desquamated skin accumulates in the retraction pocket and can enlarge, causing bony destruction most frequently of the scutum and long process of the incus, but may extend to involve the otic capsule overlying the lateral semicircular canal (Fig. 8-10B), that may be associated with symptoms of dizziness, the tegmen tympani and the tympanic facial nerve canal (causing facial palsy).

Usually the diagnosis of cholesteatoma is apparent from the otoscopic appearances of a retraction pocket in acquired and a retrotympanic 'pearl' of cholesteatoma behind an intact TM in congenital cholesteatoma

(Fig. 8-11). The clinician needs to know how extensive the cholesteatoma is, which can be assessed by the degree of ossicular or bony erosion.

In particular, answer the following questions:

- Is the bony roof (tegmen tympani or mastoideum) eroded?
- Is the otic capsule overlying the lateral semicircular canal eroded?
- Is there ossicular erosion (in particular, is the stapes eroded)?
- Does the cholesteatoma abut the tympanic facial nerve canal?
- Are there anatomical variants such as a low-lying tegmen or a lateralised sigmoid sinus that may affect the surgical approach?

A pars flaccida cholesteatoma is identified by a mass in the attic (epitympanium) lateral to the head of malleus and body of incus associated with ossicular erosion in 70%. A pars tensa cholesteatoma is identified as soft tissue in the posterior mesotympanum often extending medial to the ossicles. HRCT is used for assessing any bony involvement. Non-echo planar diffusion-weighted MR (non-EPI DWI) is increasingly used for assessing whether there is any recurrent or residual cholesteatoma in patients who have undergone canal wall preservation surgery where otoscopy provides limited visualisation. Cholesteatoma consisting of desquamated skin shows markedly restricted diffusion (Fig. 8-12) and can be differentiated from other soft tissue (granulation tissue, etc.).

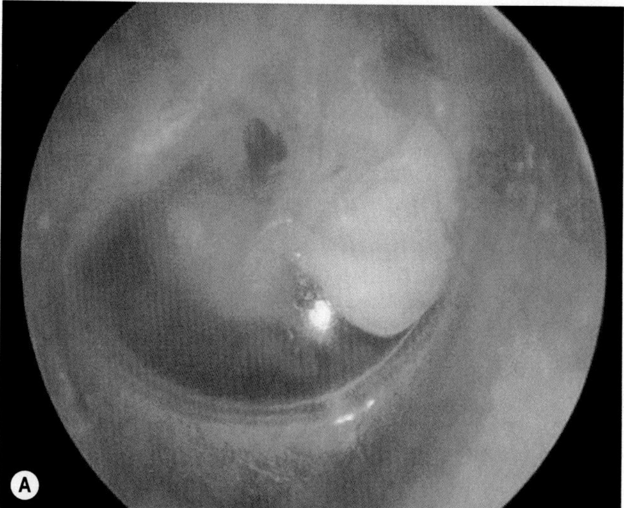

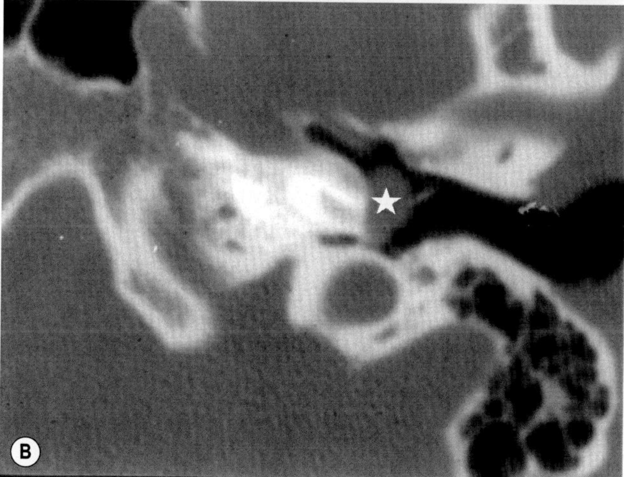

FIGURE 8-11 ■ (A) Otoscopic view of cholesteatoma (pearl) behind intact TM. (B) Star = congenital cholesteatoma overlying cochlear promontory.

Tympanosclerosis

The CT appearance is of foci of calcification, punctate or web-like in the middle ear cleft (Fig. 8-13) and tympanic membrane. Usually this is associated with a long history of otitis media (OM). The suspensory ligaments and muscles may also calcify. There is varying conductive hearing loss depending on the degree of ossicular fixation. If the tympanic membrane only is involved (calcified), the condition is known as myringosclerosis.

Otosclerosis

The diagnosis is usually suggested clinically. The hearing loss may be conductive, mixed or sensorineural. Otospongiosis is a term also used and describes the spongiform changes within the involved bone. In patients with otosclerosis the normal dense bone is replaced by foci of spongy less dense bone. Patients usually present in the third decade. The CT appearances are commonly bilateral (85%) and there may be a family history. There are two main types: fenestral and retrofenestral.

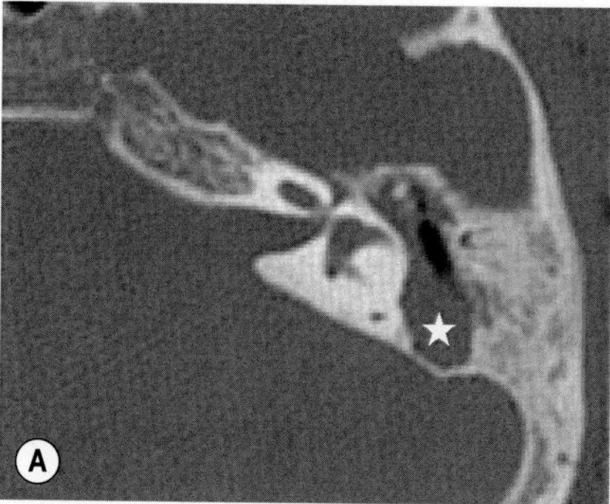

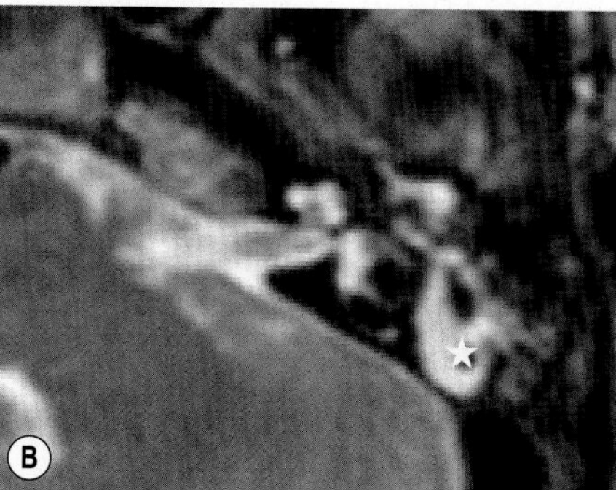

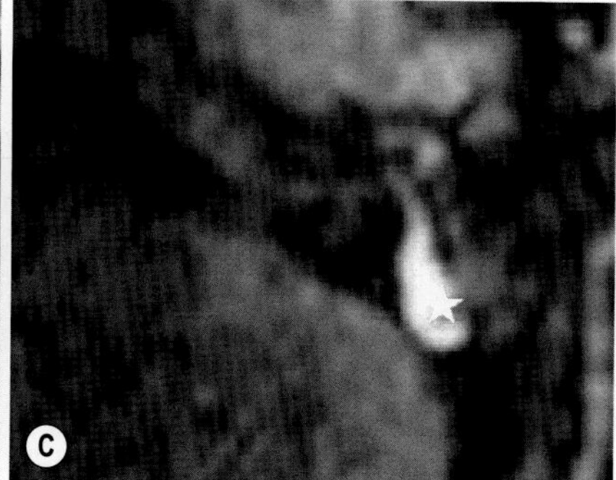

FIGURE 8-12 ■ (A) Axial CT of left petrous temporal bone and (B, C) equivalent T2W and non-EPI diffusion weighted b1000 MR images showing cholesteatoma (star) in mastoid antrum.

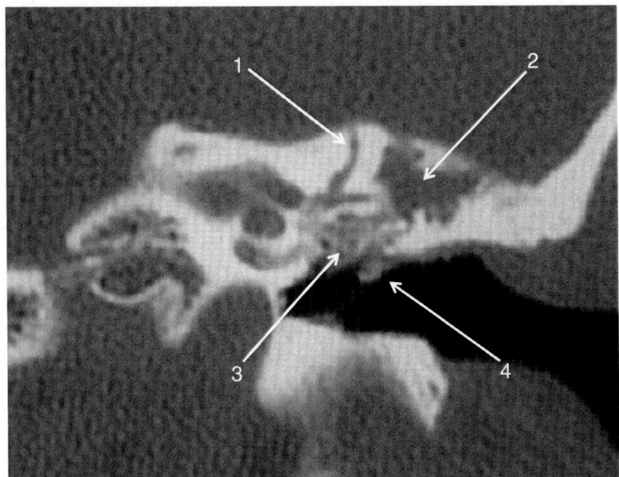

FIGURE 8-13 ■ **Coronal CT of left petrous temporal bone.** 1 = superior SCC; 2 = opacified attic; 3 = densely calcified soft tissue (tympanosclerosis) surrounding ossicles; 4 = calcified TM.

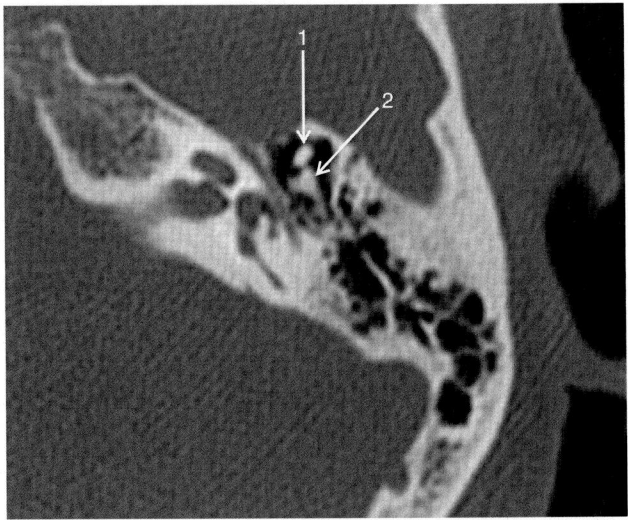

FIGURE 8-15 ■ **Axial CT of left petrous temporal bone.** 1 = head of malleus; 2 = body of incus. Note the malleoincudal separation and compare with normal anatomy in Fig. 8-9A.

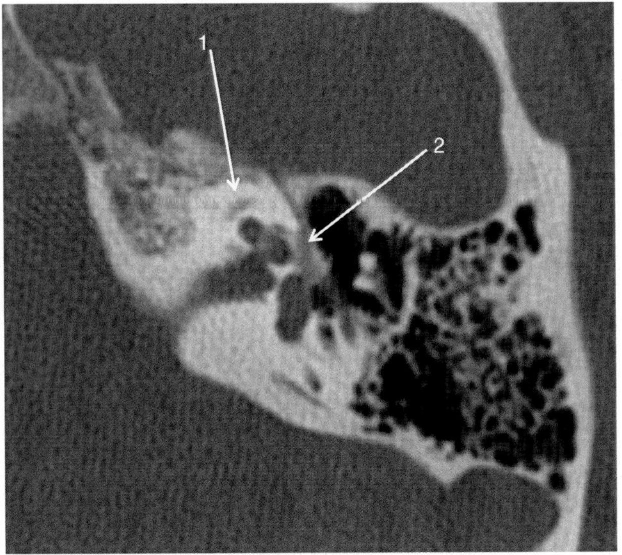

FIGURE 8-14 ■ **Axial CT of left petrous temporal bone.** 1 = pericochlear; 2 = fenestral otospongiosis.

Fenestral. The spongiotic foci occur in the lateral wall of the otic capsule in the fissula antefenestram (anterior to the oval window; Fig. 8-14) where it extends posteriorly to involve the footplate, fixing the anterior crus of the stapes causing CHL. The round window and cochlear promontory may also be involved.

Retrofenestral or Cochlear. Spongiotic foci replace the normal dense bone of the otic capsule surrounding the cochlea (Fig. 8-14) and may encroach on the cochlea and, less commonly, the vestibule and semicircular canals, causing mixed or sensorineural hearing loss. The most frequent location for a spongiotic focus is between the middle turn of the cochlea and the anterior aspect of the lateral internal auditory canal. In severe cases the cochlea is encircled, giving the appearance is of a cochlea within a cochlea. CT is used for assessing otosclerosis although the foci may be visible on MR as high signal areas on T2 that enhance post-gadolinium.

Cochlear otosclerosis is rare in the absence of fenestral disease.

Questions to answer when reviewing the CT are the following:

- Is there fenestral or pericochlear otosclerosis or both?
- Is there bilateral involvement (in 85% on CT) that may only be clinically evident on one side?
- Is the round window also involved? Round window involvement may reduce the effectiveness of surgery.
- Is the whole oval window involved and what is the depth of involvement? A markedly thickened footplate will alter the surgical technique and reduce the likelihood of a successful outcome.
- Is the facial nerve dehiscent as this may complicate surgery?

Ossicular Disruption

Nearly all ossicular disruption is associated with a temporal bone fracture. Incudostapedial joint (ISJ) disruption is the commonest derangement. Malleoincudal disruption results in loss of the normal 'ice cream cone' appearance on axial images of the head of malleus articulating with the body of the incus (Fig. 8-15). Complete dislocation of the incus is the next most common finding. Much more rarely found are fractures of the individual ossicles. The incus is the ossicle most frequently disrupted as the malleus is supported by three ligaments and the tensor tympani muscle and the stapes by the annular ligament and the stapedius muscle.

When assessing ossicular trauma, look first for the normal 'ice cream cone' appearance of the malleoincudal joint and then closely assess the alignment of the distal long process of the incus with the head of stapes at the ISJ and compare with the normal contralateral side.

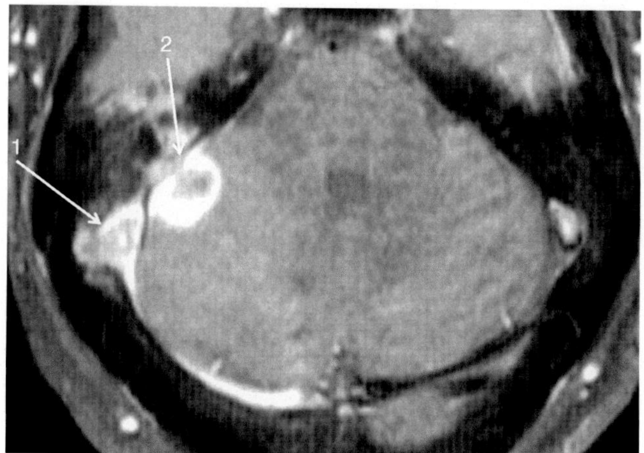

FIGURE 8-16 ■ Axial T1W MR post-gadolinium image posterior fossa. 1 = Thrombus in sigmoid sinus; 2 = epidural abscess.

Venous Sinus Thrombosis

The sigmoid sinus is an immediate posterior relation to the mastoid air cells and mastoiditis may result in sinus thrombosis with occasionally severe intracranial complications (Fig. 8-16). The transverse sinus and jugular bulb may also be involved, although the latter is usually thrombosed due to retrograde extension from the neck.

Always assess the bony dural sinus plate overlying the sigmoid sinus if adjacent air cells are opacified. If there is bony erosion, MRV or CT venography may be helpful to exclude thrombosis.

Intracranial Complications

Fortunately, intracranial complications from petromastoid infection are now rare. The commonest is extradural empyema in the posterior fossa often associated with sigmoid sinus thrombosis. Very rarely subdural empyema and intracranial abscesses may occur.

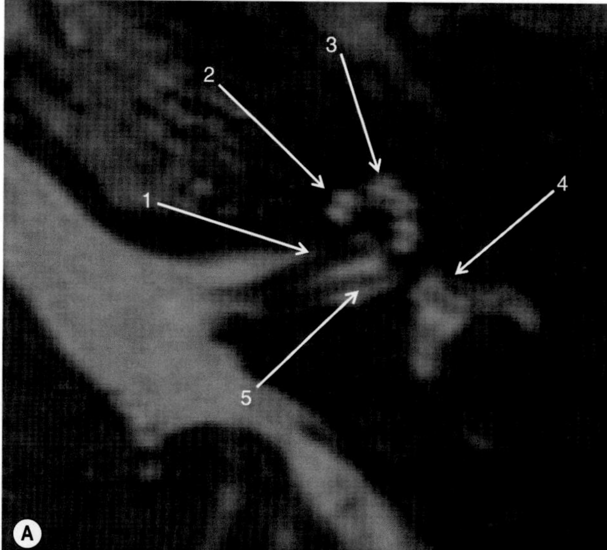

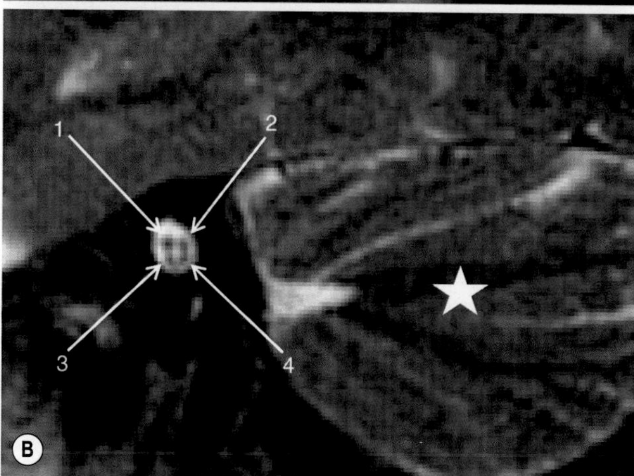

FIGURE 8-17 ■ (A) Axial T2W MR image of IAMs. Normal anatomy: 1 = cochlear nerve; 2 = cochlea (middle turn); 3 = cochlea (distal turn); 4 = vestibule; 5 = vestibular nerve (inferior). (B) Sagittal oblique T2W MR image through IAC. Star = cerebellar hemisphere; 1 = facial nerve; 2 = vestibular nerve (superior); 3 = cochlear nerve; 4 = vestibular nerve (inferior). Note 'seven-up and coke down' to remember position of nerves in IAC.

THE INNER EAR

Anatomy and Physiology

The inner ear consists of endolymph containing the functional sensory epithelium surrounded by perilymph and covered by a bony labyrinth (otic capsule). Sound is transmitted from the TM via the ossicles to the oval window. The mechanical vibrations via the vestibule then pass to the perilymph containing scala vestibuli up to the apical turn of the cochlea, returning via the perilymph containing scala tympani to the round window (Fig. 8-17A). Both perilymph scala surround the endolymphatic scala media or cochlear duct that contains the hair cell receptors of the organ of Corti. It is movement of these hair cells that generates electronic impulses in the cochlear nerve fibres. Higher frequencies up to 20 kHz are perceived in the basal turn and 20 Hz at the apex. The range of intensity of sound is huge and is expressed in alogorithmic decibel scale of 0–120 dB. A quiet whisper is 30 dB, a lawnmower is 90 dB and a jet plane take-off is 120 dB.

The electrical output of the hair cells passes to the spiral ganglion in the cochlea and then the cochlea division (Fig. 8-17B) and main trunk of the vestibulocochlear nerve to enter the brainstem in the upper lateral medulla synapsing with two cochlear nuclei, the latter forming a bulge in the lateral recess of the fourth ventricle and the foramen of Luschka. Within the brainstem, nerves pass in ipsi- and contralateral pathways to the inferior colliculus of the mid-brain, medial geniculate body of the thalamus and from there to the posterior aspect of the superior temporal gyrus. Ipsilateral hearing loss results when there is damage to the auditory pathway between the hair cells in the cochlea and the brainstem nuclei and bilateral hearing loss between the brainstem nuclei and inferior colliculi.

The semicircular canals consist of three rings, each orthogonal to the others, again containing perilymph bathing the endolymph. The superior and lateral canals are innervated by the superior vestibular nerve and the posterior by the inferior vestibular nerve. The semicircular canals form the kinetic labyrinth as they respond to rotational movement and acceleration. The dilated component of the semicircular canals called ampullae contains the hair cells forming the electronic impulses.

The vestibule consists of the utricle and macule (static labyrinth) and detects the position of the head relative to gravity.

Pathology

Vestibular Schwannoma

Vestibular schwannomas are the most common cerebellopontine angle (CPA) tumour and the most common pathology causing asymmetrical sensorineural hearing loss (SNHL). The majority are centred within the internal auditory canal, or at the porus acusticus and occur sporadically. When bilateral they indicate the diagnosis of neurofibromatosis type 2. Only a minority (approximately 2.5%) of patients who present with tinnitus or asymmetrical hearing loss have a vestibular schwanomma. There is no relationship between the size of the tumour and degree of hearing loss. The management approach is 'wait and scan' for the majority of vestibular schwannomas as approximately 60–70% do not increase in size on follow-up (MR) imaging. Those that require intervention have two options: surgery via retrosigmoid, translabyrinthine or subtemporal middle cranial fossa approach, or gamma-knife (radiation) treatment.

MRI is the imaging technique of choice when assessing patients for a possible vestibular schwannoma, but the protocols vary. A high-resolution T2-weighted imaging is the most commonly used sequence with pre- and post-gadolinium-enhanced T1-weighted sequences reserved for the small percentage of patients where a neuroma is identified and requires confirmation (Fig. 8-18) or other pathology requires clarification.

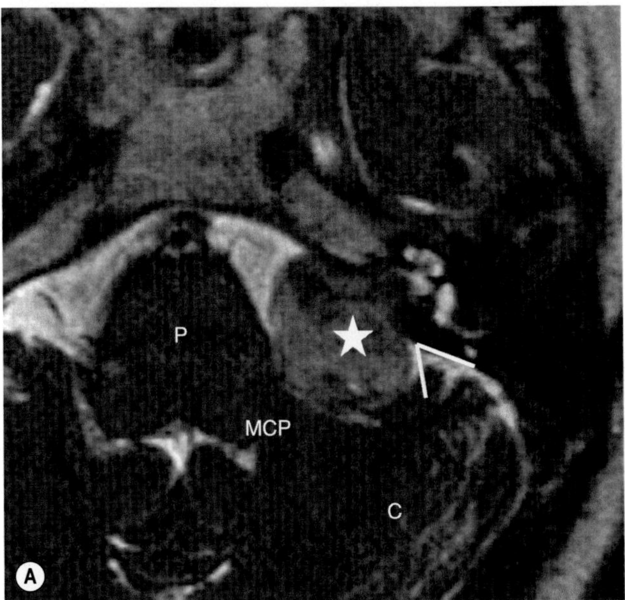

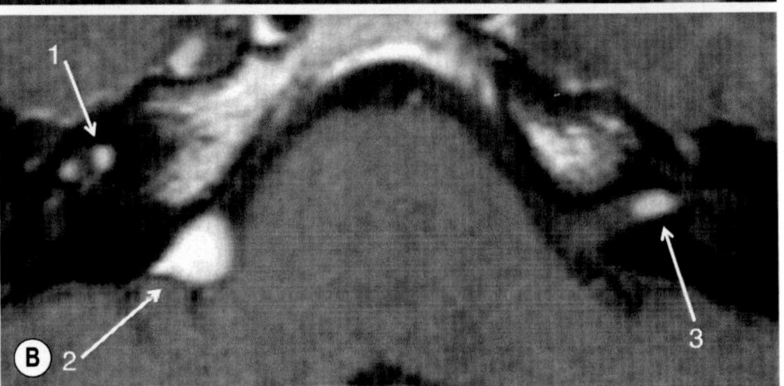

FIGURE 8-18 ■ (A) Axial T2W MR image of posterior fossa. Star = vestibular schwannoma (VS); white line shows acute angle between VS and posterior surface of petrous bone which helps differentiate between VS and posterior fossa meningioma with the latter having an obtuse angle; P = pons; MCP = middle cerebellar peduncle; C = cerebellar hemisphere. (B) Axial T1W MR post-gadolinium image of through posterior fossa. 1 = intracochlear schwannoma (in middle turn); 2 = right CPA schwannoma; 3 = left intracanalicular schwannoma.

Trauma

Skull base fractures involving the petrous bone are uncommon, but are important to identify as they may be associated with cerebrospinal fluid (CSF) otorrhoea or rhinorrhoea, facial nerve palsy or ossicular disruption.

In patients undergoing CT for head trauma HRCT reconstructions of the skull and skull base are frequently part of the routine imaging protocol. Assessing any intracranial trauma is the initial priority, but identifying skull base and, indeed, upper cervical fractures is also essential.

Classically, petrous temporal fractures have been divided broadly into transverse fractures (20%) usually secondary to occipital or frontal trauma or longitudinal fractures (80%) secondary to temporoparietal trauma. However, the fracture line frequently takes an oblique course and prognostically it is more important to accurately describe its course and the structures involved.

When reviewing the image for a possible petrous fracture, remember that transverse fractures usually start at sites of weakness such as the jugular foramen (Fig. 8-19) or vestibular aqueduct and longitudinal fractures

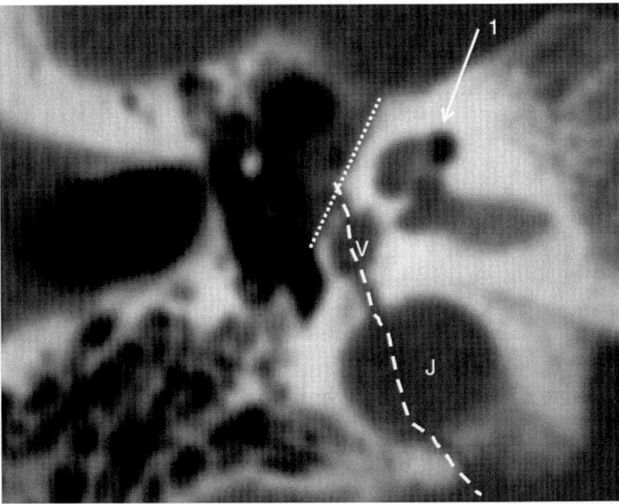

FIGURE 8-19 ■ **Axial CT of right petrous temporal bone.** Interrupted line = transverse fracture; dotted line is facial nerve (tympanic segment); 1 = air in cochlea (pneumolabyrinth); J = jugular bulb; v = vestibule.

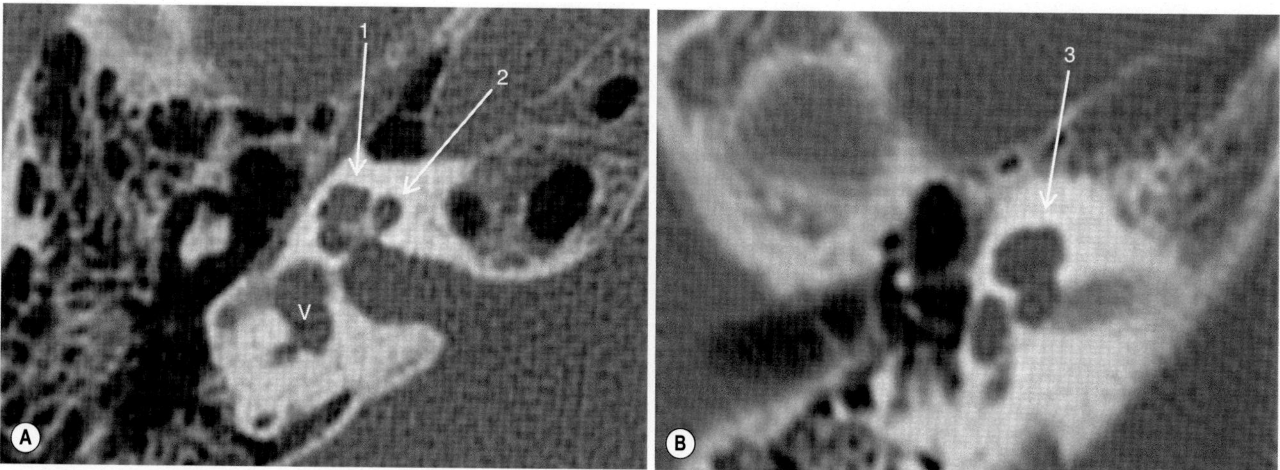

FIGURE 8-20 ■ **Axial CT of right petrous temporal bone.** (A, B) 1 and 2 = normal partitioning of distal and middle turns of cochlea, 3 = incomplete partitioning in image B; V = vestibule.

frequently involve the EAC, extending to the middle ear cleft or more inferiorly the posterior genu of the intra-petrous internal carotid artery, but usually sparing the facial nerve and inner ear structures.

Please note: CSF rhinorrhoea may be secondary to a petrous temporal fracture, with CSF passing along the eustachian tube into the postnasal space and this area should be reviewed as a recognised but rarer cause of CSF rhinorrhoea along with the anterior and central skull base and sinonasal regions. There is a 10% annual risk of meningitis in patients with CSF rhinorrhoea.

In patients with post-traumatic facial nerve palsy it is important to identify the exact site of trauma as it will alter both the surgical approach and repair technique.

As noted in the earlier section 'The Middle Ear', the commonest ossicular disruption is of the incudostapedial joint followed by the malleoincudal joint and then incus dislocation. The malleus and stapes are rarely involved as they are more firmly held in place both by a muscle (tensor tympani and stapedius) and several ligaments.

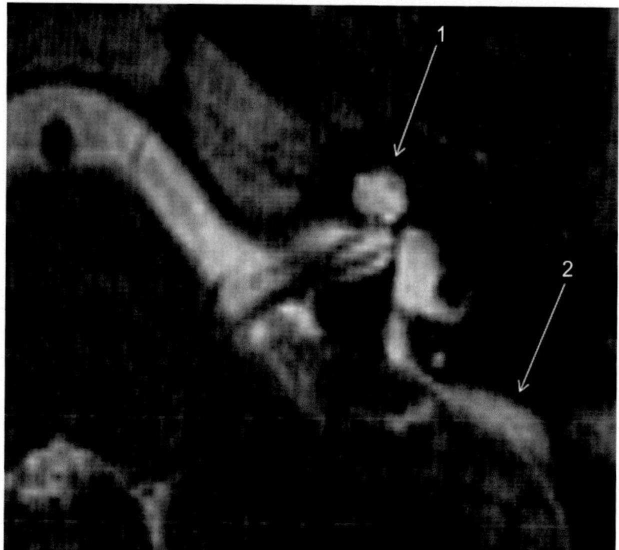

FIGURE 8-21 ■ **Axial T2W MR image of posterior fossa.** 1 = incomplete partitioning of cochlea (compare with Fig. 8-17A); 2 = enlarged vestibular aqueduct and endolymphatic sac.

Congenital Malformations

Congenital malformation of the cochlea and/or labyrinth may be genetic (alone or as part of a syndrome) or non-genetic.

The inner ear and middle/external ear have independent embryological developments, but still approximately 10% of patients with EAC atresia have inner ear deformities. The inner ear structures develop between the third and twenty-second week of intrauterine life and inner ear malformations are usually classified according to severity from the rare Michel deformity (arrest at third week and complete absence of the inner ear) to mild dysplasia of the lateral semicircular canal (twenty-second week).

CT and MR are complementary investigations and, although this subject is outside the scope of this chapter, the following checklist needs to be gone through:

- Cochlea: Is there a normal basal turn? Is the modiolus present (Fig. 8- 20)? Are there a normal number of turns?
- Vestibule: is it enlarged? Is it separate from the cochlea?
- Semicircular canals: Are they present or dysplastic?
- Oval and round windows: Are they normal, narrowed, atretic?
- Vestibular aqueduct: Is the vestibular aqueduct and endolymphatic sac enlarged? This is the most common imaging finding in patients with sensorineural hearing loss dating to infancy and is frequently missed with serious clinical consequences (Fig. 8-21).
- Cochlear nerve: Is the nerve present and of normal size?
- Facial nerve: Does the nerve take a normal course? Is it dehiscent?

Facial Palsy

Acute facial palsy is usually secondary to Bell's palsy or trauma. Bell's palsy is frequently seen clinically but is

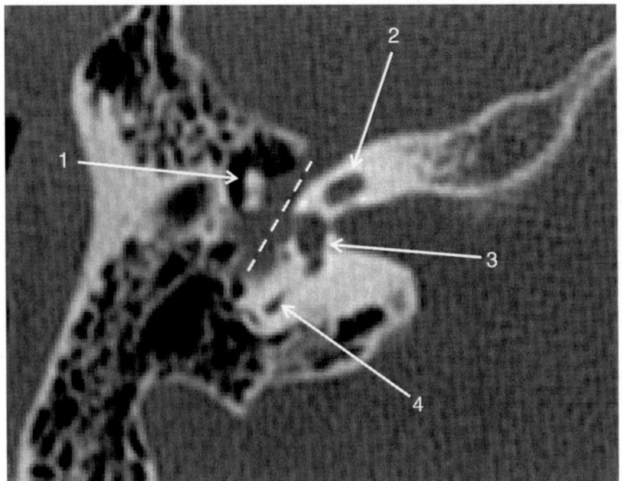

FIGURE 8-22 ■ **Axial CT of right petrous temporal bone.** There is a diffuse enlargement of the facial nerve (tympanic segment) = interrupted white line; 1 = malleus (neck); 2 = cochlea (middle turn); 3 = vestibule; 4 = posterior SCC.

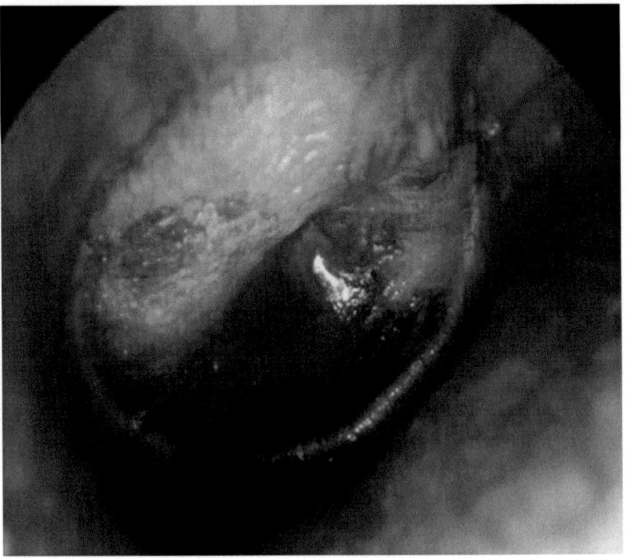

FIGURE 8-23 ■ **Otoscopic view of a retrotympanic vascular mass in a patient with a glomus tympanicum.**

uncommonly imaged. Typically the patient develops a sudden facial paralysis which recovers fully or incompletely after 2–3 months.

Imaging is mandatory for atypical cases: i.e. progressive or recurrent facial palsy (Fig. 8-22). CT and MRI are complementary. MRI is preferred but CT is usually performed if pathology such as cholesteatoma or otomastoiditis is suspected on otoscopy. Both the intra- and extracranial course of the facial nerve must be covered or pathology such as an impalpable malignant parotid tumour will be missed. On MRI, enhancement of the facial nerve within the geniculate ganglion, tympanic and mastoid segments is normal. Abnormal enhancement includes intense enhancement of the labyrinthine and mastoid segments. Enhancement of the facial nerve in the fundus of the internal auditory canal is always pathological.

Glomus Tumours (Paragangliomas)

Paragangliomas are the most common tumours causing pulsatile tinnitus and glomus tympanicum and glomus jugulotympanicum are the most common tumours of the middle ear and the second most common tumours of the temporal bone after vestibular schwannoma. It is vital to distinguish the two types. Glomus tympanicum arise on the medial wall of the middle ear cavity on the cochlear promontory and can be removed via a mastoid approach (Fig. 8-23). Glomus jugulotympanicum are tumours arising in the jugular foramen that extend into the middle ear cleft usually requiring preoperative embolisation followed by skull base surgery.

HRCT and MRI are complementary. When the tumour extends into the adjacent bone such as in a glomus jugulotympanicum or extensive glomus tympanicum, there is a characteristic permeative bony destruction seen on HRCT. MRI demonstrates an intensely enhancing tumour that on the unenhanced T1-weighted sequence may demonstrate a 'salt and pepper' appearance with the salt representing subacute haemorrhage and the pepper representing flow voids in large tumour vessels (Fig. 8-24).

Cochlear Electrode Implantation

Implantable cochlear electrodes offer a chance of hearing for some individuals, typically those whose hearing has been damaged by childhood meningitis. An array of electrodes (usually 12, 16 or 22 depending on the device) are inserted into the scala tympani of the proximal basal turn. MRI and HRCT are usually both requested preoperatively to assess for the patency of the cochlea, the size of the cochlea nerve and any malformation or anatomical variant that might alter the surgical approach or technique. Assessment of implant position can be made intraoperatively or in the early postoperative period with plain X-ray (reverse Stenver's view), HRCT or CBCT. Early studies suggest CBCT can assess whether the electrodes are within the scala tympani or vestibuli (Fig. 8-25). Cochlear implantation is now commonly bilateral and may be performed in patients with unilateral hearing loss and debilitating tinnitus.

THE PARANASAL SINUSES AND NASAL CAVITY

Anatomy and Physiology

The external nose consists of bone superiorly (frontal process of maxilla and nasal bones) and alar cartilage inferiorly. The arterial supply is via facial and ethmoidal arteries and venous drainage into the angular vein up to the medial canthus of the eye, which explains one route of how nasal sepsis can spread to involve the cavernous sinus.

The nasal cavity extends from the vestibule anteriorly to the choanae posteriorly divided by the midline nasal

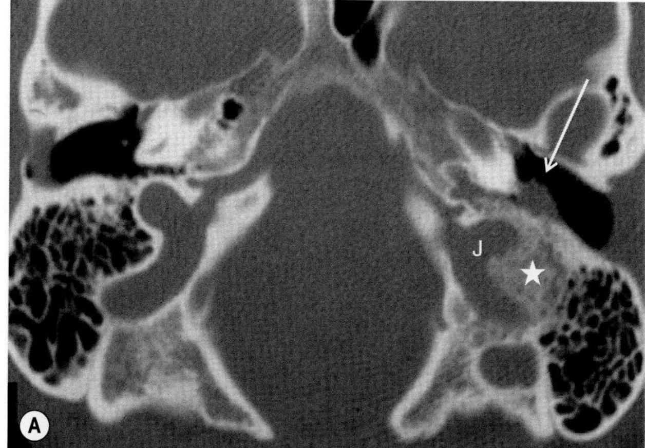

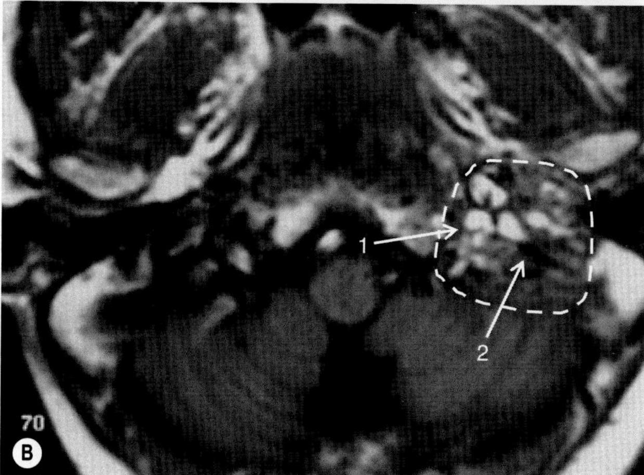

FIGURE 8-24 ■ (A) Axial CT of petrous temporal bone. Star = classic permeative appearance of a glomus tumour. Note also the loss of the dense cortical line of the jugular foramen (J). The tumour extends into the middle ear (white arrow), which is the tip of the iceberg of a large glomus jugulotympanicum (GJT). (B) Axial T1W MR image of the same patient. Interrupted white line outlines the GJT. The 'salt and pepper' appearance of the tumour is shown. 1 = T1W high signal of foci of haemorrhage; 2 = signal void of large feeding vessel.

septum. The anterior cartilaginous septum fuses posteriorly with the bony septum consisting of the vomer inferiorly and perpendicular plate of ethmoid superiorly. The roof of the nasal cavity is formed by the cribriform plate part of the anterior skull base and the floor is the hard palate. The lateral wall is more complex and supports the three turbinates (superior, middle and inferior) and their associated airway or meatus.

The middle meatus is functionally the most important and receives drainage from the maxillary sinus via the infundibulum, the anterior ethmoidal air cells via individual ostia and the frontal sinus via the frontal recess. The ostiomeatal unit is the complex anatomical region where these three mucociliary drainage pathways (frontal, anterior ethmoidal and maxillary) meet (Fig. 8-26).

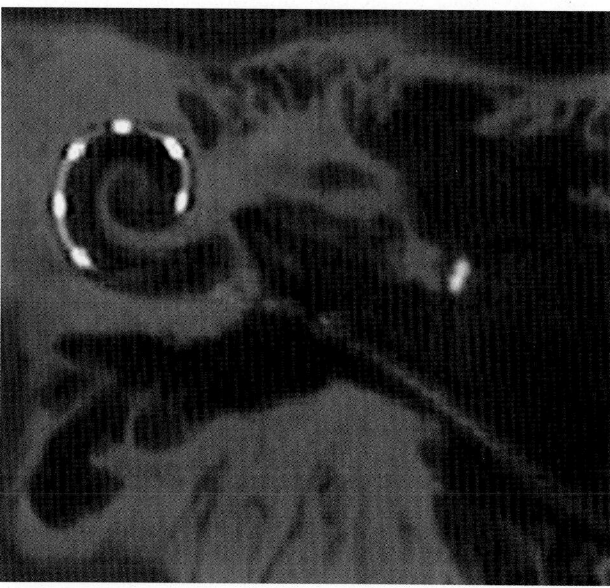

FIGURE 8-25 ■ **CBCT showing six-electrodes of the cochlear implant (CI) in the scala tympani of the cochlea.**

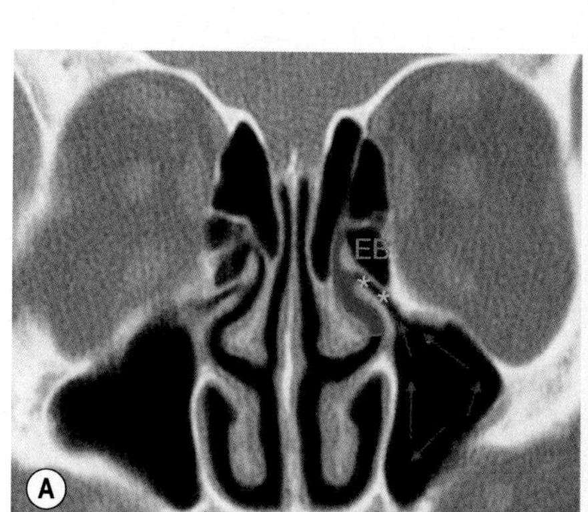

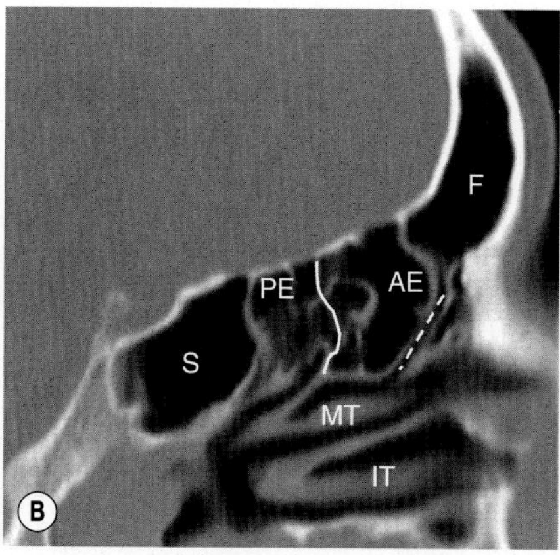

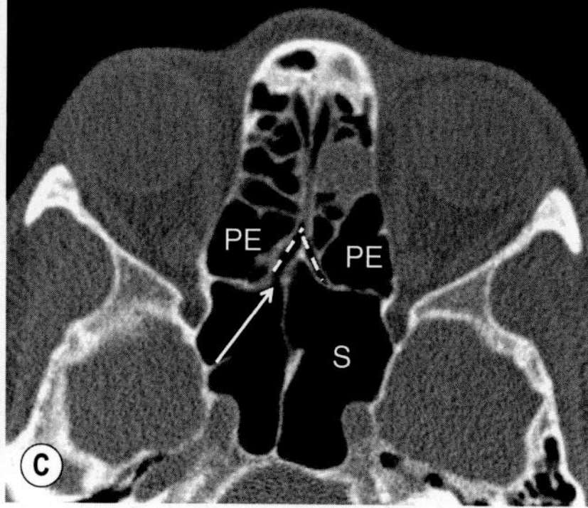

FIGURE 8-26 ■ (A) Coronal CT of paranasal sinuses and nasal cavity. Red arrows = mucociliary flow in left antrum pointing towards the infundibulum (green stars). Blue = middle meatus. EB = ethmoidal bulla (the ethmoidal air cell superior to the infundibulum or outflow). (B) Sagittal CT of paranasal sinuses and nasal cavity. F = frontal sinus; interrupted white line = frontal sinus drainage pathway; AE = anterior ethmoidal air cell; PE = posterior ethmoidal air cell; white line = basal lamella that divides AE from PE air cells; S = sphenoid sinus; MT = middle turbinate; IT = inferior turbinate. (C) Axial CT of paranasal sinuses and nasal cavity. S = sphenoid sinus; PE = posterior ethmoidal air cells; white arrow = sphenoid sinus ostium; interrupted white line = sphenoethmoidal recess (common drainage pathway for S and PE air cells).

The inferior meatus receives drainage from the nasolacrimal duct and the superior meatus the posterior ethmoidal air cells, the latter then draining into the sphenoethmoidal recess along with the sphenoid sinus.

It is important to understand the mucociliary drainage pathways and their common anatomical variants as the aim of functional endoscopic sinus surgery (FESS) is to restore these pathways.

The lining of the nose is pseudostratified ciliated columnar epithelium common to the respiratory tract. A specialised sensory epithelium lies on either side of the septum immediately beneath the cribriform plate (the olfactory niche).The specialised non-myelinated neurons connect in the olfactory niche with olfactory bulbs in the anterior cranial fossa via a perforated bone (lamina cribrosa). The commonest cause of anosmia is mucosal thickening. Other causes include frontal trauma and rarely neoplasia (olfactory neuroblastoma, subfrontal meningioma).

The sinonasal cavity serves a number of functions:

- smell;
- respiration (mouth breathing usually only required in exercise);
- air conditioning (heat exchange, humidification and cleaning);
- immune response to antigen (antibodies in nasal mucosa first line of defence); and
- sound quality (listen to anyone with a cold, the sinonasal cavity acts as a resonant chamber).

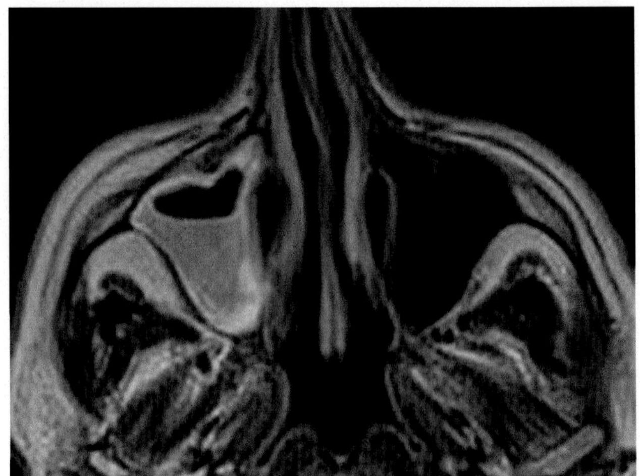

FIGURE 8-27 ■ Axial T2W MR image of the maxillary antra showing a fluid level in the right antrum and surrounding high signal mucosal thickening.

Radiology and Pathology

Low-dose CT and, increasingly, CBCT are indicated when the patient has failed medical treatment, FESS is being considered or there is an acute presentation such as orbital cellulitis or mucocoele. MRI is a problem solver and is used to differentiate tumour from inflammation, assess tumour extent and exclude non-sinonasal causes of anosmia.

Rhinosinusitis

This is an extremely common condition usually treated medically. There are a number of common causes:

- Allergic: very common and may develop into polyposis.
- Vasomotor: a disorder of autonomic regulation of mucus production.
- Infective: as in the common cold.
- Ciliary disorders: Kartagener's syndrome.
- Iatrogenic: overuse of nasal congestants.

When medical treatment has failed, surgery (FESS) is aimed at widening the mucociliary pathways with procedures such as an uncinectomy (± bullectomy) to widen the ostium of the maxillary antrum.

CT or CBCT should be performed in the axial plane with coronal and sagittal reformatted images and soft-tissue reconstruction. Radiological assessment should include the following:

- Identification of relevant anatomical variants such as deviated nasal septum and septal spur, concha bullosa or paradoxical turn to the turbinates, hypoplasia or enlargement of normal structures (maxillary antrum, frontal sinus, ethmoidal bulla, etc.) and the presence of anomalous air cells (frontoethmoidal, sphenoethmoidal and infraorbital).
- Identification of the extent of disease in relation to the mucociliary pathways. For example, does the antral inflammation extend to the ostium, infundibulum or middle meatus or is the whole ostiomeatal unit involved? Does the frontal or sphenoid sinus disease extend to the ostium or further into the frontal and sphenoethmoidal recess, respectively? Are there fluid levels to suggest an acute component (Fig. 8-27)? The extent of disease will guide the extent of surgery.
- Identification of bony thickening suggesting chronicity, or bony erosion/destruction suggesting a more aggressive process.
- Identification of dental disease that may cause a reactive inflammatory change in the overlying antra and be the underlying cause of the patient's symptoms (Fig. 8-28).
- Identification of orbital or, rarely, intracranial extension.
- Assessment of the postnasal space.
- Identification of previous surgery including extent.
- Review of soft-tissue reconstructed images in order to identify fungal disease (Fig. 8-29), desiccated secretions or tumour and pathology extending outside the sinonasal region (pre- and postantral, pterygopalatine fossa, orbit), suggesting a more aggressive process, of particular importance in immunocompromised patients.

Because of the high inherent contrast in the paranasal sinuses and nasal cavity, a low-dose technique can be used. The anterior ostiomeatal unit is best assessed in the coronal plane, the frontal sinus drainage pathway in the sagittal plane and the sphenoethmoidal recess in the axial plane (Fig. 8-26).

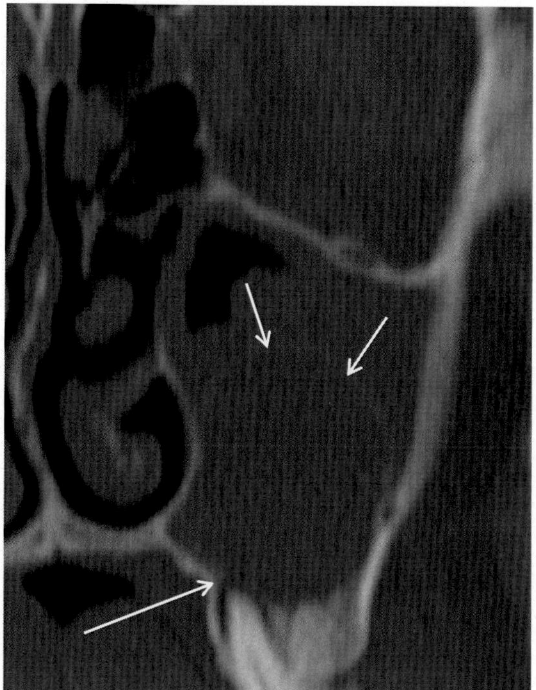

FIGURE 8-28 ■ Magnified coronal CT of left antrum. Note almost completely opacified antrum. Short white arrows = roof of radicular cyst arising from palatal root of left upper molar (long white arrow).

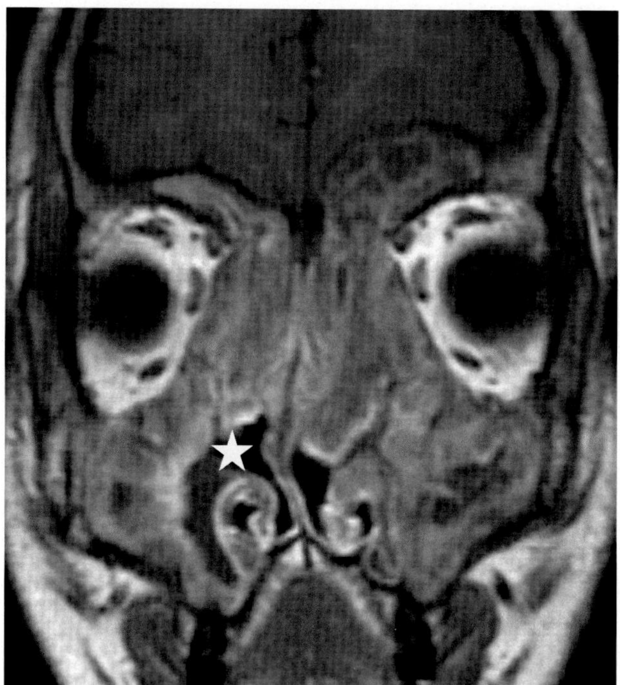

FIGURE 8-30 ■ Coronal T1W MR post-gadolinium image of the anterior osteometal unit region. Note completely opacified antra, frontal sinuses and AE air cells secondary to polypoidal mucosal thickening obstructing the outflow. Star = previous right middle meatal antrostomy.

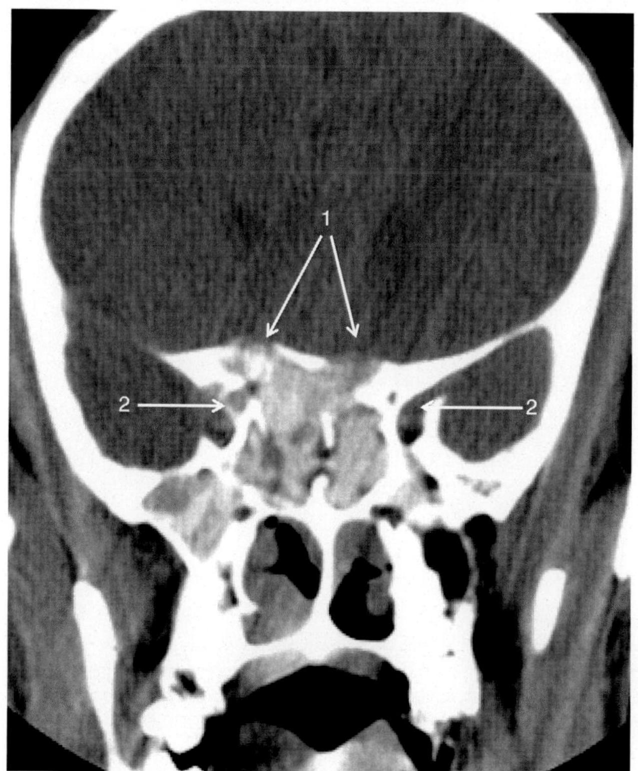

FIGURE 8-29 ■ Coronal CT of the sphenoid sinus (soft-tissue recons). Note high attenuation material filling the sphenoid sinus in keeping with fungal infection eroding the roof (1). Note close relation with the optic nerve (2).

Common problems requiring imaging include nasal polyps, antrochoanal polyp, mucocoeles, fractures, epistaxis, nasal and paranasal sinus tumours.

Nasal Polyposis

Nasal polyposis is a common condition in adults, but if seen in children cystic fibrosis should be considered as a possible cause. Nasal polyps are usually located in the middle meati, roof of nasal cavity and ethmoidal regions; they are multiple and bilateral and involve both the nasal cavity and sinuses. They are secondary to inflammatory swelling of the sinonasal mucosa which forms polyps (Fig. 8-30).

Please note that if a superior nasal cavity polyp is observed, careful review of the anterior skull base is mandatory to exclude a meningocoele or encephalocoele (Figs. 8-31 and 8-32).

Please also note that unilateral polyps require direct inspection ± biopsy to exclude neoplasia. Polyps are usually treated medically, but surgery (FESS) is frequently required.

Antrochoanal Polyp

An antrochoanal polyp is a solitary dumbbell-shaped polypoid mass that largely fills the antrum and extends through a widened accessory sinus ostium or infundibulum into the nasal cavity and from there posteriorly through the choana into the postnasal space and even the oropharynx (Fig. 8-33). These polyps are most commonly seen in young adults.

Although the imaging features and patient age are usually characteristic, nasal endoscopy is important in any patient with unilateral sinus disease to exclude underlying sinister pathology such as an inverted papilloma or other neoplasia.

Mucocoeles

The important features are a completely opacified, expanded sinus with smoothly thinned walls (Fig. 8-34). Approximately 90% occur in the frontal and ethmoidal sinuses. Mucocoeles are usually painless but present when the mass effect becomes critical. Frontal mucocoeles may present with frontal swelling or more rarely headache secondary to posterior extension into the anterior cranial fossa. Frontal and anterior ethmoidal mucocoeles may extend into the orbit, giving rise to proptosis. Mucocoeles are usually sterile but can become infected with a dramatic clinical presentation of rapid onset of pain and fever requiring urgent surgical drainage.

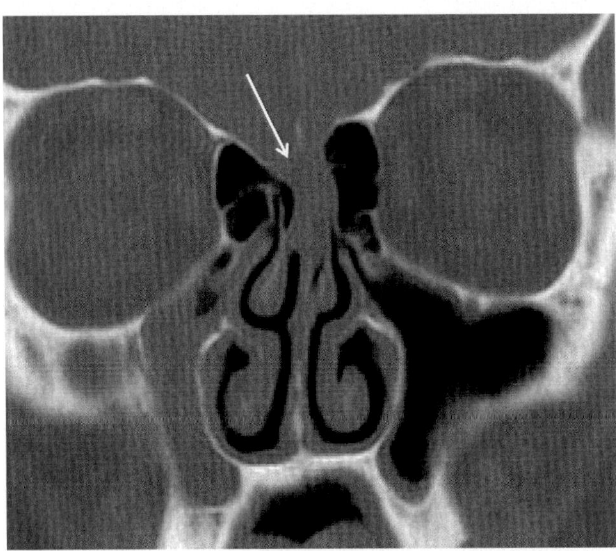

FIGURE 8-31 ■ Coronal CT of paranasal sinus and nasal cavity. Patient referred with nasal 'polyp'. Note defect in anterior skull base (white arrow). MR therefore organised (Fig. 8-32).

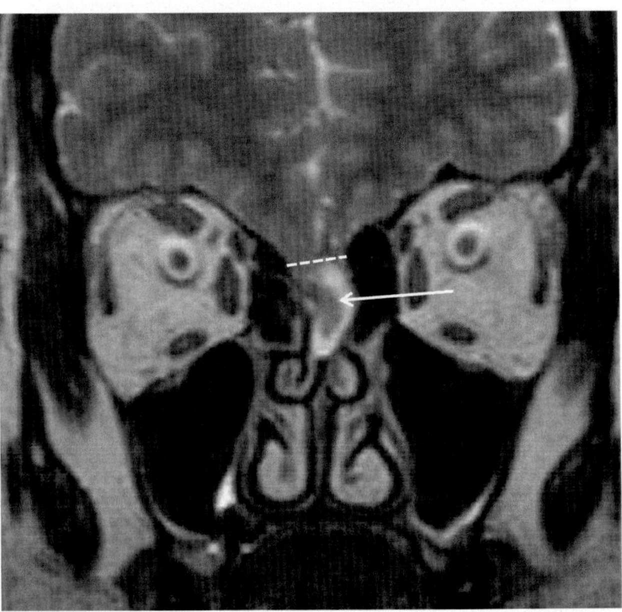

FIGURE 8-32 ■ Coronal T2W MR images of paranasal sinuses and nasal cavity. Interrupted white line = anterior skull base. Note that the 'polyp' seen in Fig. 8-31 is a meningoencephalocoele of the right gyrus rectus (white arrow).

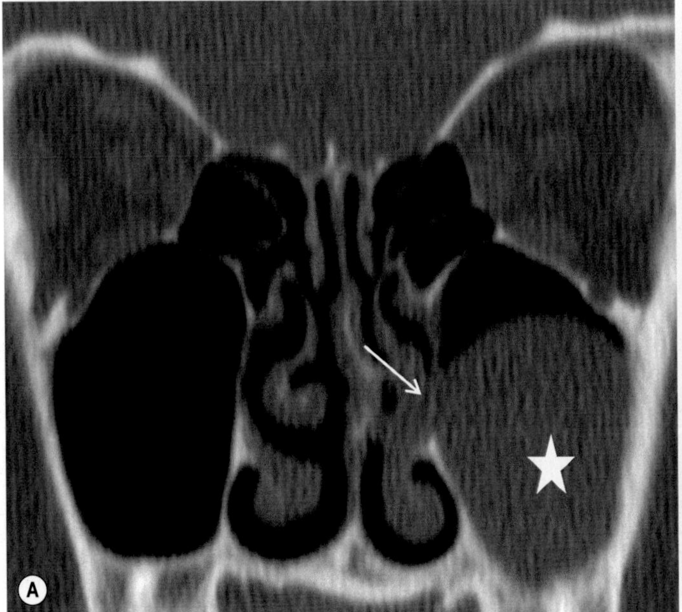

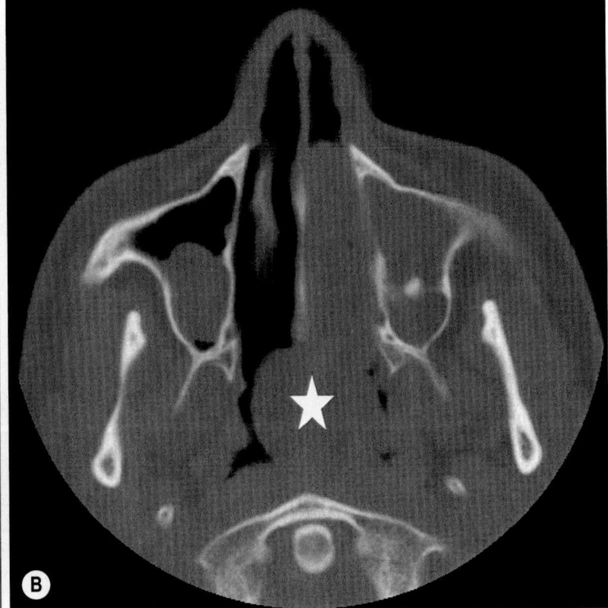

FIGURE 8-33 ■ (A) Axial CT of paranasal sinuses and nasal cavity. Star = polyp within left antrum extending through accessory sinus ostium into middle meatus (white arrow). (B) Axial CT of paranasal sinus and nasal cavity. Note polyp filling the left side of the nasal cavity and extending through the choana to fill the postnasal space (star) in keeping with an antrochoanal polyp.

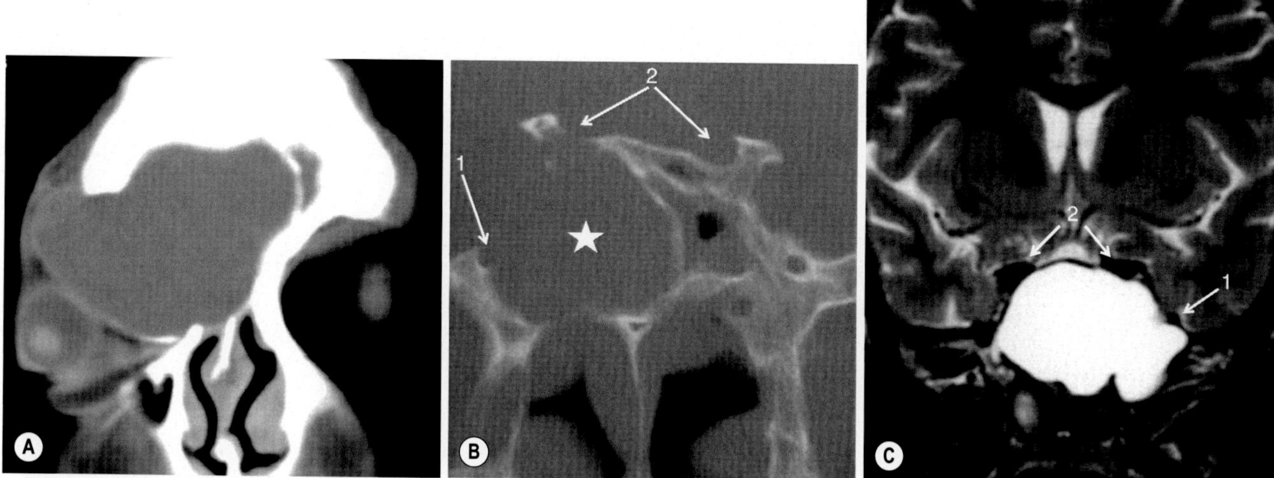

FIGURE 8-34 ■ (A) Coronal CT of frontal sinus. Note a markedly expanded and opacified right frontal sinus with extensive dehiscent inferolateral wall and secondary displacement and proptosis of the right globe in keeping with a frontal mucocoele. (B) Magnified coronal CT of sphenoid sinus. Note opacified expanded right side of the sphenoid sinus (star) with dehiscent lateral wall and close relation with the maxillary division of the trigeminal nerve (1) and the optic nerves (2). (C) Coronal T2W MR image of sphenoid sinus. Note expanded opacified sphenoid sinus filled with T2 high signal material and again the close relation to the maxillary division of the trigeminal nerve (1) and the optic nerves (2).

Epistaxis

Epistaxis does not usually require imaging, but if the bleeding is profuse or recurrent then a source for the bleeding may require investigation usually with CT post IV contrast medium performed in the arterial phase. Severe uncontrolled epistaxis may be life-threatening. Contrast angiography and selective embolisation of bleeding vessels may be life-saving.

Nasal and Paranasal Sinus Tumours

Sinonasal tumours are often advanced at presentation as the early symptoms are similar to chronic sinusitis and because tumours enlarge within hollow cavities, thus not exerting pressure effects. Early diagnosis requires a high index of suspicion in patients who have unilateral or recurrent symptoms and do not respond to medical treatment.

Early symptoms of malignancy include unilateral facial pain, nasal obstruction, unilateral nasal discharge and epistaxis. Late symptoms include altered sensation in the V2 distribution, proptosis, epiphora and trismus.

There are three main prognostic factors in sinonasal malignancy: tumour type, intracranial and orbital involvement. The radiologist's role is defining extent rather than histological diagnosis. Tumours vary from indolent to very malignant.

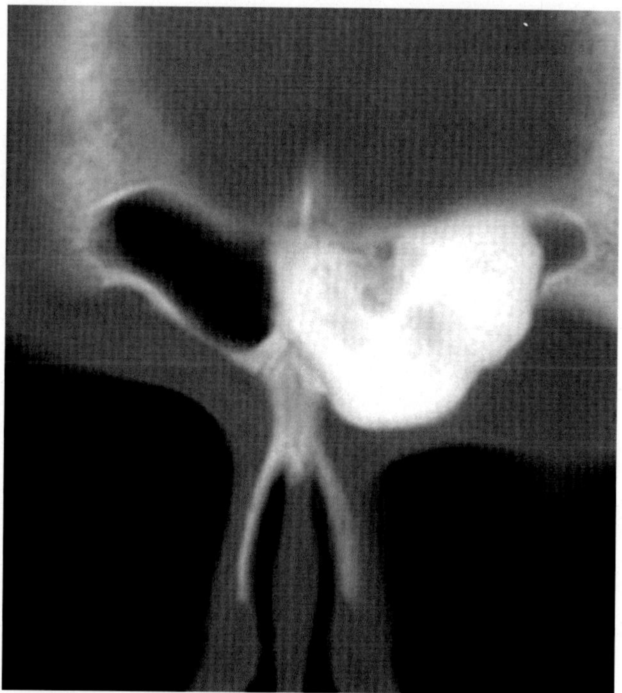

FIGURE 8-35 ■ **Coronal CT of left frontal sinus osteoma.** Note well-defined dense bony lesion filling most of left frontal sinus and bulging into the superomedial left orbit.

Osteoma

These are the most common tumour of the paranasal sinuses usually noted as an incidental finding. They are well-defined, sessile or pedunculated lesions arising from a wall of the frontal sinus (80%), ethmoidal sinus (20%) or rarely maxillary and sphenoid sinuses (Fig. 8-35). They are slow growing and often not requiring treatment although surgery is considered if the osteoma is compromising the drainage pathway or >50% of the sinus volume.

Inverted Papilloma

They are frequently present as a middle meatal mass causing unilateral nasal obstruction usually in an ostiomeatal pattern. The sex ratio is M.F 4:1. Ten per cent demonstrate calcification at the site of tumoural attachment. They have a characteristic lobulated outline on CT and a cerebriform pattern on MRI (Fig. 8-36). Surgery must include subperiosteal resection at the site of attachment to avoid recurrence. Assessment with CT is usually satisfactory, with MRI used mainly to assess recurrence.

Juvenile Angiofibroma

Adolescent boys with heavy epistaxis characterise the disease. This benign, locally invasive mass originates at the sphenopalatine foramen, widens the pterygopalatine fossa (PPF), extends into the nasal cavity and erodes the adjacent medial pterygoid plate and skull base in the region of the vidian canal aperture (Fig. 8-37).

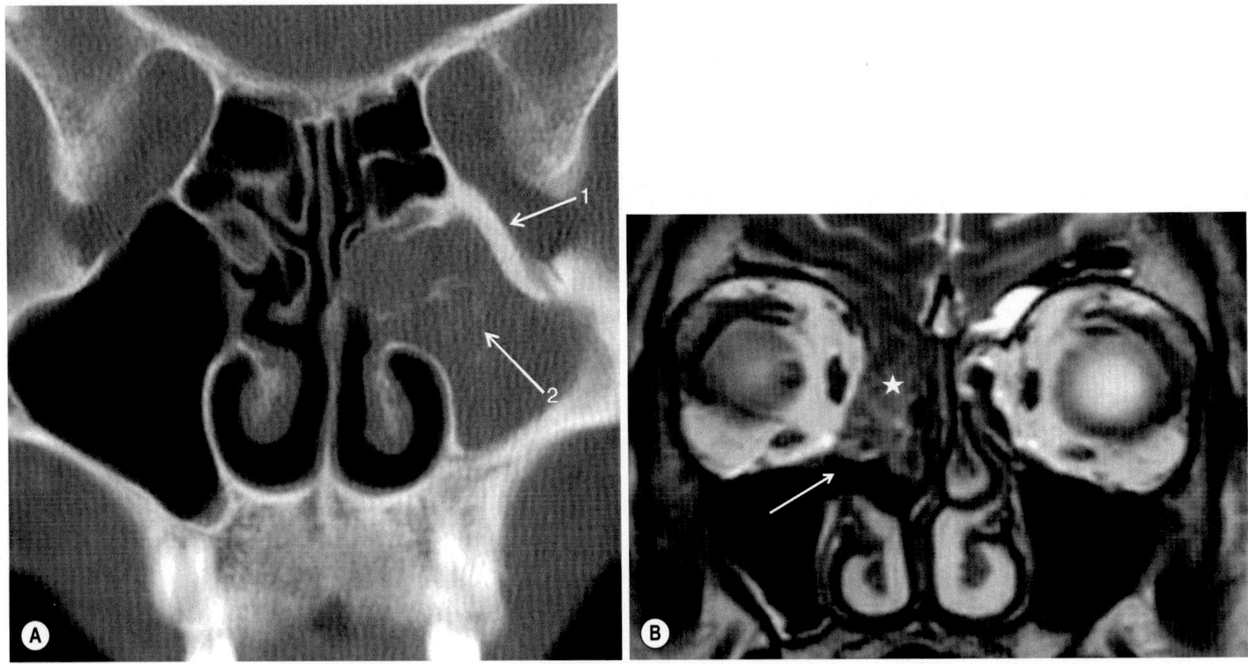

FIGURE 8-36 ■ (A) Coronal CT image of anterior osteometal unit (OMU). Note the unilateral opacified left antrum expanding into the middle meatus associated with bony thickening of the roof (1) and calcification (2). (B) Coronal T2W MR image of anterior OMU. Note (white arrow) the previous middle meatal antrostomy (MMA) and (white star) the intermediate signal of the recurrent inverted papilloma.

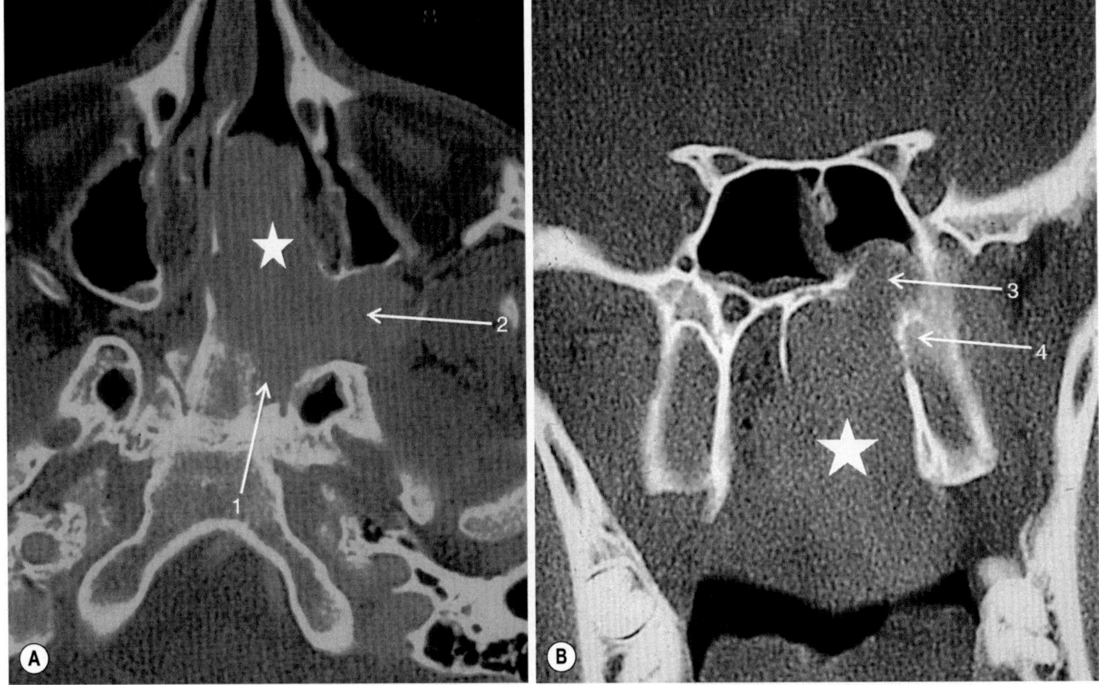

FIGURE 8-37 ■ (A) Axial and (B) coronal CT images. Note the angiofibroma (white star) filling and expanding the nasal cavity, eroding the sphenoid in the region of the vidian canal aperture (1 & 3), widening the PPF (2) and eroding the medial pterygoid plate (4).

The presence of a nasal mass and a widened PPF in an adolescent male is pathognomonic. Contrast-enhanced MR is usually required and is complementary to CT for accurate preoperative assessment. Preoperative embolisation may be used to reduce blood loss.

Sinonasal Malignancy

Sinonasal malignancy is rare and there is a wide differential; however, approximately 80% are SCC (Fig. 8-38), with adenocarcinoma, adenoid cystic carcinoma and lymphoma comprising most of the remainder. Rarer sinonasal malignancies include olfactory neuroblastoma, melanoma and sarcomas. About 30% arise in the nasal cavity and most of the remainder arise in the antroethmoidal region, with < 5% arising in the frontal or sphenoid sinuses. The role of radiology is to define the tumour extent to form the basis of any treatment planning with, in particular, careful assessment of any intracranial, orbital, PPF, palatal or nodal involvement. Multiplanar MR is the technique of choice with fat-saturated sequences post-gadolinium helpful for assessing any orbital, dural involvement or perineural extension.

When assessing the anterior skull base, it is necessary to assess whether there is any skull base erosion, dural involvement or extension through the dura (Fig. 8-39).

When assessing the orbit it is important to identify whether there is erosion of the lamina papyracea, involvement of the orbital periosteum or extension through the periosteum. The lamina papyracea may be eroded on CT, but the low signal line of the orbital periosteum still preserved on MRI (Fig. 8-40). In equivocal cases frozen sections may be performed at the time of surgery, but the tendency is towards preserving the globe.

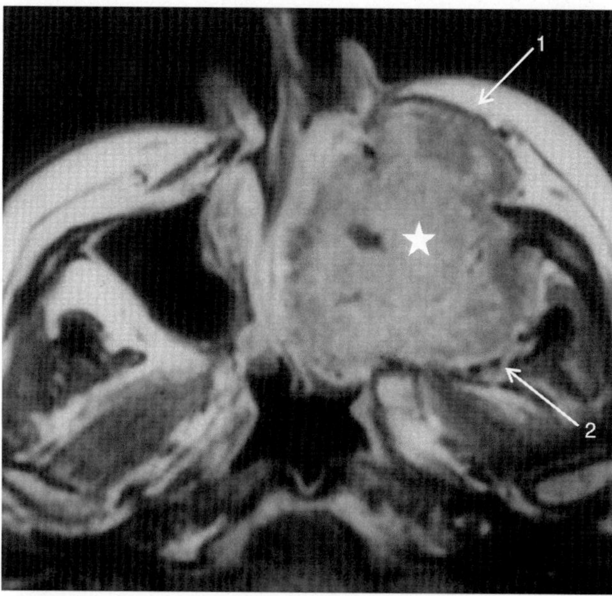

FIGURE 8-38 ■ **Axial T1W MR post-gadolinium image.** Note the expansile destructive mass (white star) centred on the left antrum extending into the pre- (1) and retroantral (2) soft tissues.

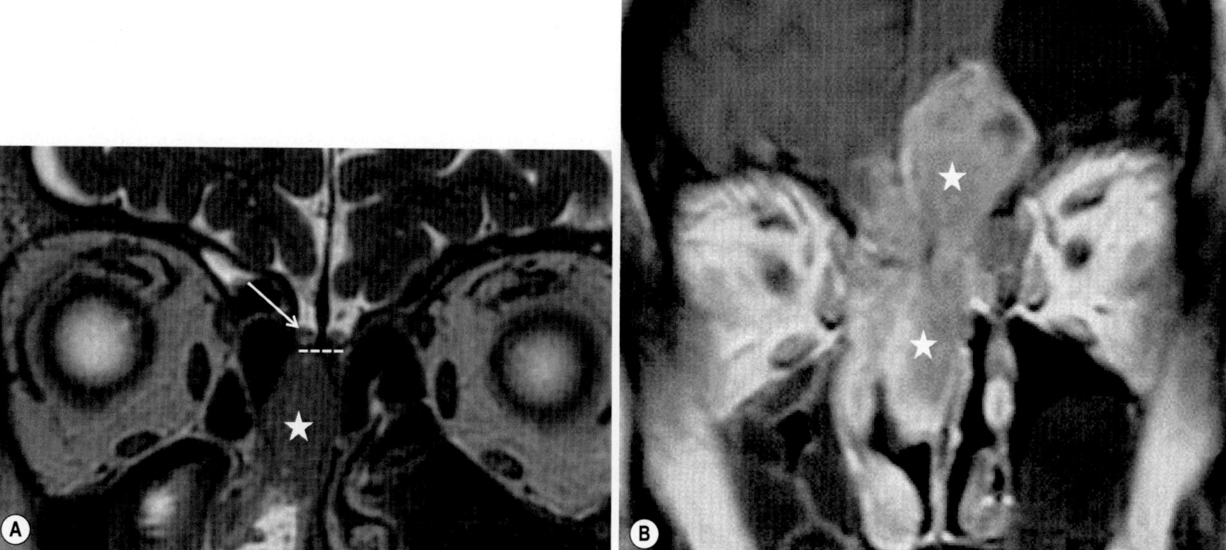

FIGURE 8-39 ■ (A) Magnified T2W coronal MR image. Note the mass (white star) filling and expanding the right olfactory niche but not eroding the cribriform plate (interrupted white line) or invading the more superior olfactory bulbs (white arrow). (B) Coronal T1 MR post-gadolinium image. There is a large dumbbell-shaped olfactory neuroblastoma (ON) (white stars), with both a large intracranial and superior nasal cavity component and a waist at the anterior skull base. Note also the peritumoural cyst occasionally seen in ON.

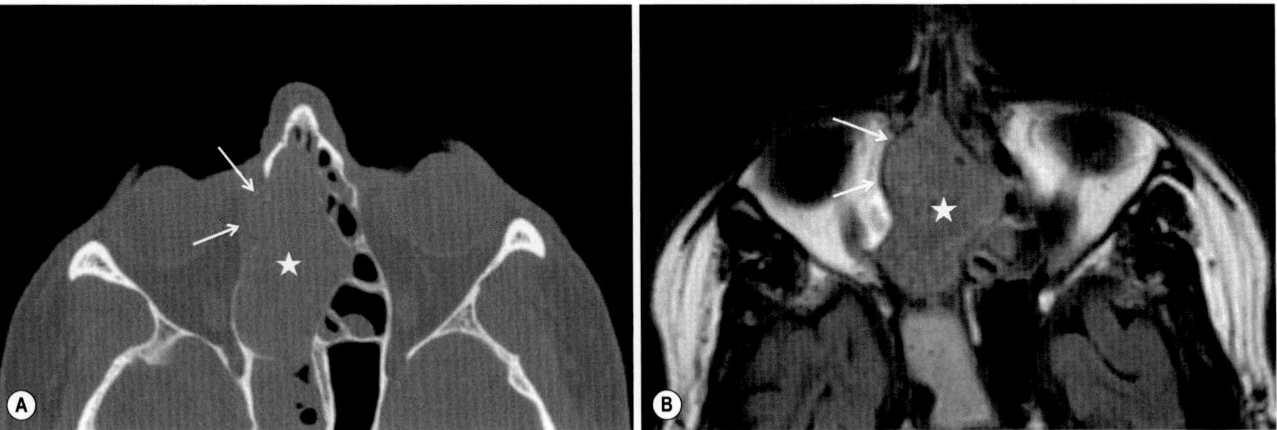

FIGURE 8-40 ■ (A) Axial CT and (B) axial T1W MR post-gadolinium images. Note the eroded lamina papyracea on CT, but the preserved orbital periosteum on MRI (white arrows). Tumour = white star.

THE NECK

THE SUPRAHYOID NECK

Anatomy

The suprahyoid neck is divided into spaces delineated by the three layers of deep cervical fascia. This is a logical method for reviewing this region as the fascial layers act as a barrier to the spread of disease and by localising the pathology to a particular space the differential diagnosis is simplified.

The following spaces in the suprahyoid neck are recognised (Fig. 8-41): the parapharyngeal space (PPS), the parotid space (PS), the retropharyngeal and danger spaces (RPS and DS), the masticator space (MS), the carotid space (CS), the pharyngeal mucosal space (PMS) and the perivertebral space (PVS).

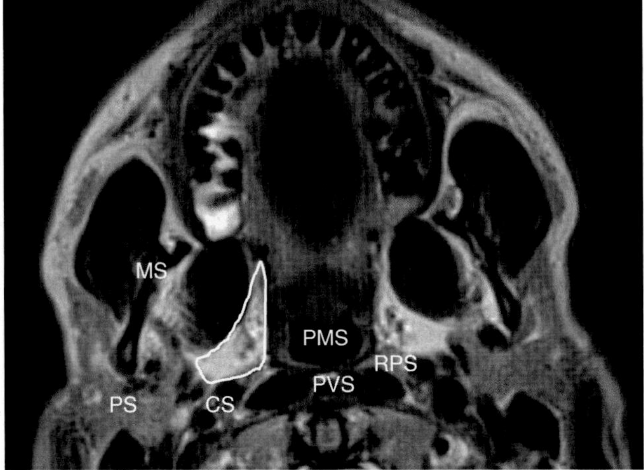

FIGURE 8-41 ■ Axial T2W MR image. Note the central location of the parapharyngeal space (outlined in white) largely filled with fat and therefore readily visible on both CT and MR relative to the other spaces of the suprahyoid neck: MS = masticator space, PS = parotid space, CS = carotid space, PVS = perivertebral space, RPS = retropharyngeal space. (The danger space (DS) has not been included as it cannot be separated on imaging from the RPS.)

The Parapharyngeal Space

The PPS is the key to the suprahyoid neck as it is centrally located and consists almost entirely of fat and therefore is easily identified on CT and MR (Fig. 8-41). This space was previously known as the prestyloid parapharyngeal space. It is rare for pathology to arise within the PPS (occasionally a salivary tumour from a salivary rest); however, the direction of displacement of the PPS fat helps the radiologist identify the adjacent suprahyoid space of origin of the pathology.

The Parotid Space

Anatomy and Radiology. The parotid space contains the parotid salivary gland, lymph nodes, facial nerve, retromandibular vein and external carotid artery enclosed by the superficial layer of deep cervical fascia (Fig. 8-42).

Ultrasound is the first-line imaging technique for salivary masses and may be combined with fine-needle aspiration cytology (FNAC). The important questions to ask on imaging are the following:

- Is the swelling arising in or adjacent to the parotid? Differentiation of an upper cervical lymph node from a tail of parotid lesion can be difficult.
- Is the swelling centred in the superficial and/or deep aspects of the gland? This is very important with regard to surgical planning and potential risk of iatrogenic facial nerve damage.
- Is the swelling ill-defined or well-defined, cystic or solid? That is, does it have features suggestive of malignancy or an inflammatory/infective process?

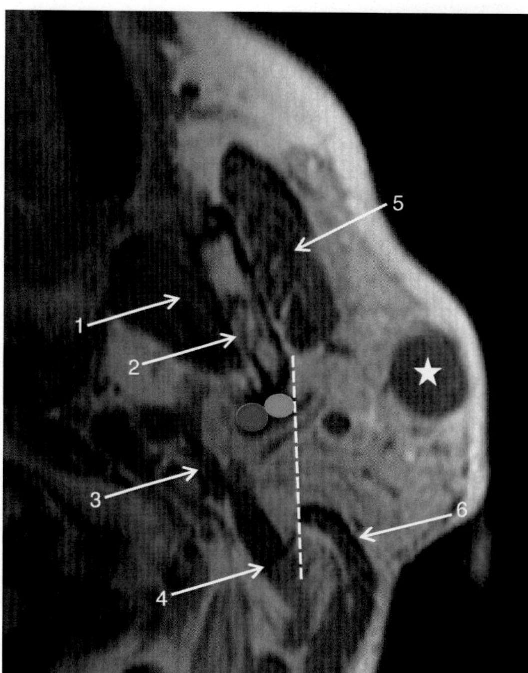

FIGURE 8-42 ■ **Axial/TW1 MR image of left parotid.** 1 = medial pterygoid muscle, 2 = inferior alveolar nerve (branch of V3), 3 = styloid process, 4 = posterior belly digastric muscle, 5 = masseter muscle, 6 = sternocleidomastoid muscle. Interrupted white line = junction of superficial and deep parotid (from lateral border of posterior belly digastric muscle to angle of mandible). Blue circle = retromandibular vein, red circle = external carotid artery (ECA), star = tumour in the superficial parotid (a pleomorphic salivary adenoma (PSA) in this patient).

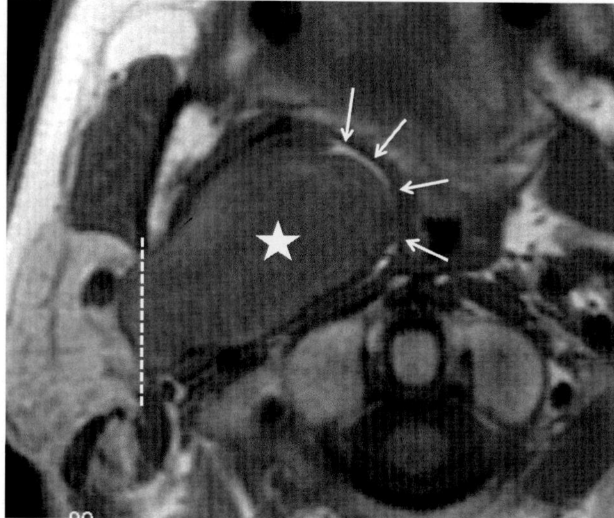

FIGURE 8-43 ■ **Axial T1W MRI of right parotid.** Interrupted white line = approximate junction superficial and deep parotid, white star = deep lobe of parotid tumour (PSA in this patient), white arrows = displaced PPS.

- Is the swelling single or multiple, unilateral or bilateral? If multiple, consider intraparotid nodes, benign lymphoepithelial lesions and chronic inflammatory pathology. If bilateral, consider the above and also a Warthin's tumour, in particular, in an elderly male smoker.
- Is there adjacent lymphadenopathy?

MRI is complementary to US and is used to assess local extent, in particular when there is proven malignancy on fine-needle aspiration (FNA) or in the parotid suspected deep lobe involvement (Fig. 8-43) or to assess perineural infiltration. Contrast-enhanced CT (CECT) does not differentiate the tumour from adjacent normal salivary tissue as clearly as MRI, but is helpful in assessing infection associated with sialolithiasis. MR sialography can be helpful in chronic inflammatory conditions such as Sjögren's syndrome (Fig. 8-44).

The Retropharyngeal and Danger Spaces (RPS and DS)

Anatomy. These are potential spaces centred posterior to the pharynx and anterior to the prevertebral muscles extending from the skull base to T4 in the superior mediastinum. The more posterior DS and RPS cannot be differentiated from each other on imaging. The importance of the RPS and DS is that disease, in particular infection in both spaces, can extend into the mediastinum.

The RPS contains a medial and lateral group of nodes from the skull base to hyoid bone, i.e. suprahyoid. Therefore, pathology in the suprahyoid RPS tends to be unilateral/asymmetrical.

Pathology. The radiological importance of the RPS is in two main areas: infection and malignancy.

The radiologist must try and differentiate between an RPS abscess that tends to distend the RPS and demonstrates wall enhancement from fluid that does not cause significant mass effect. It is important in all cases of an RPS abscess to include the superior mediastinum in the imaging field and to differentiate from pathology in the prevertebral part of the perivertebral space (PVS) by confirming that the pathology is anterior to the prevertebral muscles.

The RPS may be involved in malignancy, most frequently secondary to involved lymph nodes (in particular this region should always be reviewed when staging nasopharyngeal, oropharyngeal and the rarer posterior hypopharyngeal wall malignancy) and less commonly from direct posterior extension from the posterior pharyngeal wall (Fig. 8-45). The radiologist must try and identify whether the thin fatty density line of the RPS is preserved.

The Masticator Space

The masticator space, including the muscles of mastication, mandible and the inferior alveolar nerve (a branch of V3), is covered in the Jaw and Dental section of this chapter, as is the oral cavity.

The Carotid Space

Anatomy. The carotid space consists of the carotid arteries, internal jugular vein, sympathetic plexus and

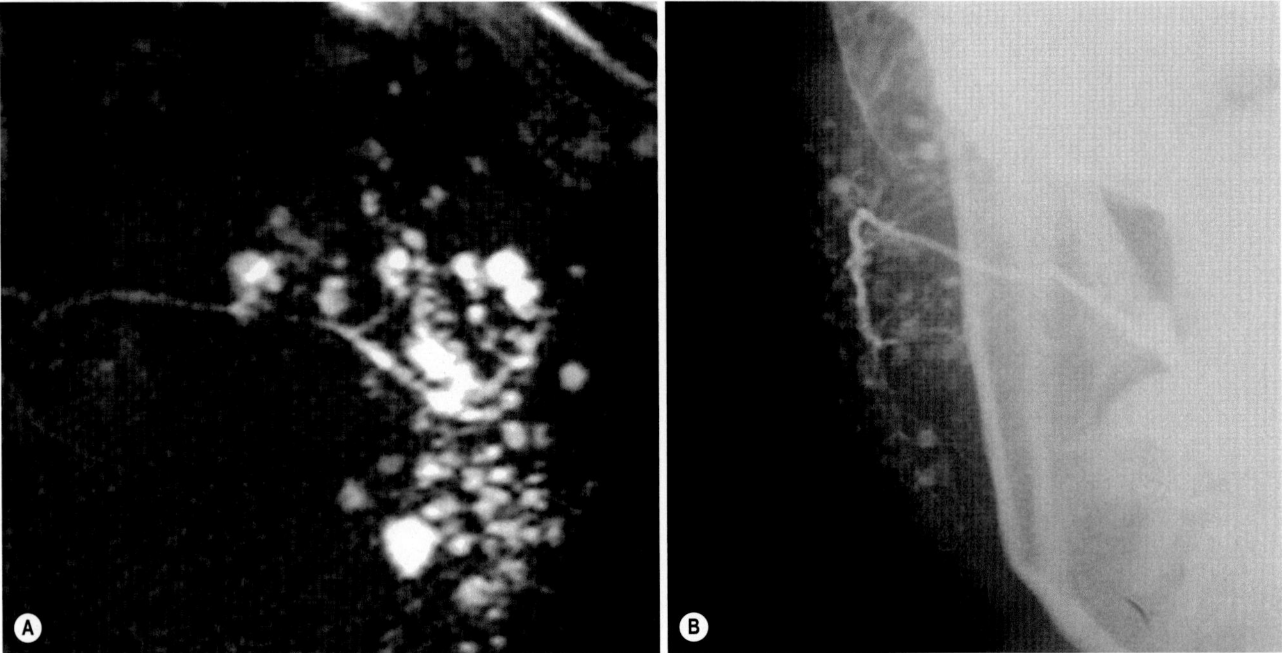

FIGURE 8-44 ■ **(A) MR and (B) conventional sialogram in a patient with Sjögren's syndrome.** Note the multiple punctate cystic spaces more marked in the MR sialogram.

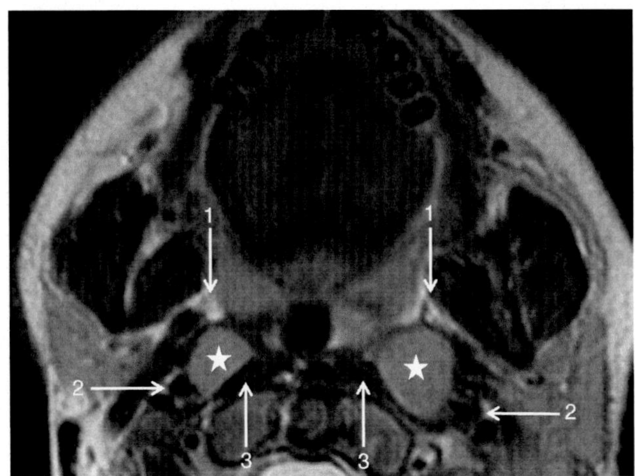

FIGURE 8-45 ■ **T1W MR post-gadolinium image at the level of the oropharynx.** Note the bilateral enlarged retrophayngeal lymph nodes (white stars) and their relation to the PPS (1), ICA (2) and prevertebral muscles (3).

cranial nerves IX–XII in the suprahyoid neck and cranial nerve X in the infrahyoid neck. It also used to be known as the retrostyloid parapharyngeal space.

The most common 'lesion' is the pseudolesion of the ectatic carotid artery or normal asymmetry of the internal jugular veins.

In infection of the deep neck it is important to exclude thrombosis of the internal jugular vein and when assessing malignant lymhadenopathy to assess whether there is invasion of the carotid or internal jugular vein. Loss of the fat plane or >180° of circumferential involvement of the carotid is suggestive of tumour involvement.

Pathology

Carotid Artery Dissection. The extracranial internal carotid artery is the most commonly involved site and is best demonstrated on axial T1 MRI with fat saturation where the intramural haematoma is of high signal.

Carotid and Vagal Paragangliomas. Paragangliomas (also known as glomus tumours) are vascular lesions that classically have a 'salt and pepper' appearance on T1 where the high signal foci represent subacute blood and the low signal flow voids from large tumour vessels. Carotid paragangliomas (or carotid body tumours) arise in the carotid bifurcation and characteristically splay the ICA and ECA (Fig. 8-46). Vagal paragangliomas are centred more superiorly posterior to and between the carotid and internal jugular vein. It is important to always review whether there is extension into the jugular foramen and whether there is a second synchronous lesion (5%–10%).

Schwannoma. These are well-defined, usually homogeneously enhancing, fusiform-shaped masses (Fig. 8-47) that occasionally, when large, demonstrate cystic change. They may, if vascular, be indistinguishable from a paraganglioma although if they extend into the jugular foramen they can be distinguished from paragangliomas as they remodel/expand the foramen rather than cause the classic permeative erosion of a paraganglioma.

The Pharyngeal Mucosal Space (PMS)

Anatomy. The PMS is deep to the middle layer of deep cervical fascia which surrounds the pharyngobasilar fascia

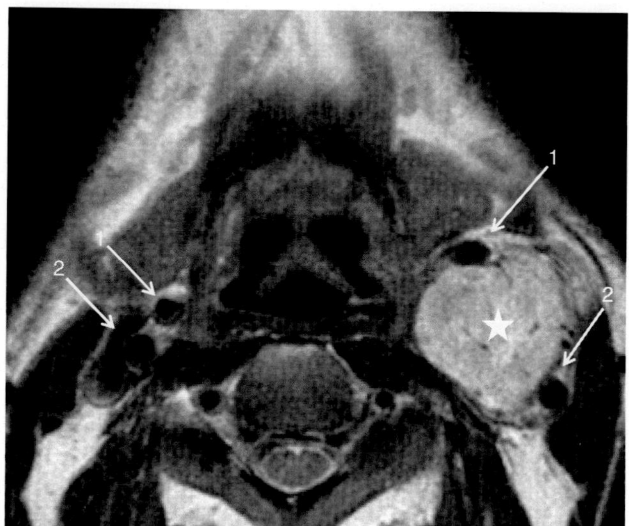

FIGURE 8-46 ■ **Axial T2W MR image.** Note the high signal carotid body tumour (white star) with flow voids splaying the ECA (1) and ICA (2) and compared to the right side. Remember up to 10% are bilateral.

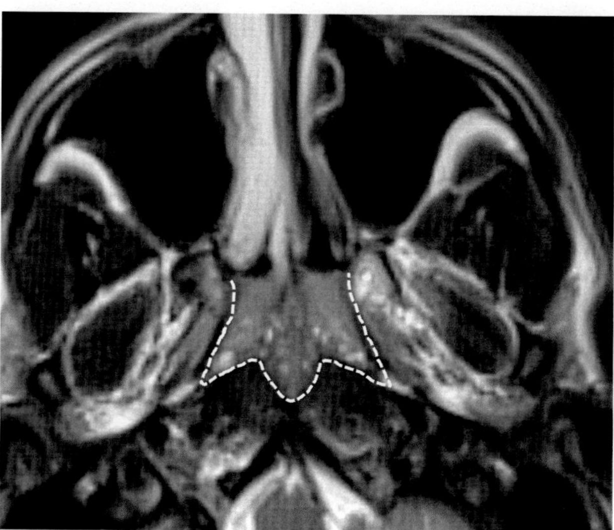

FIGURE 8-48 ■ **Axial T2W MR image.** The interrupted line outlines the pharyngobasilar fascia which has the appearance of an upturned crown. It separates the lymphoidal tissue within the PMS from the PPS laterally and the PVS posteriorly.

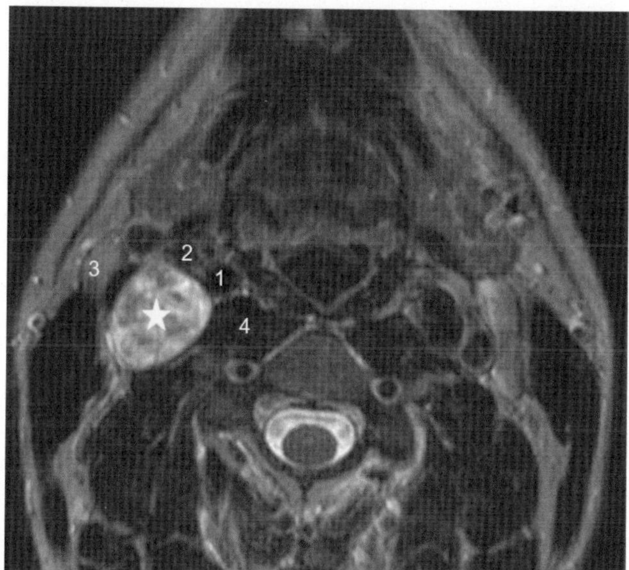

FIGURE 8-47 ■ **Axial T2W MR image.** The high signal vagal schwannoma separates the ICA (1) and ECA (2) from the compressed internal jugular vein (3) and is within the carotid space lateral to the prevertebral muscle (4).

(Fig. 8-48) and the superior and middle constrictors. The contents of the PMS include the mucosa of the nasopharynx and oropharynx (the more inferior hypopharynx is in the visceral space of the infrahyoid neck, which is an inferior continuation of the PMS), lymphatic tissue of Waldeyer's ring (in the nasopharynx adenoids and in the oropharynx faucial tonsils laterally and lingual tonsils, part of the tongue base, anteriorly) and minor salivary glands. The volume of this lymphatic tissue decreases with age.

The most important pathology in this region is SCC arising in the oropharynx and undifferentiated carcinoma in the nasopharynx.

A multidisciplinary team (MDT) approach including ENT, maxillofacial and plastic surgeons, oncologists, pathologists, cytopathologists, radiologists, radiotherapists, speech and language therapists, dietitians and specialist nurses is essential for treating malignant disease in this region. Benign disorders will also be discussed as a benign differential diagnosis is often considered even when malignant disease is suspected.

The PMS can be divided into the nasopharynx and oropharynx.

Nasopharynx

Anatomy. The nasopharynx is the superior division of the pharynx whose boundaries are the skull base superiorly, anterior arch of C1 posteriorly, the superior surface of the soft palate inferiorly, the nasal choanae anteriorly and the lateral pharyngeal wall including the prominence of the torus tubarius with anteriorly the eustachian tube opening and posteriorly the fossa of Rosenmüller.

Radiology and Pathology

Nasopharyngeal Malignancy. MR is superior to CT for assessing the nasopharynx.

Almost all nasopharyngeal malignancies are carcinomas (NPC) that are divided into keratinising, non-keratinising and undifferentiated. The differential includes non-Hodgkin's lymphoma (NHL) arising from lymphoidal tissue and minor salivary gland malignancy. The role of radiology is to define the extent for radiotherapy planning. Accurate assessment is of increasing importance with the advent of more targeted (intensity-modulated) radiotherapy or IMRT.

NPC usually arises in the lateral pharyngeal recess (of Rosenmüller). NPC is the most common tumour that

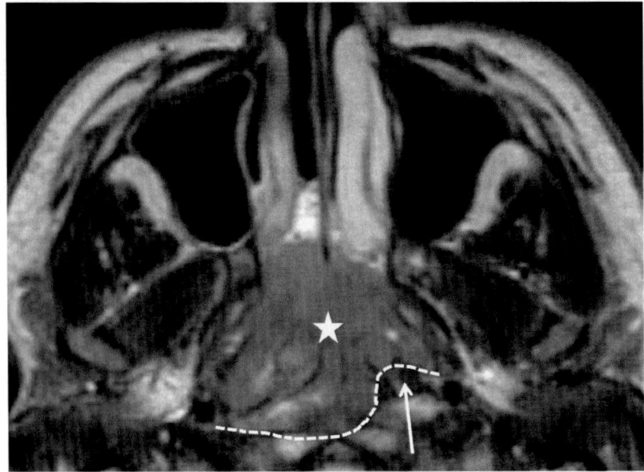

FIGURE 8-49 ■ **Axial T2W MR image.** The nasopharyngeal tumour (white star) has extended posteriorly (interrupted white line) and on the right laterally to invade the PVS and PPS. Note the remaining partially invaded left prevertebral muscle medial to the ICA (white arrow).

invades the skull base. Intracranial extension is most commonly via perineural spread through foramen ovale along the mandibular division of the trigeminal nerve (V3). Nodal metastases are present in 90% at presentation. There is a strong association with the Epstein–Barr virus (EBV) and EBV titres can be used as a marker of tumour response. NPC is the commonest cancer in Asian males. Treatment is radiotherapy or chemoradiotherapy, with surgery for recurrence following treatment.

The commonest differential of nasopharyngeal malignancy (Fig. 8-49) is adenoidal hypertrophy, which can usually be differentiated as the latter is symmetrical and contains visible folds of mucosa. Other benign pathology seen in the nasopharynx includes the Tornwaldt cyst (a benign midline developmental cyst) and a retention cyst, both of which are well defined and covered with normal mucosa. If there is still concern on nasal endoscopy, biopsy is suggested.

Oropharynx

Anatomy. The oropharynx is divided into the following subsites: the tongue base (largely comprising the lingual tonsils) and the valleculae anteriorly (the valleculae form the inferior boundary between oropharynx and hypopharynx), laterally the glosso-tonsillar sulcus and faucial tonsils, superiorly the soft palate (that separates oropharynx from nasopharynx) and posteriorly the posterior pharyngeal wall. Please note that the tongue base is included in the oropharynx and *not* the oral cavity.

Radiology and Pathology. The most common reason for imaging the oropharynx is to query tonsillar or peritonsillar abscess (quinsy). On contrast-enhanced CT (CECT) a tonsillar abscess is shown as a swollen tonsil with central low attenuation and rim enhancement. A peritonsillar abscess occurs when there is spread to adjacent spaces, commonly parapharyngeal masticator and submandibular spaces. If trismus is present, then suspect involvement of the masticator space muscles.

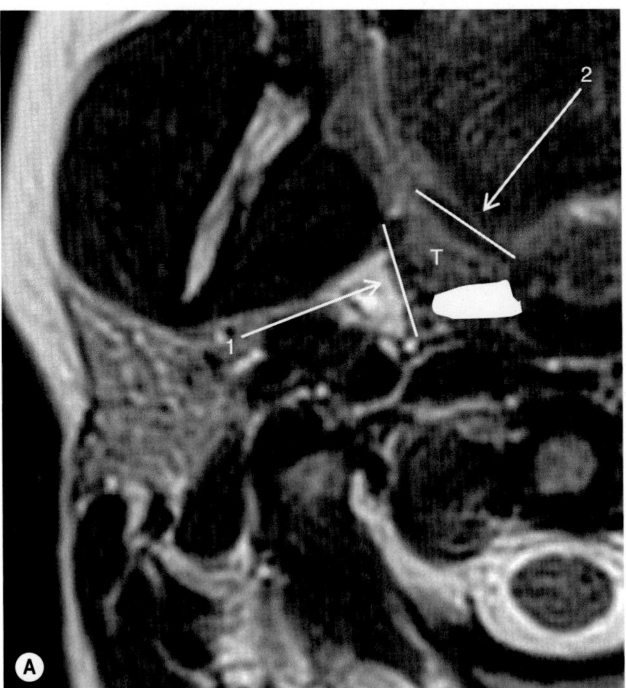

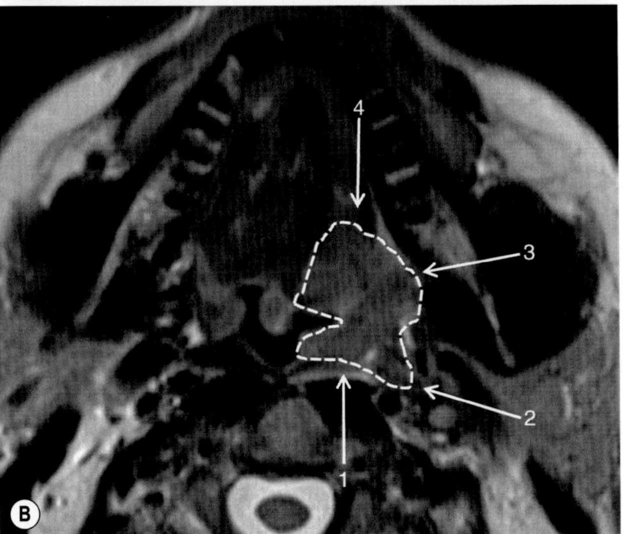

FIGURE 8-50 ■ (A) Axial T2W MR image of right faucial tonsil normal anatomy. T = faucial tonsil with the following relations: lateral border (1) = constrictors, anterior border (2) = palatoglossus muscle of the anterior tonsillar pillar and posterior border (filled in white area) = larger palatopharyngeus muscle of the posterior tonsillar pillar. (B) Axial T2W MR image of left tonsillar SCC. Note the left tonsillar SCC (interrupted white line) invading the following areas: 1 = posterior pharyngeal wall, 2 = RPS, 3 = PPS abutting the medial pterygoid muscle, 4 = tongue.

Nearly all oropharyngeal malignancy is SCC; the commonest site is the faucial tonsil and anterior tonsillar pillar (Fig. 8-50), followed by the lingual tonsil. The anterior tonsillar pillar (the palatoglossus muscle covered by mucosa) acts as a conduit for spread superiorly to the palate and inferiorly to the tongue base. MR imaging delineates oropharyngeal tumours better than CECT, but both lingual and faucial tonsillar tumours may be difficult to identify clinically and are two of the sites for an occult 'hidden' head and neck primary, the other sites being the fossa of Rosenmüller in the nasopharynx and the piriform fossa in the hypopharynx. As in the nasopharynx, rarer oropharyngeal tumours include non-Hodgkin's lymphoma (NHL) and minor salivary tumours (the latter usually arising at the junction of the hard and soft palate).

The following questions should be answered in patients with faucial tonsillar SCC:

- Is there extension laterally through the constrictors (Fig. 8-50B)?
- Is there superior extension to the palate or inferior extension to the tongue base (Fig. 8-50B)?
- Is there retropharyngeal and cervical lymphadenopathy?

The following areas should be reviewed in patients with lingual tonsillar SCC:

- Is there extension across the midline?
- What is the depth of invasion?
- Are the extrinsic tongue muscles involved?
- Is there inferior extension into the supraglottic larynx?

Fifteen per cent of patients with oropharyngeal SSC will have a second primary in the head and neck, and 60% have malignant lymphadenopathy at presentation.

Perivertebral Space (PVS)

This region is described in the neuroimaging chapters. The important point is to identify that when pathology arises in the prevertebral part of the perivertebral space it displaces the prevertebral muscles anteriorly, whereas an RPS mass is centred anterior to the prevertebral muscles, which are therefore displaced posteriorly. The commonest pathology in this region is a prevertebral abscess and metastatic disease.

THE INFRAHYOID NECK

Anatomy

As in the suprahyoid neck, the infrahyoid neck is divided into spaces defined by the layers of deep cervical fascia. There are five spaces but only one, the visceral space, is found solely in the infrahyoid neck. The other spaces are the carotid space (CS), retropharyngeal (RPS) and perivertebral spaces, which are discussed in the suprahyoid section above, and the posterior cervical space, which, as it only includes the accessory nerve, fat and lymph nodes, will not be discussed further except to note that the accessory nerve is sometimes sacrificed in neck dissection, resulting in a weak shoulder.

The visceral space includes the hypopharynx (a continuation of the pharyngeal mucosal space), the larynx and trachea, the thyroid and parathyroid glands, the recurrent laryngeal nerve and lymph nodes.

Hypopharynx

Anatomy. The hypopharynx, along with the larynx, is located within the visceral space of the infrahyoid neck and is divided into the pyriform fossae, the post-cricoid region and the posterior pharyngeal wall. The inferior aspect of the pyriform fossa is the apex. The hypopharynx and larynx are intimately associated. Surgery to the hypopharynx usually therefore involves surgery to the larynx.

Radiology and Pathology. Nearly all hypopharyngeal tumours are SCC (or very rarely minor salivary gland).

The majority arise in the pyriform fossa (Fig. 8-51A), followed by the post-cricoid area (Fig. 8-51B), and rarely the posterior hypopharyngeal wall. Patients tend to present late and approximately 50% have nodal involvement at presentation. There is a strong association with smoking and drinking. Critical observations to make are the following:

- Is there posterolateral extension into adjacent soft tissues and/or involvement of the posterior thyroid lamina?

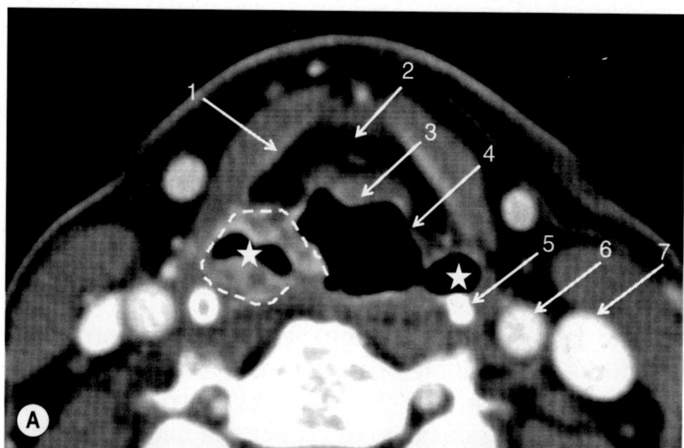

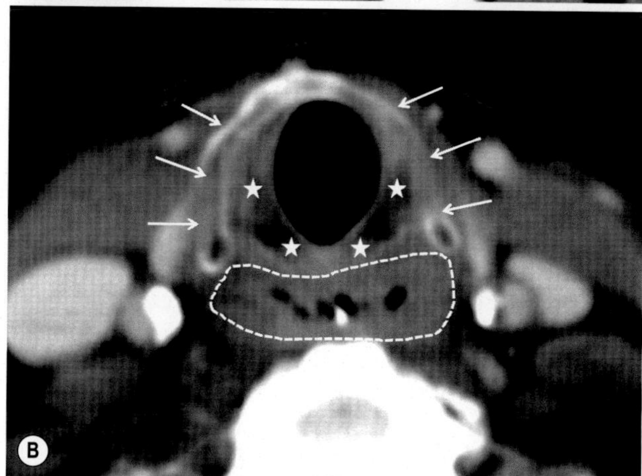

FIGURE 8-51 ■ (A) Axial CT post IV contrast through hypopharynx. Note the tumour (interrupted white line) arising in the piriform fossa (white stars). 1 = lamina of thyroid cartilage, 2 = pre-epiglottic fat, 3 = epiglottis, 4 = aryepiglottic fold, 5 = superior horn thyroid cartilage, 6 = CCA, 7 = IJV. (B) Note the circumferential post-cricoid and posterior hyppoharyngeal wall tumour (interrupted white line) containing a nasogastric tube posterior to the cricoid cartilage (white stars) and lamina of thyroid cartilage (white arrows).

- Is there inferior extension into the cervical oesophagus? Correlate with swallowing studies and endoscopic assessment.
- Is there retropharyngeal nodal involvement?

Larynx

Anatomy and Physiology. The larynx has two main functions:

1. Airway protection.
2. Sound generation.

The larynx sits on the cricoid cartilage, which resembles a signet ring with its face situated posteriorly. The larger V-shaped thyroid cartilage protects the vocal cords and consists of two lamina fused anteriorly and open posteriorly. Posteriorly there are superior and inferior extensions of the thyroid laminae called superior and inferior horns. The inferior horns articulate with the cricoid cartilage.

The arytenoid cartilages sit on the cricoid lamina protected by the thyroid laminae. The vocal cords arise from the anterior vocal processes of the arytenoid cartilage, meet anteriorly at the anterior commissure and are controlled by the intrinsic muscles of the larynx—cricoarytenoid abductors and thyroarytenoid adductors.

The epiglottis is attached inferiorly to the larynx at the petiole and to the hyoid by the hyoepiglottic ligament. It folds posteriorly over the laryngeal vestibule during swallowing, preventing aspiration.

The superior laryngeal nerve—a branch of the vagus—conveys sensation and cricothyroid motor function. All other functions are conveyed by the recurrent laryngeal nerve, also a branch of the vagus.

The larynx is divided into supraglottis, glottis and subglottis. The supraglottis extends from the epiglottic tip inferiorly to include the laryngeal ventricle and has a rich lymphatic drainage to the upper and mid deep cervical nodes. The glottis includes the true vocal cords. The subglottis extends from the undersurface of the true cords to the inferior cricoid cartilage. The glottis and subglottis have a poorer lymphatic drainage and drain to prelaryngeal, lower deep cervical and paratracheal nodes.

Radiology and Pathology

Laryngeal Malignancy. Nearly all laryngeal malignancy (98%) is SCC; other rarer tumours such as chondrosarcoma (Fig. 8-52) and adenoid cystic carcinoma will be discussed briefly. CT and MR are both useful for assessing the larynx. CT should be performed in quiet breathing with reconstructed images parallel to the true cords.

Laryngeal SCC. The role of the radiologist is to accurately stage both the primary tumour and nodal disease. Sixty per cent are glottic and usually present early due to the effect on the voice. Nodal involvement of SCC localised to the glottis is rare. Thirty per cent arise in the supraglottis and are often diagnosed late. In addition, because of the rich lymphatic network, approximately 50% of supraglottic tumours have nodal involvement at presentation. True subglottic tumours are rare. The subglottis is usually involved by inferior extension from the glottis. Transglottic tumours are so-called when tumour involves all three divisions of the larynx.

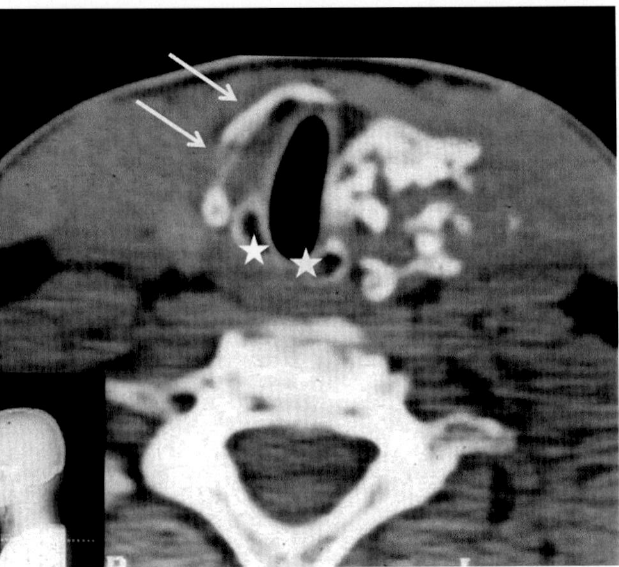

FIGURE 8-52 ■ **Axial unenhanced CT of larynx.** Note the classical coarse (popcorn) calcification of the chondrosarcoma arising from the left thyroid lamina. White arrows = right thyroid lamina, stars = cricoid cartilage.

Critical observations to make are the following:

- Does the tumour involve the anterior commissure?
- At the anterior commissure soft tissue only < 1 mm should be visible.
- Does tumour cross the midline?
- Is there subglottic extension?
- There should be no soft tissue visible within the cricoid ring.
- Is there supraglottic extension?
- In particular, is there involvement of the tongue base?
- Is there cartilage invasion?
- MRI is more sensitive than CT in difficult cases.

Chondrosarcoma. These are rare slow-growing tumours arising from laryngeal cartilage (usually cricoid); they show characteristic coarse calcification and are treated with local resection (Fig. 8-52).

Adenoid Cystic Carcinoma. These classically arise in the minor salivary glands of the subglottis and should be considered in the differential of a subglottic mass.

Laryngocoele. A laryngocoele is a dilatation of the laryngeal saccule that arises from the laryngeal ventricle and may be acquired or congenital. The laryngeal ventricle is a lateral out-pouching between the false and true cords. An internal laryngocoele is confined within the larynx and is visible as a smooth submucosal supraglottic swelling; an external laryngocoele extends through the thyrohyoid membrane at the site of the superior laryngeal vessels and may be visible as a neck swelling. The laryngocoele is usually air-filled but an air–fluid level or a completely fluid-filled structure may be present if the neck is obstructed (Fig. 8-53). It is important to exclude an obstructing SCC within the laryngeal ventricle.

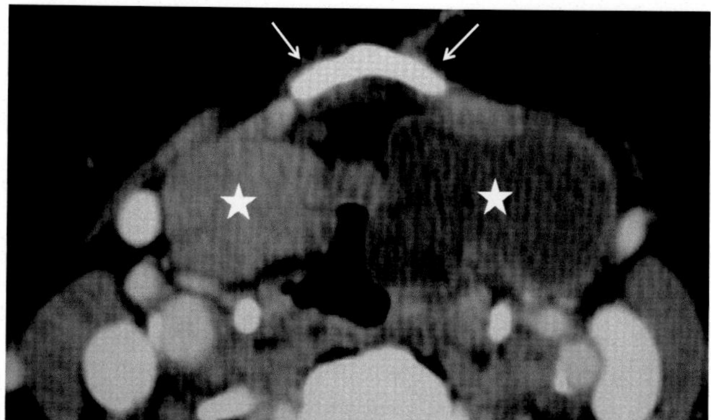

FIGURE 8-53 ■ **Axial CT post IV contrast at level of hyoid bone (white arrows).** Note the bilateral fluid-filled external laryngocoeles (white stars). The higher density of the right laryngocoele is due to its denser contents.

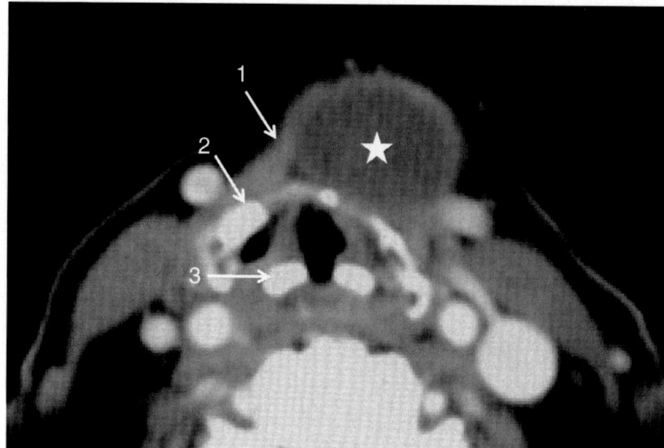

FIGURE 8-55 ■ **Axial CT post IV contrast.** Star = paramedian thyroglossal cyst centred anterior to the laminae of the thyroid cartilage (2) and elevating the sternohyoid muscle (1). 3 = arytenoid cartilage.

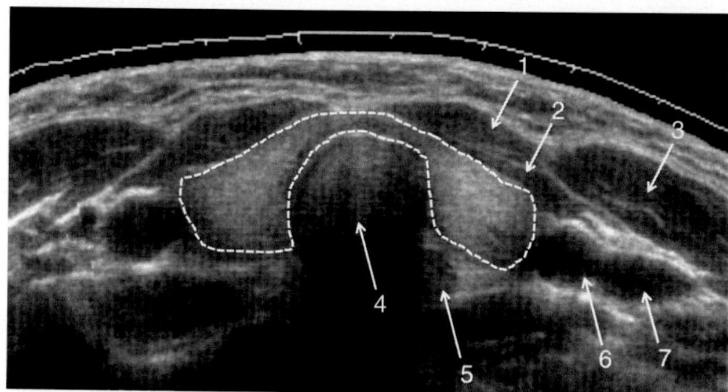

FIGURE 8-54 ■ **Panoramic transverse ultrasound image through the thyroid gland (interrupted white line).** 1 = sternohyoid muscle, 2 = sternothyroid muscle, 3 = sternocleidomastoid muscle, 4 = trachea, 5 = cervical oesophagus, 6 = CCA, 7 = IJV.

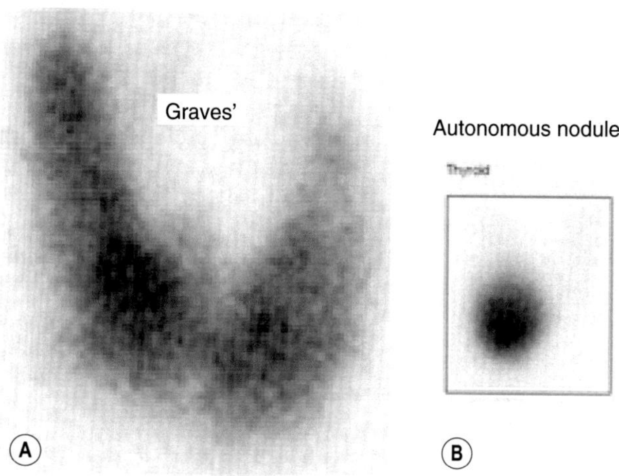

FIGURE 8-56 ■ **^{99m}Tc-pertechnetate image.** Note the diffuse increased uptake in a patient with Graves' disease (A) and the second image (B) showing an autonomous (hot) nodule.

Thyroid and Parathyroid

Anatomy. The thyroid gland is also located within the visceral space (VS) of the infrahyoid neck and consists of two lobes on either side of the proximal cervical trachea connected by an isthmus (Fig. 8-54). The thyroid gland descends during development from the foramen caecum in the midline of the tongue base. Rarely there is arrested descent, resulting in a lingual thyroid, but more commonly a pyramidal lobe persists, best demonstrated on ultrasound as a tongue of thyroid tissue extending superiorly from the isthmus sometimes as far as the hyoid bone. Occasionally a remnant remains that presents as a midline or paramedian anterior neck swelling in the thyrohyoid region usually following a cold: a thyroglossal cyst (Fig. 8-55).

There are usually four, but occasionally up to six parathyroid glands located along the thymopharyngeal tract that extends from the level of the carotid bifurcation to the lower anterior mediastinum. They are most frequently located posterior to or just inferior to the mid-to-inferior aspect of the lobes of the thyroid.

Radiology

Ultrasound. Ultrasound is the primary imaging technique for both the thyroid and parathyroid because of the superficial location of these glands and provides the highest resolution of any technique. Ultrasound also can be combined with FNAC if required.

Nuclear Medicine. Diagnostic isotope studies (usually ^{99m}Tc-pertechnetate and iodine-123) are used less frequently in thyroid imaging as anti-thyroid autoantibodies such as anti-thyroperoxidase (TPO) antibody (a non-specific test for thyroiditis) and a more specific TSH receptor antibody for Graves' disease have largely replaced their use. They are still used sometimes in two clinical scenarios: to assess for an autonomous nodule in patients with a nodular thyroid and suppressed TSH (Fig. 8-56), and in suspected thyroiditis where the blood tests have proven unhelpful. Therapeutic I-131 treatment of Graves' disease is still widely used. ^{99m}Tc-sestamibi, usually in combination with ultrasound, is used for assessing patients with primary hyperparathyroidism.

MRI and CT. Cross-sectional imaging with CT and MRI is used to assess the degree of retrosternal extension and tracheal compression in multinodular goitre or invasion of adjacent structures in thyroid malignancy. CT with intravenous contrast must not be used if a papillary carcinoma is suspected as the use of iodinated contrast will preclude radioiodine treatment for approximately 2 months.

Thyroid Pathology

Thyroiditis. Hashimoto's thyroiditis (chronic lymphocytic) is the commonest. In the early stage on ultrasound the thyroid has a heterogeneous, hypoechoic echotexture in a slightly enlarged lobulated gland. At a later stage the gland commonly decreases in size and develops echogenic linear fibrotic septae, but remains heterogeneous (Fig. 8-57). In Graves' disease patients present with a diffusely enlarged hypoechoic thyroid demonstrating markedly increased colour flow called a thyroid inferno (Fig. 8-58).

Thyroid Malignancy. A detailed description is beyond the scope of this chapter. The vast majority (90%) are differentiated carcinomas, including papillary 70–80% (Fig. 8-59) and follicular 10–20%. Medullary carcinoma compromising 5–10% of thyroid malignancy may be associated with multiple endocrine neoplasia (MEN 2A and B). Anaplastic carcinoma (1–2%) has an extremely poor prognosis and presents in the elderly as a rapidly growing mass invading adjacent structures (Fig. 8-60). Primary thyroid lymphoma (NHL) is rare but has a 70–80× increased risk in patients with thyroiditis.

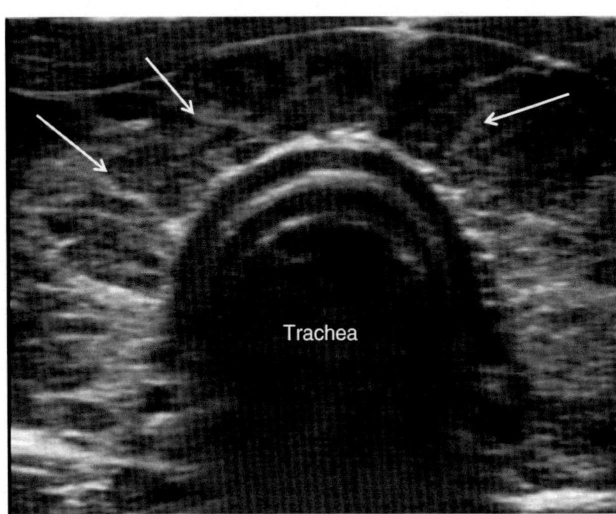

FIGURE 8-57 ■ Transverse US of thyroid. Note the diffusely heterogeneous hypoechoic (dark) thyroid containing hyperechoic lines (white arrows) in chronic thyroiditis and compare with Fig. 8-54.

Parathyroid Pathology. The most commonly clinical scenario is primary hyperparathyroidism usually investigated with a combination of ultrasound and ^{99m}Tc-sestamibi. The most frequent cause is a solitary parathyroid adenoma (80%), but parathyroid

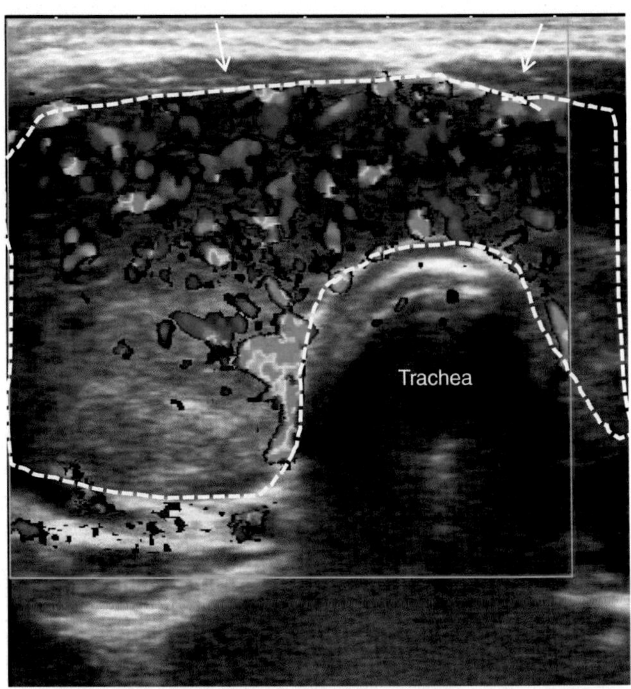

FIGURE 8-58 ■ Transverse US of thyroid. Note the swollen hypoechoic (dark) and hypervascular thyroid in Graves' disease. The appearance is called a thyroid inferno.

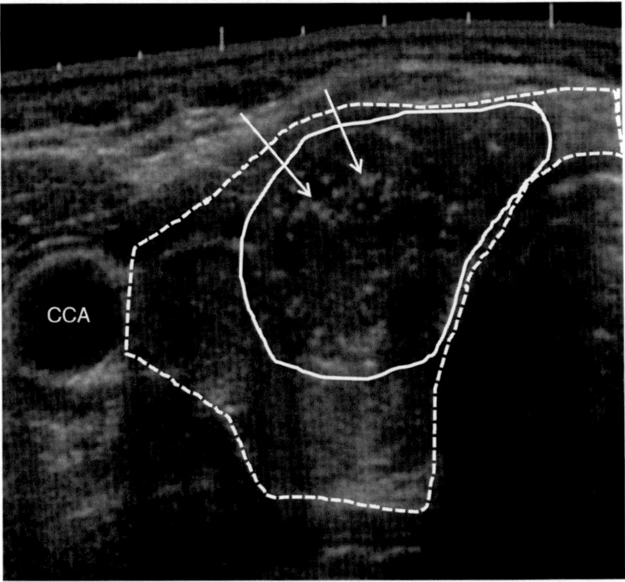

FIGURE 8-59 ■ Transverse US of right thyroid. The papillary tumour (continous white line) located within the medial right lobe of the thyroid is hypoechoic (dark) and contains characteristic echogenic foci (white arrows). Interupted white line = outline of right lobe and isthmus of the thyroid. CCA = Common carotid artery.

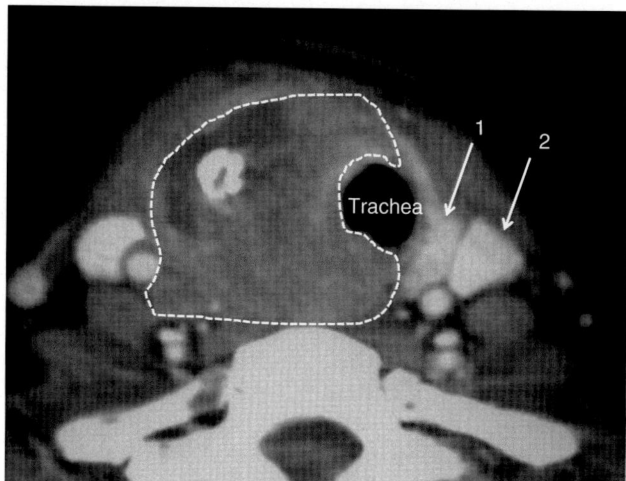

FIGURE 8-60 ■ Axial CT of thyroid post IV contrast. The ill-defined anaplastic tumour (interrupted white line) has replaced the whole right lobe and isthmus of the thyroid invading the overlying strap muscles and oesophagus. 1 = left lobe thyroid, 2 = IJV.

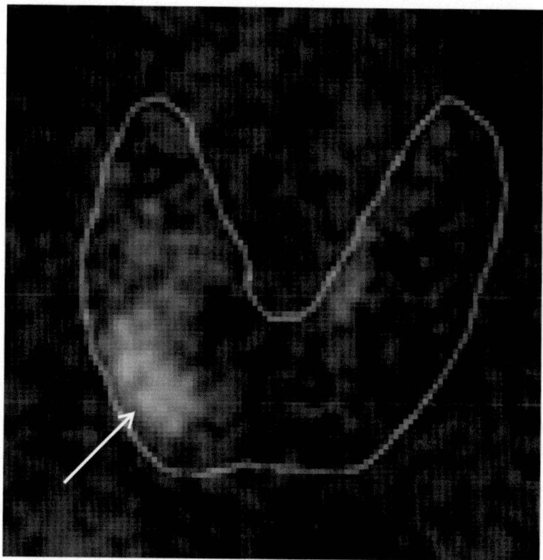

FIGURE 8-61 ■ ^{99m}Tc-sestamibi image showing focal uptake on delayed images in keeping with overactive parathyroid gland posterior to right lower pole of the thyroid.

hyperplasia is seen in 10–15%, multiple adenomas in 2–3% (Fig. 8-61) and parathyroid malignancy in approximately 1%.

The typical finding on ultrasound is a well-defined hypoechoic mass posterior or inferior to the thyroid (Fig. 8-62). Sestamibi will usually identify those adenomas not visible on ultrasound, i.e. located in the superior mediastinum or posterior to the trachea. CT, MRI and venous sampling is used in complex cases.

Recurrent Laryngeal Nerve. The course of the recurrent laryngeal nerve requires imaging when patients present with vocal cord palsy. Imaging must extend superiorly to include the medulla. On the left side the recurrent laryngeal nerve extends into the mediastinum, passing under the aortic arch, whereas on the right the recurrent laryngeal nerve remains within the neck passing under the right subclavian artery and only the neck, requires imaging.

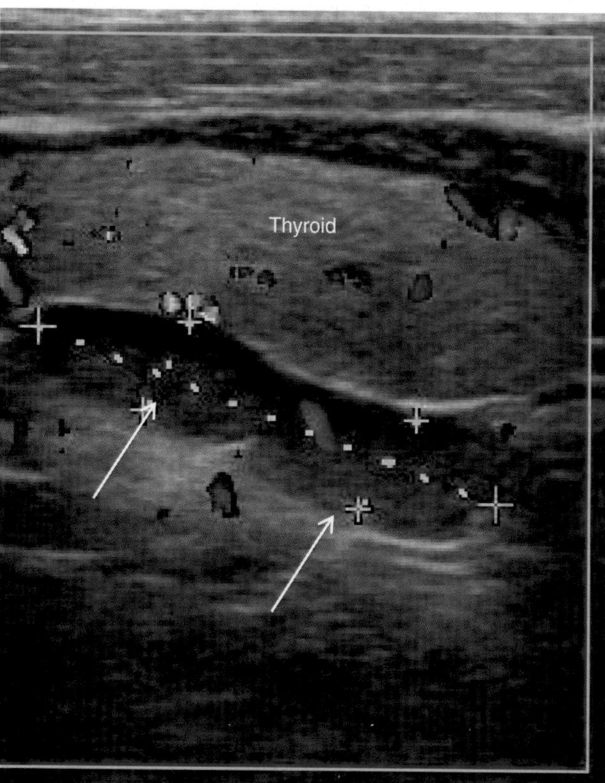

FIGURE 8-62 ■ Longitudinal US of thyroid/parathyroid. Note the two adjacent enlarged hypoechoic (dark) parathyroid glands (white arrows) posterior to the thyroid.

Cervical Lymph Nodes

Generalised lymphadenopathy is a common clinical presentation. If widespread and painful, glandular fever or other viral infections can be considered. If focal and painful, a bacterial lymphadenitis may be the aetiology. If painless spread from a head and neck malignancy, lymphoma or atypical bacterial infection may be the cause.

Radiology and Pathology. In the context of a head and neck malignancy pathological nodes are described as belonging to one of seven levels: Level 1 (a and b) submental and submandibular, 2 (a and b) upper, 3 middle and 4 lower deep cervical, 5 posterior triangle, 6 anterior cervical and 7 superior mediastinal (Fig. 8-63). These levels, however, do not include the retropharyngeal, intraparotid and facial lymph nodal groups.

Accurate nodal staging in head and neck SCC is vital for appropriate treatment and prognosis. The diagnosis

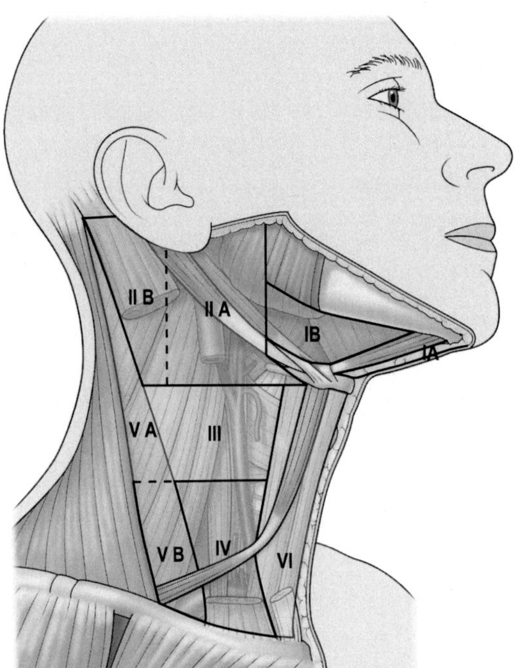

FIGURE 8-63 ■ Drawing of the right side of the neck with the sternocleidomastoid muscle and right submandibular salivary gland removed and the IJV tied off, demonstrating the nodal levels (1–6). Level 7 (superior mediastinum) has not been covered.

of an involved ipsilateral node, a contralateral node and extracapsular spread each decrease the long-term survival by 50%.

Ultrasound is the technique of choice for assessing a patient with a neck lump suspected to be secondary to lymphadenopathy and can be combined with FNAC or Tru-Cut biopsy. Often the ultrasound is performed on the same initial visit to the ENT clinic as a 'one-stop' procedure.

There are a number of imaging criteria for assessing whether a lymph node is pathological. These cannot be covered in detail in this chapter but the most important are size, shape, echotexture (on ultrasound), evidence of cystic change and abnormal or absent colour flow (ultrasound). A non-pathological lymph node should have a short axis of <1 cm and a long:short axis ratio of >2, i.e. a rugby ball rather than a round (football) shape. A darker or hypoechoic appearance on ultrasound is concerning.

DENTAL AND MAXILLOFACIAL

DISORDERS OF BONE

Developmental Disorders

Fibro-Osseous Lesions

This is a spectrum where normal bone is replaced in a benign process, extending from the purely fibrotic lesion at one end to a dysplastic bony lesion at the other. They include the ossifying fibroma, a well-defined expansile mass with a fibrous central area surrounded by a calcified rim, fibrous dysplasia and the osseous dysplasias.

Fibrous dysplasia is a localised expansile lesion in which cancellous bone is replaced initially by radiolucent fibrous tissue which matures with varying amounts of calcified tissue to a mixed-density lesion or as a radiopacity, typically with orange peel or ground-glass texture (Figs. 8-64 and 8-65). The maxilla is involved twice as frequently as the mandible. The margins blend with adjacent bone. It may displace teeth or prevent their eruption, and large lesions may cause considerable facial deformity. Seventy per cent of lesions are monostotic. Radiographically, it can resemble an ossifying fibroma, which is better defined and encapsulated, chronic sclerosing osteomyelitis and an osteosarcoma, which has ill-defined and destructive margins.

Periapical osseous dysplasia and florid osseous dysplasia are similar conditions, with the latter being the more extravagant and larger version. They mainly occur in women, particularly of Afro-Caribbean and Asian origin, after 25 years of age. Both conditions are characterised by the formation of multiple deposits around vital tooth roots, usually in the mandible. In periapical osseous dysplasia, radiolucent lesions forming at the apices of clinically sound teeth resemble periapical granulomas. Gradually, cemental-like tissue is deposited within it, becoming increasingly radiopaque and when mature is almost totally radiopaque except for a thin, peripheral radiolucent zone, which helps distinguish it from sclerosing osteitis.

Cherubism is a rare dysplasia of bone that develops during the first decade of life. It occurs bilaterally in both jaws, but more commonly affects just the mandible. It develops in the posterior aspects of the jaws as a multilocular, honeycombed, expansile radiolucency. Tooth displacement is common. It regresses spontaneously after skeletal growth ceases.

Inflammatory Disorders

Osteomyelitis of the jaws is uncommon, which is surprising considering the frequency of dental sepsis. It may

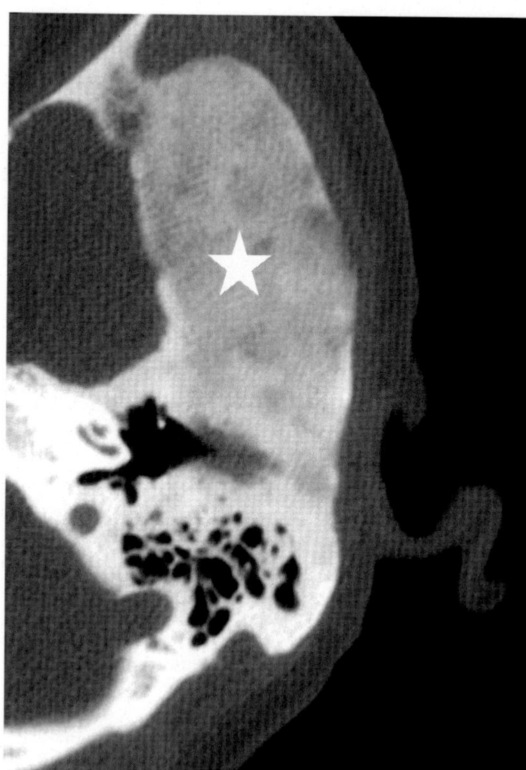

FIGURE 8-64 ■ Axial CT of left petrous temporal bone. Note markedly expanded squamous component of the temporal bone that has a ground-glass appearance in keeping with fibrous dysplasia (star).

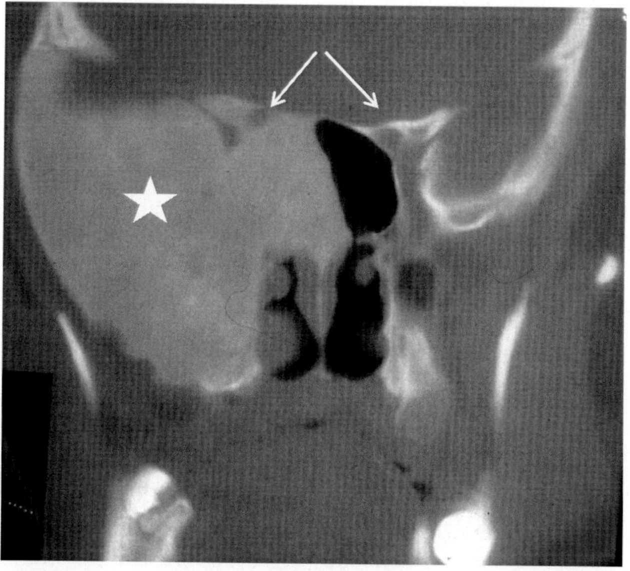

FIGURE 8-65 ■ Coronal CT through the sphenoid bone. The right side of the sphenoid is markedly expanded, with involvement of the body, greater and lesser wings, pterygoid plates, anterior clinoid process and the squamous component of the right petrous temporal bone (star). Note the close relation of the optic nerves (white arrows).

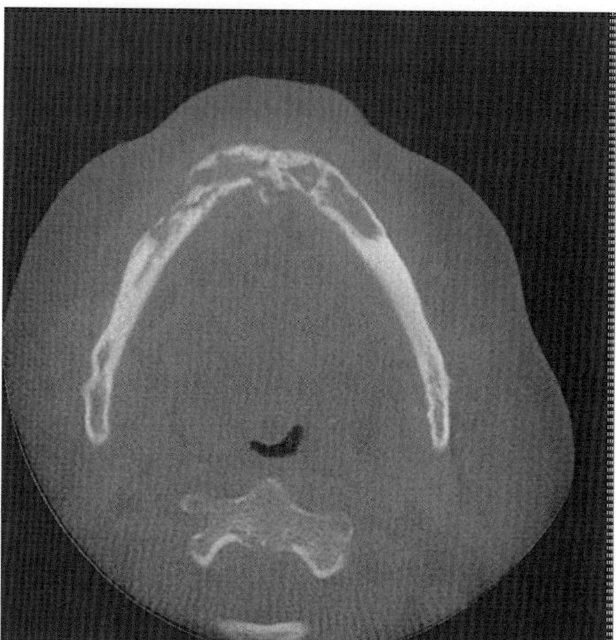

FIGURE 8-66 ■ Axial CBCT of mandible showing acute osteomyelitis of the anterior part of the mandible. The bone shows several dense bony sequestrae and lytic areas with destruction and perforation of the buccal and lingual cortical plates.

develop from a dental abscess, tooth extraction or jaw fracture. In acute osteomyelitis, there is thinning and discontinuity of the bony trabeculae to produce ill-defined, patchy areas of radiolucency. With time, bony sequestrae form and are recognised as irregularly shaped islands of bone set against a region of radiolucency (Fig. 8-66). The features of osteomyelitis are best visualised on CT or CBCT, which may also show periosteal bone formation. On MRI, the marrow usually shows a low signal intensity on T1 and high signal on T2-weighted images. If the disease becomes chronic, the bone becomes diffusely affected and extensively involved with sclerosis of the marrow spaces. CT or CBCT will demonstrate the internal structure and the presence of sequestration.

Diffuse sclerosing osteomyelitis is more common than acute osteomyelitis, from which it may develop. The bone becomes increasingly dense and radiopaque as a result of a proliferative response to low-grade infection. Bone deposition results in reduction in the size of the marrow spaces with gradual spread through the mandible; however, lytic areas are also seen. MRI shows a thickened cortex.

Bisphosphonate-Related Osteonecrosis of the Jaws (BRONJ)

This relative new condition can follow dental extraction or jaw infection of patients taking bisphophonates for osteoporosis or in the management of malignant tumours affecting the bone. Orally prescribed bisphosphonates result in a low incidence (1 in 10,000–50,000) of BRONJ, but when administered intravenously the incidence is much higher, being approximately 1 to 10%. Areas of

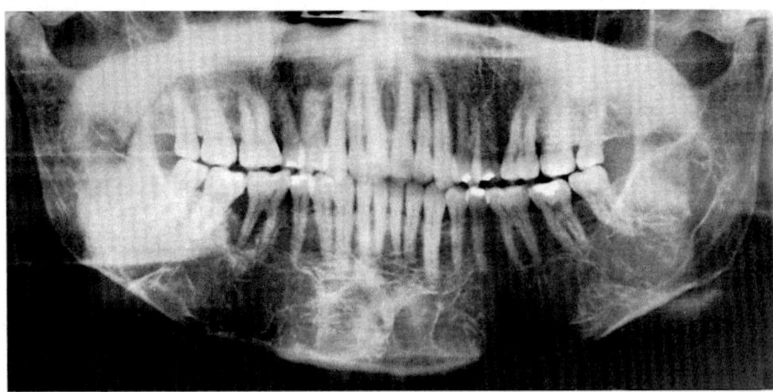

FIGURE 8-67 ■ **Panoramic radiograph of a case of thalassaemia.** There is marked increase in the height of the mandible, which is composed of coarse trabeculae enclosing large marrow spaces and the small maxillary sinuses. Note the generalised loss of the lamina dura and the periodontal abscess on the distal root of the lower right first molar.

necrotic bone develop and become exposed to the oral environment, leading to persistent chronic inflammation of the jaws. The radiographic features are of both acute and chronic osteomyelitis.

Osteoradionecrosis is an inflammatory condition that can affect the mandible if included in the radiation field after a dose of 45–50 Gy. It is a clinical diagnosis and presents as areas of exposed necrotic bone. The radiographic features resemble those of chronic osteomyelitis.

Metabolic, Endocrine and Haematological Disorders of Bone

Osteoporosis affects the jaws as elsewhere in the skeleton. The mandible becomes osteopenic, as the marrow spaces enlarge and the trabeculae thin. The cortical outline of the inferior alveolar canal becomes inconspicuous and the lower border of the mandible becomes thinner than normal, with endosseous radiolucencies.

The classical appearance of **hyperparathyroidism** is now seen less frequently because of improved diagnosis and management. However, when it affects the jaws it results in a general demineralisation of the bone, creating a ground-glass appearance, loss of the lamina dura and subperiosteal erosions at the angle. Brown tumours develop in the facial bones in approximately 15% of cases, particularly in long-standing cases and appear radiolucent and loculated, with margins that may be ill-defined or cystic.

Haematological replacement disorders may affect the jaws, the radiological manifestations depending on the severity of the condition. In moderate-to-severe thalassaemia, the jaws become radiolucent with coarse trabeculations due to marrow hyperplasia and the maxillary antrum is reduced in size (Fig. 8-8). The skull takes on a granular appearance, with thickening of the diploic spaces and occasionally a 'hair-on-end' appearance.

In sickle cell disease similar manifestations to thalassaemia are apparent; however, several sclerotic areas are seen as a consequence of dystrophic mineralisation of small thrombi.

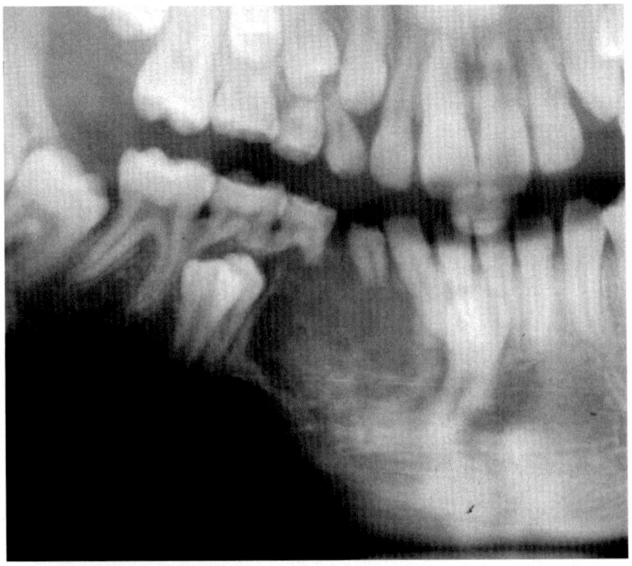

FIGURE 8-68 ■ Part of a panoramic radiograph of a **central giant-cell granuloma** of the right side of the mandible, which appears as a well-defined radiolucency containing numerous coarse bony trabeculae. There has been displacement of the premolar teeth posteriorly and the canine anteriorly.

Paget's disease of bone, a once frequently encountered disorder, is now rarely seen in the jaws, but when present affects a whole bone of the face or skull. The radiographic appearance depends on its stage of development, progressing from an initial radiolucent stage to a more granular or ground-glass appearance with loss of lamina dura. Bony trabeculae become coarse and arranged in a horizontal linear pattern and finally the bone becomes distorted and patchily radiopaque with focal collections of dense bone creating a 'cotton wool' appearance. Hypercementosis is a notable dental feature and skull changes are described as 'osteoporosis circumscripta', typically starting in the frontal bone.

Central giant cell granuloma is probably a reactive lesion and not neoplastic. It is most often detected during the first three decades of life, with twice as many being discovered in the mandible as the maxilla. The lesion is usually multilocular, is often well defined and lacks cortication, but some have ill-defined borders suggestive of a destructive lesion. Although largely radiolucent, the internal appearance varies from being almost devoid of any internal structures to those containing wispy septae (Fig. 8-68).

TUMOURS OF BONE

Ossifying fibroma is a tumour of bone but it can also be considered as a fibro-cemento-osseous lesion. Its behaviour varies from those showing slow growth to others being quite aggressive. It occurs mainly in young adults, mostly in the body of the mandible. The radiographic appearance depends on its degree of mineralisation, and typically contains a wispy or tufted bony trabecular pattern (Fig. 8-69). The lesion is encapsulated and so

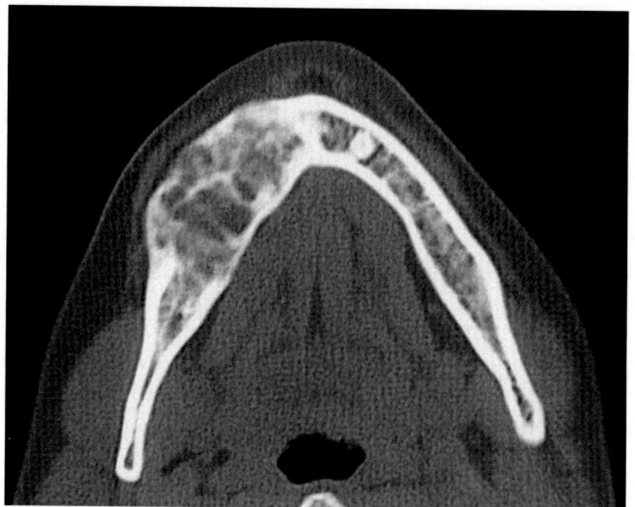

FIGURE 8-69 ■ Bone window setting of an axial CT of a **ossifying fibroma** of the mandible showing mainly buccal expansion and thinning of both cortical plates, which remain intact. The lesion is of mixed attenuation as it contains areas of fibrosis, mineralisation and coarse bony trabeculations.

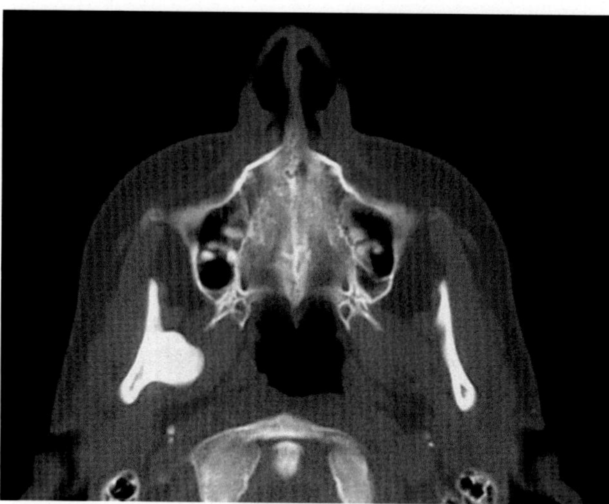

FIGURE 8-70 ■ Bone window setting of an axial CT showing a dense (compact) osteoma arising from the medial aspect of the ramus of the right mandible.

appears well defined, helping to distinguish it from fibrous dysplasia.

Osteomas of the maxillofacial bones and jaws are usually slow-growing, painless and thus discovered by chance. However, a large osteoma in the frontal sinuses may obstruct the drainage pathway and cause secondary infection. In the jaws, osteomas more commonly affect the mandible than the maxilla and, although any site can be involved, they tend to be found posteriorly on its medial aspect (Fig. 8-70). CT shows the site of origin and provides three-dimensional (3D) topographic detail. Multiple osteomas are a feature of Gardner's syndrome (familial adenomatous polyposis) and precede the formation of intestinal colonic polyposis.

Osteosarcoma is uncommon in the jaws, accounting for only 7% of all osteosarcomas. Although it can occur in early life, it most commonly presents in the jaws around 30 years of age, over 10 years later than osteosarcoma of the long bones. The mandible is more frequently affected than the maxilla. Maxillary lesions tend to arise from the alveolar ridge, and mandibular ones in the body. It has a destructive appearance and its density varies from being radiolucent, to patchily radiopaque or predominantly sclerotic. An important early dental radiographic sign is widening of the periodontal ligament space due to tumour spread along the periodontal ligament; however, this feature is also seen in other sarcomas (e.g. fibrosarcoma Ewing's sarcoma) and in a similar manner may also widen the inferior alveolar canal. Occasionally when the periosteum is elevated, a hair-on-end, sunray or onion skin appearance may be visible. CT is required to demonstrate accurately tumour calcification, bone destruction and bone reaction (Fig. 8-71), whereas MRI (T1- and T2-weighted images) will provide better information on the intramedullary and extraosseous components of the tumour.[1]

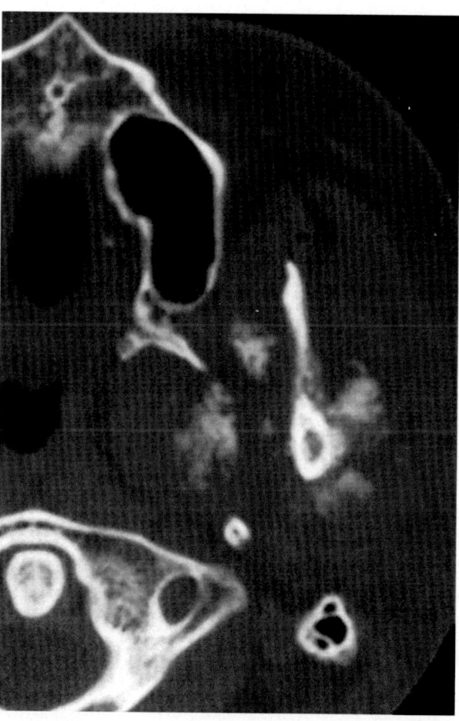

FIGURE 8-71 ■ **Bone window setting of an axial CT of osteogenic sarcoma of the left mandibular ramus.** There is bone destruction in the region of the sigmoid notch. The lesion contains areas of neoplastic bone formation and extends medially towards the lateral pterygoid plate, posteriorly to the styloid process and laterally resulting in facial swelling. (Courtesy of Mr S. Dover, Birmingham.)

Primary carcinoma of the overlying oral mucosa can invade the jaws to produce an ill-defined (but sometimes well-defined), non-corticated saucerised area of bone destruction (Fig. 8-72). Bone loss around the tooth roots may give an appearance of teeth floating in space, also

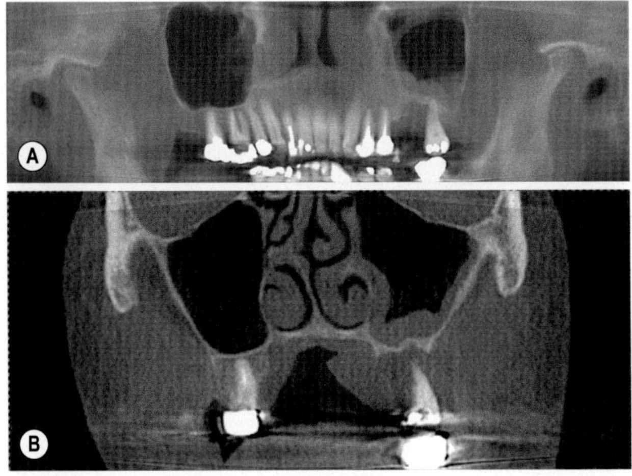

FIGURE 8-72 ■ (A) Panoramic style MPR from a CBCT and (B) coronal slice through posterior maxilla showing a primary SCC of the left maxillary palatal gingivae in the molar region in a patient presenting with a palatal swelling. It has caused alveolar bone destruction, although the antral floor remained intact. There is soft-tissue swelling in the base of the left antrum which was found to be inflammatory.

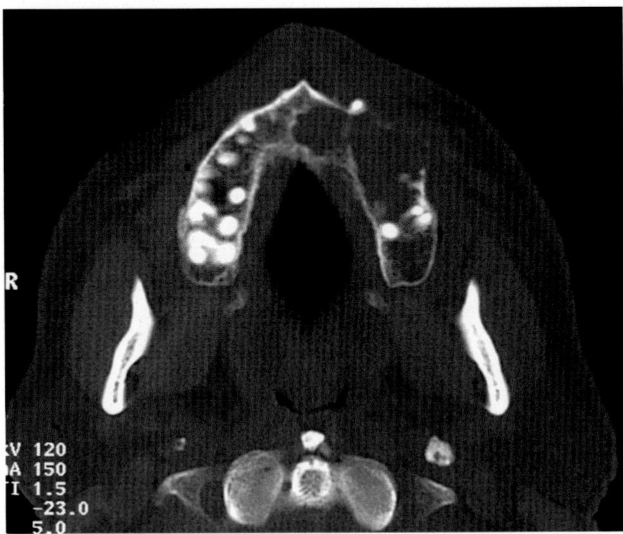

FIGURE 8-73 ■ **Extranodal lymphoma** of the maxilla shown on a bone window setting axial CT at the level of the alveolus. Although a few areas of the lesion are well defined, the overall appearance is destructive, with loss of much of the buccal alveolar plate.

seen in Langerhans' histiocytosis. Very rarely, carcinoma may arise from malignant transformation of a cyst lining or epithelial residues within the jaw bone to produce an ill-defined osteolytic lesion. It affects older patients usually in the sixth or seventh decade of life.

Metastatic tumour involvement of the jaws is uncommon, mainly arising from breast, kidney, lung, colon and prostate. They form predominantly in the posterior aspects of the mandible, resulting in loss of the outline of the inferior alveolar canal and destruction of the cortical plates. Typically their outline is moderately to poorly defined, with irregular margins that appear destructive without new bone formation. Some metastatic deposits are characterised by the development of several areas, often small, of bone destruction. Although most lesions that metastasise to the jaws are lytic, others, notably from the prostate, can produce bone and appear diffusely radiopaque.

Extranodal lymphoma may affect the head and neck, with the sinonasal area being a common site. When it affects the jaws it can mimic other diseases. It generally appears as an ill-defined non-corticated radiolucency with destruction of cortical bony outlines (Fig. 8-73). **Langerhans' cell histiocytosis**, including eosinophilic granuloma, are occasionally found in the jaws, where they may mimic dental periapical or periodontal disease. The margins are usually well-defined but lack cortication. **Multiple myeloma** is a disseminated disease particularly affecting males over the age of 60 years. About 30% of patients with multiple myeloma may have jaw lesions, with the posterior body and angle region of the mandible being the most frequent site. The typical radiographic feature is of a well-defined radiolucency that lacks a cortical margin and so appears punched out, but some have ragged margins. It usually appears destructive on CT or CBCT.

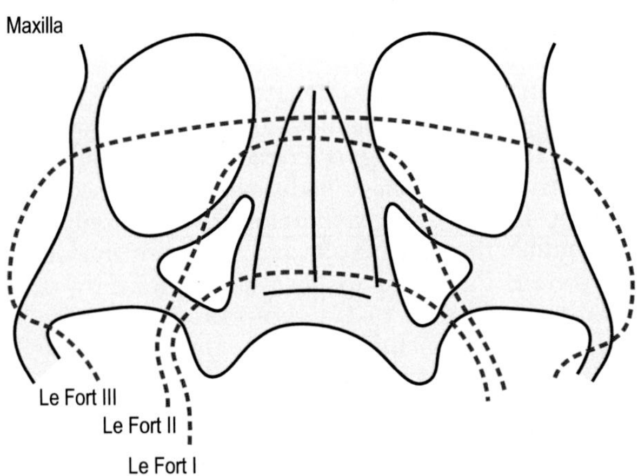

FIGURE 8-74 ■ **Fracture lines in Le Fort I, II, and III fractures.**

FRACTURES OF THE FACIAL SKELETON

The facial skeleton is a complex arrangement of bones, air cavities and soft tissues attached to the skull base. Fractures involving the facial bones are still classified according to the system described by Le Fort in 1900, who defined three principal types of fractures after applying blunt trauma to the faces of cadavers. The classification is contentious because fractures do not always follow the exact pattern he described (Fig. 8-74). Plain films form the initial assessment, but many of these injuries are complicated and require evaluation with axial and coronal CT or cone beam CT.

In **Le Fort I fracture** (Fig. 8-75), the tooth-bearing part of the maxilla is separated from the rest of the maxilla by trauma to the lower part of the face. The fracture line runs from the piriform fossa posteriorly to the pterygoid

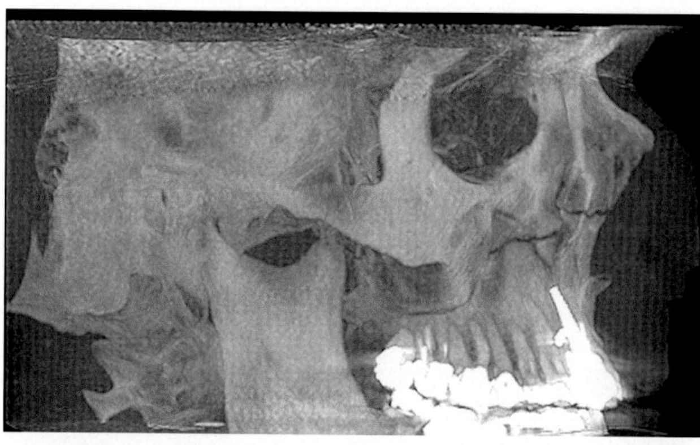

FIGURE 8-75 ■ **Le Fort I fracture.** CBCT ray-sum image of the right side showing an undisplaced fracture running from just above the piriform fossa, below the root of the zygoma to the pterygoid plate. A similar fracture was present on the left side.

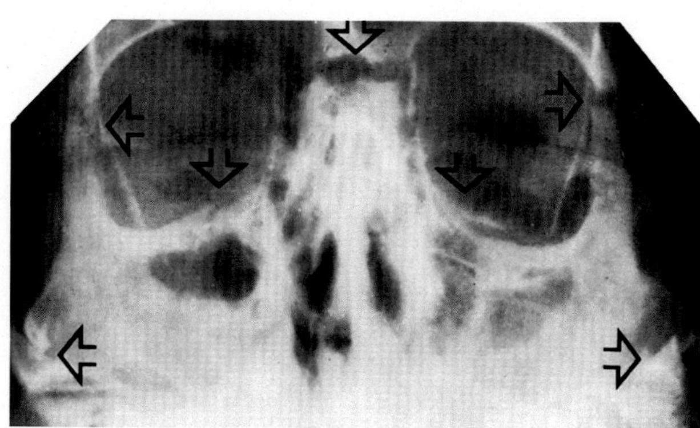

FIGURE 8-77 ■ **Combined Le Fort II and III fractures.** There are fractures of the nasal bones, lateral orbital margins, inferior orbital margins and zygomatic arches. All have been marked with arrows. There is a fluid level in the right maxillary sinus and opacification of the left maxillary sinus.

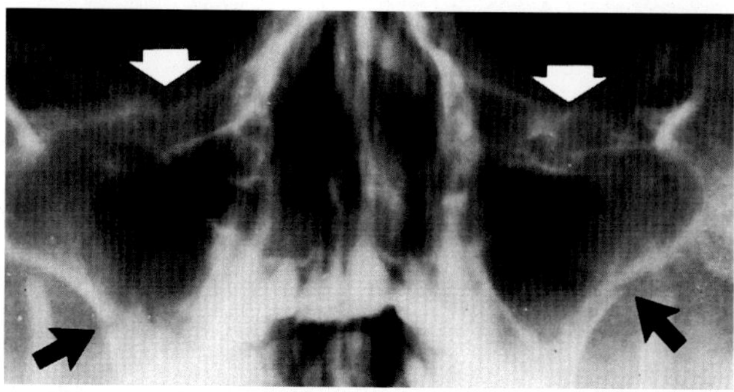

FIGURE 8-76 ■ **Le Fort II fracture.** The fractures of the inferior margins of the orbits and of the lateral walls of the maxillary sinuses have been arrowed. The fracture of the nasal bone is not visible on this projection.

plates, resulting in detachment of the dentoalveolar fragment from the remaining maxilla. The posterior portion may drop, resulting in an open bite, and this is a useful diagnostic feature, as the Le Fort I fracture can often be difficult to detect on radiographs.

Le Fort II fracture (Fig. 8-76) runs along the nasal bridge, through the lacrimal bones, across the medial orbital walls and orbital rims, to involve the anterior and posterolateral wall of the maxillary sinuses and pterygoid plates, where there may be a step deformity. The nasal septum is fractured at a variable level.

In **Le Fort III or suprazygomatic fracture** (Fig. 8-77), there is complete separation of the midface from the cranial base, resulting in clinical lengthening of the face. The fracture line runs through the nasal bones, the frontal processes of the maxilla, posterolaterally through the medial and lateral orbital walls, and through the zygomatic arches. The nasal septum is fractured superiorly.

In practice, many fractures do not exactly fit these descriptions. Fractures caused by sharp-edged objects can produce comminuted fractures of the maxilla (Fig. 8-78) without affecting the tooth-bearing alveolar bone, and some fractures are not symmetrical. For instance, Le Fort I, II and III fractures may be unilateral (Fig. 8-79), or a Le Fort I or II may coexist with a Le Fort III (Fig. 8-77). Nevertheless, the Le Fort classification is still widely used as it allows these complicated fractures to be described simply.

Fractures of the Zygomatic Complex

The zygomatic bone contributes to the lateral and inferior margins of the orbit, the lateral wall of the maxillary sinus and the anterior end of the zygomatic arch (Fig. 8-80) usually with fractures in the region of the zygomatico-frontal suture, zygomatico-temporal suture, infraorbital rim and the lateral wall of the antrum. As not all of the fractures are always visible on a single film, the presence of even one fracture should raise the suspicion that other fractures are present and, dependent upon clinical findings, further imaging may be required. CT is helpful in assessing comminuted fractures of the zygomatic complex as a result of severe trauma (Fig. 8-81). The zygomatic arch may be fractured in association with a fracture of the zygoma as described earlier, or it may be fractured alone as a result of direct trauma to the side of the head and is seen as three points of fracture (Fig. 8-81).

Orbital Blow-Out Fractures

Blunt trauma to the front of the orbit causing a blow-out leads to enophthalmos and possibly diplopia due to muscle entrapment, e.g. inferior rectus. The inward displacement of the eyeball temporarily increases orbital pressure, resulting in outward fracture of the thin bone of the orbital floor or medial wall (lamina papyracea of the ethmoid), but leaving the orbital rim intact. The orbital soft tissues herniate through the defect into the maxillary sinus. This shows as soft-tissue opacity in the upper aspect of the sinus on an occipitomental radiograph and sometimes a fluid level when blood is present. CT is helpful in defining the extent of the defect of the orbital floor and involvement of the external ocular muscles in the fracture (Fig. 8-82 and Fig. 8-83). Coronal and sagittal reformats are helpful. Orbital

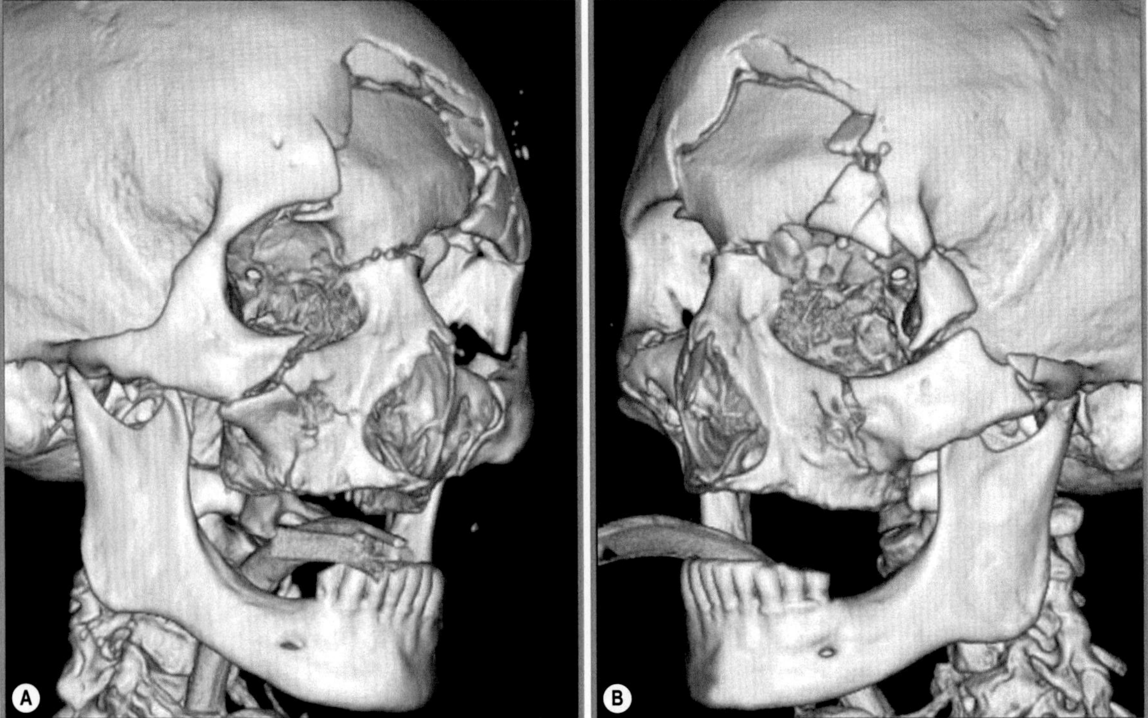

FIGURE 8-78 ■ Three-dimensional CT images showing multiple fractures of the facial bones (Le Fort II and unilateral Le Fort III) and depressed fracture of frontal ethmoidal complex. Note the asymmetrical pattern of the fractures, with the more severe injury involving the left side.

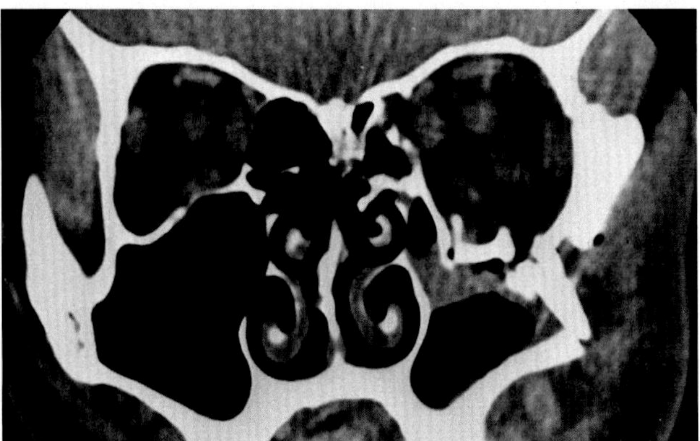

FIGURE 8-79 ■ Coronal CT of a unilateral left-sided Le Fort II fracture. There are fractures of the medial wall of the orbit, the floor and inferior rim of the orbit, and the anterior wall of the maxillary sinus.

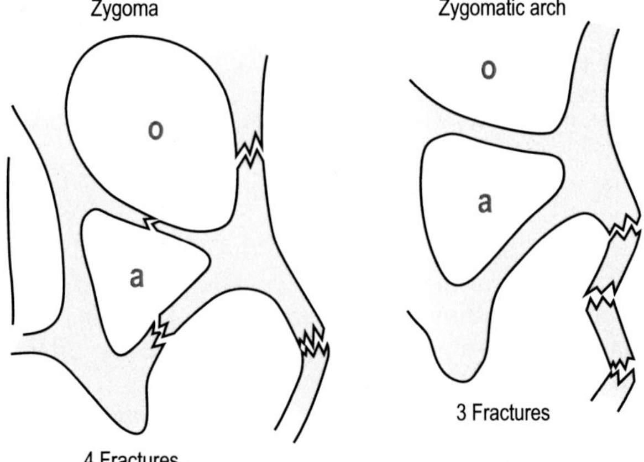

FIGURE 8-80 ■ Diagram of the usual sites of fracture of the zygoma and of the zygomatic arch. o = orbit, a = antrum.

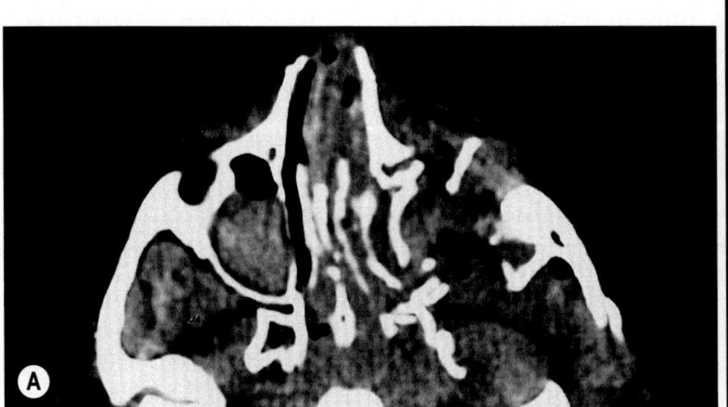

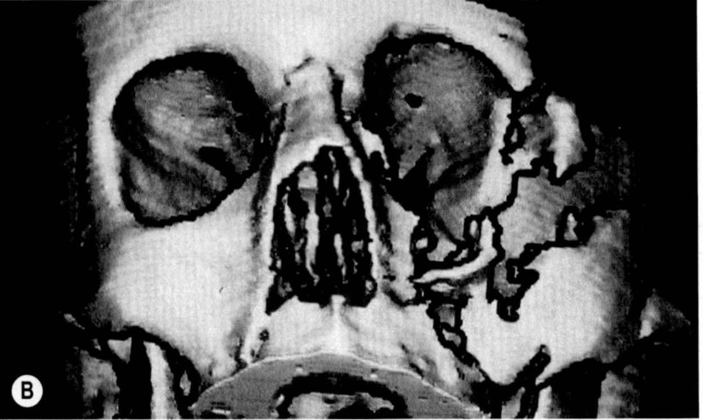

FIGURE 8-81 ■ Comminuted fracture of the left zygoma on axial CT. (A) There are multiple fractures of the anterior, posterolateral and medial walls of the maxillary sinus. There is air in the soft tissues of the cheek and infratemporal fossa. (B) Three-dimensional CT reconstruction of a comminuted fracture of the left zygoma (same case as A).

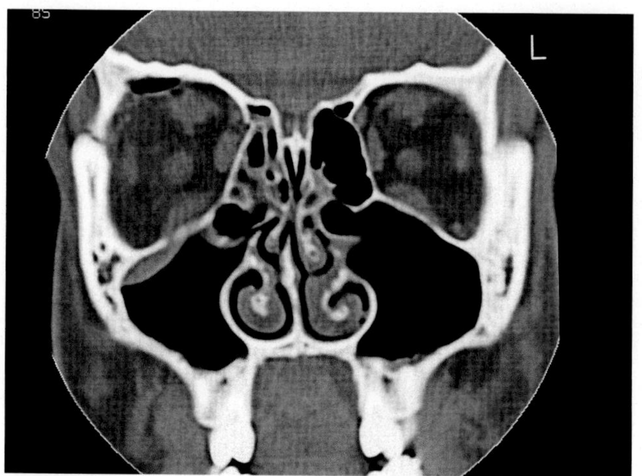

FIGURE 8-82 ■ Coronal CT showing a blow-out fracture of the floor of the right orbit. Fractures of the lamina papyracea (with blood within the ethmoid complex) and orbital floor (with herniation of orbital contents and air within orbital cavity).

ultrasound (US) may also detect orbital wall and orbital rim fractures.[2] Treatment is governed by the extent of the fracture and diplopia if it does not resolve spontaneously. Failure of recognition of a blow-out fracture or fusion of malpositioned bony fragments may lead to entrapped tissues, fibrosis and diplopia.

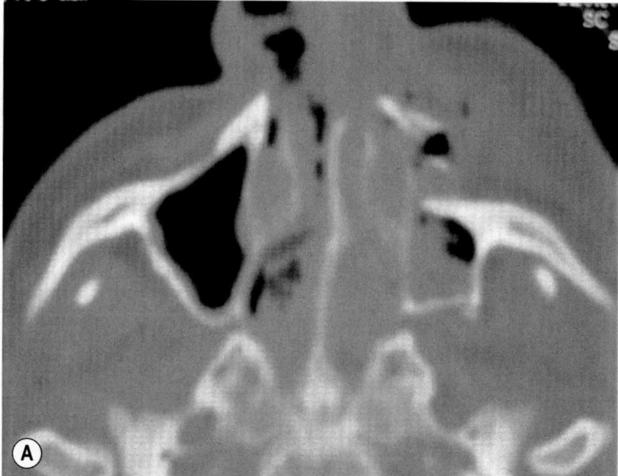

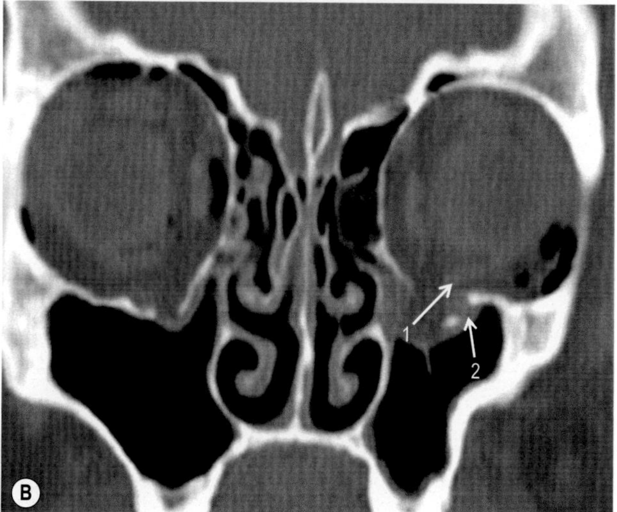

FIGURE 8-83 ■ (A) Axial CT of facial bones. Note depressed rotated left zygomatico-maxillary fracture. (B) Coronal CT of orbits. Note bilateral orbital floor fractures and orbital emphysema. 1 = inferior rectus muscle; 2 = infraorbital nerve.

RADIOLOGICAL INVESTIGATION OF MAXILLARY FRACTURES

A standard occipitomental view is initially indicated, and delayed until the patient is cooperative. Oedema may obscure fracture detail. Fractures of the zygomatic arches are usually apparent on occipitomental (OM) projections, but may be better visualised on an underpenetrated submentovertical view. These views may be supplemented by other radiographs, CBCT, or CT particularly in the more severely injured patient. In CT, thin slices are desirable for good bone detail and need not be contiguous unless 3D reconstruction is planned. CT or CBCT with 3D reconstruction can graphically demonstrate fractures of the facial skeleton (Fig. 8-78 & Fig. 8-83) and 3D data are used in modelling for repair of residual traumatic deformities that require reconstructive surgery.

Questions to answer when reviewing CT: amount of displacement or rotation of the fractured fragments, injury to the globes, optic nerve compression from bone fragments, fracture of the cribriform plate and the possible presence of foreign bodies.

Fractures of the Mandible

Fractures of the mandible tend to occur at specific sites, as shown in Fig. 8-84. They are best demonstrated on a dental panoramic radiograph (Fig. 8-85; or right and left oblique lateral mandibular views), together with a PA mandible radiograph. Parasymphyseal fractures may require intraoral views, which are also useful where the

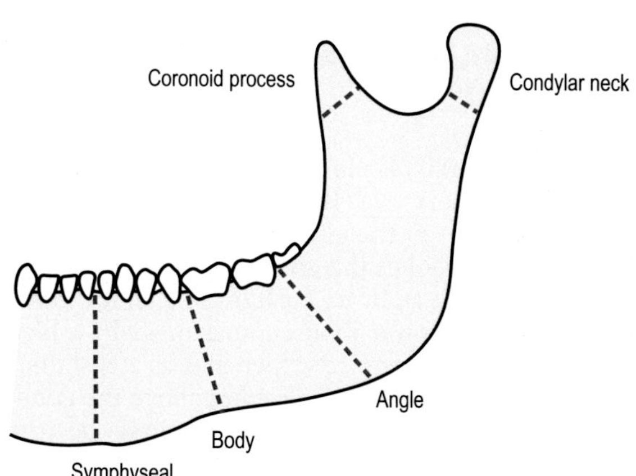

FIGURE 8-84 ■ Line diagram showing common sites of fracture of the mandible.

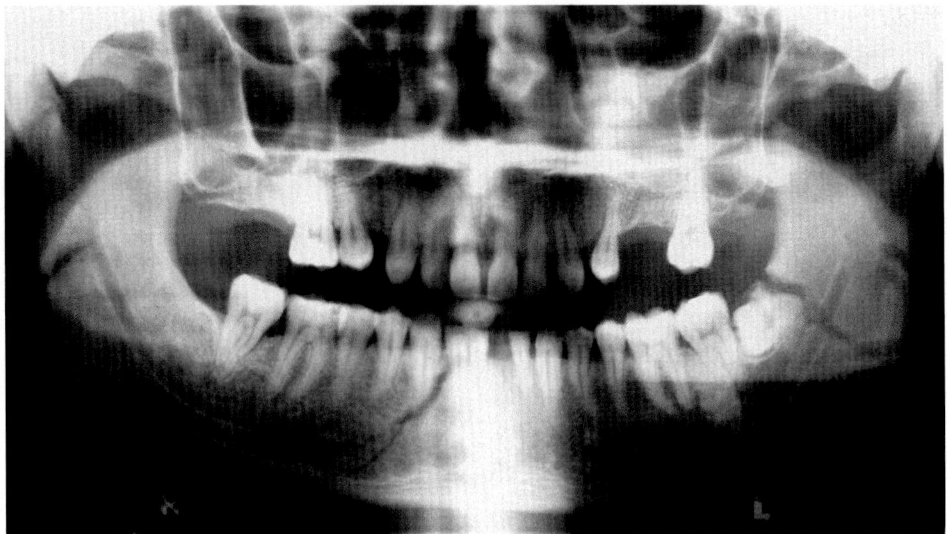

FIGURE 8-85 ■ **Panoramic radiograph showing bilateral fractures of the mandible in the right canine region and left wisdom tooth region.**

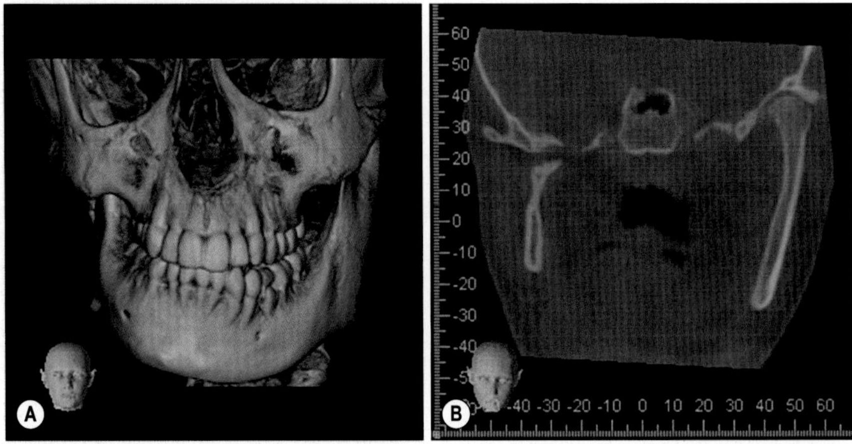

FIGURE 8-86 ■ (A, B) CBCT images of hemifacial microsomia. On the right side the ramus of the mandible and condyle is underdeveloped, resulting in flattening on the right side with facial asymmetry. The right glenoid fossa is shallow when compared with the left side.

anterior teeth are also thought to be fractured. A fracture of the body of the mandible is accompanied by a contralateral fracture in approximately 50% of cases, particularly of the condylar neck.

TEMPOROMANDIBULAR JOINT DISODERS

The temporomandibular joint (TMJ) is a complex diarthrodial, synovial joint. It contains the mandibular condyle, which sits in the glenoid fossa when the mouth is closed. Anteriorly lies the articular eminence and posteriorly the external auditory meatus. The joint is divided into an upper and lower joint compartment by a biconcave, fibrocartilagenous disc, which acts as a cushion for the mandibular condyle. The disc lies above the condyle and is attached posteriorly by fibroelastic tissue to the base of the skull, neck of the mandibular condyle and elsewhere to the fibrous joint capsule. The capsule is lined by a synovial membrane and encloses the joint. Fibres of the lateral ptergyoid muscle insert into the anterior aspect of the capsule and articular disc as well as to the anterior aspect of the condylar neck.

The TMJ is susceptible to conditions that affect other joints including developmental abnormalities, arthritic, traumatic and neoplastic disease.

Developmental Abnormalities

These usually affect the temporal and condylar components, mainly consisting of changes in size and form, and usually result in alteration in the growth of the affected side of the mandible.

Hypoplasia of the mandibular condyle is failure of the condyle to attain full size during its development. It may be confined to the joint or can be part of a local disorder such as hemifacial microsomia, which results in underdevelopment and deformity of the lower half of the face including the ears, mouth and mandible, with a reduced vertical height to the ramus on the affected side (Fig. 8-86).

Condylar hyperplasia causes enlargement of the mandibular condyle due to continued but temporary growth of the cartilaginous growth centre beyond puberty. It produces either a posterior open bite on the affected side or a centre line shift of the mandible relative to the maxilla. Radionuclide imaging may be required to demonstrate whether growth of the condylar cartilage is active prior to corrective treatment. In Hurler's syndrome (gargoylism) the articular surface of the condyle is usually concave instead of convex, an appearance thought specific for this syndrome.

Bifid condyle is believed to result from obstructed blood supply during its development or trauma at an early age. There are no clinical features but radiographically it appears as a notch or indentation of the condylar head.

Temporomandibular Joint Dysfunction

Temporomandibular joint dysfunction is a common condition and consists of myofascial pain, resulting in muscle tenderness, facial discomfort and/or internal derangement of the articular disc. Myofascial pain occurs in all age groups but is particularly common in young female patients. It presents as muscle tenderness, jaw stiffness and headaches, and is associated with stress and anxiety, tooth clenching or other parafunctional habits and occlusal disharmony. The condition is a type of fibromyalgia and as the bony tissues are not affected it has no specific radiological changes.

Internal derangement is an abnormality of the position of the articular disc, which may also show an altered morphology. The normal disc position in relation to the mandibular condyle is illustrated in Fig. 8-87. When the disc becomes displaced, it does so usually in an anteromedial, medial or sometimes lateral position relative to the condylar head. The condition may be painful and cause clicking or jaw locking; however, several studies have shown displaced discs in individuals without symptoms. Discomfort, tenderness and trismus are more prevalent in patients with disc displacement without reduction, particularly in combination with osteoarthrosis and bone marrow oedema.

The diagnosis is made from the clinical findings and in most cases the condition improves or resolves with or without non-surgical intervention. When this fails and more aggressive treatment is planned, or when the diagnosis is uncertain, the disc position can be demonstrated with MRI and the mouth in fully open and closed positions.[3]

Typically the joint is imaged using proton density (or T1) and T2 sequences using 3-mm parasagittal slices, the angulation being determined by the medial angulation of the condylar head. On MRI, the disc appears as a biconcave (bow tie-shaped) structure of low attenuation sandwiched between the anterior aspect of the articulating surface of the condyle and the glenoid fossa. Anterior disc displacement with reduction of the disc is shown in Fig. 8-88. When the mouth is opened, the anteriorly displaced disc reduces or moves back to a normal position relative to the condylar head; this manoeuvre often results

(A) Normal disc relationship

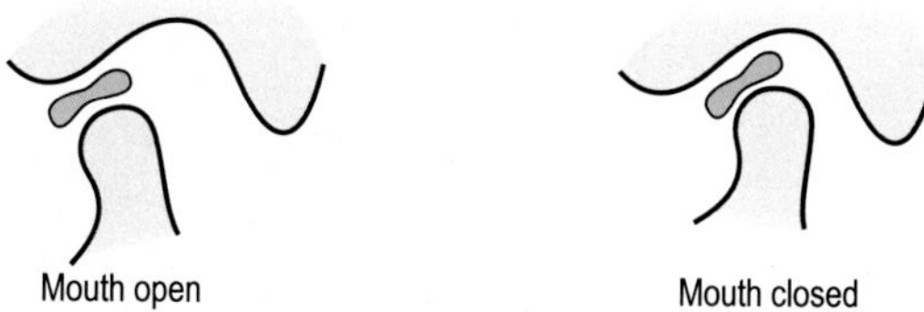

(B) Anterior disc displacement with reduction

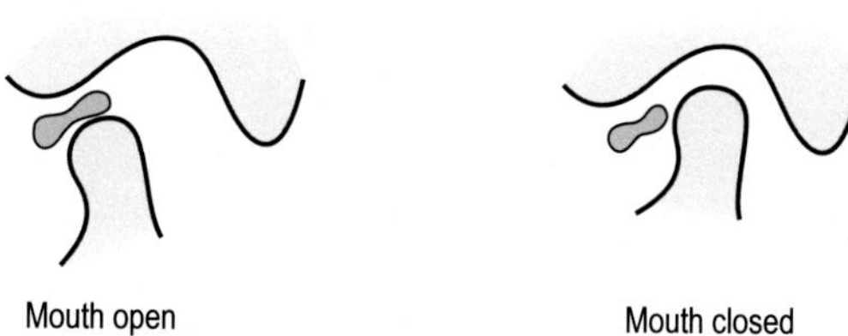

(C) Anterior disc displacement without reduction

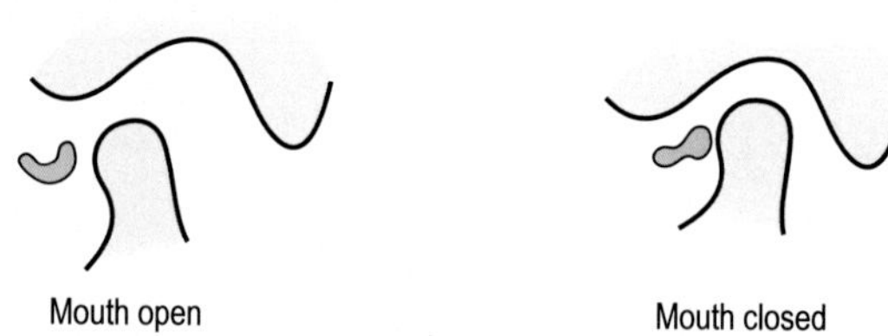

FIGURE 8-87 ■ Diagrammatic representation of the articular disc (shaded). (A) In a normal position in relationship to condylar head, (B) in an anteriorly displaced position with reduction on opening and (C) with a non-reducing disc.

in a click, which can be apparent to the patient and palpated by the clinician. However, if the disc remains anteriorly displaced (Fig. 8-89) it may interfere with forward translation of the condyle, resulting in locking and restricted mouth opening, and pressure on the disc may cause it to become distorted.

T2-weighted images can be used to show joint effusions and inflammatory change. The significance of joint effusion is controversial as it can occur in the non-painful joint. However, it is observed more often in joints with more advanced stages of disc displacement, i.e. non-reducing discs, and it is thought to represent the presence of synovitis.[4] Images taken in a coronal plane demonstrate disc displacement medially or laterally; this view is useful for showing degenerative changes to the articular surface. Using plain radiographs to assess joint space as a predictor of disc displacement has been shown to have a low predictive value.[5]

Arthritides

Degenerative joint disease (osteoarthritis) can develop at any age but its incidence increases with age. It is thought to occur when the joint is unable to adapt to remodelling forces. There may be no symptoms or there may be discomfort and joint tenderness similar to TMJ but crepitus is often present. The radiographic features are diagrammatically illustrated in Fig. 8-90, and include

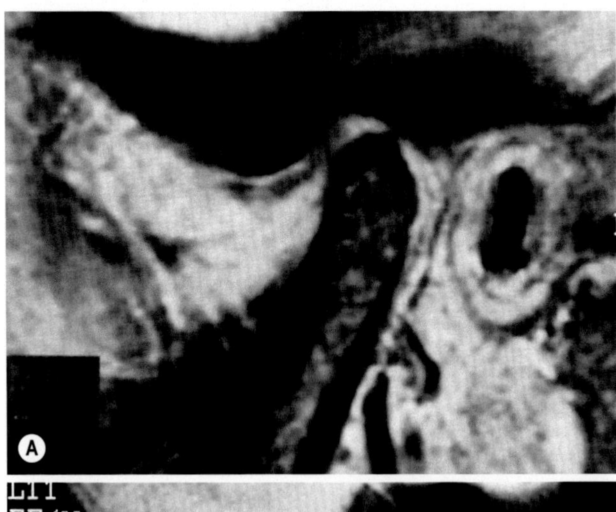

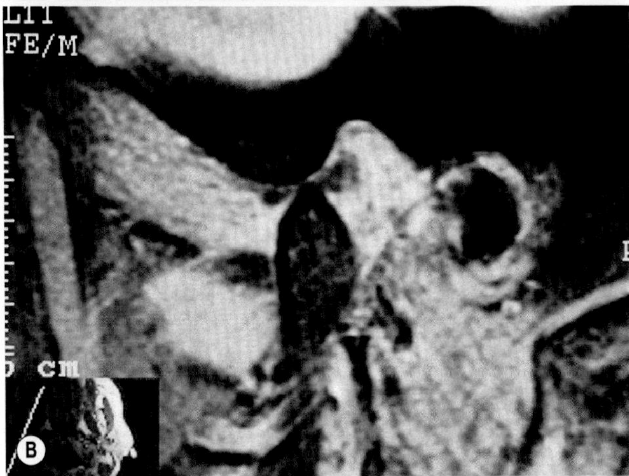

FIGURE 8-88 ■ Anterior reducible subluxation of disc. Fast-field echo (FFE) MRI parasagittal images showing an anteriorly positioned disc (A), which reduces on opening (B) to lie over the condyle.

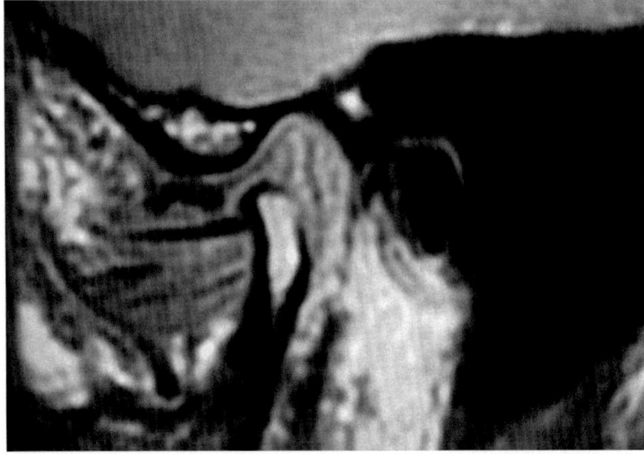

FIGURE 8-89 ■ Parasagittal T1-weighted MRI image with the mouth open showing a non-reducing, anteriorly displaced disc.

flattening and irregularity of the condylar surface, sclerosis and osteophyte formation, which is seen mainly on the anterosuperior condylar surface (Fig. 8-91). Dental panoramic radiography (OPG) demonstrates the mandibular condyles but sometime it is obscured by superimposition of the skull base. Small-volume CBCT provides excellent bony detail of the joint and may be indicated in those suspected of arthritic change not responsive to conventional management.

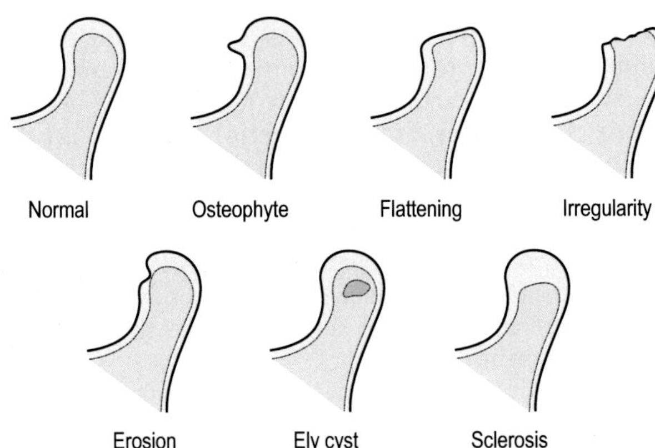

FIGURE 8-90 ■ Diagrammatic representation showing various degenerative changes that affect the mandibular condyle.

Rheumatoid arthritis (inflammatory arthritis) is a common condition in which the TMJ becomes involved in about half of cases. Symptoms include pain, swelling and jaw stiffness. Radiographic changes consist of loss of bone density and formation of erosions leading to a somewhat pointed condylar head. MRI T2-weighted coronal images are valuable for demonstrating the presence of joint inflammation. Other inflammatory arthritides may affect the joint, including systemic lupus, systemic sclerosis, psoriasis, Reiter's syndrome, juvenile chronic arthritis and synovial osteochondromatosis, which results in joint swelling and the presence of numerous loose calcific bodies (Fig. 8-92).

Juvenile chronic arthritis occurs during the first two decades of life and is characterised by intermittent synovial inflammation. It causes pain and tenderness of one or both joints and if severe will affect mandibular growth. The condyle becomes radiolucent and its surface develops erosions and irregularity.

Injury

Isolated fractures of the condylar neck can occur but often accompany fractures of the mandible, especially following a blow to the chin, and are usually visible on a dental panoramic radiograph and a PA condylar view. The slender condylar neck acts as a stress breaker, reducing the likelihood of the condyle being driven up into the middle cranial fossa. Fractures of the condylar neck may be simple and undisplaced or displaced with the condyle being pulled forwards and medially by the lateral pterygoid muscle (fracture dislocation). Intracapsular fractures are difficult to demonstrate on plain films and if suspected may require evaluation with CT if symptoms persist. Haemarthrosis and ankylosis may complicate recovery.

Acute dislocation of the TMJ occurs following a blow to the mandible when the mouth is open. It is diagnosed from the clinical presentation. The role of

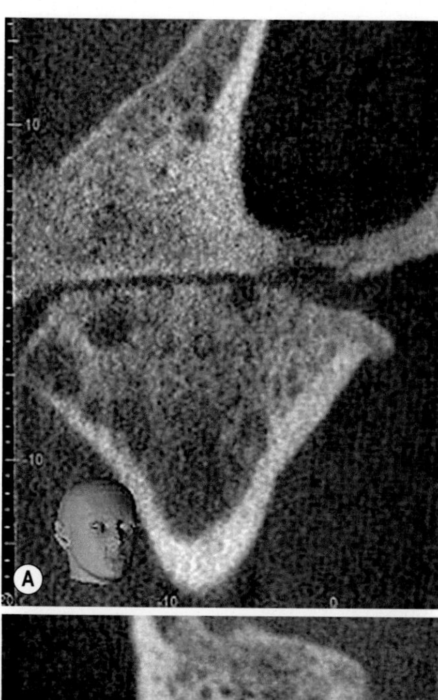

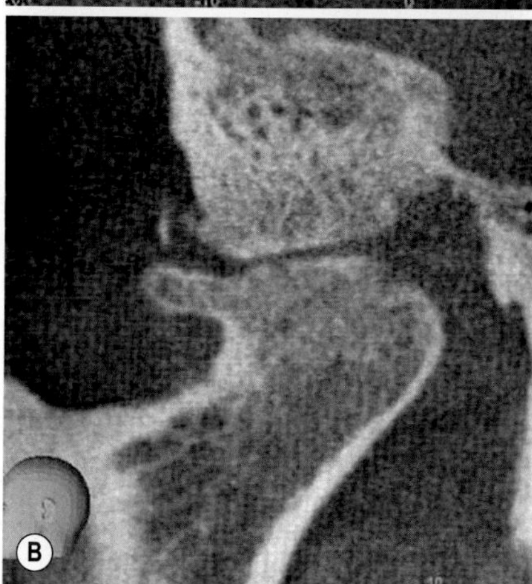

FIGURE 8-91 ■ **TMJ degenerative arthritis shown on CBCT imaging.** (A) Coronal slice and (B) parasagittal slice, both showing sclerosis of the condylar head with osteophyte formation and focal subchondral radiolucencies (Ely's cysts), slight irregularity of both articular surfaces and a narrowed joint space.

radiology is to exclude a fracture or other contributing disease. Recurrent dislocation can develop spontaneously and may be a feature of Marfan's syndrome and Ehlers–Danlos syndrome.

Ankylosis of the TMJ may follow a traumatic haemarthrosis or infective arthritis. When this happens in childhood, it may result in hypoplasia of the condyle secondary to concurrent damage to the epiphyseal growth centre. CT or CBCT is required to show the extent of the ankylosis (Fig. 8-93).

Neoplasms of the temporomandibular joint are uncommon and include osteoma, osteochondroma, chondrosarcomas and, rarely, metastatic deposits.

SALIVARY GLAND DISORDERS

There are three paired major salivary glands—the parotid, submandibular and sublingual glands—and numerous minor salivary glands supplying saliva to lubricate, cleanse and aid early digestion within the mouth.

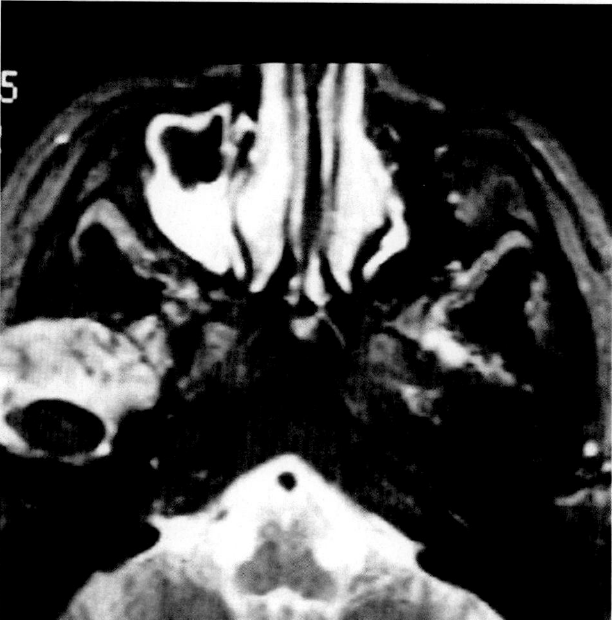

FIGURE 8-92 ■ **Osteochondromatosis of the TMJ.** Axial T2W MR view showing mass draped around the right condyle.

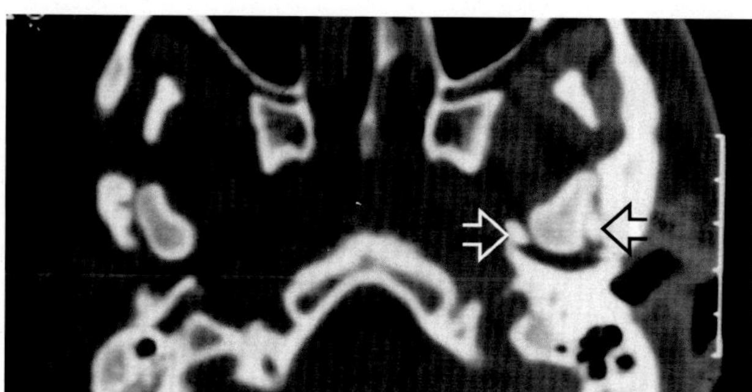

FIGURE 8-93 ■ **Bony ankylosis of the left TMJ on axial CT.** There are two bone fragments (arrows) between the mandibular condyle and the glenoid fossa, and there is partial bone union between the lateral bone fragment, the condyle and the glenoid fossa. Both mandibular condyles are rotated due to the fractures of the condylar necks. The patient had developed permanent trismus following an accident in childhood. (Courtesy of Dr Otto Chan.)

Anatomy

The **parotid gland** lies between the posterior border of the mandibular ramus and the sternomastoid muscle attaching to the mastoid process. It is enclosed in deep cervical fascia and traversed by the retromandibular vein, external carotid artery and facial nerve. The retromandibular vein is easily visible on all forms of cross-sectional imaging and indicates the plane of the dividing plexus of the facial nerve lying just laterally, which divides the gland into a larger superficial and smaller deep portion.

While tumours are more common in the superficial lobe, surgical approach to the deep lobe involves dissection of the nerve branches, with attendant risk of nerve damage. The parotid gland drains through Stensen's duct, running horizontally forward approximately 1 cm below the zygomatic arch on the surface of masseter to turn medially, perforate the buccinator muscle and emerge on a papilla on the buccal mucosa opposite the first maxillary molar tooth. The sharp sigmoid bend in the anterior portion of the parotid duct is a common site for impaction of small salivary stones and is the location of the proposed 'buccinator window anomaly', a possible obstructive phenomenon.

The **submandibular gland** wraps around the posterior free border of the mylohyoid muscle, medial to the posterior body of mandible and descends for 2–3 cm into the suprahyoid neck. The main Wharton's duct passes up from the hilum of the gland, around the posterior margin of mylohyoid, turning anteriorly in the floor of the mouth to open through a small papilla situated on either side of the lingual frenulum, behind the lower incisor teeth.

The almond-sized **sublingual glands** lie anteriorly in the floor of mouth above the mylohyoid muscle. Each gland opens by a single Bartholin's duct or by multiple ducts into the floor of mouth or terminal part of Wharton's duct.

Radiological Techniques and Their Application

Plain radiographs are of limited value in salivary gland disease. An intraoral true mandibular occlusal view detects radiopaque salivary calculi in the anterior submandibular duct, of which 60–80% are radiopaque, while an inflated or puffed out PA view of the cheek may detect the 20–40% of parotid stones that are radiopaque. A negative result does not preclude obstruction.

Sialography has limitations in demonstrating parenchymal disease but remains a highly sensitive test of ductal abnormalities. Cannulation of the parotid duct is normally straightforward but the submandibular duct orifice may be very fine and difficult to identify and usually requires a sialogogue or gland massage to release a bolus of saliva to open the duct orifice. Occasionally the sublingual duct and gland may be incidentally demonstrated on sialography. Direct visualisation of ductal filling under fluoroscopy, particularly using digital subtraction techniques (Fig. 8-94), has benefits over the traditional plain film method and water-soluble contrast media should be used to avoid the permanent foreign body reaction sometimes seen when oily media are extravasated from the ductal system. Sialography has no place in the investigation of mass lesions and is indicated primarily for symptoms directly related to the ductal system such as obstruction and sialectasis. It has the advantage of dislodging mucus plugs and so frequently brings about symptomatic relief.

Interventional sialography offers a minimally invasive alternative to formal surgical sialadenectomy or sialolithectomy. Small mobile stones may be extracted from the duct system by Dormia basket or balloon catheter, and duct strictures dilated by angioplasty balloon (Figs. 8-95 and 8-96).[6,7]

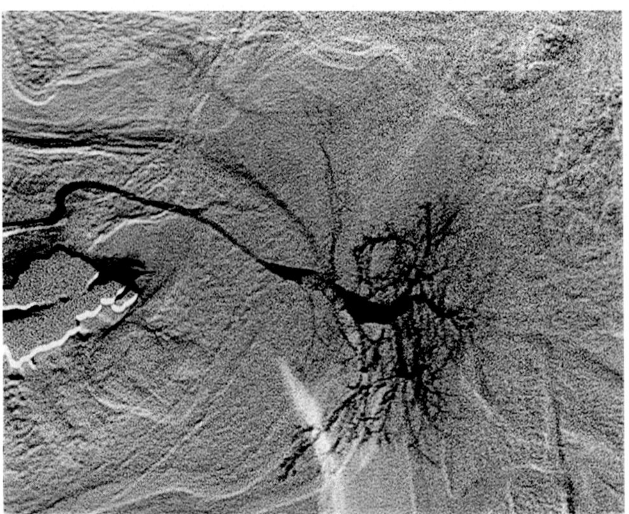

FIGURE 8-94 ■ **Collection of calculi at hilum of parotid gland.** There is minor sialectasis (irregularity of calibre of some intraglandular ducts).

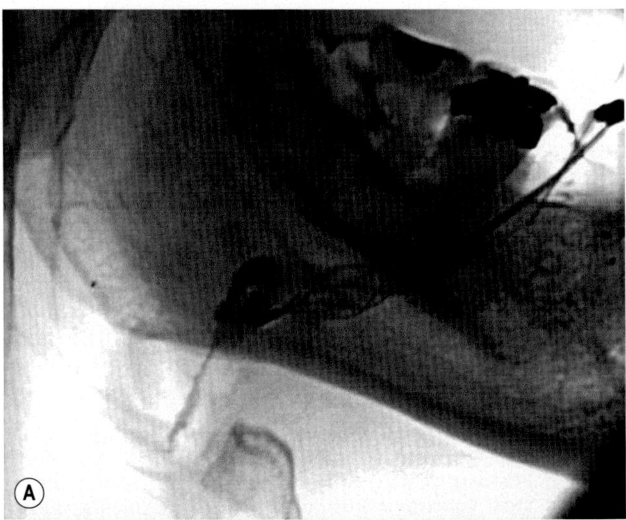

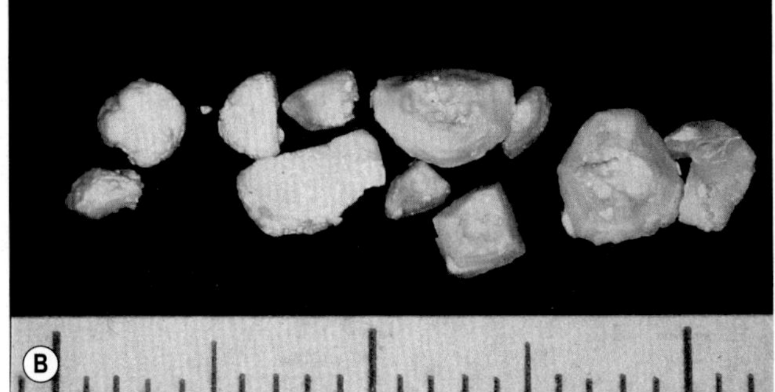

FIGURE 8-95 ■ (A) An intraoperative sialogram showing an **open Dormia basket within the submandibular duct** during removal of a salivary stone. (B) Resultant fragmented salivary stone removed from submandibular gland shown in (A).

Ultrasound (US) has become the first-line investigation for a mass within the salivary glands and for inflammatory salivary gland disease and can readily assess duct dilatation, facilitated by administering a sialogogue prior to investigation (Fig. 8-97). It is highly sensitive for

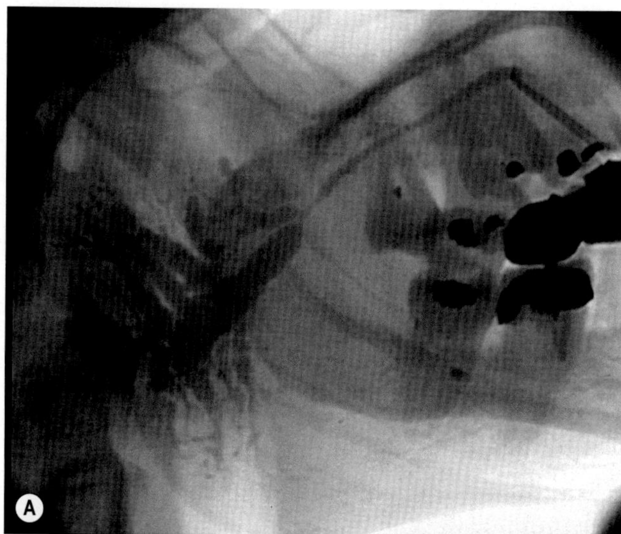

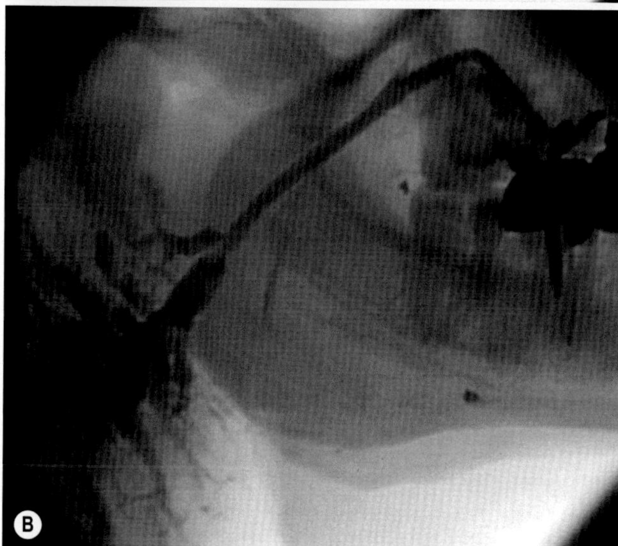

FIGURE 8-96 ■ (A) Sialogram showing a **diffuse stricture at the entrance to the hilum** of the parotid gland. (B) Postoperative sialogram showing dilatation of duct stricture following balloon ductoplasty.

the 70–80% of tumours located within the superficial parotid gland when compared with CT, though it has limitations when imaging the deep pole where a curvilinear probe may be helpful.

CT is sensitive for the detection of salivary calculi though not resolving enough to show details of duct morphology in obstruction. **MRI** has largely superseded it for tumour assessment though it can be useful in imaging early involvement of cortical bone. The technique of CT sialography has been displaced by MR sialography.

MRI has major advantages for salivary gland imaging, particularly related to its high soft-tissue contrast and multiplanar data acquisition. Gadolinium enhancement is not required in uncomplicated cases, but can be of major importance in the assessment of recurrent tumours (Fig. 8-98).

Magnetic resonance sialography using heavily T2-weighted sequences (Figs. 8-99 and 8-100) allows noninvasive assessment of obstructive disease by imaging stimulated ductal saliva and correlates well with or even

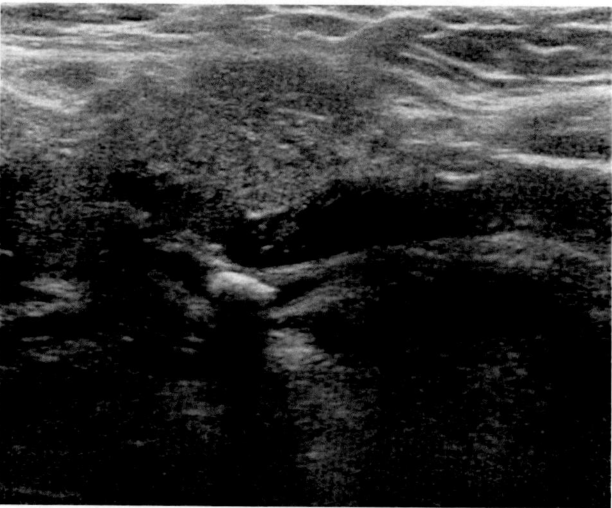

FIGURE 8-97 ■ **Ultrasound image of a salivary stone in the proximal portion of the submandibular duct.**

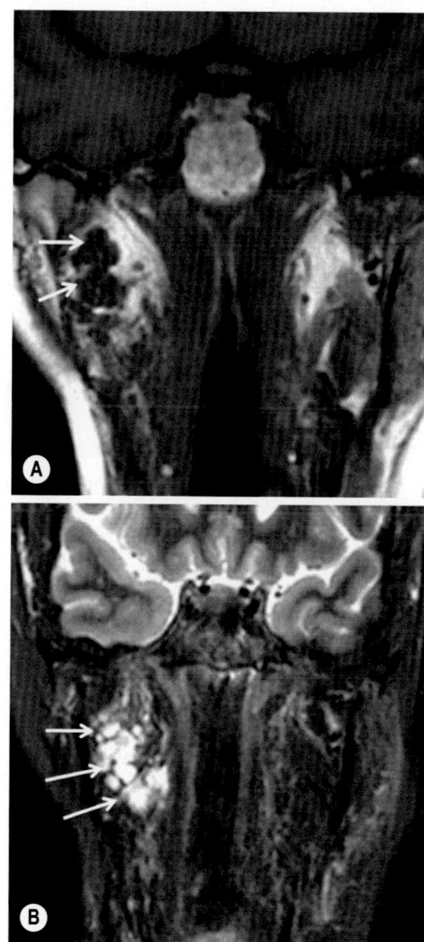

FIGURE 8-98 ■ T1W and STIR coronal MR (A and B) demonstrating multiple recurrent pleomorphic adenoma in parotid bed and parapharyngeal space (white arrows).

improves on conventional sialography in conditions such as **Sjögren's syndrome.**[8,9]

Radionuclide radiology has a limited role in salivary gland disease but may occasionally be used to assess glandular function in obstruction and inflammatory conditions. Low resolution and lack of uptake of ^{99m}Tc-sodium

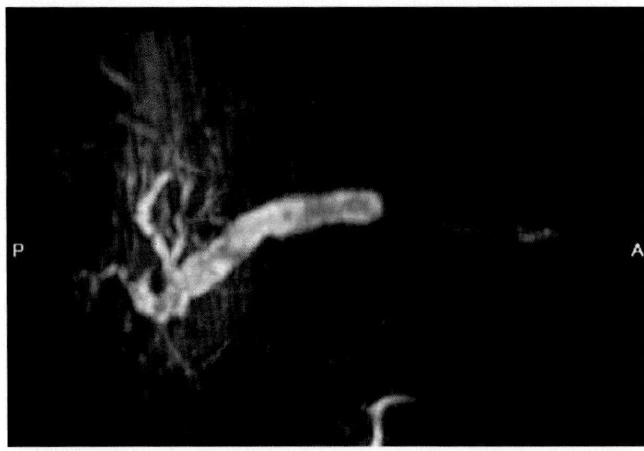

FIGURE 8-99 ■ MR sialography image showing gross dilatation of the main duct and some of the secondary ducts. Areas of low signal in the main duct are due to the presence of several large stones. The distal part of the duct is normal. (Courtesy of Dr M. Becker, Geneva.)

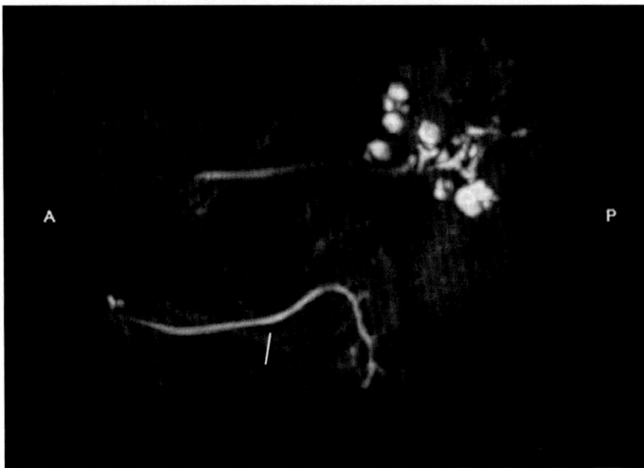

FIGURE 8-100 ■ MR sialography image showing chronic sialadenitis of the parotid gland with focal globular high signal areas of sialectasis within the parenchyma of the gland. The main duct appears normal. The submandibular duct and gland (arrow) (seen later) appear normal. (Courtesy of Dr M. Becker, Geneva.)

pertechnetate in adenolymphomas (**Warthin's tumours**) limits its value in tumour imaging.

Positron emission tomography has been used to image salivary gland tumours but, while being actively taken up by growing neoplasms, it is also concentrated in lymphoid tissue and salivary glands. It has higher uptake in both malignant tumours and in the benign Warthin's tumour.[10] The most commonly used glucose analogue is secreted in saliva, so small tumours may be missed. PET has strengths in assessing the post-treatment neck but may not distinguish tumour from acute infection or early wound healing.[11]

Calculi and Duct Strictures

Calculi cause partial obstruction of the salivary glands, typically resulting in mealtime-related swelling of the affected gland and a predisposition to infection, sialectasis and eventual gland atrophy. They are more common in the submandibular duct system (around 85%) where 60–80% are radiopaque. They may be found close to the duct opening, in the mid duct, at the genu of the submandibular duct or within the gland where they can reach a significant size. Only 20–40% of parotid calculi are radiopaque and are normally detected in the parotid hilum or main duct overlying the masseter muscle. CT is highly sensitive for small stones but US is a convenient and effective way of detecting the majority of salivary calculi (89–94% sensitivity, 100% specificity), except those lying in the most anterior parts of each duct. Single and multiple calculi may be found in dilated duct segments and may be associated with distally placed strictures. Mucus plugs also cause temporary duct obstruction but are radiolucent.

Strictures of the salivary ducts result from inflammation caused by infection or calculi and are best demonstrated by sialography or MR sialography.[12] These may appear point or diffuse with proximal dilatation of the duct system. Approximately 24% of salivary obstructions are due to strictures.[13] 'Sialadochitis' describes the combination of duct dilatation and stenosis that follows obstruction complicated by infection.

Sialectasis

Sialectasis develops in sialadenitis and radiologically demonstrates degenerative changes seen within the terminal salivary ducts and acini as a result of obstruction, infection and other conditions such as Sjögren's syndrome (see later). Progression from widened and tortuous ductules to frank cavitation is seen (cavitatory sialectasis).

Inflammatory Conditions

Infective sialadenitis of viral or bacterial origin causes generalised glandular enlargement on cross-sectional imaging with heterogeneous reduced echogenicity on US, increased uptake on contrast CT and high signal on T2-weighted MRI. Abscess formation is shown as an ill-defined hypoechoic area on US, with equivalent changes on CT and MR; acute inflammation is also evidenced by inflammatory stranding through the gland to the overlying tissues.

Focal chronic sclerosing sialadenitis (Küttner's tumour) presents as a localised area of hypoechoic tissue in the submandibular gland on US and may be mistaken for tumour.[14] Sialography is indicated in cases of recurrent infection in order to demonstrate any underlying calculus or duct stricture.

Sjögren's syndrome causes damage to intercalated salivary duct walls, allowing leakage of contrast media during sialography and creating a characteristically fine punctate sialectasis in approximately 70% of cases. This is evenly distributed throughout salivary gland tissue—normally a parotid gland is chosen to demonstrate involvement. Similar abnormalities have been described in association with other connective tissue disorders such as rheumatoid arthritis, systemic lupus erythematosus, ankylosing spondylitis, Reiter's disease, polyarteritis nodosa and scleroderma where, in the absence of clinical

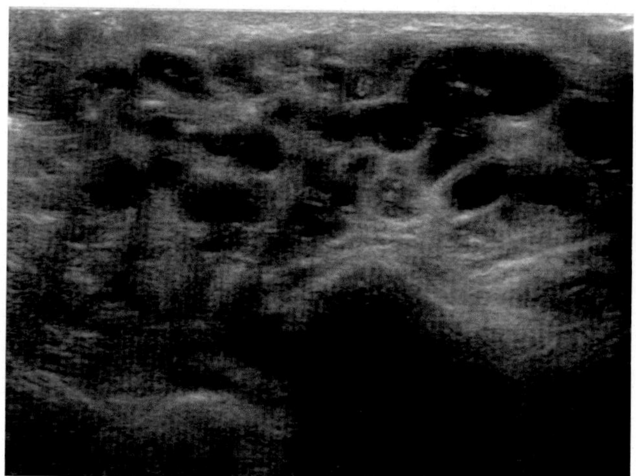

FIGURE 8-101 ■ Ultrasound image of the parotid gland showing the honeycomb pattern of hypoechogenic change in Sjögren's syndrome.

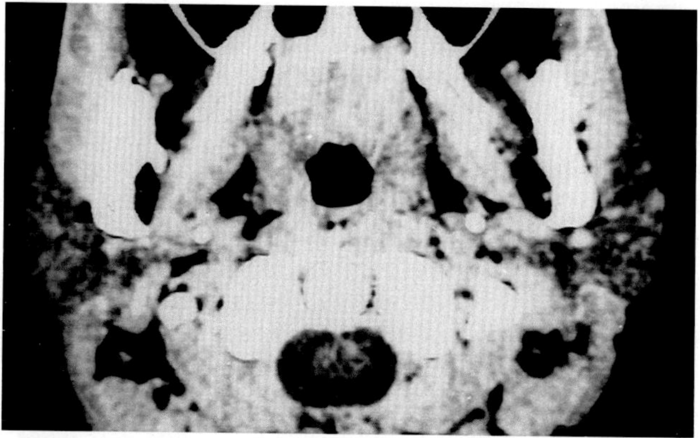

FIGURE 8-102 ■ Sarcoid of the parotid glands. There is generalised glandular enlargement and multiple small areas of decreased attenuation.

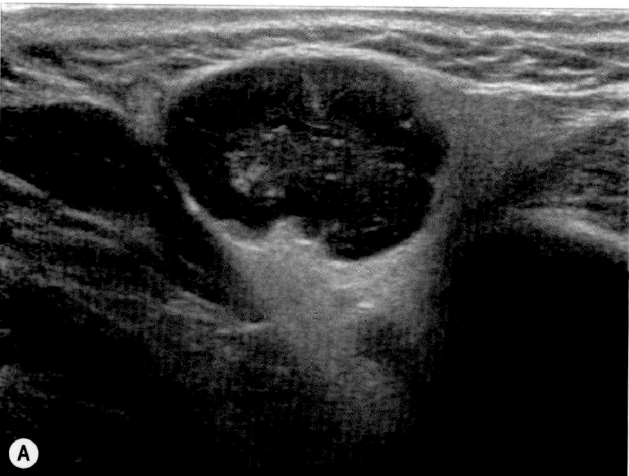

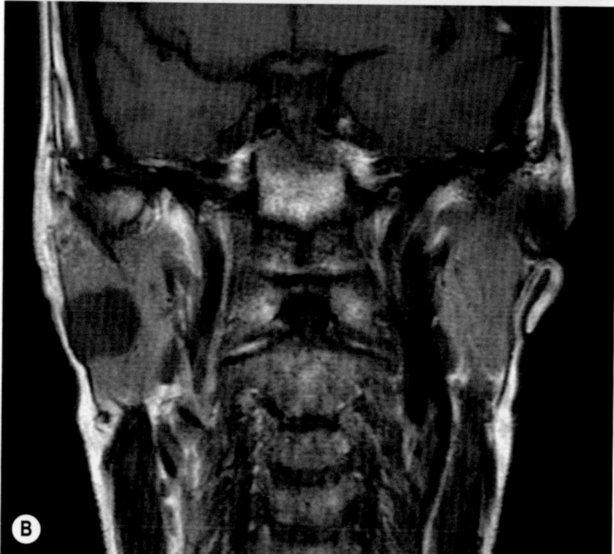

FIGURE 8-103 ■ Pleomorphic adenoma of the right parotid gland (A) on ultrasound and (B) on coronal T1W MRI.

features of Sjögren's syndrome, sialographic signs are estimated to exist in 5–15% of cases. MRI shows a speckled honeycomb appearance in moderately affected cases on both T1- and T2-weighted images, which is said to be specific and similar appearances may be found in the lacrimal glands. MR sialography has shown improved sensitivity and 100% specificity over conventional sialography in diagnosis of Sjögren's syndrome.[9] US shows a heterogeneous reticular pattern of small low-reflective foci (Fig. 8-101) and has a role in monitoring for lymphoma development, which may complicate late Sjögren's syndrome. Sjögren's syndrome sufferers have up to a 44× greater risk of developing mucosal-associated lymphoid tissue (**MALT**) lymphoma.[15]

Sarcoid results in generalised glandular enlargement with multiple small granulomatous areas of low attenuation on CT (Fig. 8-102), giving a reticular hypoechoic pattern or intraglandular nodal enlargement on US and diffuse high signal on MRI. There is, in common with all inflammatory conditions, high activity on ^{67}Ga scintigraphy.

Human immunodefiency virus (HIV)-associated salivary gland disease is a spectrum of disorders that affects approximately 20% of children and 0.5% of adults with HIV, and includes lymphoepithelial infiltration that may progress to lymphoma. The combination of multiple intraparotid cysts and cervical lymphadenopathy should alert the radiologist to this syndrome, which can occur at any stage from early post infection to full-blown acquired immune deficiency syndrome (AIDS).

Salivary Gland Tumours

Most salivary gland tumours are benign and can develop at any age. Of these tumours, 80% are found in the parotid glands, 5% in the submandibular, 1% in the sublingual and the remaining 15% in the minor salivary glands. The overall incidence of malignancy is 10–20%, and the smaller the major gland, the higher the rate of malignancy.

Benign pleomorphic adenomas (benign mixed tumours) account for around 80% of salivary tumours and typically arise in the superficial portion of the parotid gland, being most common in middle-aged women. These appear uni- or mildly loculated hypoechoic lesions on US and characteristically give a low signal on T1- but high signal on T2-weighted MRI (Fig. 8-103). Although this tumour is benign, if left untreated for many years it has a tendency to become malignant.

The commonest malignant epithelial salivary tumours are mucoepidermoid and adenoid cystic carcinomas. Mucoepidermoid carcinomas have a variable behaviour depending on their degree of differentiation (well, intermediate or poor). Adenoid cystic carcinomas, in particular, have a propensity for insidious perineural spread. MRI can usually identify the presence, but underestimates the extent, of perineural spread. Mucoepidermoid tumours are the commonest malignancy in children.

Other salivary tumours include the benign **adenolymphoma (Warthin's tumour)**, and **lipoma**, and the malignant **acinic cell carcinoma** and **NHL**. Warthin's tumours are notably found in the parotid tail of older men and may be multiple (20%) and occasionally bilateral (approximately 15%). **Lipomas** give a characteristic hypoechoic appearance with numerous layered highly reflective internal strands on US and markedly low attenuation on CT.

Distinction between benign and malignant tumours is based upon criteria, some of which are common to all cross-sectional imaging, others being specific to a particular technique. Benignity is best identified by the presence of a capsule or well-defined outline; however, notably, many salivary malignancies are relatively low grade and are well defined in the early stages. Beyond this, CT may not be particularly discriminating, since many lesions show similarly increased attenuation, though more recently MRI diffusion studies have allowed better differentiation.

MRI has a sensitivity of about 75% for identifying benign features; this can be improved by using gadolinium enhancement. Ultrasound normally depicts benign lesions as well-defined and hypoechoic without regional lymphadenopathy. Additionally, colour flow Doppler indicates vascularity and may present evidence of neoangiogenesis common in malignant tumours. Ultrasound is further used to guide FNA to accurately target nonpalpable lesions, but requires experienced cytopathology support to complete an effective diagnostic process and thus alter management.

Concurrent inflammatory change or haemorrhage can be confused with malignancy here. Contrast-enhanced MRI remains preferable for demonstrating recurrent tumour in areas that may be inaccessible to US and that give only non-specific soft-tissue change on CT. Whereas sialography is not recommended for the assessment of mass lesions, the incidental finding of distortion or amputation of intraglandular ducts should arouse concern as to the presence of a benign or malignant tumour, respectively.

Trauma

Laceration of the main parotid duct or of a larger intraglandular branch occasionally results from a penetrating facial injury, or is a rare complication of surgery. In recent injury, US may detect a fluid collection and sialography will show extravasation of contrast from the duct system into the soft tissues. Later, healing frequently results in duct stenosis.

Disorders of Function

Salivary gland function may be quantified by time–activity curves with ^{99m}Tc-pertechnetate scintigraphy and may distinguish between the functioning, the obstructed and the non-functional gland; however, the effective dose is relatively high. This may supplement sialography or be undertaken when sialography is not possible, and has been used to demonstrate recovery of salivary function following removal of an obstructing calculus.[16]

SOFT TISSUES

Effective near-field imaging, and colour flow and power Doppler ultrasound, combined with its established values of high soft-tissue contrast and use in guided biopsy, have led to US being seen as the first-line investigation for masses in the superficial soft tissues of the maxillofacial region. Some operator variability with US and difficulty in interpreting archived static images are reasons why CT remains widely used, as it demonstrates most lesions and assesses their relationship to adjacent structures, although IV contrast is often required for the accurate assessment of cervical lymphadenopathy. MRI, by virtue of its high soft-tissue contrast and multiplanar capabilities, will show most masses with similar or greater ease and has the additional advantage that different sequences may contribute information about the nature of a lesion.

US improves on the clinical examination of the parotid, submandibular and cervical regions, and is a rapid and accurate means of distinguishing between cervical lymphadenopathy, salivary and other soft-tissue neck lesions. Patterns suggestive of malignant involvement of cervical lymph nodes include a round shape (a short-axis measurement over 1 cm becoming significant), absence of hilus, irregular outline, heterogeneous internal pattern including coagulation or cystic necrosis, disorganised peripheral colour flow pattern on Doppler US, nodal clusters and fusion of nodes.[17] US has been found to be better than CT at detecting malignant cervical nodes but has the disadvantage of being unable to access deep nodes such as those within the retropharyngeal region. Identification of these features in combination with US-guided FNAC gave 100% accuracy compared with CT (77–89%), MR (88%) and US alone (83–98%).[18]

Infection in the head and neck region is characterised by spread along fascial-bound compartments (mucosal, parapharyngeal, carotid, masticator, retropharyngeal and prevertebral). CT or MRI both demonstrate such spread (Fig. 8-104).

Malignant tumours within the oral cavity and environs are predominantly squamous cell carcinomas. MRI has become the first-choice examination for imaging both the extent of the local tumour and any regional lymphadenopathy, but may be oversensitive in the assessment of recurrent disease. MRI is also useful for assessing marrow involvement and is steadily encroaching on CT's superiority in demonstrating cortical bone involvement from tumours such as those in the floor of the mouth (Fig. 8-105). The imaging of primary lesions is relatively straightforward, but controversy remains surrounding the place of imaging in the assessment of lymph node

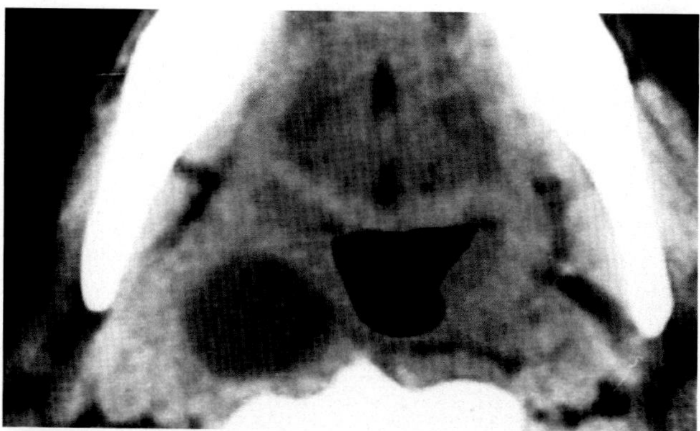

FIGURE 8-104 ■ Abscess in the right oropharyngeal region on axial CT. The patient had received antibiotic treatment for recurrent throat infections and sterile pus was subsequently aspirated from the lesion.

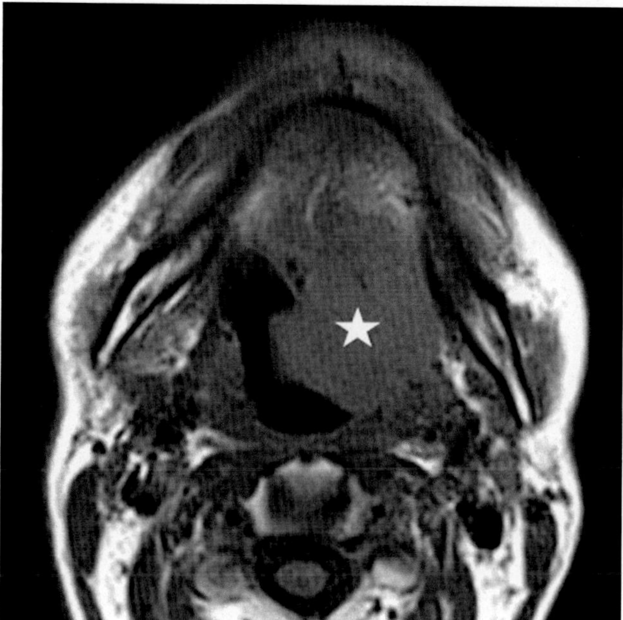

FIGURE 8-105 ■ Carcinoma of the left side of the tongue and oropharynx, T1-weighted axial MRI. The tumour (white star) extends to the midline.

involvement. Some studies state categorically that MRI lacks sufficient sensitivity and specificity to replace elective neck dissection for both staging and prognostic purposes,[19] but more recently imaging has shown increased sensitivity in detecting nodal metastases using US and combinations of PET and sentinel node biopsy. MRI has successfully predicted those patients in need of neck dissection,[20] and has successfully revealed micrometastases (described as intranodal tumour deposits of less than 2 mm diameter at any level of sectioning).[19,21] Positron emission tomography (PET), utilising either ^{18}F-fluorodeoxyglucose (FDG-PET) or ^{11}C-tyrosine (TYR-PET), has a similar sensitivity (72%) to CT (89%) for the detection of lymph node metastases, but this may be improved by co-registration with CT (96% sensitivity, 98.5% specificity), or by supplementary sentinel node biopsy.[20,22] PET and PET-CT are currently viewed as particularly promising techniques for the detection of

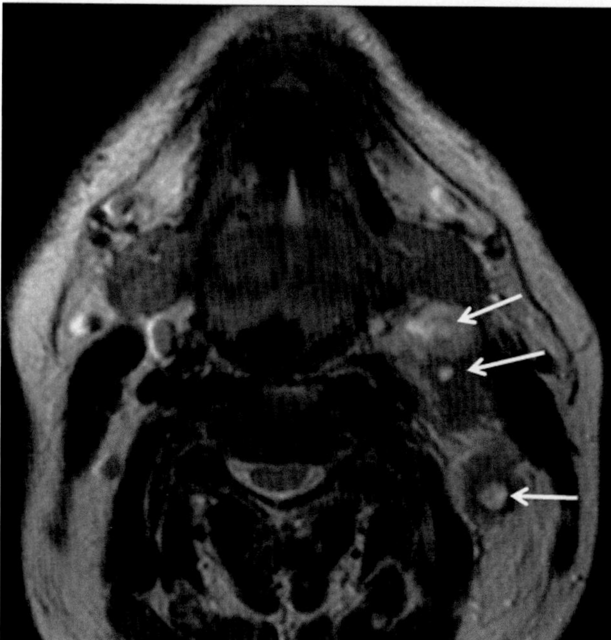

FIGURE 8-106 ■ Axial T2 MR demonstrating multifocal nodal recurrence in the left upper deep cervical region. Note the central T2 high signal in keeping with necrosis (white arrows).

occult primary lesions and along with diffusion weighted MR tumour recurrence especially in the post-radiotherapy situation. Recurrent neck disease, even when subclinical, may, however, be predicted with US and US-guided FNAC. The propensity for regional metastases from SCC to present late after treatment of the primary lesion is an indication for prolonged follow-up (Fig. 8-106). Lymphomas may arise in Waldeyer's ring and the salivary glands, including the minor glands.

Benign tumours of the soft tissues that require imaging in adults are relatively rare other than some dermoids, which present at lines of embryonic fusion; vascular abnormalities, which may grow extremely large, leading to secondary growth disturbances; and salivary gland tumours, as already discussed. Colour flow Doppler US and magnetic resonance angiography may be helpful in assessment, but conventional angiography may be necessary, particularly prior to embolisation. Phleboliths within such lesions may be apparent on plain films.

A wide spectrum of lesions present in newborns, infants and children often as benign vascular abnormalities (Figs. 8-107 and 8-108) but other hamartomas (Fig. 8-109) and malignant tumours may be seen.

Thyroglossal and branchial cysts have characteristic anatomical locations. Thyroglossal cysts arise from epithelial tissue trapped during the embryonic descent of the thyroid gland, and present as defined midline cystic structures lying on a line between the base of the tongue and the thyroid gland (Fig. 8-110). Branchial cysts arise from epithelium trapped during incorporation of the second branchial arch, and present as ovoid fluid-containing lesions lying deep to the sternomastoid muscle, protruding anterior to its anterior border.

Masseteric hypertrophy may be unilateral or bilateral, and often concurrently involves the pterygoid muscles. US is valuable for diagnosis.[23]

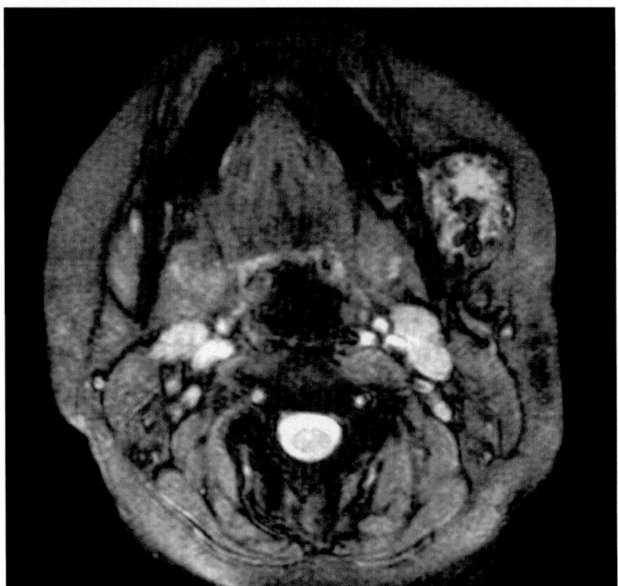

FIGURE 8-107 ■ **Axial MRI of a venous vascular malformation within the masseter muscle of a 10 year old.** Low signal areas represent calcific deposits (phleboliths).

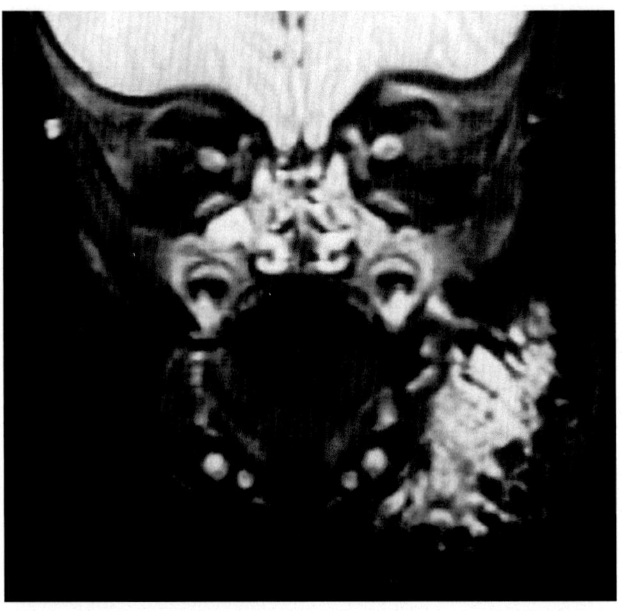

FIGURE 8-108 ■ **Lymphangioma in an infant.** Coronal STIR MRI.

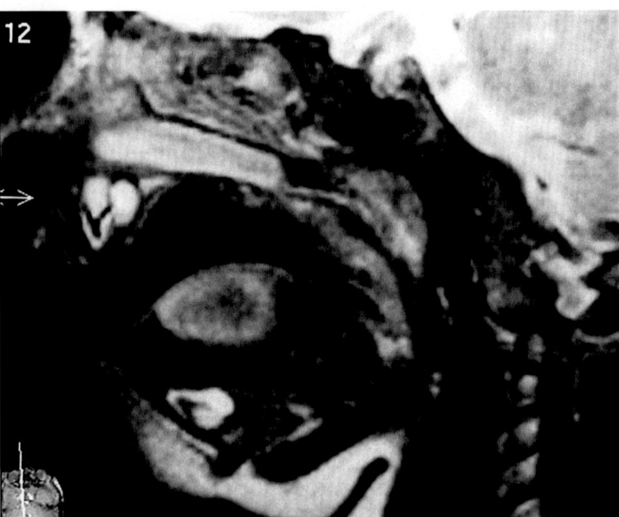

FIGURE 8-109 ■ **Fibroma of the tongue in an infant.** Sagittal T1-weighted MRI.

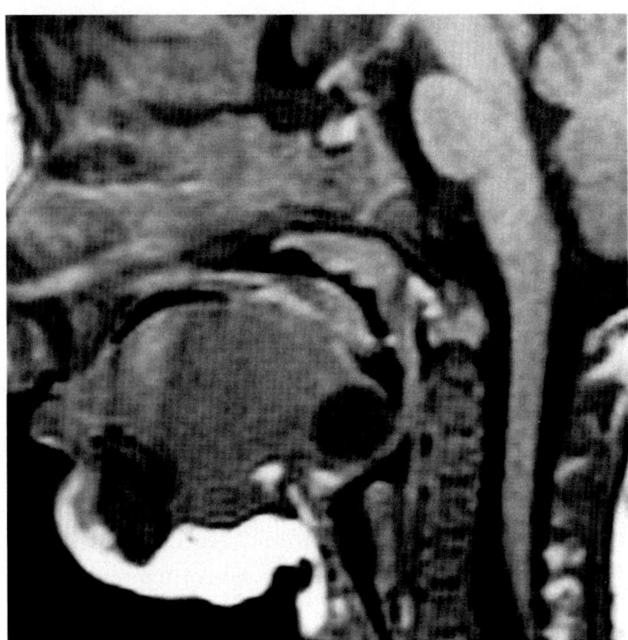

FIGURE 8-110 ■ **Thyroglossal cyst at base of tongue.** Sagittal T1-weighted MRI.

Calcification is occasionally seen in the walls of the facial and lingual arteries in patients with hypercalcaemia or renal failure. Small areas of subcutaneous calcification have been reported in Gorlin's syndrome and Ehlers–Danlos syndrome, and in acne and calcinosis cutis.

ANATOMY OF TEETH AND SUPPORTING STRUCTURES

Introduction

In the primary dentition, there are normally 20 teeth and 32 adult teeth. Both dentitons are identified using one of two systems illustrated in Table 8-1. The Zsigmondy system uses single digits for the permanent dentition and letters for the primary (deciduous) teeth, and the Fédération Dentaire Internationale (FDI) notation assigns double digits for each individual tooth (Figs. 8-111 and 8-112).[24]

Anatomy

All teeth consist of a crown and a root, which may be single or multiple (Fig. 8-113). The crown is covered with a layer of enamel, which is 97% mineral, and thus the most radiopaque tissue in the body. The bulk of the tooth consists of dentine, which is 70% mineralised. The

TABLE 8-1 The Zsigmondy (Single Digit) and FDI (Double Digit) Systems of Tooth Identification

Permanent Dentition

Upper Right								*Upper Left*							
(18)	(17)	(16)	(15)	(14)	(13)	(12)	(11)	(21)	(22)	(23)	(24)	(25)	(26)	(27)	(28)
8	7	6	5	4	3	2	1	1	2	3	4	5	6	7	8
8	7	6	5	4	3	2	1	1	2	3	4	5	6	7	8
(48)	(47)	(46)	(45)	(44)	(43)	(42)	(41)	(31)	(32)	(33)	(34)	(35)	(36)	(37)	(38)
Lower Right								*Lower Left*							

Primary Dentition

Upper Right					*Upper Left*				
(55)	(54)	(53)	(52)	(51)	(61)	(62)	(63)	(64)	(65)
E	D	C	B	A	A	B	C	D	E
E	D	C	B	A	A	B	C	D	E
(85)	(84)	(83)	(82)	(81)	(71)	(72)	(73)	(74)	(75)
Lower Right					*Lower Left*				

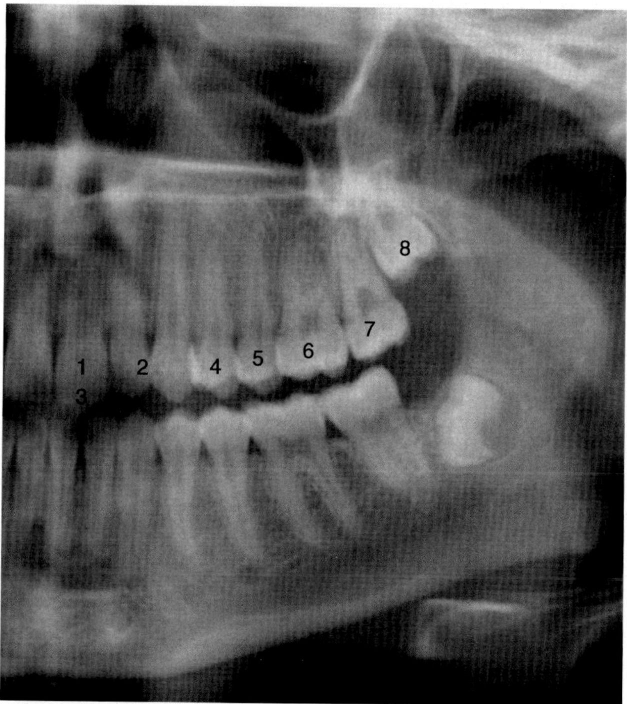

FIGURE 8-111 ■ Part of a panoramic radiograph showing the permanent dentition of a normal 18 year old. The teeth in the upper left quadrant have been numbered 1–8. The third molars are unerupted, incompletely formed and impacted.

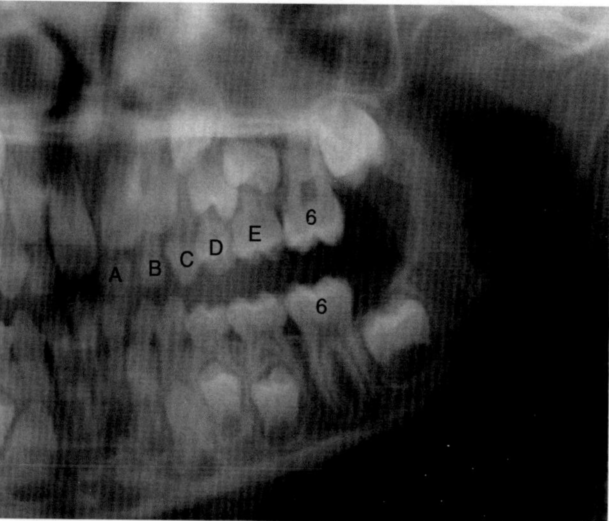

FIGURE 8-112 ■ Part of a panoramic radiograph showing the dentition in an 8 year-old child. The deciduous teeth in the upper left quadrant have been labelled A–E and the erupted first permanent molars (labelled 6).

root is covered by a thin layer of cementum, which has a radiodensity similar to that of dentine and so is indistinguishable from it. Lying within the centre of the tooth is the radiolucent soft tissue of the pulp, which runs from the pulp chamber within the crown along each root canal to the root apex, through which enter the neurovascular bundles. The tooth is supported in the jaws by the periodontal ligament, which consists largely of collagen fibres and appears as a narrow radiolucent line following the contours of the root. These fibres are inserted into a thin layer of dense cortical bone lining the tooth socket (lamina dura), which appears as a linear radiopaque structure, and is continuous with the cortical bone of the alveolar crest.

TOOTH ERUPTION

Normal Eruption

The normal eruption times are shown in Table 8-2. The primary teeth erupt between 6 and 24 months and the permanent teeth between 6 and 21 years. Root formation is not complete until 1.5–2 years and 2–3 years after eruption for the primary and permanent teeth, respectively.

Disorders of Tooth Eruption

The commonest cause for failure of full eruption is insufficient room in the dental arch to accommodate the erupting tooth. This particularly affects mandibular third molars and to a lesser extent maxillary canines. Alternatively a tooth may be prevented from erupting by, for example, a tumour, cyst or supernumerary tooth. Delayed

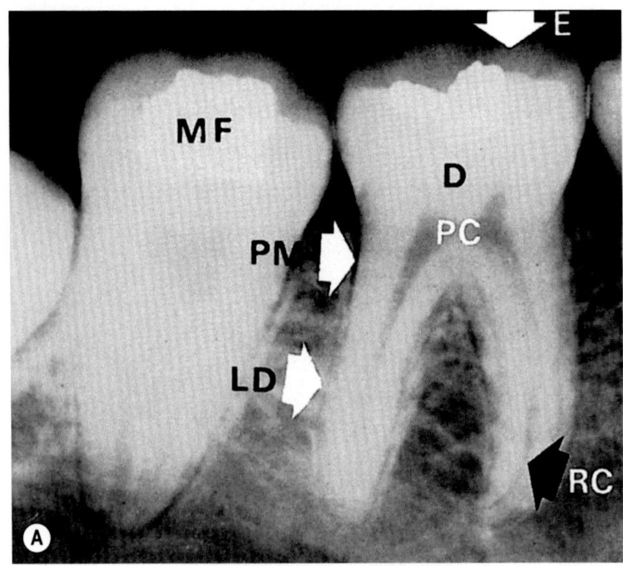

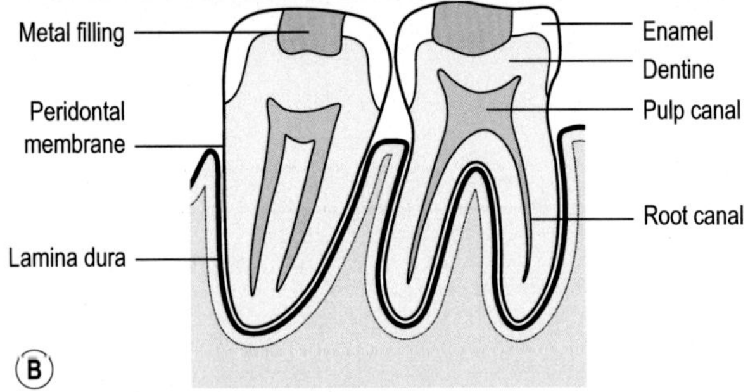

FIGURE 8-113 ■ (A) Periapical radiograph labelled to show a tooth and its supporting structures. E = enamel, D = dentine, PC = pulp chamber, RC = root canal, PM = periodontal membrane (periodontal ligament space), LD = lamina dura, MF = amalgam filling. (B) Corresponding line diagram.

TABLE 8-2 Approximate Dates of Eruption of the Primary and Permanent Teeth

Tooth	Designation	Age (months)
Primary Dentition		
Central incisors	A	6–8
Lateral incisors	B	7–10
Canines	C	16–20
First molars	D	10–14
Second molars	E	20–30
		Age (years)
Permanent Dentition		
Central incisors	1	6–7
Lateral incisors	2	7–9
Canines	3	9–12
First premolars	4	10–12
Second premolars	5	10–12
First molars	6	6–7
Second molars	7	11–13
Third molars	8	17–21

eruption occurs in certain endocrine disorders, e.g. hypothyroidism and some genetic abnormalities, e.g. Down's syndrome. Multiple failure of eruption of the permanent dentition is found in cleidocranial dysplasia (Fig. 8-114).

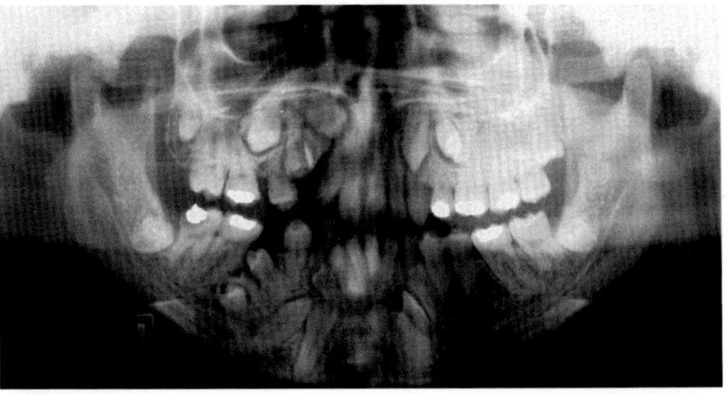

FIGURE 8-114 ■ **Panoramic radiograph of cleidocranial dysplasia in an adult.** There are numerous unerupted teeth including several supernumeraries.

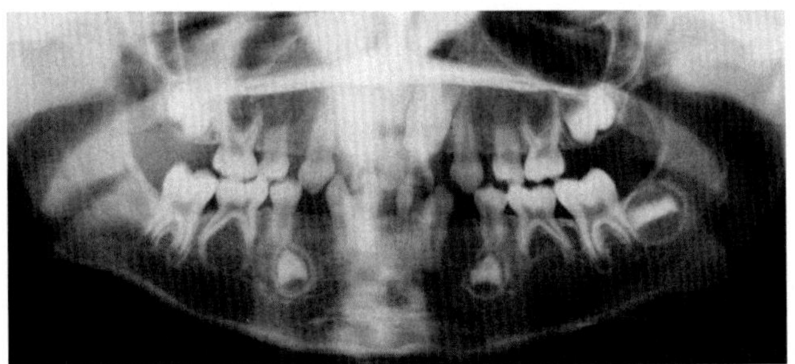

FIGURE 8-115 ■ **Panoramic radiograph showing a marked example of hypodontia involving both the primary deciduous and permanent dentitions in an 8 year-old child.** All four lateral incisors are missing from the primary deciduous dentition and 19 permanent teeth are also absent. Note that wisdom tooth formation normally starts between 9 and 13 years of age.

Disorders of Tooth Development

Variation in Tooth Number

Hypodontia is the absence of one or more teeth and anodontia (rare) where there is complete absence of teeth. Hypodontia most often affects third molars, mandibular second premolars and maxillary lateral incisors (Fig. 8-115). It is seen in association with cleft lip and palate, Ellis–van Creveld (chondroectodermal dysplasia) and facial-digital syndromes. Marked absence of teeth is seen in hypohydrotic ectodermal dysplasia.

Hyperdontia are teeth additional to the normal series and presents as either supplemental or supernumerary teeth. A supplemental tooth is an extra tooth identical in shape and form to an adjacent permanent one and is most frequently found in the lower premolar region. The commonest supernumerary teeth are mesiodens and tuberculates, which form in the maxillary midline. Mesiodens, which are small conical teeth, form chronologically after the primary upper central incisors and occasionally erupt. Tuberculate supernumeraries develop shortly after the formation of the permanent upper central incisors and usually impede their eruption. Marked hyperdontia in the permanent dentition is seen in cleidocranial dysplasia (Fig. 8-114).

Variation in Tooth Size

A tooth that is larger than normal is termed a macrodont and when smaller, a microdont, the latter being more common and typically affecting maxillary lateral incisors and upper wisdom teeth. Radiotherapy and/or chemotherapy can affect tooth development, resulting in arrested development such that they appear smaller than normal with short, spiculated roots (Fig. 8-116).

Variation of Tooth Form

Disturbance of tooth form can affect either the crown or root, or both, and may be developmental or acquired. A dens in dente is due to an infolding or invagination of the enamel into the underlying dentine towards the root, creating the appearance of a tooth within a tooth. A markedly hooked root is called dilaceration. It typically affects a maxillary central incisor either following traumatic intrusion of the primary incisor, which displaces the unerupted developing permanent incisor, or as a developmental anomaly. In taurodontism the pulp chamber is markedly elongated. A tooth that appears particularly enlarged may have split during its development (gemination) or may have become fused with an adjacent tooth.

DISTURBANCES IN STRUCTURE OF TEETH

Enamel

Enamel hypoplasia may affect a single tooth, following a localised periapical infection of its primary precursor

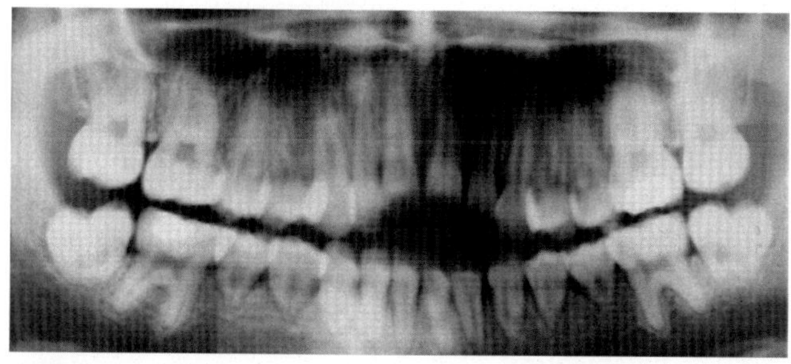

FIGURE 8-116 ■ Panoramic radiograph of a child aged 12 who received radiation to the neck for lymphoma when aged 5 years. The extent to which the roots have failed to form depends on their stage of development at the time of irradiation; thus the lower incisors, which had nearly completed root formation, are relatively unharmed. The lower first molars are slightly stunted and the premolars and second molars extensively shortened. Such teeth do not suffer from excessive mobility.

(Turner's tooth). But a more generalised form occurs as a complication of severe childhood infections or a nutritional deficiency with the manifestation depending on the time of the insult (chronological hypoplasia).

Amelogenesis imperfecta is a developmental disorder of enamel formation affecting all or most of the teeth in both dentitions. The enamel may show varying degrees of hypoplasia from being pitted (Fig. 8-117), to almost complete absence of enamel when the crown appears angular. Alternatively, the enamel may be of normal thickness but be hypomineralised such that its radiographic density is similar to that of dentine.

Dentine

Dentinogenesis imperfecta is a developmental anomaly of collagen formation that affects the dentine of both dentitions. The teeth are discoloured, having a brown or purple hue. The enamel readily chips away from the dentine so that the teeth rapidly wear down by attrition. The initial radiographic appearance shows bulbous crowns and large pulp chambers, which soon calcify with abnormal dentine formation so that little or none of the root canal is visible (Fig. 8-118). Although the teeth may appear sound, they are prone to infection, resulting in pulpal necrosis and periapical radiolucencies. The appearance of the bone of the mandible and maxilla remains normal, although type IV is associated with osteogenesis imperfecta.

Dentinal dysplasia resembles dentinogenesis imperfecta but is less common. In type I the crowns look normal in colour and shape but the roots of the primary and permanent teeth are short and abnormally shaped, and the pulp chambers become obliterated with dentine prior to eruption. In type II, loss of the pulp chamber and narrowing of the root canals occurs after tooth eruption. In some cases the pulp chambers may be thistle shaped.

Cementum

Hypercementosis describes the deposition of excessive amounts of cementum, typically around the apical half of the root so that it appears bulbous. Usually it is localised to one or two teeth as it is caused by chronic dental infection or occlusal overloading; however, it occurs in Paget's disease of the jaws (Table 8-3) and acromegaly where it is generalised.

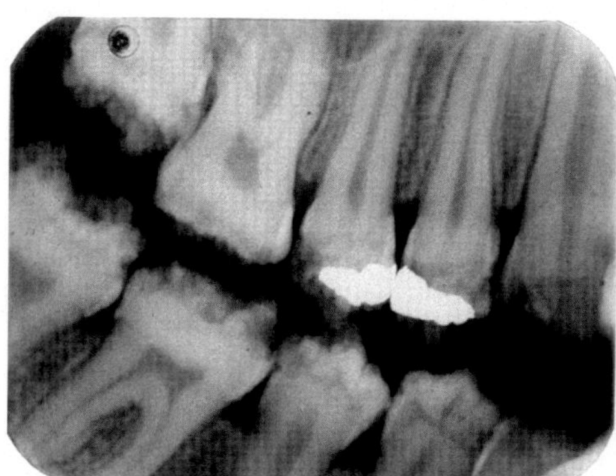

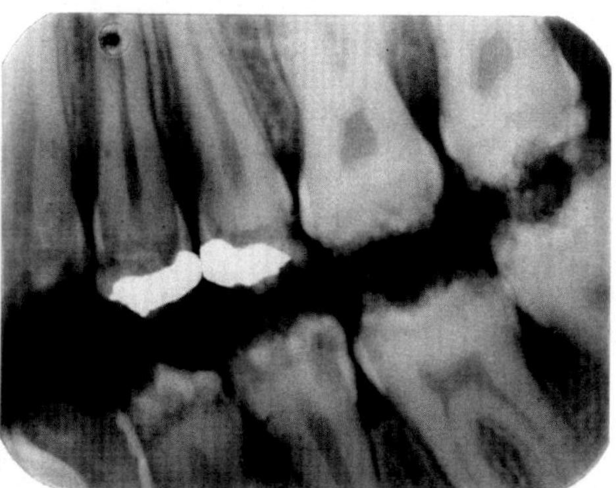

FIGURE 8-117 ■ Intraoral (bitewing) radiographs showing marked hypoplasia and pitting of the enamel, while the dentine appears normal. Several of the teeth are carious.

Miscellaneous Conditions

In **hypophosphataemia (vitamin D-resistant rickets),** the pulps of the primary and permanent teeth are enlarged with pulp horns that extend towards the enamel/dentine junction, making the pulps susceptible to infection so that the teeth frequently become abscessed. Similar dental features are noted in hypophosphatasia but there is often premature loss of the primary teeth. In both conditions the jaws usually appear osteoporotic (osteopenic).

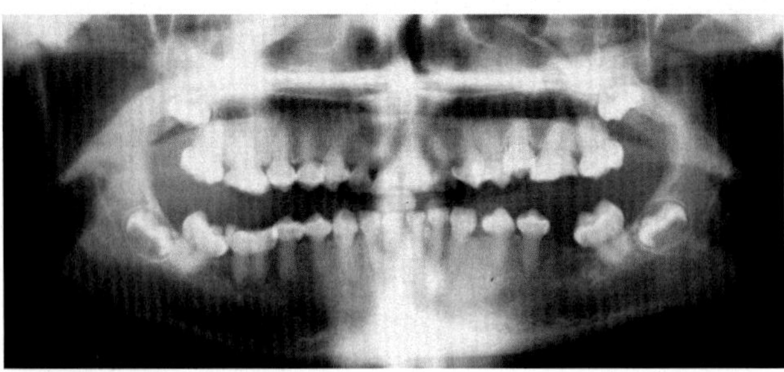

FIGURE 8-118 ■ A panoramic radiograph of a young adult with dentinogenesis imperfecta. The teeth have bulbous crowns, short stumpy roots and sclerosis of the root canals.

DENTAL CARIES

Dental caries is caused by microbial action on sugar with the formation of acid, which causes progressive demineralisation of the teeth, initially of the enamel, and then the dentine, with destruction of their organic components. If left untreated, it leads to the breakdown of the crown and subsequent bacterial infection of the pulp. It develops on the occlusal surfaces of the posterior teeth, on the approximal and cervical regions of the crown or root (if exposed), and as recurrent caries beneath restorations. The rate of mineral loss depends on a number of factors including the amount of sugar in the diet, the lack of effective oral hygiene, the presence of areas of food stagnation and

TABLE 8-3 **Differential Diagnosis of Localised Radiolucent and Radiopaque Lesions of the Jaws**

Unilocular Radiolucent	Multilocular Radiolucent	Radiopaque	Mixed Density
Common			
Alveolar abscess Apical granuloma Radicular cyst (apical) Residual cyst Dentigerous cyst Nasopalatine duct cyst Odontogenic keratocyst	Odontogenic keratocyst Central giant cell granuloma Ameloblastoma	Root fragment Dense bone island Mandibular torus Periapical sclerosing osteitis Hypercementosis Supernumerary tooth Sclerosing osteitis	Fibrous dysplasia (early) Cemento-ossifying fibroma Periapical cemento-osseous Compound odontome Complex odontome Florid cemento-osseous dysplasia Benign cementoblastoma (cementoma)
Uncommon			
Stafne's bone cavity Fibrous scar Fibrous dysplasia (early) Periapical cemento-osseous dysplasia (early) Osteomyelitis Giant cell tumour of hyperparathyroidism Central giant cell granuloma Ameloblastoma Lateral periodontal cyst Paget's disease (early) Brown's tumour of hyperparathyroidism	Giant cell tumour of hyperparathyroidism Ameloblastic fibroma Odontogenic myxoma	Fibrous dysplasia (late) Periapical cemento-osseous dysplasia Florid cemento-osseous dysplasia Ossifying fibroma (late) Complex odontome Compound odontome Paget's disease (late) Osteoma/exostosis	Chronic osteomyelitis Osteosarcoma Paget's disease
Rare			
Carcinoma Metastatic carcinoma Haemangioma Osteosarcoma Odontogenic myxoma Burkitt's lymphoma Lymphoma Eosinophilic granuloma Chondroma and chondrosarcoma Neurofibroma Neurilemmoma Odontogenic fibroma Ewing's tumour Myeloma	Aneurysmal bone cyst Haemangioma Cherubism Glandular odontogenic cyst	Metastatic carcinoma of prostate Cementoblastoma Osteosarcoma Chronic sclerosing osteomyelitis Chronic osteomyelitis Osteochondroma	Calcifying epithelial-odontogenic tumour (CEOT) Calcifying odontogenic cyst Osteoradionecrosis Adenomatoid odontogenic tumour Ameloblastic fibro-odontoma

the health of the individual. It is particularly rapid in those with reduced saliva production following radiation damage to the salivary glands.

The detection of dental decay requires images with good contrast and resolution. Bitewing radiographs are valuable in the detection and monitoring of dental decay, particularly on surfaces not easily visualised and for occult occlusal caries, which can be extensive beneath an apparently intact enamel surface. Panoramic radiographs can be used for gross and widespread dental decay.

A carious lesion appears as a radiolucent zone, corresponding to an area of demineralisation. An initial approximal lesion develops in the enamel just below the contact point with an adjacent tooth appearing as a small triangular shape with the apex pointing towards the dentine. As the lesion progresses, its advancing surface broadens as it extends along the enamel–dentine junction but also penetrates into the dentine, this margin being ill defined (Fig. 8-119). Adjacent carious lesions commonly develop on contiguous tooth surfaces. If left untreated, the caries reaches the pulp chamber and the weakened crown eventually crumbles away. A similar progression is seen on other tooth surfaces. The radiographic detection of dental caries can be difficult, particularly when the crown remains intact and the carious lesion is only marginally more radiolucent relative to the surrounding dentine.

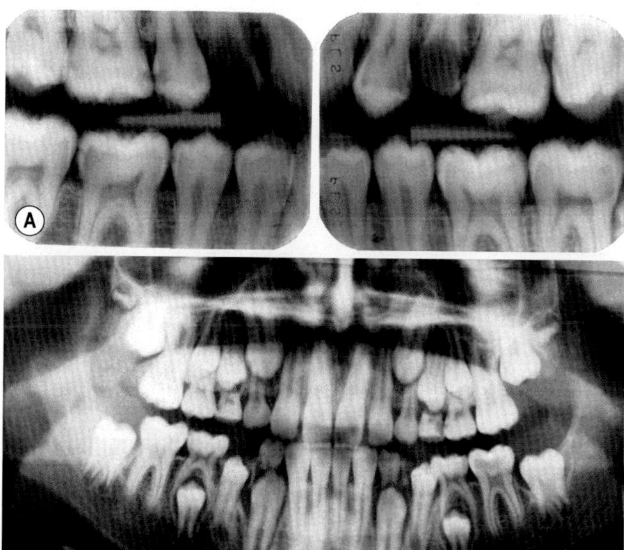

FIGURE 8-119 ■ (A) Bitewing radiographs showing gross caries with crown destruction affecting the upper right first and upper left second premolars. There is approximal caries, shown as radiolucencies of the crowns, at the contact points of the other remaining upper premolars, upper and lower right first molars and occlusal caries in the upper left first molar. (B) Panoramic radiograph of a child aged 10 in the mixed dentition. There is early approximal caries in the upper right deciduous first and second molars. There is gross caries distally in the upper left deciduous first molar, which has complete root resorption by the erupting successional premolar. The lower left permanent first molar has gross recurrent occlusal caries beneath a very small restoration. There is less extensive recurrent caries in the lower right permanent first molar. Both these teeth show periapical bone changes, most obviously the widening of the periodontal ligament space on the mesial root of the lower left permanent first molar, consistent with periapical periodontitis.

DISORDERS OF THE PULP

When dental decay extends to the pulp it usually results in acute inflammation (acute pulpitis), causing severe toothache, but has no radiological manifestations. Chronic pulpitis is much less painful or asymptomatic and results in regressive changes of the pulp due to chronic irritation such as calcific deposits (pulp stones) and sclerosis (narrowing) of the root canals. Generalised pulp sclerosis is a feature of renal osteodystrophy and prolonged corticosteroid therapy. Internal resorption of the root canal or external resorption of the outer root surface may occur following pulp death.

Periapical Periodontitis

Pulpal necrosis results from acute pulpitis (see earlier) or from dental trauma causing interruption of the pulp's blood supply. Bacterial action on the necrotic pulp within the root canal leads to the production of endotoxins, which exit the root apex and incite a periapical inflammatory response within the periodontal membrane (periodontitis) and dental abscess formation. When this is acute, the patient suffers severe discomfort and the offending tooth is tender to touch. Apical periodontitis presents as a widened periodontal ligament space, which appears more prominent than normal. However, the condition may also be chronic and continued progression of the chronic inflammatory process eventually leads to loss of the apical lamina dura and the formation of a discrete periapical radiolucency (Fig. 8-120) due to development of a focal inflammatory lesion, either a granuloma, radicular cyst or chronic abscess. When small, all three conditions have a similar radiographic appearance: i.e. a periapical radiolucency that is circular or oval, usually well defined, the outline being continuous with the remaining lamina dura around the root. Conversely, lower-grade stimulation from a non-vital tooth may result in reactive bone formation (sclerosing osteitis), which appears as an irregularly shaped, largely uniform area of dense bone at the root apex (Fig. 8-121).

CYSTS OF THE JAWS

Cysts occur in the jaws more frequently than in any other bone because of the numerous epithelial cell residues left after tooth formation. Generally they are slow growing and painless unless infected; however, some may reach a considerable size before detection.

Cysts of the jaws are divided into odontogenic, when they arise from epithelial residues of the tooth-forming tissues, or non-odontogenic, these being uncommon and mainly developmental, arising from epithelium not involved with tooth formation. The four most common

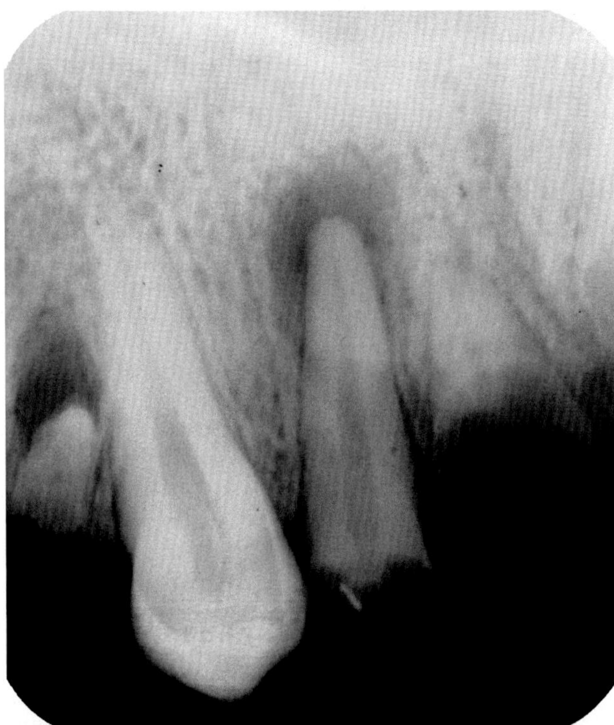

FIGURE 8-120 ■ Periapical granuloma at the apex of the grossly decayed upper right lateral incisor. Although well defined, its margins are not corticated. Note the loss of the lamina dura at the tooth apex. There is a similar but smaller lesion at the apex of the exfoliating upper right first premolar root and the upper right central incisor is markedly carious.

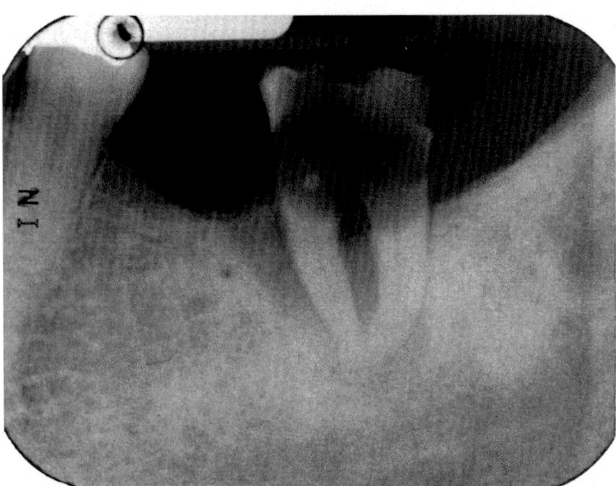

FIGURE 8-121 ■ Periapical radiograph showing sclerosing osteitis. The lower left molar is grossly decayed and its root is surrounded by a zone of radiolucency beyond which the bone is dense as shown by the lack of trabecular spaces.

odontogenic cysts are the inflammatory radicular (dental) and residual cysts, and the developmental dentigerous cyst and odontogenic keratocyst now called the keratocystic odontogenic tumour.

Odontogenic and non-odontogenic cysts have a number of radiological features in common that are characteristic of slow-growing lesions; i.e. they are radiolucent, well defined and often have a cortical margin. With the exception of the odontogenic keratocyst, they have raised intracystic pressure and expand by tissue fluid transudation, and so appear as circular or oval in shape. When large, the bony cortex of the jaws becomes thinned, expanded and then perforated. Jaw cysts tend to displace structures such as tooth roots, unerupted teeth, the inferior alveolar canal and the antral floor.

Odontogenic Cysts

Radicular cyst is the most common (over 50%) of the odontogenic cysts and develops at the apex of a non-vital tooth (see above periapical periodontitis). It arises from the cell rests of Malassez, which are epithelial remnants of root formation found in the periodontal ligament. Any tooth can be affected, but the majority are found on the permanent anterior teeth or first molars. When small (less than 15 mm in diameter) they resemble periapical granulomas but, unlike granulomas, can enlarge well beyond this size (Fig. 8-122). In the upper jaw they expand in to the maxillary sinus, displacing the antral floor.

In many cases extraction of the causative tooth brings about resolution, but when this does not happen, the cyst is then termed a **'residual cyst'**. Thus a residual cyst found in an edentulous part of the jaw has a well-defined, circular radiolucency usually with a cortical margin. A number may regress without treatment and some show dystrophic mineralisation.

Dentigerous cysts (follicular cysts) arise from the reduced enamel epithelium, the tissue which surrounds the crown of an unerupted tooth. They are thus found only on teeth that are buried, particularly mandibular third molars and maxillary canines (Fig. 8-123). Cystic enlargement of the tooth follicle produces a pericoronal radiolucency, which is attached to the tooth at its neck, with the crown appearing to lie within the cyst lumen; however, with large cysts this relationship may not be apparent.

Previously known as the **odontogenic keratocyst**, the WHO now recommend this lesion is called **keratocystic odontogenic tumour** because of its aggressive behaviour, high mitotic activity and association with chromosomal mutation of the PTCH gene. It arises from remnants of the dental lamina, the precursor of the tooth germ. The cyst is thought to enlarge by mural growth, thus behaving more like a benign neoplasm. It appears as a unilocular or multiloculated, elongated, irregularly shaped radiolucency with a scalloped, well-defined margin (Fig. 8-124). It lacks the more rounded characteristics of other odontogenic cysts appearing elongated, an important diagnostic feature. Keratocysts occur most often in the lower third molar/ramus region, where they may displace an unerupted wisdom tooth and resemble a dentigerous cyst. Recurrence is common, being 5–20%, so radiographic follow-up is necessary for at least 5 years. On non-enhanced CT, attenuation values of cyst fluid vary and although most are low the value can range from 30 to 200 Hounsfield units (HU), depending on the proteinaceous content with long-standing, multilocular cysts

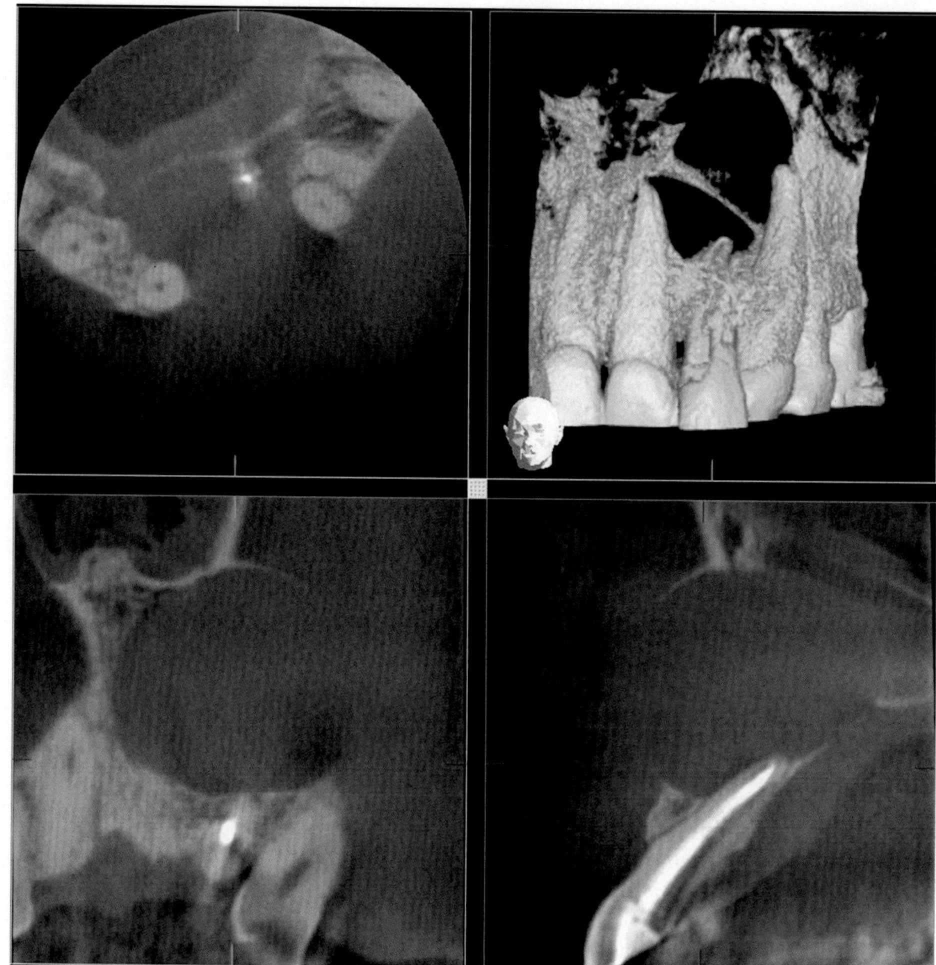

FIGURE 8-122 ■ CBCT sections in three planes showing a corticated radiolucent lesion associated with the **apex** of a root-filled upper left lateral incisor, causing expansion and thinning of the bone buccally and palatally, and of the nasal floor.

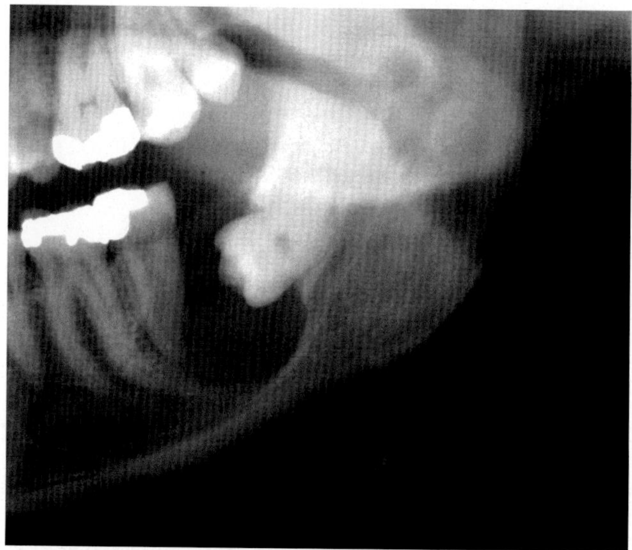

FIGURE 8-123 ■ Part of a panoramic radiograph of a dentigerous cyst arising on a lower left wisdom tooth, which is unerupted and lying horizontally. It appears as a well-defined, circular radiolucency attached to the tooth at its neck. The inferior alveolar canal has been displaced inferiorly.

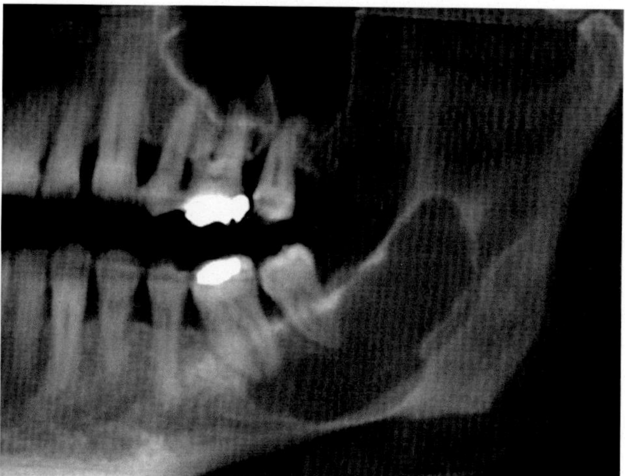

FIGURE 8-124 ■ Part of a panoramic-style MPR on CBCT of an odontogenic keratocyst which appears as an elongated, loculated radiolucency extending from the mandibular foramen to the lower first molar region. There is thinning of the bony cortices but no jaw expansion, a feature associated with odontogenic keratocysts.

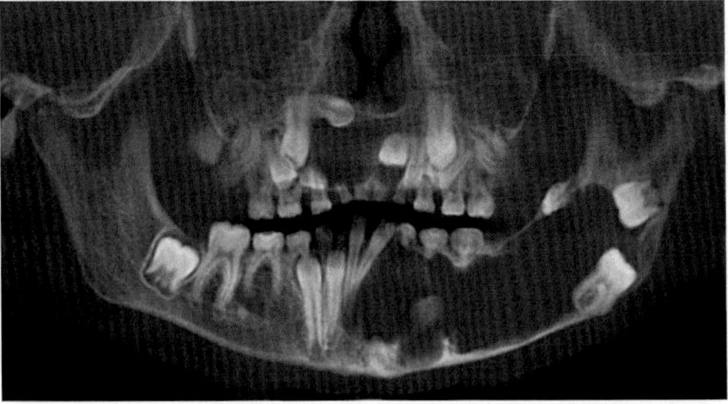

FIGURE 8-125 ■ Panoramic-style MPR on CBCT showing odontogenic keratocysts in the left mandible and anterior maxilla consistent with **Gorlin–Goltz syndrome**. There is marked displacement of teeth by the cysts, which show minimal expansion.

having the higher value.[25] On MRI the lesion has a low or intermediate signal in T1 but a high T2 signal.

Multiple odontogenic keratocysts are a feature of Gorlin–Goltz syndrome (naevoid basal cell carcinoma syndrome; Fig. 8-125), which also includes multiple basal cell naevi, calcification of the falx, bifid ribs, synostosis of the ribs, kyphoscoliosis, temporal and parietal bossing, hyperptelorism and shortening of the metacarpals.

There are several other less common odontogenic cysts. The lateral periodontal cyst is found on the lateral surface of a vital tooth root between two adjacent teeth, usually the lower incisor or canine teeth. The glandular odontogenic cyst (sialo-odontogenic cyst) mainly occurs in the anterior body of the mandible, as a multilocular or lobular, often large radiolucency that may cross the midline and has a tendency to recur.

Non-Odontogenic Cysts

The **nasopalatine cyst** is probably the commonest non-odontogenic cyst that is believed to arise from epithelial residues in the nasopalatine canal. It appears as a round, well-defined, midline radiolucency between, but not associated with, the upper central incisor teeth.

Cyst-Like Lesions

Three other lesions are now described that also resemble jaw cysts but have no epithelial lining. The solitary bone cyst occurs during the first two decades of life, mainly in the premolar/molar regions of the mandible. Its margin is less well defined than those of odontogenic cysts and its superior border typically arches up between the roots of the adjacent teeth (Fig. 8-126). Tooth displacement and root resorption is uncommon. At surgery an empty cavity is found, which subsequently heals after bleeding has been induced.

The **aneurysmal bone cyst** is considered to be a reactive lesion of bone and is characterised by a fibrous connective tissue stroma containing many cavernous blood-filled spaces. It is rare and occurs mainly in the young, with over 90% occurring before 30 years of age.

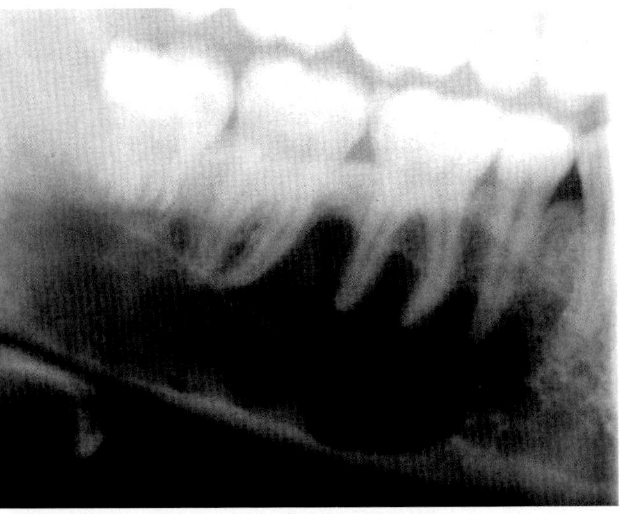

FIGURE 8-126 ■ Part of a panoramic radiograph showing a partially corticated radiolucency in the right mandible involving the apices of the second premolar and first and second molars diagnosed as a solitary bone cyst. Note the characteristic scalloping between the roots of the first and second molars.

It is typically found in the posterior region of the mandible as a well-defined, multilocular, often septated, circular radiolucency. It has a tendency to produce marked cortical expansion. On MRI it has a low-to-intermediate signal on T1- and T2-weighted images. A useful but nonexclusive feature is fluid levels due to blood-filled cavities which are more easily seen on MRI than with CT.

Stafne's bone cavity is asymptomatic and typically found in men over the age of 35 years. It forms a depression in the lingual cortex of the mandible just in front of the angle and below the inferior dental canal. Its origin is controversial and it has been postulated that it arises from pressure from the submandibular salivary gland; however, whereas some may contain salivary gland tissue, a number develop anterior to the gland. On plain radiographs, it appears as a well-defined, punched-out, dense radiolucency which rarely exceeds 2 cm in diameter (Fig. 8-127). Its appearance is characteristic and so does not require further imaging or biopsy. However, if CT or MRI is performed, the cavity is often found to contain fat.

DISEASE OF THE PERIODONTIUM

Introduction

There are several disorders that affect the support for the teeth, the **periodontium**, and these are referred to as periodontal disease. Intraoral views (bitewings and periapical films) are helpful in assessing the amount of remaining bone support for the teeth, the pattern of bone loss, the detection of subgingival calculus and local aggravating factors such as poorly contoured dental restorations. Dental panoramic radiography can be used for widespread advanced disease, although it does not demonstrate the anterior teeth particularly well.

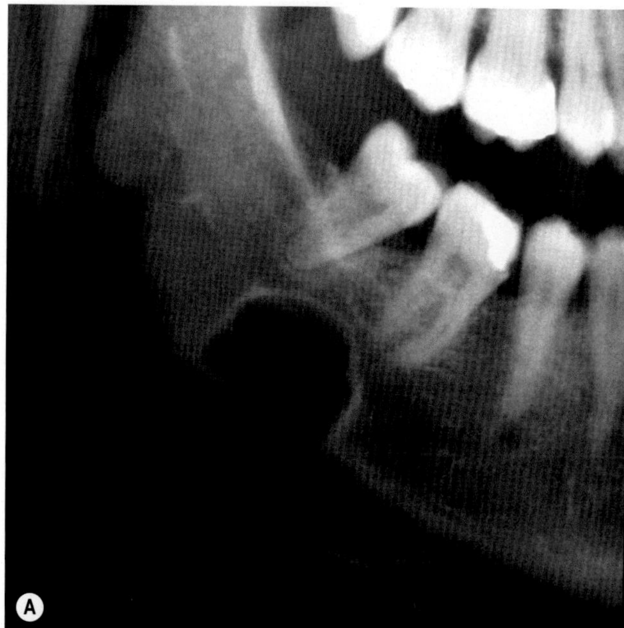
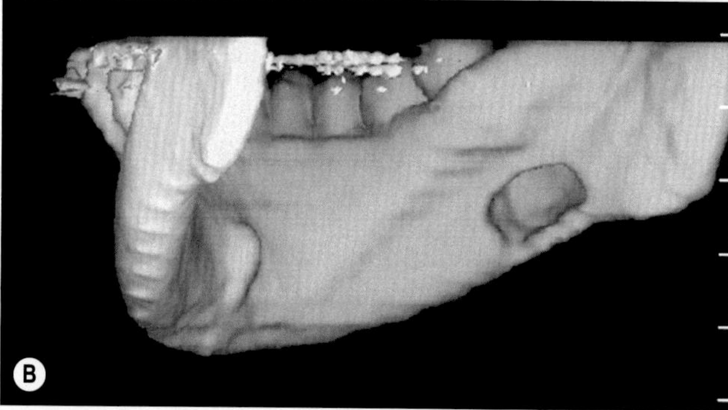

FIGURE 8-127 ■ (A) Part of a panoramic radiograph showing a corticated radiolucency between the inferior alveolar canal and the lower border of the mandible due to the presence of a Stafne's bone cavity. The 3D CT (B) shows the depression on the lingual aspect of the mandible.

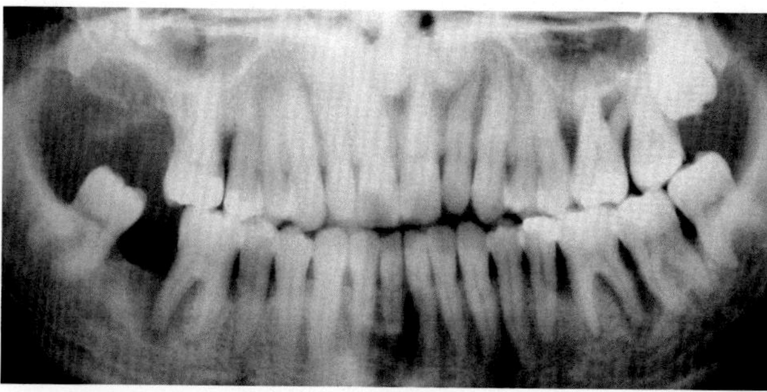

FIGURE 8-128 ■ **Part of a panoramic radiograph of a man aged 40 with smoking-related aggressive chronic periodontal disease.** There is furcation involvement of the upper left first molar and loss of up to 70% of the bony attachment between the upper right first molar and second premolar and similarly on the upper left side. Combined periodontal–endodontic lesions affect both lower first molars.

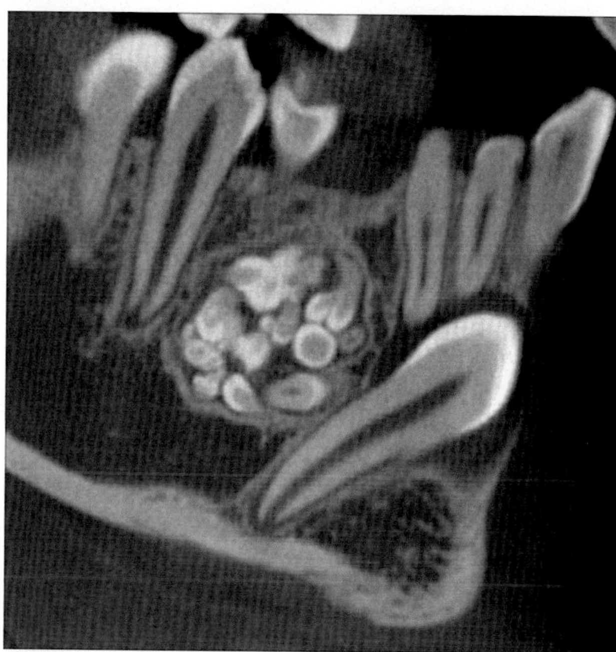

FIGURE 8-129 ■ **CBCT parasagittal slice showing a compound odontome consisting of numerous small teeth (denticles).** The odontome has displaced and prevented the lower right canine from erupting.

Chronic periodontitis results from the accumulation of dental plaque on the teeth, initially causing low-grade inflammation of the gingivae (gingivitis) with subsequent progression to involve the periodontal tissues. Gingivitis, which causes bleeding of the gums during tooth brushing, has no radiological features. Chronic periodontitis is a painless condition that affects almost all adults to a greater or lesser extent and results in slow but gradual horizontal bone loss from the alveolar crest so that the teeth lose their support. Advanced periodontitis affects 10–15% of the population, with smoking and poor oral hygiene being specific risk factors. A particularly aggressive form called rapidly progressive periodontitis occurs in young adults, where several teeth are affected by vertical bone loss resulting in angular bony defects that extend down towards the tooth apex (Fig. 8-128). Symmetrical widening of the periodontal ligament space affecting several teeth is sometimes seen in progressive systemic sclerosis or as irregular localised widening as an early feature of osteosarcoma of the jaws.

ODONTOMES AND ODONTOGENIC TUMOURS

As a generalisation, odontogenic disorders occur or are centred upon the tooth-bearing parts of the jaws, whereas lesions not involving the jaw alveolus, e.g. those lying predominantly below the inferior dental canal, are usually non-odontogenic.

Odontomes are developmental malformations or hamartomas consisting of dental hard tissues or tooth-like structures. Most are diagnosed in the second decade of life and frequently impede tooth eruption. There are two main types. The compound odontome consists of a collection of small discrete teeth called denticles (Fig. 8-129) and is found typically in the anterior region of the

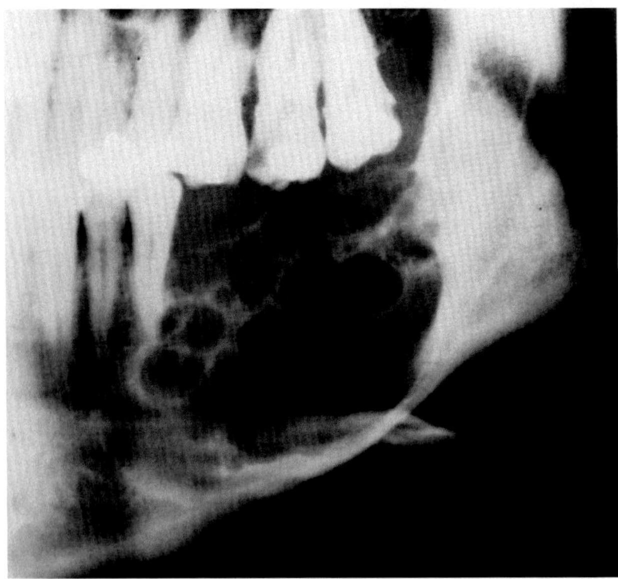

FIGURE 8-130 ■ Part of a panoramic radiograph showing an ameloblastoma, which appears as an expansile, multilocular radiolucency involving the left body of the mandible.

FIGURE 8-131 ■ An axial CT on bone window settings of a large cystic ameloblastoma of the right side of the mandible showing marked thinning and expansion of the bone. Note the presence of root resorption.

maxilla, whereas the complex odontome consists of a randomly arranged mass of enamel, dentine and cementum and is found mostly in the lower premolar/molar region. Both types are densely radiopaque due to the presence of tooth enamel and are surrounded by a thin radiolucent capsular space and radiopaque cortical margin. There are several minor developmental anomalies also classified as odontomes that can resemble teeth.

Odontogenic tumours are uncommon, mostly benign and arise either from the odontogenic epithelium, odontogenic epithelium and ectomesenchyme, or primarily from ectomesenchyme. The **ameloblastoma** accounts for 11% of all odontogenic tumours. It occurs mainly in patients between 30 and 50 years of age, with most (80%) forming in the molar/ramus region of the mandible. When the maxilla is involved, it has the potential to spread insidiously to involve the infratemporal fossa, orbit and skull base; thus a thorough assessment is essential. The ameloblastoma has a variable radiographic appearance, being a unilocular or multilocular radiolucency, but typically contains septa or locules of variable size to produce a soap bubble appearance (Fig. 8-130). The margin is well defined, often corticated but, when large, produces jaw expansion with perforation of the bony cortex. A useful diagnostic feature is knife-edge resorption of the tooth roots by the tumour, which can be quite marked.

The lesion is locally aggressive and requires a wide excisional margin, so accurate presurgical assessment of the bone integrity is necessary. Contrast-enhanced CT will show the tumour–bone interface but has poor soft-tissue delineation. Multislice CT can be used to differentiate ameloblastoma from keratocystic odontogenic tumours which they resemble, because of higher-density increase during the arterial phase.[26] On T1-weighted images with gadolinium enhancement and T2-weighted images, there is good conspicuity of the tumour margin with the soft tissues, the lesion having a moderate-to-high signal. There is a rare malignant variety in which the ameloblastoma probably undergoes malignant transformation, with metastases most often occurring in the lungs.[27] The unicystic ameloblastoma occurs around the age of 20 years and often causes marked bony expansion (Fig. 8-131).

The **odontogenic myxoma** is a benign but locally aggressive tumour of odontogenic mesenchyme occurring mainly in those younger than 45 years of age. Most occur in the mandible in the premolar/molar region. The lesion is usually well defined, is unilocular and contains a variable number of straight internal coarse trabeculations to produce a reticular pattern.

There are many types of odontogenic tumour; however, two lesions that are well defined and contain variable amounts of focal mineral deposits are the calcifying epithelial odontogenic tumour and the adenomatoid odontogenic tumour. The former is more common in men, occurs in middle life and is found mainly in the premolar/molar region of the mandible. The latter mainly affects females in the second decade of life and typically occurs anteriorly, especially in the maxilla, and is associated with an unerupted tooth. The cementoblastoma is the only neoplasm of cementum; it is rare and mainly affects young males. It appears as an encapsulated radiopaque mass attached to the root, usually of a lower posterior tooth.

IMAGING IN IMPLANTOLOGY

Dental implants are placed into the jaws to replace missing teeth or give anchorage for dental prostheses. These have gained considerable popularity since the discovery, by Branemark, that endosseous titanium implants

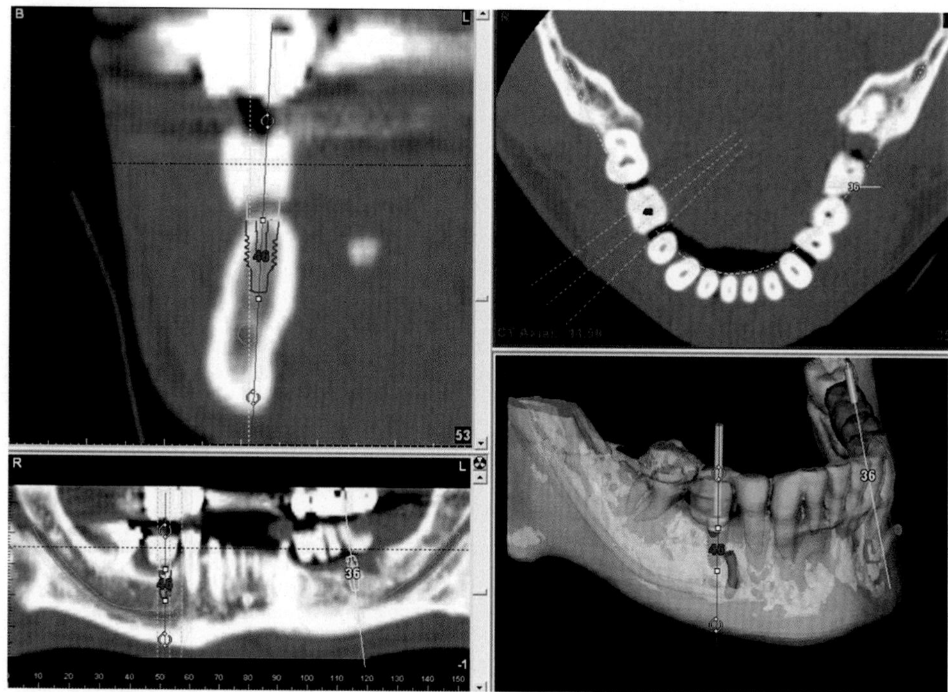

FIGURE 8-132 ■ Images reconstructed from fine axial CT slices of an implant site within the mandible (SimPlant). An original axial slice is cross-referenced with a cross-sectional slice, a panoramic-like reconstruction and 3D surface-rendered views. The software allows precise planning of implant placement to avoid injury to adjacent structures and helps predict the aesthetic outcome. (Courtesy of Mr Sean Goldner.)

could successfully integrate with bone. Imaging plays an essential role in pre-implant assessment, defining the volume and quality of recipient bone, identifying the location of relevant anatomical structures such as the inferior dental canal, the floor of the nose and maxillary antrum, and in assessing the status of adjacent teeth. Postoperatively, imaging is necessary to examine the degree of healing and monitor osseointegration.[28]

Intraoral periapical and dental panoramic radiography are valuable for initial preoperative assessment but cannot identify volume of a recipient bone site or accurately localise key structures and are prone to distortion. Cross-sectional imaging provides accurate information in all three planes and is particularly indicated in complex cases. CT data from multiple contiguous 1- to 2-mm slices taken parallel to the maxillary hard palate or lower border of mandible are reformatted by dedicated multi-planar reconstruction programmes to give cross-sectional slices cross-referenced with axial plan views of the dental arch. CBCT offers a similar imaging capability but with better resolution and substantially lower radiation exposure, due to use of exclusively hard tissue imaging parameters. Dedicated software packages depict the course of the inferior alveolar canal and allow 'trial placement of virtual implants' to assist with optimum implant location (Fig. 8-132). National and European selection or referral guidelines are available for the use of CBCT and implant assessment.[29,30] MRI has also been shown to be a feasible alternative to CT.[31] A radiographic localisation plate (stent) is generally needed for any form of cross-sectional imaging to indicate chosen implant sites—this may be metallic (tomography), gutta percha or brass (CT) or gadolinium (MRI).

In the postoperative phase intraoral periapical radiographs taken perpendicular to the implant, are most useful, monitoring osseointegration and identifying peri-implant bone loss, especially at the neck, which may indicate early failure of integration.

TRAUMA

Teeth

The teeth, particularly the upper incisors, are frequently involved in traumatic injuries to the face. They may be partially or completely avulsed or the crowns or roots may be fractured. Crown fractures may just involve the enamel, or the enamel and dentine, or if at a lower level expose the pulp. Root fractures occur less frequently and if undisplaced can be difficult to detect on radiographs when two different angled views may be required. Dental trauma can be associated with a localised dento-alveolar fracture in which a block of bone becomes detached containing several teeth. Intraoral radiographs best demonstrate traumatic injuries of the teeth.

REFERENCES

1. Lee YY, van Tassel P, Nauert C, et al. Craniofacial osteosarcomas: plain film, CT, and MRI findings in 46 cases. Am J Roentgenol 1988;150:1397–402.
2. Jank S, Emshoff R, Etzelsdorfer M, et al. Ultrasound versus computed tomography in the imaging of orbital floor fractures. J Oral Maxillofac Surg 2004;62:150–4.
3. iRefer. Making the Best Use of Clinical Radiology. 7th ed. Royal College of Radiologists; 2012.

4. Larheim TA. Role of magnetic resonance imaging in the clinical diagnosis of the temporomandibular joint. Cells Tissues Organs 2005;180(1):6–21.
5. Wilson DJ. Imaging. In: de B Norman JE, Bramley P, editors. A Textbook and Colour Atlas of the Temporomandibular Joint. London: Wolfe; 1990. pp. 90–109.
6. Brown JE, Drage NA, Escudier MP, et al. Minimally invasive radiologically guided intervention for the treatment of salivary calculi. Cardiovasc Intervent Radiol 2002;25:352–5.
7. Drage NA, Brown JE, Escudier MP, et al. Balloon dilatation of salivary duct strictures—report on 36 treated glands. Cardiovasc Intervent Radiol 2002;25:356–9.
8. Niemela RK, Takalo R, Paakko E, et al. Ultrasonography of salivary glands in primary Sjögren's syndrome. A comparison with magnetic resonance imaging and magnetic resonance sialography of parotid glands. Rheumatology 2004;43:875–9.
9. Ohbayashi N, Yamada I, Yoshino N, Sasaki T. Sjögren syndrome: comparison at assessments with MR sialography and conventional sialography. Radiology 1998;209:683–8.
10. Uchida Y, Minoshima S, Kawata T, et al. Diagnostic value of FDG PET and salivary gland scintigraphy for parotid tumors. Clin Nucl Med 2005;30:170–6.
11. Jones J, Farag I, Hain SF, McGurk M. Positron emission tomography (PET) in the management of oro-pharyngeal cancer. Eur J Surg Oncol 2005;31:170–6.
12. Becker M, Marchal F, Becker CD, et al. Sialolithiasis and salivary ductal stenosis: diagnostic accuracy of MR sialography with a three-dimensional extended-phase conjugate symmetry rapid spin-echo sequence. Radiology 2000;217:347–58.
13. Ngu RK, Brown JE, Whaites EJ, et al. Salivary duct strictures: nature and incidence in benign salivary obstruction. Dentomaxillofac Radiol 2007;36(2):63–7.
14. Ahuja AT, Richards PS, Wong KT, et al. Kuttner tumour (chronic sclerosing sialadenitis) of the submandibular gland: sonographic appearances. Ultrasound Med Biol 2003;29:913–19.
15. Voulgarelis M, Moutsopoulos HM. Mucosa-associated lymphoid tissue lymphoma in Sjögren's syndrome: risks, management, and prognosis. Rheum Dis Clin North Am 2008;34(4):921–33, viii.
16. Makdissi J, Escudier MP, Brown JE, et al. Glandular function after intraoral removal of salivary calculi from the hilum of the submandibular gland. Br J Oral Maxillofac Surg 2004;42: 538–41.
17. Evans RM, Ahuja A, Rhys Williams S, et al. Ultrasound and ultrasound guided fine needle aspiration in cervical lymphadenopathy. Br J Radiol 1991;64(P):58.
18. Ying M, Ahuja A, Brooks F. Accuracy of sonographic vascular features in differentiating different causes of cervical lymphadenopathy. Ultrasound Med Biol 2004;30:441–7.
19. Wide JM, White DW, Woolgar JA, et al. Magnetic resonance imaging in the assessment of cervical nodal metastases in oral squamous cell carcinoma. Clin Radiol 1999;54:90–4.
20. Kovacs AF, Dobert N, Gaa J, et al. Positron emission tomography in combination with sentinal node biopsy reduces the rate of elective neck dissections in the treatment of oral and oropharyngeal cancer. J Clin Oncol 2004;22:3973–80.
21. El-Sayed IH, Singer MI, Civantos F. Sentinel lymph node biopsy in head and neck cancer. Otolaryngol Clin North Am 2005;38:145–60, ix–x.
22. Schwartz DL, Ford E, Rajendran J, et al. FGD-PET/CT imaging for preradiotherapy staging of head-and-neck squamous cell carcinoma. Int J Radiat Oncol Biol Phys 2005;61:129–36.
23. Morse M, Brown EF. Ultrasonic diagnosis of masseteric hypertrophy. Dentomaxillofacial Radiol 1990;19:18–20.
24. Browne RM, Edmondson HD, Rout PGJ. Atlas of Dental and Maxillofacial Radiology. London: Mosby-Wolfe; 1995.
25. Yoshiura K, Higuchi Y, Ariji Y, et al. Increased attenuation in odontogenic keratocysts with computed tomography: a new finding. Dentomaxillofac Radiol 1994;23:138–42.
26. Kawai T, Murakami S, Kishino M, et al. Diagnostic imaging in two cases of recurrent maxillary ameloblastoma: comparative evaluation of plain radiographs, CT and MR images Br J Oral Maxillofac Surg 1998;36:304–10.
27. Verneuil A, Sapp P, Huang C, et al. Malignant ameloblastoma: classification, diagnostic, and therapeutic challenges. Am J Otolaryngol 2002;23:44–8.
28. Faculty of General Dental Practitioners (UK). Selection Criteria for Dental Radiography. 2nd ed. London: Royal College of Surgeons of England; 2004.
29. European Commission. Radiation Protection 172. Evidence Based Guidelines on Cone Beam CT for Dental and Maxillofacial Radiology. Office for Official Publications of the European Communities, Luxembourg. Available at: <http://ec.europa.eu/energy/nuclear/radiation_protection/publications_en.htm>. Accessed 13 March 2012.
30. Health Protection Agency. Guidance on the Safe Use Of Dental Cone Beam Computed Tomography (CBCT) Equipment 2010.
31. Gray C, Redpath TW, Smith FW. Low-field magnetic resonance imaging for implant dentistry. Dentomaxillofacial Radiol 1998;27: 225–9.

Subject Index

Page numbers followed by '*f*' indicate figures, '*t*' indicate tables, and '*b*' indicate boxes.

Notes

To simplify the index, the main terms of imaging techniques (e.g. computed tomography, magnetic resonance imaging etc.) are concerned only with the technology and general applications. Users are advised to look for specific anatomical features and diseases/disorders for individual imaging techniques used.

vs. indicates a comparison or differential diagnosis.

To save space in the index, the following abbreviations have been used:

CHD—congenital heart disease
CMR—cardiac magnetic resonance
CT—computed tomography
CXR—chest X-ray
DECT—dual-energy computed tomography
DWI-MRI—diffusion weighted imaging-magnetic resonance imaging
ERCP—endoscopic retrograde cholangiopancreatography
EUS—endoscopic ultrasound
FDG-PET—fluorodeoxyglucose positron emission tomography
HRCT—high-resolution computed tomography
MDCT—multidetector computed tomography
MRA—magnetic resonance angiography
MRCP—magnetic resonance cholangiopancreatography
MRI—magnetic resonance imaging
MRS—magnetic resonance spectroscopy
PET—positron emission tomography
PTC—percutaneous transhepatic cholangiography
SPECT—single photon emission computed tomography
US—ultrasound

A

D

E

J

K

L

M

Printed in the United States
By Bookmasters